Essential Paediatric Surgery

With this timely practical textbook encompassing the full range of clinical conditions within paediatric surgery, surgeons-in-training will be delighted to discover that the book offers them a concise outline of paediatric surgical practice, thus ensuring that they are wholly familiar with a wide range of clinical scenarios.

Key topics are included within sections on neonatal surgical conditions, surgical disorders of infancy, surgical conditions in childhood and adolescence, head and neck, hepatobiliary and pancreatic disorders, preparation of the child for surgery, malignant disorders, urology, neurosurgery and trauma. Short chapters complemented by clinical photography, schematic figures and tables splendidly enable the reader to understand key concepts with confidence.

Author-experts throughout the world have generously contributed to this textbook, ensuring that the contents reflect 'real-world' practice. A wide range of readers, notably surgeons-in-training, members of the paediatric surgery care team, including nursing staff, postgraduates seeking core knowledge of paediatric surgery for board examinations and surgeons planning to specialise in paediatric surgery, will benefit greatly from this practical guide.

Essential Paediatric Surgery
A Practical Guide

Edited by

Paul D. Losty, MD, FRCSI, FRCS (Ed), FRCS (Eng), FRCS (Paed), FEBPS
Professor of Paediatric Surgery
Institute of Systems and Molecular Biology
University of Liverpool, UK

Visiting and Distinguished Professor of Paediatric Surgery
Ramathibodi Hospital
Mahidol University
Bangkok, Thailand

Professor Martin T. Corbally, MB, BCh, BAO, MCh, FRCSI, FRCSEd, FRCS (Paed Surgery), MRCPI (Assoc), FEBPS, Grad Dip (Risk Management), CCST (Paed Surgery)
Chief of Staff and Consultant Paediatric Surgeon
King Hamad University Hospital
Kingdom of Bahrain, Bahrain

Professor and Chairman
Department of Surgery
Royal College of Surgeons of Ireland – Medical University of Bahrain
Kingdom of Bahrain, Bahrain

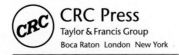

CRC Press
Taylor & Francis Group
Boca Raton London New York

CRC Press is an imprint of the
Taylor & Francis Group, an **informa** business

Cover image: Shutterstock ID 251585578

First edition published 2024
by CRC Press
2385 NW Executive Center Drive, Suite 320, Boca Raton FL 33431

and by CRC Press
4 Park Square, Milton Park, Abingdon, Oxon, OX14 4RN

CRC Press is an imprint of Taylor & Francis Group, LLC

Library of Congress Cataloging-in-Publication Data

Names: Losty, Paul D., editor. | Corbally, Martin T., editor.
Title: Essential paediatric surgery : a practical guide / edited by Paul D Losty, Professor Martin T Corbally.
Description: First edition. | Boca Raton, FL : CRC Press, 2024. | Includes bibliographical references and index.
Identifiers: LCCN 2023039719 (print) | LCCN 2023039720 (ebook) | ISBN 9781032005737 (paperback) | ISBN 9781032021928 (hardback) | ISBN 9781003182290 (ebook)
Subjects: MESH: Surgical Procedures, Operative--methods | Child | Infant | Diagnostic Techniques, Surgical
Classification: LCC RD31.4 (print) | LCC RD31.4 (ebook) | NLM WO 925 |
DDC 617.083--dc23/eng/20240126
LC record available at https://lccn.loc.gov/2023039719
LC ebook record available at https://lccn.loc.gov/2023039720

ISBN: 978-1-032-02192-8 (hbk)
ISBN: 978-1-032-00573-7 (pbk)
ISBN: 978-1-003-18229-0 (ebk)

DOI: 10.1201/9781003182290

Typeset in Minion Pro
by KnowledgeWorks Global Ltd.

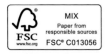

MIX
Paper from responsible sources
FSC
www.fsc.org FSC® C013056

Printed and bound in Great Britain by
TJ Books Limited, Padstow, Cornwall

Contents

Preface

Essential Paediatric Surgery: A Practical Guide is a new living textbook designed, steered, focused and aimed in a stepwise systematic manner to explore core knowledge and decision making in paediatric surgery. The textbook is subdivided into assigned sections beginning with the opening chapter – 'I want to be a paediatric surgeon' set out to help navigate and guide 'early years' young surgeons seeking career guidance with regard to the speciality, i.e. 'how to get started'. Subsequent textbook chapter sections are devoted to neonatal surgery, fetal medicine, surgical disorders of infancy and childhood, head and neck, hepatobiliary and pancreatic disorders, preparation of the child for surgery including patient safety, ethics, and consent with the latter sections covering malignancy, urology and trauma. The textbook is splendidly illustrated with clinical photography, radiology, schematic figures and tables appropriate to each section and chapters. The international guest authors were all carefully chosen and selected by the editors-in-chief for their vast expertise and wealth of knowledge in the speciality fields. We thank them enormously for devoting their time, efforts and many excellent chapters.

We sincerely hope the textbook will be a very practical reference guide and knowledge portal for surgeons-in-training, including those who are preparing for paediatric surgery board examinations, medical students seeking a wider knowledge of paediatric surgery and nursing staff caring for babies, infants and children with surgical disorders.

Special thanks must be shared with Daina Habdankaite, Georgia Thompson and Hudson Greig of the Taylor & Francis Group, who worked tirelessly with the editors-in-chief. Enormous gratitude, of course, is finally owed to Miranda Bromage at Taylor & Francis Group for her unfailing support at all times with the project and the ultimate publication of the textbook.

Paul D. Losty
Martin T. Corbally

Editor biographies

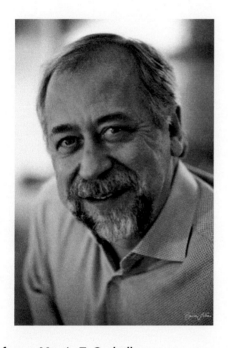

Professor Martin T. Corbally

He is a consultant paediatric surgeon and chief of staff at the Royal Medical Services – King Hamad University Hospital, Kingdom of Bahrain. An Ainsworth scholar, he has completed training in paediatric surgical oncology at Memorial Sloan Kettering Cancer Center, New York City, liver transplantation at Kings College Hospital, London, and is a former senior registrar at Great Ormond St. Hospital and Our Lady's Children's Hospital Crumlin, Dublin. He is the professor and head of the Department of Surgery at the Royal College of Surgeons – Medical University of Bahrain. He has a major interest in surgical education and global paediatric surgery and is the founder and programme director of Operation Childlife – an Irish registered global charity.

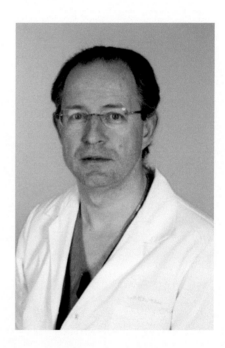

Professor Paul. D Losty

He has served as a professor of paediatric surgery at Alder Hey Children's Hospital Liverpool, one of the largest children's hospitals in the UK and Europe. Professor Losty trained in general surgery and paediatric surgery in the major university teaching hospitals affiliated with the Royal College of Surgeons (RCSI) in Ireland, Massachusetts General Hospital, Harvard Medical School Boston, Massachusetts, and Alder Hey Children's Hospital Liverpool. Working as a university academic surgeon at the University of Liverpool for almost 30 years, Professor Losty delivered clinical and faculty leadership in academic paediatric surgery. He has major interests in surgical research, education and teaching, mentorship and leadership and has helped train generations of young paediatric surgeons in the clinic, operating room and science laboratory. Professor Losty is now currently serving as a distinguished and visiting professor of surgery at Ramathibodi Hospital Mahidol University, Bangkok, Thailand, and is a volunteer surgeon with Operation Child Life – an Irish global charitable organisation providing surgical health care to low- and middle-income countries.

Contributors

Simone de Campos Vieira Abib
Head of Pediatric Surgical Oncology
Pediatric Oncology Institute - GRAACC -
    Federal University of São Paulo
São Paolo, Brazil

N. Scott Adzick
Surgeon-in-Chief
Children's Hospital of Philadelphia
University of Pennsylvania
Pennsylvania, USA

Talal Almayman
Consultant Neurosurgeon
Royal Medical Services
King Hamad University
    Hospital
Kingdom of Bahrain, Bahrain

Faisal M. Almutairi
Royal Manchester Children's
    Hospital
Manchester, England

Mohammed Amin Al Awadhi
Consultant Paediatric Surgeon
Royal Medical Services
King Hamad University Hospital
Kingdom of Bahrain, Bahrain

Marion Arnold
Paediatric Surgeon
Red Cross War Memorial Children's Hospital
University of Cape Town
Cape Town, South Africa

Nabeel Asheeri
Consultant Paediatric Surgeon
Salmanya Hospital
Kingdom of Bahrain, Bahrain

Olugbenga Awolaran
Paediatric Surgeon
St George's University Hospitals
    NHS Trust
London, UK

Pietro Bagolan
Head of Department
Bambino Gesù Children's Hospital, Italy
AOU Meyer and University of Florence
University of Rome "Tor Vergata"
Rome, Italy

Lisa Barneto
Consultant Anaesthetist, Wellington Regional
    Hospital
Capital, Coast and Hutt Valley, New Zealand

Fabio Bartoli
Professor and Chief of Paediatric Surgery
Department of Medical and Surgical Sciences,
    Policlinico "Ospedali Riuniti"
University of Foggia
Foggia, Italy

Spencer W. Beasley
Professor of Paediatric Surgery
University of Otago, Otago, New Zealand
Christchurch Hospital
Te Whatu Ora Health, New Zealand

Cara Berkowitz
Surgery Research Fellow
The Children's Hospital of Philadelphia
Philadelphia, Pennsylvania

Kejd Bici
Meyer Children's Hospital
University of Florence
Florence, Italy

Ampaipan Boonthai
Paediatric Surgeon
Ramathibodi Hospital
Mahidol University
Bangkok Thailand

Rocio Boudou
Hospital Italiano de Buenos Aires
Buenos Aires, Argentina

Georgina Bough
Paediatric Surgery Specialist Registrar
University Hospital Southampton
Southampton, England

Sarah Braungart
Locum Consultant
Leeds Teaching Hospitals
	NHS Trust
Liverpool, UK

Oliver Burdall
University Hospitals Bristol and Weston NHS
	Foundation Trust
Bristol and Weston, UK

Abraham Cherian
Consultant Paediatric Urologist
Great Ormond Street Hospital for Children
	NHS Foundation Trust
London, UK

Jennifer Mou Wai Cheung
Clinical Assistant Professor
CUHK Medical Centre
Ma Li Shui, Hong Kong

Alexander Cho
Consultant Paediatric Urologist
Great Ormond Street Hospital for Children
	NHS Foundation Trust
London, UK

Chan Hon Chui
Paediatric surgeon
Mount Elizabeth Medical Centre
Singapore City, Singapore

Patrick Chung
Clinical Assistant Professor
Department of Paediatric Surgery
Queen Mary's Hospital
Hong Kong University
Hong Kong, China

Riccardo Coletta
Consultant in Paediatric Surgery
Meyer Children's Hospital
University of Florence
Florence, Italy
and
University of Salford
Manchester, England

Andrea Conforti
Paediatric Surgeon
Bambino Gesù Children's Hospital -
	Research Institute
Rome, Italy

Sharon Cox
Charles F. M. Saint Professor of Paediatric Surgery
Red Cross War Memorial Children's Hospital
University of Cape Town
Cape Town, South Africa

Alessandro Crocoli
Chief of Surgical Oncology Unit
Bambino Gesù Children's Hospital -
	Research Institute
Rome, Italy

Peter Cuckow
Consultant Paediatric Urologist
Great Ormond Street Hospital for Children NHS
	Foundation Trust
London, UK

Paul S. Cullis
Consultant Paediatric and Neonatal Surgeon
Department of Paediatric Surgery
Royal Hospital for Children and Young People
Edinburgh, UK

Mark Davenport
Consultant Paediatric Surgeon
Kings College Hospital
London, UK

Diane De Caluwé
Chelsea and Westminster and Imperial
	College Hospitals
London, UK

Paolo De Coppi
Consultant Paediatric Surgeon
Zayed Centre for Research
Great Ormond Street Institute of Child Health
London, UK

Belinda H. Dickie
Harvard Medical School
Boston Children's Hospital
Massachusetts, USA

Adam J. Donne
Consultant Paediatric ENT Surgeon
Alder Hey Children's Hospital
Liverpool, UK

Steve Donnell
Paediatric Surgeon
Alder Hey Children's Hospital
Liverpool, UK

Natalie Durkin
Zayed Centre for Research
Great Ormond Street Institute of
    Child Health
London, UK

Simon Eaton
Associate Professor
Department of Paediatric Surgery
    and Metabolic Biochemistry
UCL Great Ormond Street Institute of
    Child Health and Great Ormond
    Street Hospital
London, UK

Abdulla Fakhro
Consultant Plastic Surgeon
Department of Plastic and
    Reconstructive Surgery
King Hamad University Hospital
Medical University of Bahrain
Kingdom of Bahrain, Bahrain

Abeer Farhan
Junior Resident in Paediatric Surgery
Royal Medical Services
King Hamad University Hospital
Kingdom of Bahrain, Bahrain

Marie-Klaire Farrugia
Consultant Paediatric Urologist
Chelsea and Westminster and Imperial
    College Hospitals
Westminster, UK

Adel Fattah
Alder Hey Children's Hospital
Liverpool, UK

Steven J. Fishman
Professor of Surgery
Harvard Medical School
Boston Children's Hospital
Massachusetts, USA

Semiu Eniola Folaranmi
Consultant Paediatric Surgeon
University Hospital of Wales
University Hospital Cardiff
Wales, UK

Hany Gabra
Consultant Paediatric Surgeon
Great North Children's Hospital
Newcastle, UK

Anju Goyal
Consultant Paediatric Urologist
Royal Manchester Children's Hospital
Manchester, England

Ahmed T. Hadidi
Head of Hypospadias Center and
    Paediatric Surgery Department
San Offenbach Teaching Hospital
Goethe University, Germany

Hussein Ahmed Hamdy
Consultant Paediatric Surgeon
Women's and Childrens Hospital
Kingdom of Bahrain, Bahrain

Andrew J. A. Holland
Professor of Paediatric Surgery
The Children's Hospital at Westmead
    Clinical School
The University of Sydney
Sydney, Australia

Zeni Haveliwala
Great Ormond Street Hospital for Children
    NHS Foundation Trust
London, UK

Alessandro Inserra
Chief General Pediatric Surgeon
Bambino Gesu Hospital
University Roma Tor Vergata
Rome, Italy

Bruce Jaffray
Consultant Paediatric Surgeon
The Great North Children's Hospital
Newcastle upon Tyne, UK

Rong Khaw
Plastic Surgery Registrar
Alder Hey Children's Hospital
Liverpool, UK

Neetu Kumar
Paediatric Urology Fellow
Great Ormond Street Hospital for Children
    NHS Foundation Trust
London, UK

Pablo Laje
Paediatric Surgeon
Children's Hospital of
    Philadelphia
University of Pennsylvania
Philadelphia, Pennsylvania

Bronagh Lang
Childrens Health Ireland
Crumlin, Ireland

Nick Lansdale
Consultant Paediatric and
    Neonatal Surgeon
Royal Manchester Children's
    Hospital
Manchester, Engalnd

Katherine Lau
Consultant Paediatric Anaesthetist
Alder Hey Children's Hospital
Liverpool, UK

Marc A. Levitt
Chief, Division of Colorectal & Pelvic
    Reconstruction
Children's National Hospital
Washington, DC

Pablo A. Lobos
Pediatric surgeon
Hospital Italiano de Buenos
    Aires
Instituto Universitario HIBA
International Society of Pediatric Surgical
    Oncology (IPSO)
Buenos Aires, Argentina

Anna McGuire
Boston Children's Hospital
Massachusetts, Boston

Rania Mehanna
Consultant in ENT Surgery
Childrens Health Ireland
Crumlin, Ireland

Antonino Morabito
Consultant Paediatric Surgeon
Meyer Children's Hospital
University of Florence
Florence, Italy

Francesco Morini
Paediatric Surgeon
AOU Meyer and University of
    Florence
Florence, Italy

Dhanya Mullassery
Consultant Neonatal and Paediatric Surgeon
Great Ormond Street Hospital
London, UK

Annika Mutanen
Paediatric Surgeon
The New Children's Hospital
University of Helsinki and Helsinki
    University Hospital
Helsinki, Finland

Gerlin Naidoo
Paediatric & Neonatal Surgery Registrar
Nuffield Department of Surgical Sciences
University of Oxford, UK

Iain J. Nixon
Consultant ENT Surgeon
NHS Lothian
University of Edinburgh
Edinburgh, UK

Elizabeth O'Connor
Consultant
Great North Children's Hospital
Newcastle, UK

Bruce Okoye
Consultant Paediatric Surgeon
St George's University Hospitals
    NHS Trust
London, UK

Claire A. Ostertag-Hill
Pediatric Surgery Research Fellow
Boston Children's Hospital
Boston, Massachusetts

Mikko P. Pakarinen
The New Children's Hospital
University of Helsinki and Helsinki University
    Hospital
Helsinki, Finland

William H. Peranteau
Pediatric Surgeon
The Children's Hospital of Philadelphia
Philadelphia, Pennsylvania

Laura Phillips
Great North Children's Hospital,
    Newcastle, UK

Agostino Pierro
Pediatric Surgeon
Hospital for Sick Children
University of Toronto
Toronto, Canada

Sabrina de los A. Pintos
Hospital Italiano de Buenos Aires
Buenos Aires, Argentina

Luca Pio
Bicêtre Hospital, Paris-Saclay University
GHU Paris Saclay Assistance Publique
    Hôpitaux de Paris (AP-HP)
Le Kremlin Bicêtre, France

Agata Plonczak
Alder Hey Children's Hospital
Liverpool, UK

Nisha Rahman
Consultant Paediatric Surgeon and Urologist
Chelsea and Westminster and Imperial
    College Hospitals
London, UK

Prince Raj
Chief Resident in Paediatric Surgery
King Hamad University Hospital
Kingdom of Bahrain, Bahrain

Mark Redmond
Consultant Paediatric Cardiothoracic
    Surgeon
Children's Health Ireland at Crumlin
Dublin, Ireland
and
Mater Misericordiae University Hospital
Dublin, Ireland

Timothy N. Rodgers
University Hospitals Bristol and Weston NHS
    Foundation Trust
Bristol, UK

John Russell
Consultant Paediatric Otolaryngologist
Childrens Health Ireland
Crumlin, Ireland

Elke Ruttenstock
Research Fellow
Hospital for Sick Children
University of Toronto
Toronto, Canada

Hesham Yusuf Saad
Consultant Otolaryngologist
King Hamad University Hospital
Kingdom of Bahrain, Bahrain

Payam Saadai
Paediatric Surgeon
University of California, Davis and
    Shriners Hospitals for Children-
    Northern California
Sacramento, USA

Omar Sabra
Consultant Head and Neck Surgeon
King Hamad University Hospital
Kingdom of Bahrain, Bahrain
and
Senior Lecturer
Royal College of Surgeons of Ireland Medical
    School of Bahrain
Kingdom of Bahrain, Bahrain

Mohammed Shalaby
Consultant Paediatric Surgery
    and Urology
Bristol Royal Hospital for Children
Bristol, UK

Raghu Shankar
Chief Resident in Paediatric Surgery
King Hamad University Hospital
Kingdom of Bahrain, Bahrain

Alok Sharma
Consultant Otolaryngologist
Department of Otolaryngology Head
    and Neck Surgery
Royal Hospital for Children and
    Young People
Edinburgh, UK

Emma Sidebotham
Consultant Paediatric Surgeon
Leeds Teaching Hospitals
    NHS Trust
Leeds, UK

Michael Stanton
Consultant Paediatric Surgeon
University Hospital Southampton
Southampton, UK

Mark D. Stringer
Paediatric Surgeon
Wellington Children's Hospital
University of Otago
Wellington, New Zealand

Paul Tam
Macau University of Science
    and Technology
Macau City, Macau and
and
University of Hong Kong
Hong Kong City, Hong Kong

Ryo Tamura
Great North Children's Hospital
Newcastle, UK

Martin Van Carlen
Alder Hey Children's Hospital
Liverpool, UK

David Vondrys
Children's Health Ireland at Crumlin
Dublin, Ireland

Emma J. Whitehall
Alder Hey Children's Hospital
Liverpool, UK

Cara Williams
Consultant Gynaecologist
Alder Hey Children's Hospital
Liverpool, UK
and
Liverpool Women's Hospital
Liverpool, UK

Vicky Wong
Hong Kong Children's Hospital
Hong Kong City, Hong Kong
and
Prince of Wales Hospital
The Chinese University of
    Hong Kong
Hong Kong City, Hong Kong

Iain Yardley
Consultant Paediatric Surgeon
Department of Paediatric Surgery
Evelina Children's Hospital
London, UK

Hind Zaidan
Senior Resident in Paediatric
    Surgery
Department of Paediatric Surgery
Royal Medical Services
King Hamad University Hospital
Kingdom of Bahrain, Bahrain

Augusto Zani
Neonatal and Paediatric Surgeon
Division of General and
    Thoracic Surgery
Hospital for Sick Children
Toronto, Canada

I want to be a paediatric surgeon …

PAUL D. LOSTY AND MARTIN T. CORBALLY

INTRODUCTION

There can be little doubt that many medical graduates and young trainee surgeons can find it difficult to settle on a chosen specialty career. In writing an introductory chapter that extols the speciality of paediatric surgery, we are drawing on a combined experience over approximately 80 years and spread over several world continents. The editors-in-chief have been privileged to have trained and worked with some of the 'movies stars and giants' in surgery, paediatrics and paediatric surgery.

If you are reading this textbook, it is possible you are considering a career in paediatric surgery. The range and depth of a busy clinical practice certainly guarantee that paediatric surgery will constantly amaze you. Training and being mentored in the best hospitals and residency programmes with inspiring surgeons is key to life skills proficiency while developing resilience together with a 'never quit' attitude. You're going to need these skill sets and tools ready to hand when you graduate from your training programme going forward to serve the most vulnerable patients across our world nations for the next 30–35 years or so, when you become a consultant surgeon. Whilst perhaps not for the faint-hearted, surgeons who thrive and enjoy paediatric surgery never wish to retire!

WHERE TO START AND HOW TO TRAIN...

It is sometimes said a person was 'born to be a surgeon'. Whilst we believe this is true, you have to get yourself fully trained. Entry into paediatric surgery is highly competitive. Basic surgical training rotating through general surgery, vascular surgery, thoracic, urology, trauma and oncology services sets your compass map on course, as ALL these specialties are wedded to interplay with paediatric surgery. You will need to steadily progress in your formative early surgical training years with an internship and obtain a general surgery membership exam, e.g. MRCS (as in the UK and Ireland), etc., to move forward to the next phase of higher surgical training. Many countries may have a similar style of examination operational at this career point.

Research fellowships (MD, PhD), particularly in North American programmes, add significant credits to your training portfolio, making the surgeon candidate applicant competitive for the national residency matching programmes. Other countries, notably the UK and Ireland, value research fellowship training, and indeed points are scored and credited at UK paediatric surgery national selection recruitment linked to the prospective applicant's CV with evidence of a higher degree (e.g. MD, PhD, MCh, MPhil) and peer review publications at final interview. Surgical research is 'alive and well' – thank you. Don't therefore let anyone put you off undertaking a research fellowship just because they have not been to the surgical laboratory! Your career and pathway trajectory to be a paediatric surgeon are your own personal goals and journey, no one else's.

TRANSITING TO THE NEXT PHASE …

You should be familiar with the rules and requirements of your own country, and when you have undertaken and successfully passed basic surgical training with a membership or fellowship-type examination, then the stage is set to apply for and hopefully gain entry to paediatric surgery training. There is a universal language here, as the applicant's CV – if competitive – will speak loud and clear. Know when the national selection training programmes are announced and advertised in your own country – be prepared and ready! Have your CV portfolio always up to date. In the UK as a worked example, paediatric surgery training is co-ordinated through national consortia networks, with surgeons-in-training rotating through at least two major surgical centres in 6 years (ST3–ST8) to acquire paediatric general surgery and subspecialist training. The intercollegiate paediatric surgery boards examination (FRCS Paed) is typically sat for in the final years of training in paediatric surgery (ST6–ST8) and followed then (subject to training consortia approval and sign-off) by the acquisition of a CCT certificate of completion of training (ST8) with the General Medical Council (GMC) signifying licence eligibility registration as a specialty paediatric surgeon. Reaching this milestone indicates that the surgeon can apply to hospitals seeking to recruit consultant paediatric surgeons. For surgeons training and working outside the UK and Ireland, you will wish to check and be familiar, with your nation's regulations and training requirements for attending consultant appointments.

ARE YOU READY FOR PAEDIATRIC SURGERY?

Undertaking a surgical fellowship after the completion of higher training in a subspecialist area of practice, e.g. oncology, thoracic, hepatobiliary surgery, transplantation or urology, will be greatly beneficial to your working life and career as a paediatric surgeon. Surgeons should actively seek out these much-sought-after fellowships which will often entail international travel to world centres of excellence typically located in North America, Canada, Europe, Australia and New Zealand. Some nations have their own fellowship schemes available for trainees, e.g. UK paediatric urology. Reflect on your achievements and aim to 'give back' to a wider society by teaching, promoting research and contributing your special skills to training surgical teams in low- and middle-income nations.

LIFE AS A CONSULTANT ATTENDING PAEDIATRIC SURGEON – THE NEXT 30–35 YEARS …

You must enjoy paediatric surgery as a vocation to thrive and own it. Working in a supportive and nurturing environment in the best hospitals you can find is crucial. You will experience great days and days perhaps 'best not to remember', for that is the real world, as they say. Continue to advance, learn and acquire new skills (e.g. surgical robotics). Research, write and publish – be always enquiring. Get to the many international congress meetings, network, meet new friends and colleagues. Finally, the children and families you care for will likely never forget you – always remember that!

'Paediatric surgery – The best job in the world'

BIBLIOGRAPHY

1. O'Donnell B. Training in paediatric surgery. World J Surg 1985; 9: 316–320.
2. Spitz L. So You want to train in paediatric surgery. Br J Hosp Med. 1996;56(6):281–3.
3. Beasley SW. The challenges facing training in pediatric surgery worldwide. Front Pediatr. 2013 Sep 11,1:24.
4. Schmedding A, Rolle U, Czauderna P. European pediatric surgical training. Eur J Pediatr Surg. 2017;27(3):245–250.
5. O'Neill Jr JA. Key factors in the establishment of pediatric surgery: Who did it and how? J Pediatr Surg. 2020 Jan;55S:38–42.
6. Rode H, Millar AJW. Our surgical heritage; the role of the Department of Paediatric Surgery in the development of paediatric surgery in Cape Town, in Africa, and around the world. S Afr Med J. 2012 Mar23;102(6):409–11.
7. Beasley SW. Understanding the responsibilities and obligations of the modern paediatric surgeon. J Pediatr Surg. 2015;50(2): 223–31.
8. Chung Ho Yu P, Tam Kwong Hang P. Academic leadership in and beyond pediatric surgery - A view from Hong Kong. Semin Pediatr Surg. 2021 Feb;30(1):151024.
9. Losty PD. Academic paediatric surgery – Why not? Semin Pediatr Surg. 2021;30:151021.
10. Donahoe PK. Sustained inquiry: In the clinic and at the bench. J Pediatr Surg. 2004;39(11):1601–6.

PART 1

Neonatal Surgery

Congenital diaphragmatic hernia and eventration of the diaphragm

RAGHU SHANKAR
King Hamad University Hospital, Kingdom of Bahrain, Bahrain

MARTIN T. CORBALLY
King Hamad University Hospital, Al Sayh, Bahrain and Royal College of Surgeons of Ireland, Medical University of Bahrain, Adliya, Bahrain

PAUL D. LOSTY
Institute of Systems and Molecular Biology, University of Liverpool, Liverpool, UK and Ramathibodi Hospital, Mahidol University, Bangkok, Thailand

Scenario: A full-term male newborn is noted to have respiratory distress at two hours after birth. On examination, oxygen (O_2) saturation records 75% (oximeter probe on left thumb). The newborn infant has decreased air entry on auscultation of the left chest. Breath sounds are reduced with muffled gurgles. Heart sounds are noted to be more prominent on the right side of the thorax. The abdomen appears scaphoid on closer inspection (see figure above).

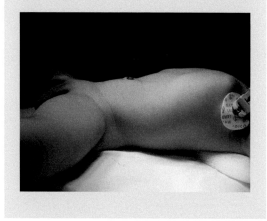

Question: What are the possible differential diagnoses in this emergency scenario?

Answer: There are two main possible causes of this acute clinical scenario, notably (a) congenital diaphragmatic hernia (CDH) or (b) eventration of the diaphragm. CDH is the more likely diagnosis given the early newborn presentation and associated severe hypoxia. Significant mediastinal displacement (note – heart sounds displaced in the right thorax), scaphoid 'empty' abdomen and hypoxia make an eventration unlikely. The gurgling sounds heard on chest auscultation are due to herniated bowel in the chest cavity displacing and pushing the heart and mediastinum to the contralateral side. Significant mediastinal displacement can reduce venous return to the

DOI: 10.1201/9781003182290-2

heart and impair cardiac output. Diaphragm eventration may cause newborn respiratory distress but generally not to the same severe degree and not usually associated with such severe hypoxia at birth. The presence of herniated viscera (gut, liver and spleen) in the chest cavity during fetal life impairs lung development leading to hypoplastic growth of the lung and the pulmonary vasculature, with abnormal arterial medial wall hypertrophy and thickened adventitia. This in conjunction with abnormal vascular smooth muscle reactivity in response to hypoxia and acidosis, causes significant pulmonary hypertension, which is a physiological emergency and the main leading cause of CDH mortality.

So taken together all these findings suggest a working diagnosis of CHD or, less likely, diaphragmatic eventration.

Question: What is the pathophysiology cycle of persistent hypoxemia in a newborn with CDH?
Answer: Persistent pulmonary hypertension of the newborn (PPHN) is linked to co-existent lung hypoplasia with excessive precocious muscularisation of the pulmonary arterial vasculature system. This leads to right-to-left shunting of blood with persistent fetal circulation and refractory hypoxemia.

Question: How may we confirm the diagnosis?
Answer: A plain X-ray of the chest (**Figure 1.1**) including a view of the abdomen would offer confirmatory diagnosis in almost all cases.

However, in some rare situations the diagnosis may perhaps be challenging preoperatively, with notable eventration of the diaphragm (**Figure 1.2**) and only confirmed during the operation.

Exercise: Compare the findings here with the normal chest X-ray in a neonate (**Figure 1.3**).

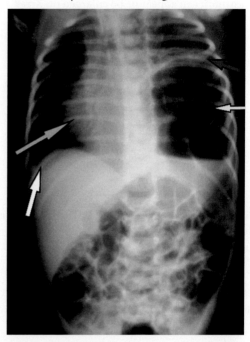

Figure 1.2 The red arrow demonstrates the intact left hemi-diaphragm. The yellow arrow shows the intestine pushed against the eventrating hemi-diaphragm. The blue arrow shows the heart shadow pushed to the right. The white arrow shows the normal right hemi-diaphragm.

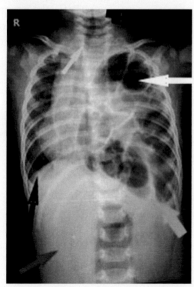

Figure 1.1 The yellow arrow shows displaced trachea. The white arrow shows the multiple gas filled shadows in the hemithorax. The blue arrow shows bowel herniating into the chest. The red arrow shows the liver in its normal positron.

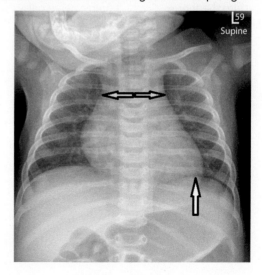

Figure 1.3 Blue arrows show thymic shadow. White arrow shows normal hemi-diaphragm.

The left hemidiaphragm (white arrow) is always a little lower than the right because of the liver.

Also note the widened mediastinum (blue arrows).

1. Do you know any reason(s) why the mediastinum can appear or be enlarged on X-ray examination (widened)?
   - Thymus shadow (normal enlargement until what age?)
   - Trauma (unrestrained vehicle passenger with rupture of the thoracic aorta, though very unusual in a newborn)
   - *Tumour*: Lymphoma and germ cell tumours
   - Foregut duplication (check and search for associated vertebral anomalies like hemivertebra)

Question: How is CDH different from eventration?
Answer:

Congenital diaphragmatic hernia	Diaphragm eventration
1. There is a defect (abnormal opening) in the diaphragm through which the abdominal contents herniate into the thorax.	The diaphragm is intact (no abnormal opening) but very attenuated, thinned out and 'floppy' due to a congenital or birth trauma–related phrenic nerve palsy, thereby having a raised dome and allowing the abdominal contents to migrate cephalad towards the thorax (**Figure 1.2**).
Eighty per cent of defects are in the posterolateral hemidiaphragm, known as Bochdalek CDH, and occur in the left thorax vs the right thorax. The other lesion encountered is a Morgagni hernia, where the defect is seen in the anterior diaphragm.	

2. Hypoplasia of the lung (reduced absolute total number of respiratory bronchioles and terminal alveoli) with abnormally thickened smooth muscle pulmonary arterioles involving the gas-exchanging portions of the lungs leading to impaired oxygenation and pulmonary hypertension (PPH). — Lung development is often grossly normal. Lower lung lobar segments may be collapsed from impaired ventilation resulting from diaphragm palsy. Hence, this is a 'milder clinical problem' with no associated pulmonary hypertension.

3. Despite effective surgical repair, newborn survival approaches 80% of index cases, and the prognosis must be cautiously guarded. The clinical outcome depends on the severity/degree of pulmonary hypoplasia. — An elevated 'raised' hemidiaphragm may not always require surgical correction. Those with degrees of moderate-to-severe respiratory distress due to significantly elevated floppy hemidiaphragm require surgery. Following surgical repair, the prognosis is usually excellent.

Question: How is CDH classified?
Answer: See **Figure 1.4**.

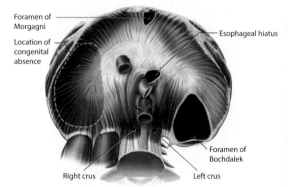

Foramen of Morgagni

Location of congenital absence

Esophageal hiatus

Foramen of Bochdalek

Right crus

Left crus

Figure 1.4 Anatomical location of normal and abnormal diaphragmatic structures.

Bochdalek hernia

- Most common CDH defect (80% of index cases).
- 85% involve the left hemithorax.
- Defect located in the posterolateral regions of the diaphragm.

Morgagni's hernia

- Rare (2%). May be encountered with trisomy 21 (Down's syndrome).
- Defect in the diaphragm is anteromedial in anatomical location.
- *Paraoesophageal hernia (15%–20%)*: Not a newborn emergency/Gastroesophageal reflux (GER) feeding issues predominate.
- *Complete agenesis* of the hemidiaphragm (1%–2%, extremely rare lesion).

Question: With the chest X-ray showing abnormal 'gas shadows' (as seen in Figure 1.2) in the hemithorax instead of normal lung parenchyma, which other congenital condition should be thought of? (*Note*: Approximately 50%–80% of CDH index cases are diagnosed with high-quality antenatal ultrasound imaging.)
Answer: *Congenital cystic malformation of the lung (CPAM)*: CPAM can mimic intestinal gas shadows on plain film imaging (**Figure 1.5**). If the diaphragm cannot be clearly defined and abdominal contents are not observed herniating into the thorax film, a CT scan may be needed to fully differentiate between these two conditions.

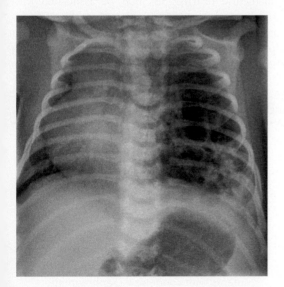

Figure 1.5 Chest X-Ray showing multiple fluid filled cysts and intact diaphragm of CPAM-Compare with Figure 1.2.

MANAGEMENT OF CDH

Chest radiography is suggestive of CDH in this newborn (**Figure 1.2**). Since the baby is in severe respiratory distress, how would you then proceed with newborn clinical management?

At the outset, it is essential to consider that CDH is a 'medical physiologic emergency' and not a surgical emergency. Severe respiratory distress is due to the combination of two key pathology factors, notably lung hypoplasia and pulmonary hypertension.

Emergent resuscitation should begin with prompt endotracheal intubation and insertion of a nasogastric tube (with frequent aspiration) to avert pulmonary aspiration and over-inflation of the intestine. Avoid hypothermia by keeping the infant warm and stable, and ensure the baby is sedated, avoiding where possible further hypoxia stressors. Secure vascular access is required with insertion of preductal and postductal monitoring. Inotrope support for cardiovascular blood pressure control is required with additional therapy adjuncts (vide infra).

Aggressive ventilation with face mask and Ambu bag is contraindicated in all newborns suspected as having CDH, as it causes gross distension of the stomach and intestines, which are herniated in the thorax, and will further compromise ventilation and hemodynamic stability due to increasing pathological mediastinal shift.

What is the current best treatment strategy?
'Gentle' ventilation, best termed permissive hypercapnia or pressure-limited ventilation. This greatly reduces pulmonary barotrauma and iatrogenic lung injury.

Other ventilatory strategies that may be employed if conventional ventilation fails to reverse hypoxia and hypercapnia include high-frequency oscillatory ventilation (HFOV) with inhaled nitric oxide (iNO – a pulmonary vasodilator used to treat persistent pulmonary hypertension). Extracorporeal membrane oxygenation (ECMO) is reserved for the sickest and most severe CDH patients failing all conventional ventilation strategies.

SURGERY

The CDH EURO consortium currently recommends delayed/CDH elective operative repair to be performed after adequate clinical stabilization.

The classical operation often utilises a subcostal incision. Thoracotomy is occasionally deployed by some paediatric surgeons to repair a right-sided CDH (RCDH). Minimal invasive surgery (MIS) is often best reserved for the most physiologically stable newborns with smaller CDH defects (CDH International Study Group Grades A and B), where primary repair (without a patch) is wholly feasible.

With an open classical operation, the surgeon gently manually reduces the herniated thoracic contents to the abdomen with excision of the hernia sac where present (less than 20% cases) with a primary closure of the diaphragmatic defect using non-absorbable Ethibond sutures. Large defects (C and D grades) require Gore-Tex prosthetic patch/or mesh placement.

Abdominal wall closure may be difficult in the large defect in severe CDH cases (grades C and D) where there is 'loss of domain' i.e., not enough adequate space in the abdominal cavity to safely accommodate reduced herniated viscera at normal abdominal pressures from the thoracic cavity. Primary abdominal wall closure here may likely lead to abdominal compartment syndrome (ACS), so to avert this scenario, a prosthetic (synthetic or biological) patch may be incorporated with the fascia musculature layers with final skin closure. Alternatively, a 'skin silo' as with a gastroschis or omphalocele to create a ventral hernia can also be undertaken with delayed musculofascial component repair at a later date. Non-fixation rotation disorders of the intestines may often be seen in CDH. Ladd's procedure is frequently unnecessary.

FETAL THERAPY

Current fetal therapy (FETO) – from the NEJM 2021 TOTAL RCT trial – is based on the concept(s) of temporary tracheal occlusion to accelerate lung growth in the 'high risk' isolated CDH fetus (without other co-existent anomalies) as best defined by a low O/E LHR (<25%) and those with thorax liver herniation, termed 'liver up' cases. Percutaneously with ultrasound guidance – in brief – a balloon device is delivered to occlude the fetal trachea at around 27–29 weeks, which is later deflated and/or retrieved by 34 weeks. Survival benefits as reported by the 2021 NEJM TOTAL trial in the 'severe CDH' fetus must always be counterbalanced in terms of counselling 'risk vs benefits' to expectant parents and a fetus with precipitated delivery and co-morbidity expected health outcomes vs elective near-term delivery with postnatal care at high-volume specialist CDH centres who are reporting >85% survival with antenatally diagnosed CDH.

LONG-TERM OUTCOMES: SURVIVORSHIP

Respiratory function in CDH survivors may be impaired due to the combination(s) of pulmonary hypoplasia and ventilator-induced barotrauma. Studies have shown that pulmonary function, perhaps better termed 'lung health', may improve for many survivors as they reach adolescence and adulthood.

Cardiovascular health and pulmonary hypertension with O_2 dependency/medications is linked to CDH disease severity and co-existent congenital heart disease.

Gastro-oesophageal reflux disease (GERD) is also common in CDH survivors. Aggressive GERD medical management at specialist CDH clinics with multidisciplinary teams has shown that 10% of patients may require fundoplication (+/– feeding gastrostomy).

Long-term follow-up studies report varying degrees of neurodevelopmental delay in some 30%–70% of surviving patients. This may be linked to neonatal hypoxia events, aggressive mechanical ventilation and/or ECMO. Deafness with sensorineural hearing loss may be associated with mechanical ventilation and/or use of aminoglycoside antibiotic therapy. Autism in more recent published studies is now reported increasingly in approximately 10% of survivors.

BIBLIOGRAPHY

1. Losty PD. Congenital diaphragmatic hernia: where and what is the evidence? Semin Pediatr Surg. 2014 Oct;23(5):278–82.
2. Losty PD. Congenital diaphragmatic hernia. In: PD Losty, AW Flake, RJ Rintala, JM Hutson, N Iwai (Eds.). Rickham's Neonatal Surgery. Springer Publishers 2018.
3. Snoek KG, Reiss IKM, Greenough A, et al. Standardized postnatal management of infants with congenital diaphragmatic

hernia in Europe: The CDH EURO Consortium Consensus – 2015 Update. Neonatology 2016;110(1):66–74.

4. Deprest JA, Nicolaides KH, Benachi A, et al. Randomized trial of fetal surgery for severe left diaphragmatic hernia. NEJM 2021 Jul 8;385(2):107–118.

5. Stolar CJH, Flake AW, Losty PD. Fetal surgery for severe left diaphragmatic hernia. NEJM 2021 Nov 25;385(22):2111–2112.

6. Lewis L, Sinha I, Losty PD. Clinical trials and outcome reporting in congenital diaphragmatic hernia overlook long-term health and functional outcomes – a plea for core outcomes. Acta Paediatr 2022 Aug;111(8):1481–1489.

7. Lewis L, Sinha I, Losty PD. Long term outcomes in CDH: cardiopulmonary outcomes and health related quality of life. J Pediatr Surg 2022 Nov; 57(11): 501–509.

2

Oesophageal atresia and tracheo-oesophageal fistula and allied congenital oesophageal disorders

RAGHU SHANKAR AND MARTIN T. CORBALLY
King Hamad University Hospital, Kingdom of Bahrain, Bahrain

PAUL D. LOSTY
University of Liverpool, UK

Scenario: A newborn male with a birth weight of 2.8 kg is noted to have frothy oral secretions, coughing with choking and gagging apparent when receiving his first feed.

Questions:

1. **What is the most likely congenital anomaly with this newborn male?**
2. **Why is the baby choking and gagging?**
3. **How do we proceed to confirm the diagnosis?**

Answers:

1. The combination of frothy oral secretions and choking with feeds makes the diagnosis almost certainly to be oesophageal atresia with or without trachea-oesophageal fistula (OA-TOF) until proved otherwise.
2. Feeds cannot reach the infant's stomach, as there is no oesophageal luminal continuity (atresia), and the baby thus regurgitates. Since the oral cavity is overwhelmed, a majority of the feed may be aspirated into the major airway, causing choking. The infant may also become distressed and cyanosed. Even when not fed, the baby is also notably unable to swallow his or her own saliva, leading to overwhelming choking and aspiration with pulmonary soiling that will progress to pneumonitis with pneumonia.

    Ideally every newborn in a hospital should not be fed unless you rule out this major anomaly by using a simple infant feeding tube (IFT) which, if passed easily into the stomach, confirms oesophageal continuity.
3. A simple bedside procedure will also help make our suspicion much stronger by introducing an IFT size Fr 8 (stiffer than size 6) via the oral cavity. There will be firm resistance felt at approximately 10 cm from the mouth opening, as the tube cannot be advanced farther into the stomach. The tube may subsequently coil and come back out of the infant's nose or mouth, and a chest X-ray (CXR) obtained will show the tube coiled in the proximal blind-ending upper oesophageal pouch (**Figure 2.1**). (*Note*: There is absolutely no need for an oral contrast study or further sophisticated imaging studies.)

DOI: 10.1201/9781003182290-3

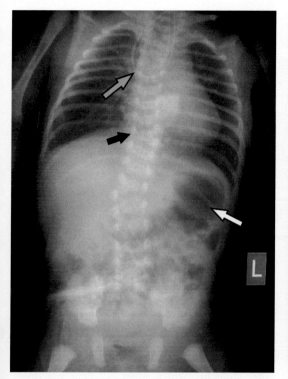

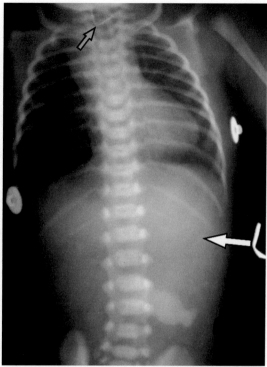

Figure 2.1 X-ray showing a coiled Oro-gastric tube in the proximal oesophagus (blue arrow). White arrow shows air in stomach-outruling a pure atresia. Black arrow shows vertebral anomalies.

Figure 2.2 X Ray showing absent intestinal gas shadows - Pre oesophageal atresia without fistula. TYPE A.

There are other major anomalies that may be associated with oesophageal atresia, and they must be excluded in every case. The most well-known and common include VACTERL syndrome, i.e., *v*ertebral, *a*no-rectal, *c*ardiac, *c*hromosomal, *t*racheo-oesophageal, *r*enal and *l*imb reduction defects. Others can include CHARGE sequence, i.e., *c*oloboma (iris), *h*ypogonadism, mental *r*etardation, *e*xomphalos.

With this typical classical presentation, the CXR and the association with other coexistent malformations (if present), the diagnosis is thus confirmed. We now know that the oesophagus is not formed normally, and we must now confirm whether or not there is also an abnormal fistula communication (tracheoesophageal fistula [TEF]) with the trachea. A CXR will readily depict an air shadow within the stomach, and this confirms that an abnormal fistula tract connects the trachea by way of the fistula to the distal oesophageal segment leading to the stomach. If no air is seen in the stomach on plain imaging, then the diagnosis here is most likely pure (no communicating fistula) oesophageal atresia (**Figure 2.2**).

There are therefore major variant types of OA-TOF as defined by the Gross classification (**Figure 2.3**).

Exercise: Examine the different variant lesions (**Figure 2.3**) and decide which type(s) would show air in the stomach on plain X-ray imaging and which ones would not.

If the plain abdominal radiograph shows an air shadow in the stomach, it informs us of the coexistence of a TEF, as seen in Gross type C – the most common variant anomaly observed in 85% of index cases – or Gross type D (1% of index cases).

Complete absence of the stomach gas shadow, i.e., a featureless abdominal X-ray study, indicates there is no TEF fistula, i.e., diagnosis is pure oesophageal atresia – (**Figure 2.2**) Gross type A – 6% of index cases – or perhaps the rarer variant where only an upper oesophageal pouch fistula may exist – Gross type B – 2% of index cases.

After we establish this major diagnosis, we must always ensure that no further pulmonary aspiration occurs.

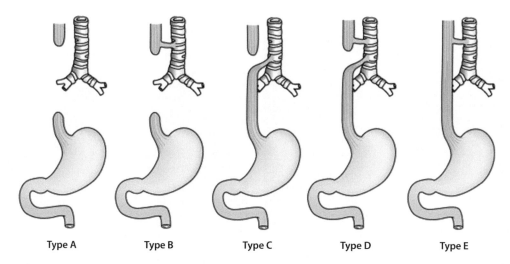

Figure 2.3 TEF classification as per Gross.

Question: What bedside measures can be used to prevent aspiration prior to undertaking a corrective operation?

Answers:

1. Stop all oral feeds.
2. Elevate the head end of the baby's nursing cot by about 30°. This simple measure can prevent reflux of gastric content into the lungs with the Gross type C lesion – 85% of index cases.
3. Provide continuous regular suctioning of the oral cavity with a low-pressure pharyngeal tube, i.e., a Replogle sump tube is often best if available on the newborn baby unit, which prevents aspiration of saliva.
4. Never undertake an oral radiology contrast screening study. This may be permissible only in the infant with a rare, suspected H type OA-TEF lesion, which presents in the first few days of life (not within 24 hours of birth) or the older infant and child with a history of recurrent chest infections and intermittent oral feeding crisis.
5. Investigate and rule out associated VACTERL anomalies (echocardiography is most important), etc.
6. Arrange for transfer when adequately stabilised to a paediatric surgical service for emergent definitive operation.

OPERATION

Classical surgery traditionally involves a muscle-sparing thoracotomy identification and corrective repair of the TEF and primary end-to-end anastomosis of the disconnected upper and lower oesophageal segments over a trans-anastomotic tube (TAT) for feeding (Gross variant types C, B and D). Aesthetic options with the classical operation include an axillary skin crease incision (after Bianchi), which gives excellent outcomes. Minimally invasive surgery (MIS) and robotic oesophageal atresia repair utilising thoracoscopy is increasingly practiced in advanced MIS centres requiring advanced expert skills and training.

Surgery must ideally be performed within 24 hours of life to minimise respiratory morbidity.

For Gross type A variants and OA-TOF long gap atresia, delayed primary repair may be scheduled to allow a period for the two disconnected segments of the oesophagus to 'grow closer' to each other. Other innovative approaches to achieve success with 'long gap OA' have been described by Foker, Kimura and Hendren.

In rare instances the native oesophagus may have to be replaced with gastric, jejunal or colonic graft as a staged operative procedure.

Question: What are the major complications of surgery?

Answer: Immediate complications include a major anastomotic leak with empyema, sepsis and recurrent TEF fistula.

Early, medium and long-term complications include an anastomotic stricture requiring serial balloon dilatation(s), oral feeding aversion and gastro-oesophageal reflux disease (GERD) – treated with proton pump inhibitors or antireflux surgery (e.g., Nissen, Thal, Toupet fundoplication).

Airway malacia (tracheomalacia), associated with postoperative infant ventilator dependency from recurrent tracheal airway collapse and 'blue dying spells', is a result of insufficient and deficient cartilage tissue support and may require an aortopexy.

Late complications include oesophageal cancer; this is a low-risk association (<1% risk) but underscores the need for GI endoscopy health surveillance and transition of care to adult surgical services. This is now crucially important for lifelong after-care follow-up.

Question: What are the major determinants of survival?
Answer: See the Spitz Prognostic Classification (**Table 2.1**).

Apart from birth weight, the presence of major cardiac defects and significant postoperative leakage (with sepsis) are considered to be independent prognostic factors.

Table 2.1 Spitz prognostic classification

Group	Features	Survival
I	Birth Weight > 1,500 g, no major cardiac anomaly	97%
II	Birth Weight <1,500 g or major cardiac anomaly	59%
III	Birth Weight <1,500 g and major cardiac anomaly	22%

Question: Which variant type of OA-TOF may not be readily detected in the immediate newborn period?
Answer: Patients with H type fistula (Gross E classification) are typically diagnosed beyond the immediate newborn period, as they are readily able to swallow and feed because the oesophagus lumen is patent. Troublesome later symptoms include 'recurrent chest infections' from occult aspiration events via an H fistula tract to the trachea.

Infants and older children (Gross D classification) with a 'missed' upper pouch fistula (i.e. born with a double fistula anomaly) may also similarly present late with aspiration and chest infections.

Question: If a baby with an oesophageal atresia cannot adequately swallow in utero, what may the mother have experienced during the course of pregnancy?
Answer: Polyhydramnios (with or without preterm birth delivery, with premature rupture of membranes) due to the inability of the fetus to swallow liquor.

Other congenital anomalies of the oesophagus may include:

1. *Congenital oesophageal stenosis*: 1 in 25,000–30,000 live births. The lesion typically occurs at the junction of the middle and distal thirds of the oesophagus. Three variant types are noted: (i) tracheobronchial remnant, (ii) oesophageal webs or diaphragms and (iii) diffuse fibrosis of the muscularis and submucosa. Children with this condition often become symptomatic typically by 4–10 months of age when they are weaned on to solid foods. Some variant lesions are amenable to serial dilatations, while others require surgical resection of the stenotic disease segment with end-to-end anastomosis.

2. *Oesophageal duplication cysts*: Often present with respiratory symptoms or regurgitation of feeds in infancy. Some of these lesions may rarely communicate with the spinal cord, i.e., as neurenteric cysts. All duplication cysts require surgical excision.

3. *Oesophageal achalasia*: Rare in children. This abnormality is characterised by failure of the lower oesophageal sphincter to relax during swallowing. Achalasia may present in infancy with a troublesome history of recurrent regurgitation and pneumonia due to aspiration, but more often is encountered in the older teenage age groups as progressive dysphagia. Heller's balloon dilatation provides effective temporary relief of symptoms. Definitive therapy involves Heller's myotomy accomplished by a classical or MIS operation. An added antireflux operation, notably a loose wrap fundoplication, acts to prevent reflux oesophagitis. POEM – *per oral endoscopic myotomy* – is gaining increasingly popularity, particularly in Asia.

BIBLIOGRAPHY

1. Losty PD. Esophageal atresia and tracheoesophageal fistula. Rickham's Neonatal Surgery Springer Publishers 2018. Eds. PD Losty, AW Flake, RJ Rintala, JM Hutson, N Iwai.

2. Sampat K, Losty PD. Diagnostic and management strategies for congenital H-type tracheoesphageal fistula: A systematic review. Pediatr Surg Int 2021;37(5):539–47.

3. Spitz L. Esophageal atresia. Lessons I have learned in a 40-year experience. J Pediatr Surg 2006;41(10):1635–40.
4. Corbally MT, Spitz L, Kiely E, Brereton RJ, Drake DP. Aortopexy for tracheomalacia in oesophageal anomalies. Eur J Pediatr Surg 1993;3(5):264–6.
5. Bruch SW, Coran AG. Congenital esophageal pathology. Rickham's Neonatal Surgery Springer Publishers 2018. Eds. PD Losty, AW Flake, RJ Rintala, JM Hutson, N Iwai.
6. Yeung F, Wong K, Tam P. Achalasia. Pediatric Surgery Diagnosis and Management Springer Publishers 2023. Eds. P Puri, ME Hoellworth.
7. Sampat K, Losty PD. Transitional care and paediatric surgery. Br J Surg 2016;103(3): 163–4.

3

Neonatal mediastinal mass lesions

RYO TAMURA AND HANY GABRA
Great North Children's Hospital, Newcastle, UK

Scenario: Neonatal mediastinal mass lesions are relatively rare, with an incidence of 1 in 20,000–30,000 live births (1). Their pathogenesis may be of neoplastic, developmental, inflammatory, or traumatic origin, with neoplasia the most common likely cause. Thirty-four percent of mediastinal masses encountered in the pediatric population are neurogenic tumors followed by lymphomas, germ cell, and mesenchymal tumors, which account for approximately 24%, 11%, and 7% cases, respectively. Thymic masses and vascular anomalies comprise up to 6% and 4% of all mediastinal masses, respectively (2). Approximately 70%–75% of mediastinal masses in childhood are malignant (3, 4).

Question: What is the differential diagnosis of a neonatal mediastinal mass?

Answer: The mediastinum is subdivided into three main compartments: Anterior, middle, and posterior regions (**Figure 3.1**) (5). The anterior compartment is demarcated by the sternum anteriorly and the pericardium posteriorly. This space harbours the thymus gland and lymphatic tissues. Common neonatal pathologies arising in this compartment are thymic hyperplasia and teratomas (**Table 3.1**). The middle compartment is the space delineated by the anterior border of the pericardium and a line drawn 1 cm posteriorly to the anterior border of the vertebral bodies. Major structures in this

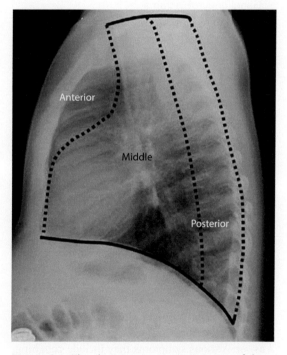

Figure 3.1 The three main compartments of the mediastinum: Lateral chest X-ray film (5).

compartment are the heart, great vessels, tracheobronchial tree, esophagus, and lymph nodes. The posterior mediastinum is located behind a line drawn 1 cm posteriorly to the anterior border of the vertebral bodies and contains the paravertebral autonomic nervous system chain, intercostal nerves, thoracic vertebral column, and again lymph nodes. In infants and young children aged

Table 3.1 Primary mediastinal masses encountered in infancy (0–2 years): Location and prevalence (5)

Location/Type of mass	Prevalence (%)
Anterior	
Thymic hyperplasia	6
Teratoma	2
Others including	16
Subtotal	24
Middle	
Duplication cysts including bronchogenic cyst or esophageal duplication cyst	4
Others including	8
Subtotal	12
Posterior	
Neuroblastoma	13
Ganglioneuroblastoma	2
Plexiform neurofibroma	1
Others or mixed neurogenic masses	33
Subtotal	49
Other miscellaneous	
Angiomatous malformations and lymphangiomas	4
Undifferentiated sarcoma	1
Other	10
Subtotal	15
Total	100

between 0 and 2 years old, the posterior mediastinum region may harbour 49% of all mediastinal mass lesions, while the anterior and middle mediastinum account for 24% and 12%, respectively (5).

Question: What clinical signs may suggest the presence of mediastinal masses?
Answer: Various symptoms may include coughing, dyspnea, dysphagia, superior vena cava syndrome, and Horner's syndrome. These varied symptoms may be caused by extrinsic compression of the airway, great vessels, esophagus, or the sympathetic nerve chain ganglia from the mediastinal mass (6). At the same time, nearly half of all mediastinal masses, in particular those termed posterior lesions, are incidentally detected on imaging examinations often performed for other medical reasons (5). Spinal cord infiltration may notably cause symptoms of cord compression, and this is perhaps the one single

example to be aware of with posterior mediastinal tumors, which largely tend to be initially asymptomatic. Cord compression is observed in some 12% of infants and children with neurogenic tumors of the posterior mediastinum (7).

Question: How can a diagnosis be established?
Answer: Diagnostic workup is aided by laboratory studies and imaging. Some malignant neurogenic neoplasms such as neuroblastoma actively secrete catecholamines, so homovanillic acid and vanillylmandelic acid urinary metabolite collection and analysis are key. Germ cell tumors such as immature teratomas or yolk sac tumor will result in significant elevations in serum alpha-fetoprotein (AFP), whereas choriocarcinoma will be associated with raised beta-human chorionic gonadotropin (HCG). AFP levels should be interpreted against normative age-matched control values, since AFP is typically elevated in the neonatal to infant age group.

Imaging studies should include plain film chest X-ray – posteroanterior and lateral views. This examination is highly sensitive in terms of showing an abnormal mediastinal shadow suggesting a mediastinal mass (8). However, plain film radiography is rarely specific enough to reach a definitive diagnosis, and cross-sectional imaging, including computed tomography (CT) and/or magnetic resonance imaging (MRI), are far superior and are part of the standard work-up (9). Ultrasound may be useful for evaluation of the thymus, which lies within the anterior mediastinal compartment, and this is typically depicted on chest X-ray as an abnormal shadow. Note: In infants the thymus is relatively large in the first year of life. The non-ossified sternum in young infants allows ultrasound to depict the normal thymus and differentiate it from a pathological mass in the anterior mediastinum. CT has many advantages and can be performed without sedation in neonates and infants. CT imaging is readily able to delineate lung parenchymal disease involvement and calcification within a mass, which are all important clues in confirming and detecting lung metastasis and teratomas (10). MRI with minimal radiation burden is increasingly performed in a 'feed and wrap manner' in neonates, thereby avoiding general anesthesia, and may better establish diagnosis of the mediastinal mass. For instance, in case of a duplication cyst, which may sometimes appear as a solid mass on CT, MRI can depict its cystic components accurately (11). MRI may show in greater detail the presence of intraspinal tumor extension, noted to occur in approximately 8%–12% of patients with posterior mediastinal neurogenic tumor (12, 13). Histological and biogenetic information is vital to decide on the appropriate management strategy, i.e. medical – 'watchful waiting' vs. surgical in certain selected tumors, e.g. ganglioneuroma, low- and intermediate-risk neuroblastoma, or lesions of undetermined pathology. A multidisciplinary discussion will then be required to assist the decision to proceed to biopsy for tissue diagnosis. Biopsy may be readily facilitated by interventional radiological image guidance methods, i.e. ultrasound or CT.

Question: What treatment strategies are deployed for a mediastinal mass?

Answer: Treatment is dependent on anatomical site and location and the expected and confirmed pathology of the mediastinal mass. Tumor board meetings facilitate decision-making pathways. For instance, if the mass requires surgical resection, the operative approach may be best selected based on the anatomical location of the mass. Thymus and anterior mediastinal lesions (e.g. teratomas) may be approached via a median sternotomy, while thoracotomy (left or right) is more suitable for posterior mediastinal masses. Apical lesions pose a considerable challenge owing to their proximity to vascular and neural structures and are not easily or safely approached by a standard thoracotomy. A trapdoor approach provides a safer approach (14). A conservative approach – 'watchful waiting' – can be adopted for some patients where the lesion is expected to involute, e.g. neonatal neuroblastomas and ganglioneuromas. In patients with spinal cord disease involvement and neurological signs, urgent and active discussion with neurosurgery is essential, as operative cord decompression as up-front primary management may be crucial or may be secondary to failure of the initial medical treatment.

SUMMARY

1. **Anterior mediastinal mass**
   1.1. Teratomas and germ cell tumors
   1.2. Thymic tumors
2. **Middle mediastinal mass**
   2.1. Esophageal duplications
   2.2. Bronchogenic cyst
3. **Posterior mediastinal mass**
   3.1. Neurogenic tumors
4. **Other**
   4.1. Lymphangiomas
   4.2. Vascular malformations

BIBLIOGRAPHY

1. Bush A. Prenatal presentation and postnatal management of congenital thoracic malformations. Early Human Development. 2009;85(11):679–84.
2. Lima M, Maffi M. Mediastinal masses. Neonatal Surgery. 2019. 139–49.
3. Grosfeld JL, Skinner MA, Rescorla FJ, West KW, Scherer L. Mediastinal tumors in children: Experience with 196 cases. Annals of Surgical Oncology. 1994;1(2):121–7.
4. Gun F, Erginel B, Ünüvar A, Kebudi R, Salman T, Celik A. Mediastinal masses in children: Experience with 120 cases. Pediatric Hematology and Oncology. 2012;29(2):141–7.
5. Lee EY. Imaging evaluation of mediastinal masses in infants and children. Evidence-Based Imaging in Pediatrics. Springer; 2010. pp. 381–99.
6. Ranganath SH, Lee EY, Restrepo R, Eisenberg RL. Mediastinal masses in children. American Journal of Roentgenology. 2012;198(3):W197–W216.
7. Ribet ME, Cardot GR. Neurogenic tumors of the thorax. The Annals of Thoracic Surgery. 1994;58(4):1091–5.
8. Harris GJ, Harman PK, Trinkle JK, Grover FL. Standard biplane roentgenography is highly sensitive in documenting mediastinal masses. The Annals of Thoracic Surgery. 1987;44(3):238–41.
9. Ahn JM, Lee KS, Goo JM, Song KS, Kim SJ, Im J-G. Predicting the histology of anterior mediastinal masses: Comparison of chest radiography and CT. Journal of Thoracic Imaging. 1996;11(4):265–71.
10. Siegel M, Sagel S, Reed K. The value of computed tomography in the diagnosis and management of pediatric mediastinal abnormalities. Radiology. 1982;142(1):149–55.
11. Williams H, Alton H. Imaging of paediatric mediastinal abnormalities. Paediatric Respiratory Reviews. 2003;4(1):55–66.

12. Akwari O, Payne WS, Onofrio B, Dines D, Muhm J, editors. Dumbbell neurogenic tumors of the mediastinum. Diagnosis and management. Mayo Clinic Proceedings; 1978.

13. Slovis T, Meza MP, Cushing B, Elkowitz SS, Leonidas JC, Festa R, et al. Thoracic neuroblastoma: What is the best imaging modality for evaluating extent of disease? Pediatric Radiology. 1997;27(3): 273–5.

14. McMahon SV, Memon S, McDowell DT, Yeap BH, Russell J, Corbally MT. The use of the trapdoor incision for access to thoracic inlet pathology in children. Journal of Paediatric Surgery. 2013;48:1147–51.

4

Neonatal pulmonary barotrauma: Surgical aspects

RAGHU SHANKAR AND MARTIN T. CORBALLY
King Hamad University Hospital, Kingdom of Bahrain, Bahrain

Scenario: A 27-week male newborn with a birth weight of 845 grams was intubated for respiratory distress on day 1 of life. The baby had received two doses of surfactant on the same day. The baby had a 'normal for gestational age' chest X-ray taken when intubated. By the second week of ventilation, progressive radiological changes in the right lung were noted which involved the left lung also. The baby could not be weaned off the ventilator (see below figures).

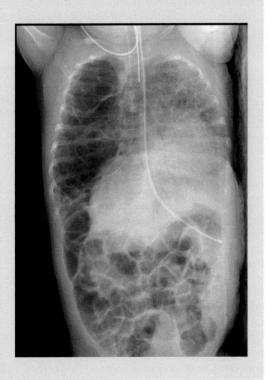

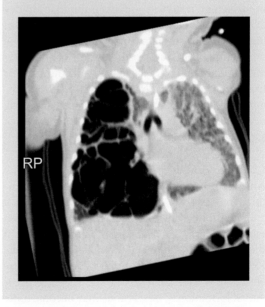

DOI: 10.1201/9781003182290-5

Question: What is the most likely diagnosis in this neonate?

Answer: The newborn is preterm and has respiratory distress syndrome (RDS) of the newborn because of the early delivery and for which surfactant has been administered and the baby subsequently ventilated. Chest X-ray during the initial 2 weeks was relatively normal, and changes developed thereafter. It therefore appears that lung changes developing after a period of prolonged ventilation are now most likely representative of pulmonary interstitial emphysema (PIE). Another potential differential diagnosis may include a congenital pulmonary airway malformation (CPAM).

Question: What are the outcomes of barotrauma in the newborn?

Answer: Complications of barotrauma in the premature newborn are air leak syndromes – notably pneumothorax and PIE. In pneumothorax, the air leak is extrapulmonary into the pleural space, whereas in PIE, the air leaks into the pulmonary interstitial tissues.

Question: What is the aetiology and pathogenesis of PIE?

Answer: The currently accepted aetiology of persistent PIE (PPIE) is considered multifactorial. The use of intermittent positive pressure ventilation (IPPV) in the immature lungs, which are deficient in surfactant, results in ongoing pulmonary injury due to a combination of barotrauma and a local increase in inflammatory mediators and cytokine production. This leads to disruption of the basement membranes of the alveolar wall, allowing air to then enter into the interstitial space. The communication between the alveolus and the lung interstitium allows for air to subsequently track along the bronchovascular bundles.

Question: How does PIE affect the newborn?

Answer: In acute PIE air tracks from the interstitium into adjacent spaces, which can result in a pneumothorax, pneumomediastinum or a pneumopericardium. In PPIE, air remains trapped in the lung interstitium and doesn't track outside. PPIE may then lead to a choke-valve-type airway obstruction with air trapping and multiple pseudocyst formation. Cystic lesions may become quite large, likely due to the relationship between intraluminal pressure and wall tension.

Question: How does PIE differ from CPAM?
Answer: See the following table.

PIE	CPAM
Pulmonary interstitial emphysema (PIE) is a rare, acquired condition that occurs in preterm infants with respiratory distress syndrome and usually as a complication of assisted mechanical ventilation.	This is a type of bronchopulmonary congenital malformation. Usually detected in the antenatal period.
Usually bilateral lung changes.	Usually unilateral and confined to single lung lobe.

Question: What investigations should be undertaken to diagnose barotrauma?

Answer: Plain chest X-ray film would be sufficient to diagnose pneumothorax.

In PIE a chest X-ray will demonstrate cystic changes; however, CT scan imaging will aid the definitive diagnosis where the bronchovascular bundles appear as soft tissue attenuation nodules or dots in the centre of air-filled cysts (**Figure 4.1**).

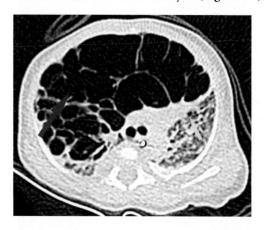

Figure 4.1 Red arrow shows the large cystic emphysematous changes in the right middle lobe and arrow (yellow) shows less marked emphysematous changes in the left lung.

Question: What strategies are used to prevent or minimise barotrauma in a ventilated neonate?

Answer: Use of exogenous surfactant therapy and deployment of 'gentle' ventilation techniques like high-frequency oscillation ventilation (HFOV) have minimised the incidence (%) of barotrauma.

Question: What are the treatment options in such cases?

Answer: Pneumothorax is promptly managed by inserting a chest tube drain and connecting it to an underwater seal apparatus. For PIE, treatment is mainly conservative, which may include any and/or all of these measures: Selective intubation of the contralateral main bronchus, selective ipsilateral bronchial occlusion, steroids, surfactant and lateral decubitus patient positioning. For severely ill neonates with PIE, HFOV and extracorporeal membrane oxygenation (ECMO) have been deployed.

Question: When may surgical intervention be indicated in PIE?

Answer: Surgical intervention is required in very rare instances when the neonate cannot be weaned off the ventilator because of the 'pressure effects' of the large acquired cystic changes in a lung lobe compressing lesser affected lobes. Hence, operation may entail thoracotomy and lobectomy. Resecting the most affected diseases lobe, i.e. removing the 'space-occupying lesion' and its pressure effect then hopefully allows the rest of the lung to heal spontaneously by means of continued conservative treatments. The overall prognosis for these neonates appears good despite lobectomy, which is probably reflective of the innate ability for compensatory alveolar growth in children.

BIBLIOGRAPHY

1. Miller DJ, Carlo WA. Pulmonary complications of mechanical ventilation in neonates. Clin Perinatol 2008;35:273–81.
2. Hussain N, Noce T, Sharma P, Jagjivan B, et al. Pneumatoceles in preterm infants incidence and outcome in the post-surfactant era. J Perinatol 2010;30:330–6.
3. Shankar R, Hussein A, Farhan A, Corbally M. Ventilator-induced pulmonary interstitial emphysema treated with lobectomy in a preterm infant. J Pediatr Surg Case Rep 2020. https://doi.org/10.1016/j.epsc.2020.101566
4. Matta R, Matta J, Hage P, Nassif Y, Mansour N, Diab N. Diffuse persistent pulmonary emphysema treated by lobectomy. Ann Thorac Surg 2011;92:e73e5.
5. Pursnani SK, Amodio JB, Guo H, Greco MA, Nadler EP. Localized persistent interstitial pulmonary emphysema presenting as a spontaneous tension pneumothorax in a full term infant. Pediatr Surg Int 2006;22:613–6.

5

Congenital lung malformations

GEORGINA BOUGH AND MICHAEL STANTON
University Hospital Southampton, England, UK

Scenario: The neonatal unit calls you to refer a 36-week-gestation male baby who has been born with an antenatal diagnosis of a left lower lobe lung malformation. The malformation was diagnosed at the 20-week anomaly scan. There have been regular surveillance fetal scans during pregnancy but no antenatal intervention. The baby is currently asymptomatic.

Question: What are the possible diagnoses that should be considered?

Answer: Congenital cystic adenomatous lung malformations (CCAMs) and broncho-pulmonary sequestrations (BPSs) are the most prevalent antenatally diagnosed congenital lung malformations (CLM) [1] and should be considered first. Both arise from anomalies during fetal lung development, and postnatal management continues to cause significant debate. CCAMs are discrete intrapulmonary mass lesions formed of cysts of various sizes. Pulmonary sequestrations are areas of lung tissue without connection to the tracheo-bronchial tree and with a typical anomalous aortic blood supply. It is now recognised that 'hybrid' lesions with histological features of both CCAM and BPS are relatively common but are usually diagnosed only after resection.

The differential diagnosis for this baby also includes other, less common, primary respiratory tract lesions such as congenital lobar emphysema and bronchogenic cyst, as well as lesions arising from other thoracic structures, e.g. foregut duplication cysts, mediastinal teratoma, neuroblastoma and hamartoma. Pathology arising from other anatomic regions is important to exclude, particularly congenital diaphragmatic hernia (CDH), as the implications for prognosis and management are significant.

The anatomical location of the lesion can provide clues to diagnosis: Bronchogenic cysts, foregut duplication cysts and teratomas are typically mediastinal; congenital lobar emphysema often occurs in the upper lung lobes; and CCAM/BPS is found in the lower lobes [2, 3]. Antenatal imaging usually provides a working diagnosis, which is confirmed or clarified on postnatal cross-sectional imaging.

Question: What antenatal investigations/interventions may have been considered?

Answer: Sonographic assessment is the first antenatal investigation. Ultrasound delineates the size, anatomical location and nature of any lung lesion. Ultrasound will also determine whether the lesion is unifocal or multifocal and identify the presence or absence of complications. Serial ultrasound monitors the progression of the lesion and development of complications – lesions often increase in size but may then reduce in size in the third trimester, or even completely resolve [4–6]. Fetal MRI may be a useful adjunct if there are significant concerns about either the clinical prognosis or

DOI: 10.1201/9781003182290-6

diagnosis of the lesion and antenatal intervention is being considered.

Options for antenatal intervention depend on the type of lesion and the size of any cysts. Maternal steroids often have a significant impact on microcystic CCAMs and (less commonly) on macrocystic CCAMs [7]. CCAMs with a dominant cyst may be amenable to thoraco-amniotic shunt insertion. Fetal lung resection, ex utero intrapartum therapy (EXIT) procedures and laser ablation are utilised less frequently [8].

The decision whether to intervene depends on the clinical impact of the lesion on the fetus. The main concern is *hydrops fetalis*, effectively, fetal heart failure. Hydrops is defined as abnormal fluid in two or more body compartments (ascites, pleural effusion, skin oedema, pericardial effusion), and if untreated, the expected mortality approaches 100% [5]. Large CCAMs can cause hydrops by compressing the heart or major vessels, whereas pulmonary sequestrations cause hydrops by shunt – abnormal blood flow through the lesion increases cardiac workload. Other potential complications include polyhydramnios, mediastinal shift and maternal mirror syndrome.

In fetuses with CCAM, the size of the lesion can be used to predict the development of hydrops. Size is expressed as a ratio of the volume of the lesion to the baby's head circumference – CCAM volume ratio (CVR). CVR greater than 1.6 is associated with a higher rate of hydrops and fetal demise and may be used as an indication for intervention [5]. Postnatally, CCAMs can be classified using the histological Stocker classification, published in 1977 [9] and modified in 2002 [10], but as this requires surgical resection, it is not practical antenatally. Prior to resection, the distinction between microcystic, macrocystic and mixed lesions is more helpful [11].

There is currently no prognostication model for BPS, and intervention in the form of resection or embolisation is performed on the basis of clinical progress. Sequestrations can also be classified as intra-lobar or extra-lobar, which may or may not be determined antenatally.

The majority of congenital lung lesions are not associated with other congenital anomalies. Genetic testing via amniocentesis or chorionic villus sampling is not typically performed unless there are other indications.

Question: How would you assess and manage this child in the neonatal period?

Answer: The most important focus is to rule out respiratory or cardiovascular distress by clinical assessment. The diagnosis of CCAM or BPS needs to be confirmed. It is ideal (but not always possible) to view the antenatal images and reports. Clinical examination of the respiratory system includes observation for nasal flaring, intercostal or subcostal recession and recognition of tachycardia, tachypnoea and desaturation. Chest X-ray on the first day of life is routine practice, although the malformation is often not visible on plain X-ray (**Figure 5.1**).

With a left lower lobe lesion, CDH may remain in the differential working diagnosis. A lateral chest X-ray (looking for herniation of bowel into the chest, typically posteriorly) or antero-posterior film with a nasogastric tube in situ (looking for passage of the tip of the nasogastric tube into the hemithorax) can help clarify the situation. If concern remains, ultrasound can delineate the integrity of the diaphragm, but other modalities such as a contrast study or cross-sectional imaging may be preferred.

The majority of neonates with CCAM and sequestration remain asymptomatic [12] and are discharged home after a period of observation with a plan for outpatient cross-sectional imaging and clinic follow-up.

A neonate with respiratory or cardiovascular distress requires close collaboration between the surgical and neonatal teams. Babies with mild or moderate symptoms should be admitted to the neonatal unit for close observation, chest X-ray and echocardiography. Ideally, positive pressure ventilation and intubation are avoided in CCAMs, as this worsens air trapping. Definitive management is surgical resection for both CCAM and BPS if symptoms persist.

Life-threatening deterioration may occur secondary to significant air trapping within a CCAM, causing a picture similar to a tension pneumothorax (**Figure 5.2**). A vascular shunt may cause heart failure or pulmonary hypertension. If in extremis, the baby should be intubated and ventilated, potentially advancing the tube into the bronchus of the unaffected lung or angling the bevel of the tube in this direction [13]. A drain may be placed into a dominant cyst as a temporising measure to

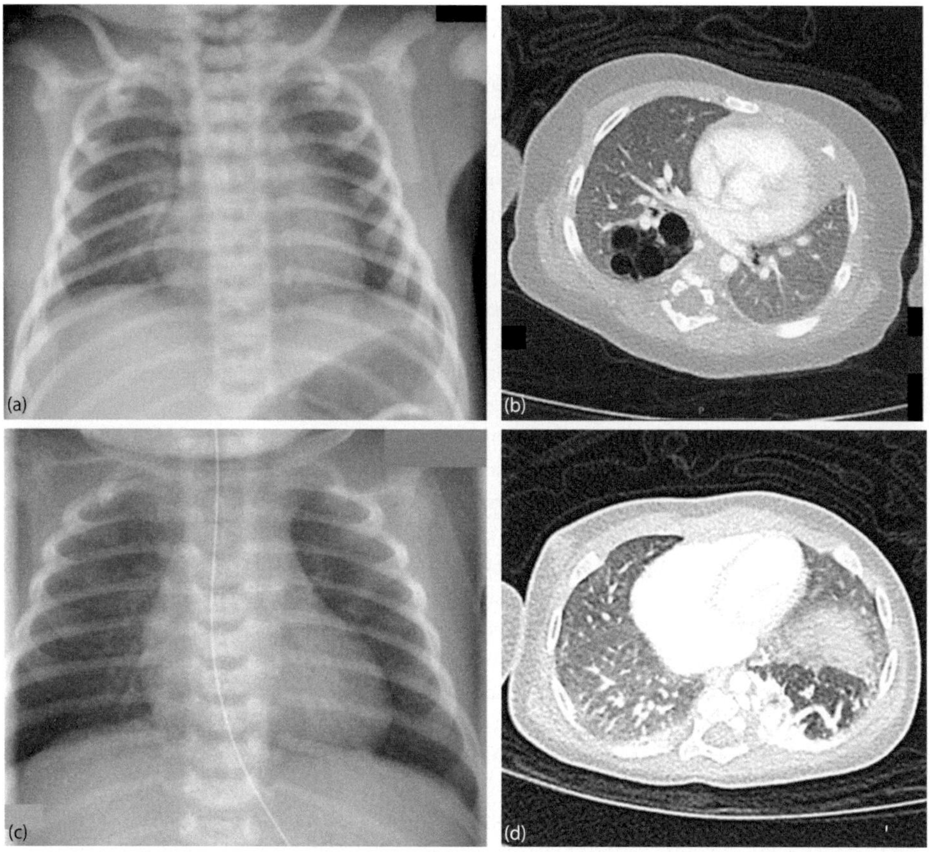

Figure 5.1 Chest (a) X-ray and (b) contrast CT of an asymptomatic infant with a small right lower lobe CCAM. The right heart border stands out clearly on X-ray. Chest (c) X-ray and (d) contrast CT of an asymptomatic infant with a left lower lobe pulmonary sequestration with arterial supply from the thoracic aorta.

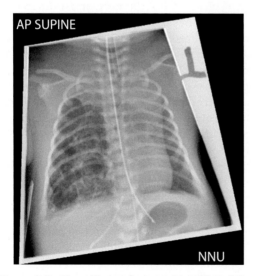

Figure 5.2 Chest X-ray of a neonate with a right lower lobe CCAM, respiratory distress and pulmonary hypertension. Note hyper-expansion of the right lung field, flattening of the diaphragm and mediastinal shift.

decompress the cyst, thus reducing intra-thoracic pressure, easing ventilation and improving venous return to the heart [14]. There is a concern that drain placement may result in preferential ventilation through the chest drain and worsen respiratory parameters.

Urgent or emergent thoracotomy is required in this scenario – a challenging operation for the anaesthetist and surgeon with a significant risk of difficult ventilation, poor visualisation of the anatomy and major haemorrhage [15, 16]. Babies with pulmonary hypertension may benefit from a period of lung stabilisation prior to surgery [17].

Question: The baby's parents would like to talk about management options and whether surgery is necessary; what are the options for intervention and areas of debate?

Answer: Conservative and surgical management are the main management options. Surgical excision of a CCAM, BPS or hybrid lesion is performed via

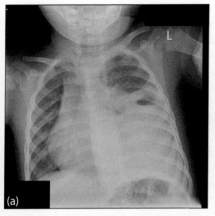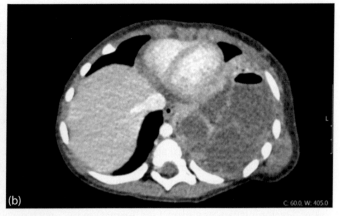

Figure 5.3 Chest (a) X-ray and (b) CT of a child with abscess formation within a left lower lobe CCAM.

either thoracotomy or thoracoscopy. Preoperative CT provides a guide to the origin of the lesion and the vascular anatomy. Excision is performed by lobectomy or segmentectomy, with the risk of recurrence or incomplete excision being higher if segmentectomy is undertaken [16]. Complications of surgery include bleeding, infection, damage to remaining lobes, persistent air leak, recurrence and chest wall deformity (less common with minimally invasive resection) [18]. There is no current interventional radiological management option for CCAM.

In a child with a pulmonary sequestration, surgery may be facilitated by preoperative embolisation, particularly if there is evidence of heart strain. Embolisation may resolve the symptoms and obviate the need for surgery [19].

The main area of controversy is the indication for intervention, particularly in the management of asymptomatic children. Symptomatic children – those with recurrent chest infections, pneumonia with abscess formation within the lesion (see **Figure 5.3**) or those who develop heart strain or haemoptysis – should be offered operation. For those with milder symptoms, indication for intervention is more difficult to determine; it remains controversial as to whether other common symptoms of infancy such as wheeze should be considered to be related to a CLM.

Asymptomatic lung lesions are more complex, and consensus has yet to be obtained. Advocates of prophylactic resection cite prevention of complications of conservative management such as infection and concerns about impairment of growth of adjacent lung tissue, lower surgical complication rates in asymptomatic lesions [16] and the potential for compensatory lung growth of the residual lung if resection is performed in early childhood [20, 21].

For proponents of conservative management, the large (and increasing) majority of children with CLM would have remained undetected under previous screening regimens and would likely have not come to harm. A policy of blanket intervention for CLM exposes these children to the risks of invasive surgery for a lesion that is very unlikely to be pathological (potentially never causing symptoms).

Question: The parents ask specifically about the long-term risk of malignancy. How would you address this?
Answer: Malignancy risk in CCAM is both controversial and understandably extremely emotive for families, surgeons and physicians [20, 22, 23]. The literature is subject to bias and interpreted differently by advocates of prophylactic resection and proponents of conservative management.

There are two main concerns: Whether a lesion assumed to be a CCAM could contain a congenital/ neonatal-onset malignancy (pleuropulmonary blastoma [PPB]) and whether there is an increased chance of developing cancer in the atypical lung tissue as the child grows up (mainly bronchoalveolar carcinoma) [24, 25].

PPB is a very rare, DICER-1 mutation–associated tumour of infancy with an incidence of around 1 in 300,000 [26]. Suspicion of PPB is increased by a family history suggesting DICER-1 mutation, postnatal diagnosis or atypical imaging of the malformation [21]. Atypical imaging features include multifocality, increase in size postnatally, effusion and pneumothorax [27]. Determining the incidence of PPB in CCAM is complex – there are case reports and published series [6, 21] of PPB detected within lesions that were thought to be CCAM prior to resection and many series of pro-phylactically resected CCAMs that contain no his-topathological evidence of malignancy and other series of conservatively managed patients who remain well without evidence of cancer [28–31].

Case reports of bronchoalveolar carcinoma (which in general has a median age of diagnosis of >60 years) and other tumours have been reported in association with congenital lung lesions both in childhood and adulthood [20, 32]. The relative risk of developing cancer within a malformation in comparison with the risk in normally formed lung tissue is currently unquantified.

For advocates of prophylactic resection, his-topathological certainty about the presence or absence of cancer is often the decisive point in dis-cussion with families [20]. For proponents of con-servative management, the risk of malignancy in asymptomatic patients with no DICER-1 mutation and without atypical findings on imaging is con-sidered extremely low and not enough to justify resection [23].

Parental anxiety is not commonly mentioned in the literature as an indication for surgery, but can be a significant factor when managing children with CLMs.

Question: What is the likelihood that an infant who is initially asymptomatic will develop symptoms?
Answer: There is currently no 'true' answer to this question, as the denominator is unknown and attribution of symptoms to the congenital lung lesion is sometimes difficult. As antenatal detec-tion improves, the apparent incidence of congeni-tal lung lesions is increasing (currently around 1 in 2,200) [33]. It is likely that as antenatal detection improves, the chance of any individual with this diagnosis later developing symptoms will decrease – this makes it difficult to prognosticate for a newly diagnosed infant on the basis of historical cohorts.

It is also difficult to provide a complete answer to this question given that many lesions are rou-tinely resected based on surgeon preference or parental request. Cook et al. reported a single-centre UK series of cystic lung lesions covering patients born between 1996 and 2009 [28]. They found 111 patients who did not require neonatal surgery – of these, 11% underwent surgery after

becoming symptomatic within a median follow-up of 9.9 years. Median age at surgery for recur-rent respiratory tract infections was 1.6 years, and no patient underwent surgery for a symptomatic lesion over the age of 5. However, 28% of their cohort also underwent surgery outside the neona-tal period for other reasons, most commonly fol-lowing medical advice.

Question: How would you remove this lesion?
Answer: After careful review of the preoperative imaging, single-lung ventilation is employed and the patient is placed in the lateral decubitus position with a roll under the ribs. Once secured in place, access to the chest can be gained through thoracos-copy, thoracotomy or a hybrid approach [34]:

- *Thoracoscopic*: Two 3–5 mm ports and one larger port are often placed. The first is placed in the fifth to sixth intercostal space, mid-axillary line; the second is determined by the anatomy, but typically more posterior; and the larger port is placed near the anterior axillary line, seventh intercostal space, for extraction of the specimen and potentially introduction of a larger stapling device. Pressure and flow depend on the size of the patient, but a starting pressure of 4–6 mmHg and flow of 1 L/min is likely appropriate [35–37].
- *Open*: A postero-lateral thoracotomy is sited at the 4th – 6th rib space, and the muscles are split, preserving the latissimus dorsi and ser-ratus anterior along with their nerve supply. The rib space is entered inferiorly to avoid the neurovascular bundle, and a self-retaining retractor is placed [3].
- Hybrid approaches utilise a video-assisted technique to minimise the size of the thora-cotomy wound.

Once access to the chest has been secured, the anatomy is assessed, the pulmonary ligaments divided and the fissure completed if required. The lesion can be removed by lobectomy or lung-sparing resection, e.g. segmentectomy, wedge resection or other non-segmental resection. For lobectomy, the lobar vessels are identified and skeletalised, ensur-ing adequate length for safe ligation. The vein, artery and bronchus are divided and the specimen removed. A chest drain is usually left in place, the remaining lung reinflated and the chest closed.

Question: What are the complications of surgical resection?

Answer: Early complications of surgical resection include infection, bleeding, air leak, respiratory failure and damage to surrounding structures, including the oesophagus, phrenic nerve and thoracic duct. Late complications include residual disease, chest wall abnormality and recurrent pneumonia. Death is a recognised risk of resection, and some degree of scarring is inevitable.

The extent of surgical risk depends on the clinical context and surgical approach [16, 31, 38, 39]. Risk of death and significant bleeding is higher in small, unstable infants undergoing emergency surgery but is not limited to this group. Risk of early complications is higher in symptomatic patients than in asymptomatic patients. The extent of scarring and risk of chest wall deformity is greater following open surgery than thoracoscopic surgery, but the risk of early postoperative complications appears roughly equivalent between the two approaches, potentially even lower in the thoracoscopic group. Lung-sparing resection carries a higher risk of air leak and residual disease than lobectomy.

BIBLIOGRAPHY

1. Zobel M, Gologorsky R, Lee H, Vu L (2019) Congenital lung lesions. Semin Pediatr Surg 28:150821. https://doi.org/10.1053/j.sempedsurg.2019.07.004

2. Mani H, Suarez E, Stocker JT (2004) The morphologic spectrum of infantile lobar emphysema: A study of 33 cases. Paediatr Respir Rev 5. https://doi.org/10.1016/S1526-0542(04)90056-5

3. Islam S, Geiger JD (2013) Lung surgery. In: Spitz L, Coran AC (eds) Operative Pediatric Surgery, 7th ed. CRC Press, pp. 207–216.

4. Calvert JK, Boyd PA, Chamberlain PC, et al (2006) Outcome of antenatally suspected congenital cystic adenomatoid malformation of the lung: 10 Years' experience 1991–2001. Arch Dis Child Fetal Neonatal Ed 91:26–29. https://doi.org/10.1136/adc.2004.068866

5. Crombleholme TM, Coleman B, Hedrick H, et al (2002) Cystic adenomatoid malformation volume ratio predicts outcome in prenatally diagnosed cystic adenomatoid malformation of the lung. J Pediatr Surg 37:331–338. https://doi.org/10.1053/jpsu.2002.30832

6. Cavoretto P, Molina F, Poggi S, et al (2008) Prenatal diagnosis and outcome of echogenic fetal lung lesions. Ultrasound Obstet Gynecol 32:769–783. https://doi.org/10.1002/uog.6218

7. Curran PF, Jelin EB, Rand L, et al (2010) Prenatal steroids for microcystic congenital cystic adenomatoid malformations. J Pediatr Surg 45:145–150. https://doi.org/10.1016/j.jpedsurg.2009.10.025

8. Kotecha S, Barbato A, Bush A, et al (2012) Antenatal and postnatal management of congenital cystic adenomatoid malformation. Paediatr Respir Rev 13:162–171. https://doi.org/10.1016/j.prrv.2012.01.002

9. Stocker JT, Madewell JE, Drake RM (1977) Congenital cystic adenomatoid malformation of the lung: Classification and morphologic spectrum *. Hum Pathol 8:155–171.

10. Stocker J (2002) Non-neoplastic lung disease. Histopathology 41:424–458.

11. Scott Adzick N, Harrison MR, Glick PL, et al (1985) Fetal cystic adenomatoid malformation: Prenatal diagnosis and natural history. J Pediatr Surg 20:483–488. https://doi.org/10.1016/S0022-3468(85)80470-X

12. Ruchonnet-Metrailler I, Leroy-Terquem E, Stirnemann J, et al (2014) Neonatal outcomes of prenatally diagnosed congenital pulmonary malformations. Pediatrics 133. https://doi.org/10.1542/peds.2013-2986

13. Ho AMH, Flavin MP, Fleming ML, Mizubuti GB (2018) Selective left mainstem bronchial intubation in the neonatal intensive care unit. Brazilian J Anesthesiol (English Ed 68:318–321. https://doi.org/10.1016/j.bjane.2017.04.007

14. Oh SH, Kim CY, Lee BS, et al (2017) Transthoracic catheter drainage for large symptomatic congenital pulmonary airway malformation. Pediatr Pulmonol 52:1572–1577. https://doi.org/10.1002/ppul.23835

15. Dias R (2019) Anaesthesia recommendations for Congenital Pulmonary Airway Malformation. 1–8

16. Stanton M, Njere I, Ade-Ajayi N, et al (2009) Systematic review and meta-analysis of the postnatal management of congenital cystic lung lesions. J Pediatr Surg 44:1027–1033. https://doi.org/10.1016/j.jpedsurg.2008.10.118

17. Parikh D, Samuel M (2005) Pulmonary stabilisation followed by delayed surgery results in favourable outcome in congenital cystic lung lesions with pulmonary hypertension. Eur J Cardio-thoracic Surg 28:607–610. https://doi.org/10.1016/j.ejcts.2005.06.036

18. Leblanc C, Baron M, Desselas E, et al (2017) Congenital pulmonary airway malformations: state-of-the-art review for pediatrician's use. Eur J Pediatr 176:1559–1571. https://doi.org/10.1007/s00431-017-3032-7

19. Cho MJ, Kim DY, Kim SC, et al (2012) Embolization versus surgical resection of pulmonary sequestration: Clinical experiences with a thoracoscopic approach. J Pediatr Surg 47:2228–2233. https://doi.org/10.1016/j.jpedsurg.2012.09.013

20. Singh R, Davenport M (2015) The argument for operative approach to asymptomatic lung lesions. Semin Pediatr Surg 24:187–195. https://doi.org/10.1053/j.sempedsurg.2015.02.003

21. Nasr A, Himidan S, Pastor AC, et al (2010) Is congenital cystic adenomatoid malformation a premalignant lesion for pleuropulmonary blastoma? J Pediatr Surg 45:1086–1089. https://doi.org/10.1016/j.jpedsurg.2010.02.067

22. Bush A (2017) Evidence-based approach to congenital thoracic malformations. Arch Dis Child 102:1095. https://doi.org/10.1136/archdischild-2017-313708

23. Stanton M (2015) The argument for a non-operative approach to asymptomatic lung lesions. Semin Pediatr Surg 24:183–186. https://doi.org/10.1053/j.sempedsurg.2015.01.014

24. Dusmet M (2015) Adult lung tumours of childhood origin. Semin Pediatr Surg 24:196–200. https://doi.org/10.1053/j.sempedsurg.2015.01.015

25. Hartman GE, Shochat SJ (1983) Primary pulmonary neoplasms of childhood: A review. Ann Thorac Surg 36:108–119. https://doi.org/10.1016/S0003-4975(10)60664-9

26. Messinger YH, Stewart DR, Priest JR, et al (2015) Pleuropulmonary blastoma: A report on 350 central pathology– confirmed pleuropulmonary blastoma cases by the international pleuropulmonary blastoma registry. Cancer 121:276–285. https://doi.org/10.1002/cncr.29032.

27. Feinberg A, Hall NJ, Williams GM, et al (2016) Can congenital pulmonary airway malformation be distinguished from Type i pleuropulmonary blastoma based on clinical and radiological features? J Pediatr Surg 51:33–37. https://doi.org/10.1016/j.jpedsurg.2015.10.019

28. Cook J, Chitty LS, De Coppi P, et al (2017) The natural history of prenatally diagnosed congenital cystic lung lesions: Long-term follow-up of 119 cases. Arch Dis Child 102:798–803. https://doi.org/10.1136/archdischild-2016-311233

29. Kunisaki SM, Lal DR, Saito JM, et al (2021) Pleuropulmonary blastoma in pediatric lung lesions. Pediatrics 147. https://doi.org/10.1542/peds.2020-028357

30. Thompson AJ, Sidebotham EL, Chetcuti PAJ, Crabbe DCG (2018) Prenatally diagnosed congenital lung malformations—A long-term outcome study. Pediatr Pulmonol 53: 1442–1446. https://doi.org/10.1002/ppul.24119

31. Khan H, Kurup M, Saikia S, et al (2021) Morbidity after thoracoscopic resection of congenital pulmonary airway malformations (CPAM): Single center experience over a decade. Pediatr Surg Int 37:549–554. https://doi.org/10.1007/s00383-020-04801-1

32. Durell J, Thakkar H, Gould S, et al (2016) Pathology of asymptomatic, prenatally diagnosed cystic lung malformations. J Pediatr Surg 51:231–235. https://doi.org/10.1016/j.jpedsurg.2015.10.061

33. Stocker LJ, Wellesley DG, Stanton MP, et al (2015) The increasing incidence of foetal echogenic congenital lung malformations: An observational study. Prenat Diagn 35:148–153. https://doi.org/10.1002/pd.4507

34. Moyer J, Lee H, Vu L (2017) Thoracoscopic Lobectomy for Congenital Lung Lesions. Clin Perinatol 44:781–794. https://doi.org/10.1016/j.clp.2017.08.003

35. Rothenberg SS (2008) First decade's experience with thoracoscopic lobectomy in infants and children. J Pediatr Surg 43:40–45. https://doi.org/10.1016/j.jpedsurg.2007.09.015

36. Rothenberg SS (2007) Thoracoscopic pulmonary surgery. Semin Pediatr Surg 16:231–237. https://doi.org/10.1053/j.sempedsurg.2007.06.004

37. Lai SW, Rothenberg SS (2019) Culture of safety and error traps in pediatric thoracoscopy. Semin Pediatr Surg 28: 178–182. https://doi.org/10.1053/j.sempedsurg.2019.04.021

38. Downard CD, Calkins CM, Williams RF, et al (2017) Treatment of congenital pulmonary airway malformations: A systematic review from the APSA outcomes and evidence based practice committee. Pediatr Surg Int 33:939–953. https://doi.org/10.1007/s00383-017-4098-z

39. Adams S, Jobson M, Sangnawakij P, et al (2017) Does thoracoscopy have advantages over open surgery for asymptomatic congenital lung malformations? An analysis of 1626 resections. J Pediatr Surg 52:247–251. https://doi.org/10.1016/j.jpedsurg.2016.11.014

40. Kersten CM, Hermelijn SM, Dossche LW, Muthialu N, Losty PD, et al. (2023). Collaborative Neonatal Network for the first European CPAM Trial (Connect): A study protocol for a randomised controlled trial. BMJ Open 13(3):e071989.

6

Exomphalos and gastroschisis

RAGHU SHANKAR AND MARTIN T. CORBALLY
King Hamad University Hospital, Kingdom of Bahrain, Bahrain

PAUL D. LOSTY
University of Liverpool, UK

Scenario: A newborn female is transferred emergently to your hospital with the intestine and liver exposed and lying outside the abdominal cavity. The anomaly seems to be centred in the umbilical region. A thin membrane sac is seen covering the exposed intestines with the umbilical cord emanating from it (**Figure 6.1**).

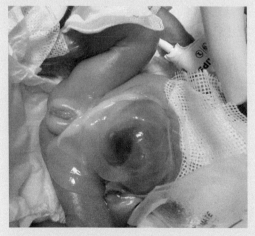

Figure 6.1

Question: What is the diagnosis in this newborn?
Answer: This is exomphalos, also termed omphalocoele

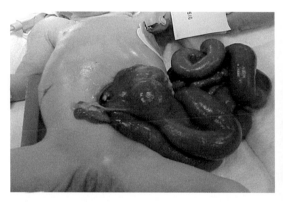

Figure 6.2 Malformation (sac like covering) is easily distinguished from other abdominal wall defects.

The fact that the malformation has a sac-like covering easily distinguishes it from other abdominal wall defects (**Figure 6.2**). The sac covering the underlying viscera and liver consists of amnion, Wharton's jelly and peritoneum.

Question: What would the diagnosis be if the malformation had a similar newborn presentation but the intestines were found lying totally exposed without any sac layer covering and the gut was lying to the right side of a normally situated umbilical cord (Figure 6.2)?
Answer: This malformation is termed gastroschisis.

Both of these birth defects can be readily detected antenatally with ultrasonography, often done

DOI: 10.1201/9781003182290-7

at the 20-week fetal anomaly scan. If an antenatal diagnosis of omphalocoele is made, then detailed antenatal screening for associated major coexistent anomalies is essential. The most common anomalies are cardiac (atrial septal defect [ASD], ventral septal defect [VSD], tetralogy of Fallot) and central nervous system malformations (corpus callosum agenesis, hydrocephalus, meningomyelocoele). Severe associated defects that will impact prognosis and survival will require prenatal counselling by the multidisciplinary fetal medicine team, and options with regard to termination of pregnancy can be considered.

Question: How are these two abdominal wall birth defects different from one another?
Answer: Please see the following table.

Omphalocoele	Gastroschisis
• Malformation covered with sac	• No sac covering – intestines are exposed
• Defect central location on the abdominal wall with the umbilical cord arising from its apex	• Defect is located to the right side of the umbilicus. Umbilical cord is distinct and separate from the defect
• Aetiology-pathogenesis – Defect with failure of the viscera to return to the abdominal cavity during fetal development	• Failure of migration of the lateral folds of mesoderm (more frequent on the right side)
• Herniation of intestine with or without liver	• Herniation of the intestines only
• Associated anomalies are common (50%) – chromosomal, cardiac, neural, renal lesions	• Associated anomalies are uncommon (10%) – most notably intestinal atresia
• Underlying bowel beneath sac coverings often healthy	• Thickened exposed bowel with peel may have coexisting intestinal atresia
• Surgical management is individualised with staged operative procedures	• Surgical management = Urgent

Question: What is the immediate management of a newborn with these malformations?
Answer: The exposed viscera should be protected and kept moist to avoid desiccation. Jelonet (paraffin gauze tulle) or saline-soaked gauze may be placed over the exposed sac in omphalocoele or used to cover the eviscerated intestines in infants with gastroschisis, together with a plastic 'cling film' torso wrap. These measures help prevent fluid and heat loss in the newborn. The potential for fluid and heat loss is significantly greater in gastroschisis, as there is no protective membrane sac covering the exposed viscera.

A nasogastric tube should be inserted and placed on free drainage with regular aspiration to prevent pneumonitis and bowel distension. IV fluids are administered by peripheral venous access. Infants with gastroschisis will require total parenteral nutrition (TPN) support, as return of normal gut physiologic function may take days to weeks.

In newborns with omphalocoele, the baby should be further evaluated for associated anomalies and echocardiography and renal tract ultrasound studies undertaken.

Question: What are the management strategy options in newborns with omphalocoele?
Answer: Varied approaches have been used in omphalocoele management, which are individualised dependent on the clinical circumstances of the newborn and mostly according to the size of the defect (major or minor), gestational age/birth weight and presence of associated anomalies.

IMMEDIATE PRIMARY CLOSURE

Defects less than 1.5 cm are often referred to by the term 'hernia of the umbilical cord' (**Figure 6.3**). These are easily repaired in the newborn period and rarely associated with a major anomaly.

Be cognizant of omphalomesenteric duct remnants that may exist with cord hernia. Defects which are larger omphalocoele minor variants (between 2 and 5 cm) can also be closed primarily in the newborn period, as there is minimal 'loss of abdominal domain'.

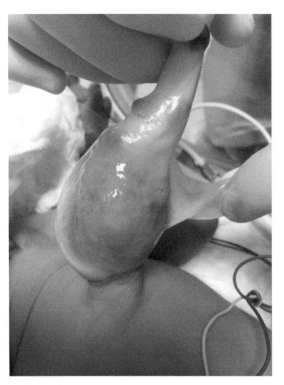

Figure 6.3 Hernia of the umbilical cord.

Questions: What complication(s) would you anticipate if you attempt to reduce the bowel and liver into the abdomen with a larger omphalocoele anomaly and closed the abdominal wall? What strategies may be deployed if problems do arise when primary closure is undertaken?

Answer: Abdominal compartment syndrome (ACS) is the major risk to life with overzealous efforts to obtain a primary closure. Elevated intra-abdominal pressures (as measured by either urinary bladder catheter placement or gastric pressure assessment) are detrimental to splanchnic blood flow circulation, which will severely compromise renal and intestinal perfusion with recorded pressures of 10–15 mm Hg. To best avoid it, a silo pouch should be secured by the operating surgeon, described later in the subsequent section (dealing with large defects). Another less popular option used by some surgeons is to create a skin silo, securing closure only of the skin over the defect and not muscle or fascia. This will give the patient a ventral hernia, which can be repaired later in infancy. Prosthetic materials, e.g. Gore-Tex, can also be used either primarily at time of the first repair or electively later (during staged ventral hernia repair) to secure closure of the abdominal wall without tension.

STAGED CLOSURE (SILO)

Large omphalocoele defects termed 'major 'lesions (greater than 5 cm or those containing the liver in the sac) are best managed with staged closure.

The omphalocoele sac may be excised (or if it has ruptured spontaneously) and a silastic pouch (silo) sutured to the full thickness of the abdominal wall fascia layer or a preformed spring-loaded silo (**Figure 6.4**) considered. Graded reduction is achieved by 'tightening' the top of the silo bag every few days with folding sutures or umbilical tape. Final delayed closure of the abdominal wall may be undertaken some weeks later in the anaesthetised patient in the operating room, observing all the precautions for compartment syndrome as listed before.

DELAYED CLOSURE

When the defect is massive, often termed 'giant omphalocoele' and considered too large (>5 cm) and the newborn has coexistent significant cardiac or respiratory issues, epithelialisation of the sac with wound healing promoted by secondary intention is an option. Various topical agents (silver sulphadiazine, medical-grade manuka honey) are particularly useful with an intact omphalocoele sac. The eschar epithelialises over time (4–10 weeks), leaving the patient with a ventral scarred defect (similar to a hernia), which will be repaired later in childhood.

LONG-TERM OUTCOMES

In newborns with omphalocoeles long-term medical problems may include prolonged ventilator dependency with diaphragm dysfunction, need for tracheostomy, home ventilation, reactive airway disease/bronchomalacia and calorie malnutrition with gastro-oesophageal reflux disease (GERD). A significant number of males later require operations for undescended testes.

Intestinal rotational and fixation anomalies (variant degrees of malrotation/non-rotation) exist universally in almost all newborns with omphalocoele. Only a small percentage (1%–2%) subsequently risk developing midgut volvulus. However, any such child with intermittent/recurrent bile-stained vomiting should be thoroughly screened and investigated for malrotation and undergo Ladd's procedure where indicated. At present,

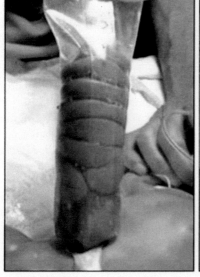
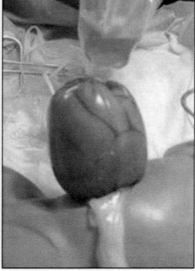

Figure 6.4

however, there is no compelling evidence to undertake a Ladd's procedure during the initial closure of an omphalocoele.

Question: What is the surgical management strategy in gastroschisis?
Answer: Newborns with gastroschisis need to be dealt with urgently and emergent operation scheduled by the surgeon. Primary closure with umbilicoplasty can be achieved in approximately 75% of cases, and timely inter-hospital transfer to the paediatric surgical centre facilitates good outcomes. In 25% of gastroschisis patients there is a serious risk of loss of abdominal domain with aggressive

'forced' closure and subsequent risk of ACS. These are best managed by creation of a silo and staged closure over a few days.

1. Primary closure – 75% of index cases.
2. Temporary silo placement with serial reduction followed by surgical closure – 25% of index cases. Often these patients may have matted bowel with thickened peel and may be termed 'complex gastroschisis'.

General principles: At operation the surgeon should always carefully inspect the bowel and note any obstructing bands, atresia or perforation.

Bands should be lysed and any perforation closed. Consideration of temporary diverting stomas, even if silo placement is undertaken, is best. It is not advisable to seek to correct an associated atresia at the time of primary closure and far better to schedule atresia repair after 2–3 weeks when the inflammatory intestinal oedema has hopefully settled down. In the intervening time the baby is supported by TPN (consider central venous access at an early stage).

LONG-TERM OUTCOMES

Infants with gastroschisis are generally considered to have excellent outcomes with survival in >95% of index cases in the modern era of care. Early-years survivors are often small in height and weight (<25th percentile) but often 'catch up' in terms of growth and development as they approach adolescence. Males may have undescended testes that later undergo spontaneous descent in the early years. Orchidopexy – unlike with omphalocoele patients – is required less often.

Complex gastroschisis patients, notably those with loss of bowel due to ischemic gangrene from compartment syndrome, gut atresia(s) or from acquiring necrotising enterocolitis (NEC) as neonates – may develop intestinal failure (short bowel syndrome).

BIBLIOGRAPHY

1. Gamba P, Midrioa P. Abdominal wall defects: Prenatal diagnosis, newborn management, and long-term outcomes. Semin Pediatr Surg. 2014;23:283–90.
2. Islam S. Congenital abdominal wall defects. In Holcomb III GW, Murphy JP and St. Peter SD eds. Holcomb Ascraft's Pediatric Surgery (seventh edition). Elsevier 2020: 763–79.
3. Khalil BA, Losty PD. Gastroschisis and exomphalos. In Losty PD, Flake A W, Rintala RJ, Hutson JM, and Iwai N eds. Rickham's Neonatal Surgery. Springer Publishers 2018.
4. Murphy FL, Mazlan, TA, Tarheen F, Corbally MT, Puri P. Gastroschisis and exomphalos in Ireland 1998–2004. Does antenatal diagnosis impact on outcome? Pediatr Surg Int. 2007;23(11):1059–1063. https://doi.org/10.1007/S00383-007-2001-Z
5. Ledbetter DJ. Congenital abdominal wall defects and reconstruction in pediatric surgery: Gastroschisis and omphalocele. Surg Clin North Am. 2012;92(3):713–27. x. https://doi.org/10.1016/j.suc.2012.03.010. Epub 2012 Apr 17. PMID: 22595717.
6. Skarsgard E D. Immediate versus staged repair of omphaloceles. Semin Pediatr Surg. 2019;28:89–94. https://doi.org/10.1053/j.sempedsurg.2019.04.010
7. Pacilli M, Spitz L, Kiely EM, Curry J, Pierro A. Staged repair of giant omphalocele in the neonatal period. J Pediatr Surg. 2005;40:785–8.
8. Adam AS, Corbally MT, Fitzgerald RJ. Evaluation of conservative therapy for exomphalos. Surg Gynecol Obstet. 1991;172(5):394–6.
9. Yardley IE, Bostock E, Jones MO, Turnock RR, Corbett HJ, Losty PD. Congenital abdominal wall defects and testicular maldescent – a ten year single center experience. J Pediatr Surg. 2012;47(6):1118–1122.

7

Intestinal atresia: Duodenal-jejunal-ileal-colonic disorders

MARION ARNOLD AND SHARON COX
University of Cape Town, Western Cape, South Africa

DUODENAL ATRESIA

Scenario: A 13-week-gestation fetal antenatal scan shows mild polyhydramnios, a dilated stomach and fluid-filled distended duodenum ('double bubble').

Question: What information should be conveyed on counselling the parent(s)?
Answer: This is the appearance of duodenal atresia (DA), which has an incidence of 1–2 per 10,000 births and is apparent antenatally in about two thirds of cases (1). It results from an embryologic event at 8–10 weeks of gestation but has no known etiological factors. Polyhydramnios is present in 30%–60% of cases. Trisomy 21 (T21) is present in about a third of DA cases. Proximal jejunal atresia is a differential diagnosis if T21 is ruled out with a detailed fetal nuchal translucency scan and amniocentesis. DA is associated with cardiovascular anomalies in 20%–30% of patients. Other rare associations include heterotaxy (with malrotation [10%–15%]), VACTERL-associated anomalies (renal [5%], oesophageal atresia [5%], anorectal malformation [3%]) and, very rarely, other bowel atresias (7% – mainly seen with type III DA) (2, 3).

Scenario: The mother declines further fetal assessment for T21. The baby is born at 37 weeks of gestation weighing 2.4 kg and presents at 15 hours with bile-stained vomiting. Other than mild epigastric distension the rest of the examination is normal.

Question: If you did not have the earlier information from the antenatal ultrasound, what would your differential diagnosis now be?
Answer: This would now include malrotation with volvulus, DA or web, annular pancreas, jejuno-ileal atresia, meconium ileus/plug, Hirschsprung's disease (HD), anorectal malformation, small left colon syndrome, anorectal malformation and sepsis; however, increased abdominal distension is expected with more distal intestinal obstructive causes.

Scenario: The baby is stable on 10% dextrose-containing crystalloid intravenous maintenance fluids. An orogastric tube is placed; losses over 10 mL/kg are replaced intravenously with appropriate fluid.

DOI: 10.1201/9781003182290-8

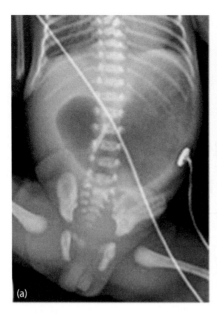
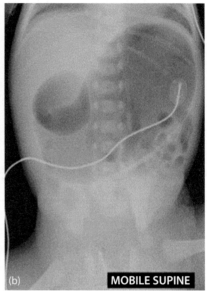

Figure 7.1 (a) plain-film abdominal X-ray showing grossly dilated stomach and proximal duodenum with a rounded configuration and no distal gas in duodenal atresia. (b) Abdominal X-ray with dilated stomach and duodenal 'double bubbles'. Distal bowel gas indicates a possible fenestrated web, complete atresia with bifid pancreatic duct or midgut volvulus.

Question: What workup would confirm the diagnosis?
Answer:

- *Bloods*: Routine blood chemistry and full blood count.
- *Abdominal X-ray (consider deferring to >18 hours after birth)*: Typical DA will show a large stomach bubble, rounded proximal duodenum and gasless rest of abdomen. Some distal gas is seen with a fenestrated duodenal web/windsock or bifid pancreatic duct (**Figure 7.1**).
- Upper gastrointestinal contrast is indicated if there is distal gas or the second bubble tapers (not rounded), suggesting a less severe degree of chronic distension.
- Features of Down's syndrome (T21) or clinical indication of a cardiac anomaly requires preoperative echocardiogram.
- Genetic testing (T21) if suggestive clinical features.

Question: How is DA classified?
Answer:

Type I (92%): Membranous obstruction (with or without fenestration).
Type II (1%): Fibrous cord joining the two ends of the duodenum (**Figure 7.2**).

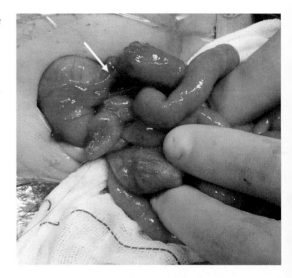

Figure 7.2 Type II duodenal atresia: A fibrous cord (*white arrow*) joins the proximal dilated duodenum and the distal duodenum.

Type III (7%): Complete interruption of duodenal continuity.
You make a diagnosis of DA and proceed to surgery.

Question: Describe the basic operative steps.
Answer: A transverse upper abdominal laparotomy incision is performed. The proximal and distal duodenal ends are mobilized. Via transverse proximal

and longitudinal distal enterotomy, a 'windsock' of prolapsed mucosa obstructing the lumen is excluded by easy passage of a catheter and a 'diamond-shaped' (Kimura) duodeno-duodenostomy is commonly performed. Alternatives include endoscopic balloon dilatation or incision for a fenestrated web or a duodenojejunostomy for a more distal DA. A transanastomotic feeding tube is useful in low-resource settings without parenteral nutrition access but risks the tube causing anastomotic breakdown or or pressure necrosis of the bowel wall. A laparoscopic approach is technically demanding but delivers equivalent outcomes despite a longer operating time, fairly high conversion rate and some cases of missed malrotation or Ladd's bands (4).

Scenario: The operations proceed without complications, and the baby is transferred to the neonatal unit.

Question: Discuss your postoperative management and the baby's subsequent course.

Answer: The mean time to achieve full feeds is 10 days. Parenteral nutrition is generally weaned as enteral feeds are built up. The rate of progression of enteral feeds is guided by the orogastric tube effluent volume and colour.

Genetic counselling is required if there is associated T21, heterotaxy or microdeletion syndromes.

Potential complications include anastomotic leak, stenosis, adhesions, wound infection and biliary tract injury. Long-term problems include obstruction from anastomotic stenosis and a dysmotile megaduodenum, which may require tapering duodenoplasty (risk is minimized by the initial anastomosis being performed in the most distal portion of the proximal bulbous end region).

Overall, the prognosis is excellent, and mortality is often related to associated cardiac anomaly (5).

JEJUNAL AND ILEAL ATRESIA

Scenario: A 37-week-gestation 2.4-kg infant vomits bile 18 hours after birth. Upper abdominal distension progresses to a scaphoid abdomen on passing an orogastric tube and aspiration of dark green fluid. Systemic examination is otherwise normal. A small white mucus plug is passed per rectum.

Question: What is the most likely diagnosis in this newborn?

Answer: Bilious vomiting in a newborn is usually due to bowel obstruction distal to the ampulla of Vater. Other causes include systemic sepsis and necrotizing enterocolitis. Infectious markers and radiology help with differentiation. Epigastric distension suggests proximal bowel obstruction (duodenal atresia, jejuno-ileal atresia, midgut volvulus) versus distal causes (HD, meconium plug, small left colon syndrome, meconium ileus and rectal or colonic atresia). White meconium (shed intestinal cells and mucus, lacking bile pigments) strongly suggests jejuno-ileal atresia, although most babies will pass no meconium. Intestinal atresia causes a third to half of all newborn bowel obstruction cases (6). Preterm birth and low birth weight suggest nutritional impairment from reduced fetal amniotic fluid gut absorption.

Question: The 20-week antenatal ultrasound was normal. What other causes of bowel obstruction should be considered?

Answer: Under half of jejunoileal atresia cases are detected on antenatal ultrasound (7). Dilated, thickened, fluid-filled bowel loops are typically only noted towards the end of the second trimester. Polyhydramnios suggests proximal bowel obstruction, including DA, which is more likely to be detected antenatally and presents similarly to jejunoileal atresia. Acquired bowel obstruction (e.g. malrotation with midgut volvulus, incarcerated inguinal hernia) needs to be considered, especially in the absence of findings related to chromosomal anomalies or VACTERL associations.

Question: What immediate management should be undertaken?
Answer:

- Intravenous fluid resuscitation if fluid depleted: Baseline blood gas and electrolyte measurements guide intravascular volume restoration.
- Intravenous access:
  - *Peripheral venous cannula*: Fluids and antibiotics.
  - *Peripherally inserted central cannula (PICC)*: For expected parenteral nutrition.
- Gastric decompression and intravenous replacement of gastric losses greater than 10 mL/kg.
- NPO, monitor blood glucose levels.
- Keep infant warm.

Question: What radiological investigations will aid diagnosis?

Answer:

- Plain abdominal film X-ray taken after 12–24 hours from birth (in conjunction with 20–40 mL air bolus through the orogastric tube directly before performance of X-ray if antenatal diagnosis is suspected) (**Figure 7.3**).
- *Upper GI contrast study*: Consider an upper gastrointestinal study with duodenal C-loop follow-through course if the diagnosis is unclear or there are distal gas locules to differentiate atresia from a fenestrated luminal web or malrotation. Use of air contrast often avoids this.
- *Lower GI contrast study*: Perform to exclude associated distal colonic atresias, 1% incidence (6), especially if minimally invasive surgery, including mini-laparotomy, is considered (**Figure 7.3**).

> **Scenario:** You diagnose jejunal atresia and are asked about the cause and any related diagnoses.

Question: What maternal and infant associations are found with this diagnosis?

Answer: Half of jejuno-ileal atresia cases appear to be due to an antenatal mechanical event disrupting the local blood supply (8), e.g. malrotation with antenatal midgut volvulus (10%), limited volvulus of small intestine associated with inspissated meconium in cystic fibrosis (5% in Caucasian populations) and gastroschisis (from obstruction of blood supply at para-umbilical defect level) (6). Smoking and vasoactive drug use are loosely associated. Sporadic genetic mutations affecting endodermal signalling pathways play a role (9), and multiple intestinal atresias (type IV; 10%–15%) (6) are occasionally seen as part of a hereditary genetic syndrome with an associated immune disorder (10) (**Table 7.1**).

> **Scenario:** The mother is concerned about a large scar on her baby's abdomen.

Question: What minimally invasive operative approaches options are available, and what caveats apply?

Answer: Cosmetic approaches include a peri-umbilical laparotomy incision and laparoscopic-assisted

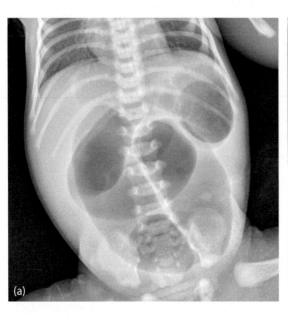
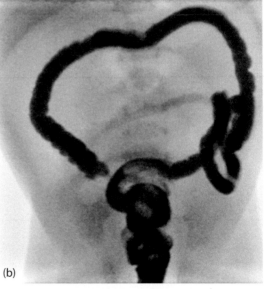

(a) (b)

Figure 7.3 (a) Plain abdominal X-ray showing dilated gas-filled stomach and two other grossly dilated gas-filled loops of bowel with a paucity of distal bowel gas, typical for proximal bowel obstruction as seen in jejunal atresia. Note absence of calcification (associated with antenatal perforation) or free air (postnatal perforation). (b) Contrast enema in a patient with jejunal atresia; note the patent microcolon with background proximal bowel obstruction and normal rectosigmoid ratio.

Table 7.1 Small bowel classification (10)

Type	I	II	IIIa	IIIb	IV
Bowel lumen	Simple obstructive web (may be fenestrated)	Interrupted bowel mucosal and serosal continuity			Multiple atresias (may be various combinations of types I, II and III)
Bowel mesentery	Intact	Intact	Defect	Wide defect with distal bowel spiralled around single supplying marginal vessel, usually in association with intestinal malrotation	May have multiple mesenteric defects in keeping with atresia types
Picture					
Association	Sporadic endodermal signalling pathway defect	Antenatal micro thrombo-embolic event/ sporadic endodermal signalling pathway defect	Antenatal macrovascular thrombo-embolic event Cystic fibrosis with local volvulus	Antenatal midgut volvulus/ malrotation	Antenatal micro thrombo-embolic event Sporadic/familial endodermal signalling pathway defect, may have arthrogryposes

techniques with intra- or extra-corporeal anastomosis. Both create difficulties in evaluation of the distal bowel for additional atresias. A 5-mm stapling device to facilitate laparoscopic bowel anastomosis has been described (11). Endoscopic balloon dilation of an isolated proximal jejunal fenestrated web is also described (12).

Question: When should operative management proceed?

Answer: Operation can be deferred up to 24–48 hours after birth. Ensure fluid and electrolyte status is optimized. Give preoperative vitamin K. With delayed diagnosis and sepsis from gut bacterial

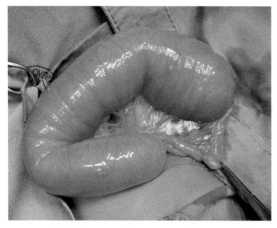

Figure 7.4 Type 1 jejunal atresia.

translocation, first treat the sepsis then check for and correct any coagulopathy preoperatively.

> **Scenario:** You proceed with a peri-umbilical approach. At laparotomy, a massively dilated, thick-walled loop of proximal jejunum in serosal continuity with distal collapsed bowel is found (**Figure 7.4**).

Question: How is this operative finding classified?

Answer: Grosfeld et al. (13) classified jejunoileal atresia according to the luminal continuity and presence and configuration of an associated mesenteric defect. The four variant types have distinct clinical implications (**Table 7.1**).

> **Scenario:** You are now able to assess the bowel fully and decide how to proceed surgically.

Question: Describe the operative technique used for the best outcome.

Answer: Resect 10–15 cm of the dilated bowel proximal to the atresia and 2 cm of bowel distal to the atresia or fenestrated web, with tapering (stapled or handsewn) of the remaining proximal dilated bowel to allow for an end-to-end anastomosis with interrupted sutures (**Figure 7.5**). Spatulate the distal lumen for a wider anastomosis. De-rotation of

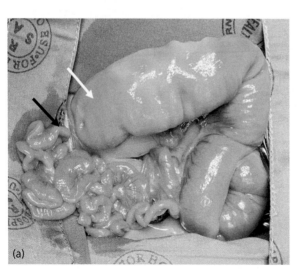
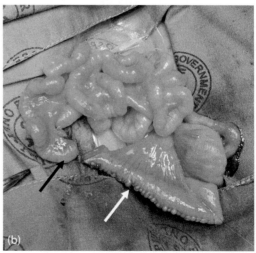

Figure 7.5 (a) Type I jejunal atresia with a large blind-ending proximal dilated loop of bowel (*white arrow*) (10 cm of which was later resected) adjacent to the blind end of the normal length of the distal collapsed disused bowel (*black arrow*). (b) The same patient after resection of 10 cm of the distal end of the dilated loop and hand-sewn tapering of the residual dilatation (*white arrow*), ready to perform an end-to-end anastomosis with the distal jejunum (*black arrow*).

the small bowel with take-down of the ligament of Treitz may be required for a very high proximal atresia. Inadequate resection of proximal dilated bowel is associated with poor gut motility, related to histopathological features of muscle fibrosis (14). It may be necessary to retain this segment in patients with type III or type IV atresia to prevent short bowel syndrome.

Prior to the anastomosis, flushing the distal bowel with saline rules out additional atresias and evacuates distal meconium plugs, which may delay postoperative stool function.

A trans-anastomotic nasojejunal feeding tube may be placed if access to parenteral nutrition is limited, but can place the anastomosis at risk if 'bowstrung' tension develops.

Question: What postoperative care is required?
Answer: Postoperative care involves optimization of fluid status, management of jaundice and sepsis if present and parenteral nutritional support until the postoperative ileus resolves, followed by a gradual introduction of enteral feeds. Progression to full enteral feeds can take 1–2 weeks. Prophylactic antibiotics can be stopped if septic markers and vital signs are normal with 24 hours of surgery. The

average length of hospital stay, assuming an uncomplicated hospital course, is 2–3 weeks (15).

> **Scenario:** The baby is stable but just not progressing with feeds as you would have wished.

Question: What are the possible complications and long-term problems?
Answer: Surgical considerations include adhesive bowel obstruction, pre-anastomotic ulcer (associated with short bowel syndrome), anastomotic leak or stenosis, wound infection and poor motility due to inadequate tapering and/or resection of dilated bowel. These are rare, occurring in 5–10% of cases. Adhesive bowel obstruction, foreign body lodgement at the anastomotic site and left-sided appendicitis related to de-rotation of the bowel occasionally occur long-term. In general, the long-term outcome with jejunoileal atresia is considered excellent.

> **Scenario:** Another two patients present with a similar clinical picture. Operative findings for the cases are shown in **Figure 7.6**.

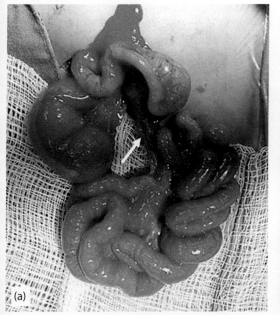 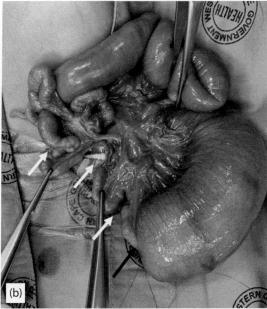

Figure 7.6 (a) Patient 1: Type IIIb 'apple-peel/Christmas-tree' deformity of distal bowel associated with a single distal marginal artery (*white arrow*) supplied from the middle colic and/or terminal ileal vessels. (b) Patient 2: Type IV jejunal atresia (proximal type I [*white arrow*]) with subsequent type II, type IIIa and another type II atresia (*white arrows*), with minimal residual bowel length.

Question: How does your operative management differ in these cases?

Answer: Operative strategies include possible de-rotation if required, proximal bowel tapering, confirming distal patency and anastomosis, as previously discussed. However, short bowel length related to type III or IV atresia may mandate retention of most of the dilated proximal segment, even though this is associated with poor motility. Tapering the dilated bowel may mitigate against dysmotility. In patient 1, do not attempt to unravel the spiral configuration of the bowel, even though this may result in the anastomosis not aligning on the mesenteric sides of the bowel, and ensure the distal bowel is not tightly wound around the precarious supplying marginal artery. The mesenteric defect often cannot be closed without compromising bowel. There is no risk for bowel herniation through the defect. In patient 2, multiple end-to-end anastomoses are required, preserving as much bowel length as possible.

Question: What is the long-term outcome in this case?

Answer: The most important determinants of long-term outcome in these cases are the total bowel length. Intestinal length in type IIIb and IV atresia can cause short bowel syndrome in about 10% of cases (13). This may require long-term parenteral nutritional support, intestinal rehabilitation and possible later consideration of intestinal lengthening. Even if length is normal, bowel ischaemia related to partial occlusion of the single vascular pedicle can lead to malabsorption and poor motility (**Figure 7.7**). Common causes of death include intestinal failure, even in high-income settings, and central line complications and sepsis in low- and middle-income settings.

COLONIC ATRESIA

Scenario: A day 2 term baby presents with gross abdominal distension and vomiting of feculent material. The child has not passed meconium. Examination reveals an increased capillary refill time (delayed) and a tachycardia. The abdomen is markedly distended but soft and non-tender with obstructive bowel sounds.

Question: What further information would assist diagnosis?
Answer:

- *Family history*: Cystic fibrosis, HD, maternal diabetes?
- *Antenatal history*: Polyhydramnios? Distended/Thickened bowel loops?
- *Examination*: Hernial orifice sites, perineal examination findings.
- *Abdominal X-ray*: Distended air-filled loops? Calcifications? Ground glass appearance of meconium?

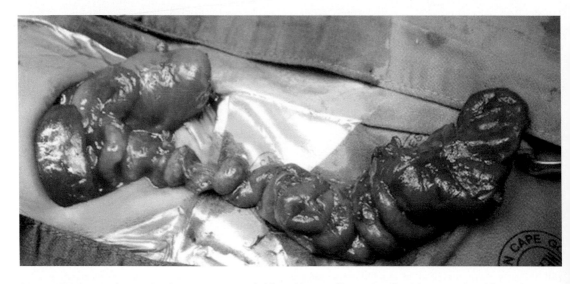

Figure 7.7 Type IIIb atresia showing proximal dilated loop of bowel with ischaemic distal bowel in a spiral configuration wound around a single blood vessel.

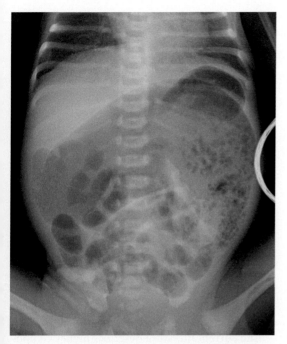

Figure 7.8 Abdominal X-ray typical of colonic atresia showing an extremely dilated loop of bowel. This is the dilated segment of colon proximal to the atresia, where bowel gas is trapped between the atresia and ileocecal valve.

Scenario: There is no relevant family or maternal history. The antenatal ultrasound showed polyhydramnios and a dilated loop of bowel. Hernial sites and perineal examination are normal with no gush of air or explosive passage of stool on rectal probing. An abdominal X-ray (**Figure 7.8**) reveals many dilated loops of bowel with one disproportionately large, dilated loop.

This is a clinical and radiological picture of distal bowel obstruction.

Question: What is the differential diagnosis of distal bowel obstruction in a neonate, and how would you rule these out in this child? Answer:

- *Anorectal malformation*: Ruled out by the normal patent anus.
- *Jejuno-ileal atresia*: Possible – more distal atresias show increased abdominal distension and a greater number of distended loops of bowel.
- *HD*: Possible – proximal aganglionosis may not have explosive release of stool on rectal manipulation.

- *Meconium ileus/Peritonitis*: Unlikely as no X-ray ground-glass appearance, calcification or free air.
- *Meconium plug syndrome*: No meconium on the X-ray; such dilated bowel is uncommon in this diagnosis.
- *Small left colon*: Rare without maternal history of diabetes.
- *Congenital pouch colon*: Associated with anorectal malformations especially in India and Asia.
- *Colonic atresia*: Possible due to polyhydramnios, antenatal evidence of dilated bowel and gross abdominal distension together with the disproportionately large gas-filled loop on abdominal X-ray.

Atresia of the colon comprises less than 5% of all bowel atresias and has an incidence of 1:40 000–1:60 000 live births (16). There is no gender or racial predilection, but it is associated with HD, cloacal exstrophy, gastroschisis (**Figure 7.9**), malrotation/non-fixation of the bowel and a more proximal atresia of the small bowel (16). Common aetiologies of an intrauterine vascular insult, including volvulus and closing umbilical ring, explain why these latter entities are associated with each other (17, 18).

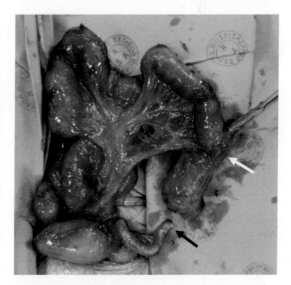

Figure 7.9 Colonic atresia in a patient with gastroschisis. This patient initially had an inflammatory exudate on the bowel, precluding management of the atresia. Here the bowel was reduced intra-abdominally, and operative atresia correction took place at 4 weeks of age with distal patency confirmation and a normal rectal biopsy. The image shows the ileo-caecal junction (*white arrow*), a few centimetres of dilated blind-ending colon and the distal disused colon (*black arrow*).

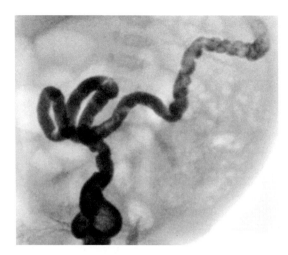

Figure 7.10 Contrast enema of a patient with colonic atresia showing a collapsed, disused distal colon with an atresia at the level of the splenic flexure on a background of dilated loops of proximal bowel.

Subtypes I, II or IIIa atresia(s) – which are the most common – occur in any part of the colon (16, 18, 19).

Scenario: After fluid resuscitation, the baby is haemodynamically stable with normal electrolytes. A nasogastric tube has been placed, and the baby is nil by mouth.

Question: What is your plan?
Answer: In clinically suspected distal bowel obstruction, contrast enema should be carried out before surgery to either diagnose colonic atresia or investigate other differential causes, including small left colon syndrome and meconium plug syndrome, and assess for an inverted rectosigmoid ratio or a transition zone that would prompt a biopsy to rule out HD (19, 20).

Scenario: The contrast enema is performed and shows a disused distal colon with contrast cut-off (**Figure 7.10**).

Question: What is your operative strategy?
Answer: The gross discrepancy between the proximal and distal bowel diameters and the association with HD render the management strategies used in small bowel atresia less useful (17).

The current literature describes higher complication rates in patients with primary anastomosis, usually due to undiagnosed distal pathology, and improved outcomes in cases where initial stoma creation has been performed.

Stomas are required if distal patency has not been confirmed, there is a large diameter discrepancy (**Figure 7.11**) between the proximal and distal end and HD has not been ruled out. Tapering

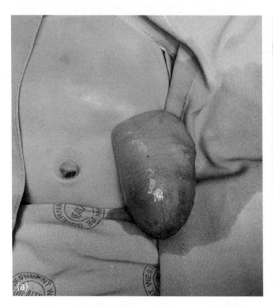

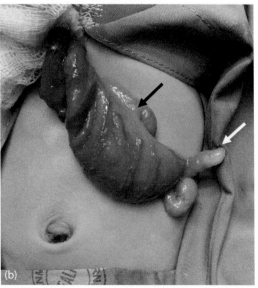

Figure 7.11 (a) Operative image of the distal dilated descending colon just proximal to the atresia. This loop of bowel prolapsed as the left-sided abdominal wall incision was opened. (b) Operative image of the same patient in (a). Note the calibre difference of the now fully exteriorized, extremely dilated proximal bowel (*black arrow*) and the disused narrow sigmoid colon (*white arrow*). This patient had a type IIIa atresia.

of the grossly distended colon to produce a more manageable stoma may be required.

Stoma closure would then occur later when the baby is stable and thriving and results of investigations on the distal bowel are known and cleared. It is important to resect a few centimetres of adjacent bowel proximally and distally because this may have abnormal innervation and vascularity. Primary resection and anastomosis can be performed in selected cases, provided the distal bowel is normal and patent.

A rapid progression to full feeds can occur in well patients with an isolated colonic atresia with a stoma, while in patients with multiple atresias and the possibility of short bowel, slower build-up of oral feeds, on a background of parenteral nutrition, is advised.

The outcome after surgery for colonic atresias is determined by coexistent pathology such as further atresias and short bowel syndrome, as well as the initial surgery. Outcomes in general are considered good.

BIBLIOGRAPHY

1. Turkbay D, Canpolat FE, Derme T, Altug N, Yilmaz Y. The birth prevalence of selected major congenital anomalies: Six-year's experience in a tertiary care maternity hospital. Turk Pediatri Ars. 2020;55(4): 393–400.
2. Bishop JC, McCormick B, Johnson CT, Miller J, Jelin E, Blakemore K, et al. The double bubble sign: Duodenal atresia and associated genetic etiologies. Fetal Diagn Ther. 2020;47(2):98–103.
3. Miscia ME, Lauriti G, Lelli Chiesa P, Zani A. Duodenal atresia and associated intestinal atresia: A cohort study and review of the literature. Pediatr Surg Int. 2019;35(1):151–7.
4. Mentessidou A, Saxena AK. Laparoscopic repair of duodenal atresia: Systematic review and meta-analysis. World J Surg. 2017;41(8):2178–84.
5. Kimura K, Mukohara N, Nishijima E, Muraji T, Tsugawa C, Matsumoto Y. Diamond-shaped anastomosis for duodenal atresia: An experience with 44 patients over 15 years. J Pediatr Surg. 1990;25(9): 977–9.
6. Verma A, Rattan KN, Yadav R. Neonatal intestinal obstruction: A 15 year experience in a tertiary care hospital. J Clin Diagn Res. 2016;10(2):SC10–3.
7. Wax JR, Hamilton T, Cartin A, Dudley J, Pinette MG, Blackstone J. Congenital jejunal and ileal atresia: Natural prenatal sonographic history and association with neonatal outcome. J Ultrasound Med. 2006;25(3):337–42.
8. Louw JH, Barnard CN. Congenital intestinal atresia observations on its origin. The Lancet. 1955;266(6899): 1065–7.
9. Nichol PF, Reeder A, Botham R. Humans, mice, and mechanisms of intestinal atresias: A window into understanding early intestinal development. J Gastrointest Surg. 2011;15(4):694–700.
10. Cole C, Freitas A, Clifton MS, Durham MM. Hereditary multiple intestinal atresias: 2 new cases and review of the literature. J Pediatr Surg. 2010;45(4):E21–4.
11. Rothenberg S. Laparoscopic Jejunal atresia repair technique 2018 [Available from: https://videolibrary.globalcastmd.com/.
12. Mochizuki K, Obatake M, Kosaka T, Tokunaga T, Eguchi S, Kanematsu T. Endoscopic balloon dilatation for congenital membranous stenosis in the jejunum in an infant. Pediatr Surg Int. 2011;27(1):91–3.
13. Grosfeld JL, Ballantine TVN, Shoemaker R. Operative management of intestinal atresia and stenosis based on pathologic findings. J Pediatr Surg. 1979;14(3):368–75.
14. Tyagi P, Mandal MB, Gangopadhyay AN, Patne SC. A functional study on small intestinal smooth muscles in jejunal atresia. J Indian Assoc Pediatr Surg. 2016;21(1):19–23.
15. Piper HG, Alesbury J, Waterford SD, Zurakowski D, Jaksic T. Intestinal atresias: Factors affecting clinical outcomes. J Pediatr Surg. 2008;43(7):1244–8.
16. El-Asmar KM, Abdel-Latif M, El-Kassaby AA, Soliman MH, El-Behery MM. Colonic atresia: Association with other anomalies. J Neonatal Surg. 2016;5(4):47.

17. Moore SW, Rode H, Millar AJW, Cywes S. Intestinal atresia and Hirschsprung's disease. Pediatr Surg Int. 1990;3(5):182–4.

18. Baglaj M, Carachi R, MacCormack B. Colonic atresia: A clinicopathological insight into its etiology. Eur J Pediatr Surg. 2010;20(2):102–5.

19. Cox SG, Numanoglu A, Millar AJ, Rode H. Colonic atresia: Spectrum of presentation and pitfalls in management. A review of 14 cases. Pediatr Surg Int. 2005;21(10): 813–8.

20. Dalla Vecchia LK, Grosfeld JL, West KW, Rescorla FJ, Scherer LR, Engum SA. Intestinal atresia and stenosis: A 25-year experience with 277 cases. Arch Surg. 1998;133(5):490–6; discussion 6–7.

8

Malrotation and heterotaxy disorders

PABLO A. LOBOS, SABRINA DE LOS A. PINTOS, AND ROCIO BOUDOU
Hospital Italiano de Buenos Aires, Buenos Aires, Argentina

INTESTINAL MALROTATION

Scenario: A 2-day-old, 35-week-gestation female patient, with a prenatal scan diagnosis of a double-bubble anomaly and history of maternal polyhydramnios presents with increasing irritability. Physical exam reveals progressive abdominal distension, with visible bowel loops. An orogastric tube was placed, obtaining abundant bilious fluid output.

Question: Do you suspect any particular condition? Is there something characteristic that warrants your immediate attention?

Answer: The prenatal scan finding of polyhydramnios and neonatal bilious vomiting point to the diagnosis of an intestinal obstruction disorder. The double-bubble fetal scan image is typically characteristic of congenital duodenal obstruction. Its most frequent cause is duodenal atresia, though the postnatal clinical picture with worsening abdominal distension and irritability is not a hallmark consistent with this diagnosis. Thus intestinal malrotation must be considered as an alternative working diagnosis.

Question: A plain abdominal X-ray is performed, which is illustrated in Figure 8.1. What findings will guide you toward the possible differential diagnoses?

Answer: Although plain film radiological findings are usually non-specific, the first study we

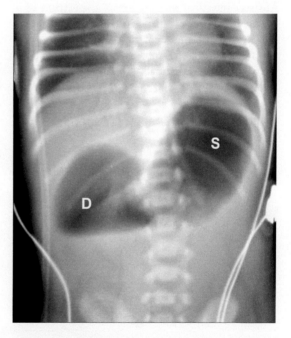

Figure 8.1 Plain abdominal X-ray showing gastric (s) and duodenal (D) distension (double-bubble image) with no air in the rest of the abdomen.

should request is an abdominal radiograph. If foregut obstruction is suspected, the sensitivity of the study can be increased by delivering 20 cc of air through the orogastric tube. The double-bubble image (distension of the stomach and first portion of the duodenum) confirms the suspicion of duodenal obstruction. The absence of air distally may be secondary to duodenal or jejunal atresia, but this diagnosis does not readily explain the marked abdominal distension presented by the sick patient, since air/fluid contents from the gastrointestinal tract distal to the site of obstruction are usually very scarce with congenital duodenal anomalies.

Question: How could this radiograph image be better explained if the patient presents with intestinal malrotation?

Answer: The double-bubble sign can also be seen as a consequence of compression of the second portion of the duodenum by Ladd's bands, and the abdominal distension may also be related to an associated midgut intestinal volvulus. These are discussed next.

Question: How is intestinal malrotation defined? What is its pathophysiology?

Answer: Intestinal malrotation is a spectrum of a disease that is a consequence of an abnormal alteration in the anatomical rotation and fixation of the intestines. During the embryonic period, the midgut intestinal loops leave the abdominal cavity as a result of its rapid growth and enter the extraembryonic coelom (**Figure 8.2a**) where it then makes a first 90° rotation counterclockwise in relation to the major axis of the superior mesenteric artery (SMA) (**Figure 8.2b**). Around the tenth week of gestation, a second 90° rotation occurs (**Figure 8.2c**) and then a third one once the gut loops return to the abdominal cavity, thus completing a full 270° rotation (**Figure 8.2d**). This rotational process results in the normal anatomical position of the intestine, notably the duodenum positioned on the right, the duodeno-jejunal (DJ) flexure on the left of the vertebral column, and the cecum and ascending colon situated on the right, with the base of the intestinal mesentery extending from left to right and from top to bottom (**Figure 8.2e** and **f**) toward the right iliac fossa.

Any alteration during this developmental process will generate an abnormal anatomical position of the midgut. The cecum is thus usually located in an abnormal position close to the duodenum in such a way that the mesenteric root is shortened. In addition, abnormal band adhesions termed Ladd's bands are formed between the cecum (in its elevated position) and the abdominal wall at the right flank,

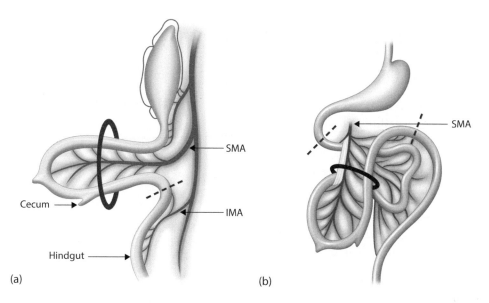

(a)   (b)

Figure 8.2 Diagram representing the sequence of rotation and fixation of the intestine during embryonic development. (a) As a result of rapid growth, most of the bowel leaves the abdominal cavity at the level of the base of the umbilical cord. (b) The elongated intestine loop makes a first rotation of 90° counterclockwise in such a way that the posterior intestine is displaced to the left of the abdomen. (c) Around the tenth week of gestation, the intestinal loop performs a second 90° rotation. At this moment the entire digestive tube is inside the abdomen. (d) Once inside the abdominal cavity, the intestine then performs a third rotation, thus completing a 270° rotation. *(Continued)*

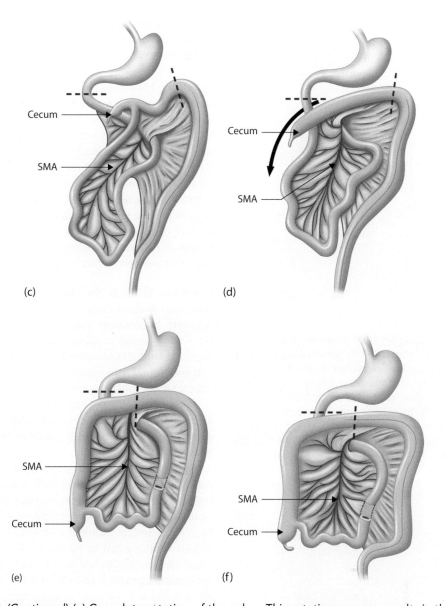

Figure 8.2 *(Continued)* (e) Complete rotation of the colon. This rotation process results in the final position of the intestine: The duodenum sited on the right, the duodeno-jejunal flexure on the left, and the cecum and ascending colon on the right, with the base of the mesentery extended from left to right and from top to bottom. (f) Final phase of mesenteric adhesions: The ascending and descending colon fuse at the posterior abdominal wall. *Abbreviations*: SMA: Superior mesenteric artery, IMA: Inferior mesenteric artery.

compressing the anterior wall of the second portion of the duodenum (**Figure 8.3**). The bands cause compression, which can result in varying degrees of duodenal obstruction, which may thus explain the prenatal scan findings in the sick patient. The shortening of the mesenteric root facilitates volvulus of the midgut on its axis, which provokes gut ischemia by compressing (twisting of the SMA) the vascular territories nourished by the SMA, from the first jejunal loop to the proximal right half of the colon as far as the midportion of the transverse colon (**Figure 8.4**).

The findings in our patient can thus be explained by the combination of duodenal compression by

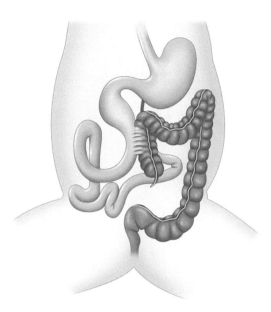

Figure 8.3 Representative diagram of a malrotation anomaly. Note that the cecum is abnormally located in a position close to the duodenum in such a way that the mesenteric root is foreshortened. In addition, abnormal adhesions – Ladd's bands – are formed between the cecum and the abdominal wall at the right flank, thus compressing the anterior wall of the second portion of the duodenum.

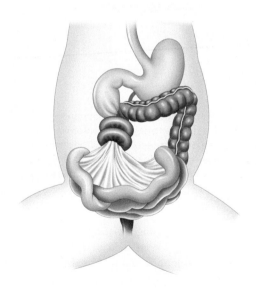

Figure 8.4 Representative diagram of a midgut volvulus over the axis of the SMA. *Abbreviation*: SMA: Superior mesenteric artery.

Ladd's bands and a midgut volvulus causing abdominal distension and irritability due to pain secondary to gut ischemia.

Question: How frequent is intestinal malrotation in the newborn period?

Answer: A prevalence of malrotation of 3.9 per 10,000 live births has been estimated, while other studies suggest a prevalence as high as 1 in 500 live births (1, 2). We should mention that other congenital malformation entities like omphalocele, gastroschisis and congenital diaphragmatic hernia can present with "gut non-rotation" anomalies as part of their pathophysiology, which must be clearly distinguished from the classical "malrotation" that we refer to here in this chapter.

Question: What is the clinical presentation of intestinal malrotation?

Answer: Malrotation can present in two ways: (1) a non-specific clinical picture with recurrent vomiting (bilious) associated or not with intermittent abdominal pain symptoms or (2) the devastating picture of midgut volvulus.

In the first scenario, what we observe are the visible manifestations of duodenal sub-occlusion, which may or may not be associated with an intermittent intestinal volvulus, although without significant arterial vascular insufficiency or compromise. The patient may therefore present with sporadic vomiting (may be of gastric content but more characteristically bilious), sudden abdominal pain (evidenced by crying) and/or transient abdominal distension. Bilious vomiting can be readily explained by duodenal obstruction secondary to Ladd's bands, the concomitant presence of a duodenal atresia anomaly or intestinal volvulus, in which case, the symptoms and physical examination could vary greatly depending on the time of evolution of the injury. These symptoms may be exacerbated by feeding.

In the second form listed, i.e. those cases presenting with midgut volvulus, patients may appear very irritable with severe abdominal pain, erythema/inflammation of the abdominal wall with hematemesis and even bloody stools. In these catastrophic cases, there is often a rapid deterioration of the patient's general condition that leads to profound shock in only a matter of a few hours due to the massive intestinal necrosis that is taking place.

There are also cases encountered in which malrotation remains virtually asymptomatic until adulthood, and it may be diagnosed incidentally in the context of a screening radiology study for another suspected condition or due to non-specific symptoms such as occasional vomiting, recurrent abdominal pain and/or lack of gain in weight and height milestones.

Question: Given the clinical suspicions of intestinal malrotation, what imaging studies can assist in the diagnosis?
Answer: We should distinguish here between the diagnosis of intestinal malrotation and a diagnosis of midgut volvulus.

As discussed earlier, a plain abdominal X-ray should be requested as the first initial study.

In an emergent case scenario secondary to intestinal volvulus, gastric distension will be observed followed by a paucity of widespread intestinal gaseous distension and even pneumatosis (**Figure 8.5**). It is therefore important to mention that in non-complicated intestinal malrotation, a normal gas pattern may be seen with surprisingly no marked abnormalities in the abdominal plain X-ray (**Figure 8.6a and b**).

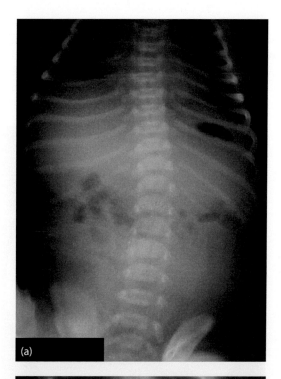
(a)

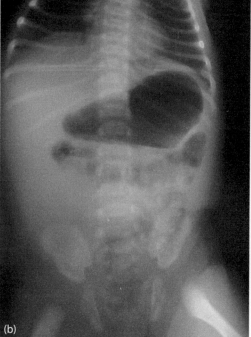
(b)

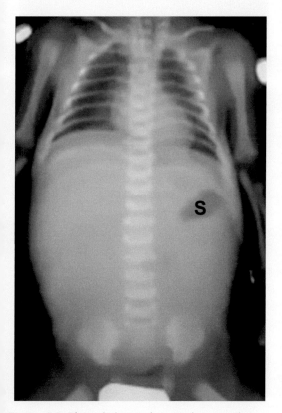

Figure 8.5 Plain abdominal X-ray showing the gastric shadow(s) and absence of air in the rest of the abdominal cavity.

Figure 8.6 (a and b) Plain abdominal X-ray images in a patient with intestinal malrotation. *Note*: We recommend performing the upper GI series using barium as contrast media. Besides allowing for better definition of images, it is then possible to do a follow-up contrast study with delayed X-rays some hours later. This may better clearly display the position of the cecum.

A contrast enema study can be useful to show the position of the colon and the suspected level of intestinal obstruction. It will provide clear and pathognomonic images of malrotation such as the cecum abnormally sited in a subhepatic location (**Figure 8.7a–c**). However, a high cecum is not always indicative of a malrotation.

In those patients with chronic, intermittent bilious vomiting who may perhaps attend a regular clinic visit on an outpatient basis, an oral

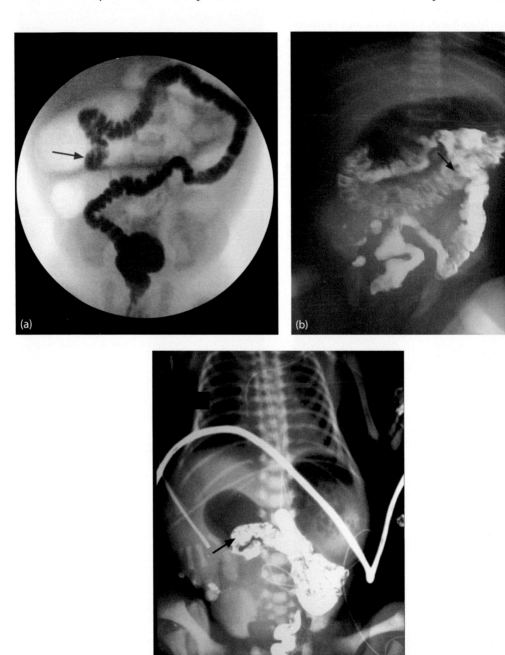

Figure 8.7 (a–c) Images of a contrast enema in a patient with intestinal malrotation. Note the abnormal position of the cecum (*black arrow*) due to the rotation anomaly.

signifies the presence of intestinal volvulus with high specificity, although sonography does not replace a foregut contrast study as a gold-standard diagnostic method. It is operator dependent, and it may be difficult to view the superior mesenteric vein (SMV) lateral to the DJ flexure/junction.

Question: Once a diagnosis of intestinal malrotation is made, what treatment would you plan for the patient?
Answer: Due to the risks of catastrophic intestinal necrosis secondary to midgut volvulus, intestinal malrotation requires operation. Ladd's operation is scheduled on an urgent or semi-urgent basis in patients without associated volvulus (**Figure 8.9a–d**), whereas suspected or confirmed volvulus requires immediate surgical intervention.

Ladd's procedure (3, 4, 13) includes the following key steps:

1. Intestinal de-rotation in a counterclockwise fashion.
2. Division of Ladd's bands (if present) to relieve duodenal compression and release the cecum from its abnormal subhepatic location.
3. The right colon is mobilized by division of all adhesions and progressively moving it toward the left upper quadrant.
4. Straightening the loop of the duodenum, widening the root of the mesentery and then placing the small bowel to the right side of the abdomen and the colon to the left. Great care is needed not to damage the SMV, which will be exposed during this maneuver.
5. Appendectomy may be undertaken, as the colon will be abnormally located to the left of the abdominal cavity with a Ladd's operation. This may be achieved using an inversion technique.

In the event that the patient presents with acute intestinal volvulus, it is crucial to expedite volume resuscitation and electrolyte acid-base imbalance and secure prompt placement of a decompressive nasogastric tube.

The surgeon must assess viability of the midgut after untwisting the volvulus (**Figure 8.10a and b**). If there are dubious signs of gut viability recovery, it is acceptable surgical practice to

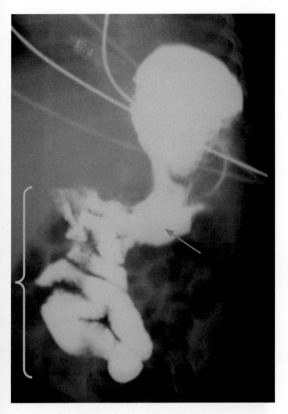

Figure 8.8 Image of an upper GI series in a patient with intestinal malrotation. The position of the duodenal-jejunal junction can be seen on the right (*arrow*) and a "corkscrew" image associated with the intestinal volvulus (*curly bracket*).

contrast study may be used to diagnose intestinal malrotation.

The upper GI series is the study of choice to confirm the diagnosis. The contrast study will show evidence of a dilated duodenum secondary to obstruction by Ladd's bands (megaduodenum) and also clearly identify the anatomical position of the DJ junction. Malrotation is confirmed when the DJ junction is located to the right of the vertebral spine. If the patient has an associated volvulus, the classic corkscrew image of the small intestine may be diagnostic (**Figure 8.8**).

Some authors advocate abdominal ultrasound imaging as another possible diagnostic tool if the abnormal position of the SMA and vein can be clearly identified or if a "whirlpool effect" is shown during Doppler examination. The whirlpool sign

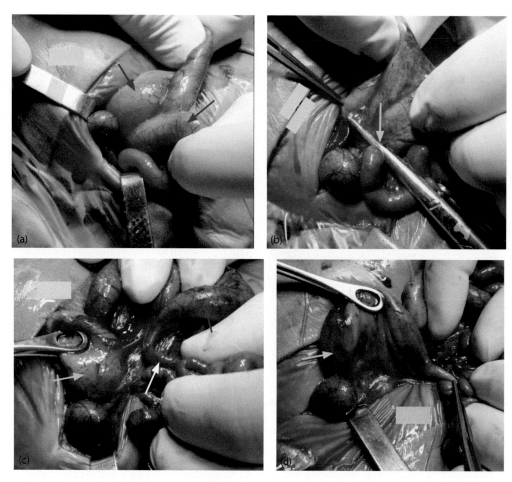

Figure 8.9 Surgical photo images of a patient with intestinal malrotation during Ladd's procedure. (a) The cecum is located at the epigastrium (*blue arrow*), to the left of the gallbladder; note also the terminal ileum (*red arrow*). (b) Release of Ladd's bands (*light blue arrow*) with duodenal exposure. (c) Dissection and verticalization of the dilated duodenum (*green arrow*), separating it from the cecum (*blue arrow*) and the appendix (*white arrow*). (d) Exposure of the dilated duodenum, confirming a caliber change distally (with congenital duodenal atresia co-associated anomaly).

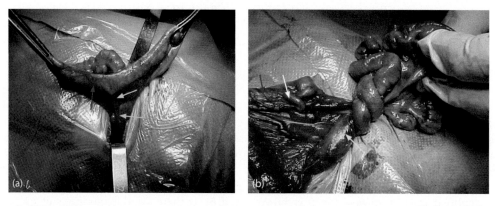

Figure 8.10 Photographs representing the intraoperative findings of a malrotated patient with a midgut volvulus. (a) When the abdominal contents are exteriorized, Ladd's bands (*light blue arrow*) are seen here found between the colon (*blue arrow*) and the duodenum (*green arrow*). (b) Midgut volvulus with two twisting turns on its vascular axis (*yellow arrow*). The change in color of the volvulated loops can be clearly observed, which suggests compromise of their vascular flow.

adopt a "watchful waiting" approach before contemplating an up-front massive intestinal resection by temporarily closing the abdomen and scheduling re-exploring within the next 24 hours in a second-stage operation.

Question: The patient had an initial good early postoperative recovery, but persistent bilious output persists after 11 days since surgery. For this reason, an abdominal X-ray is requested, where a non-obstructive intestinal gas pattern is verified. Enteral feeds are restarted with good response. What is the prognosis of intestinal malrotation?

Answer: Intestinal malrotation, when diagnosed and treated in a timely manner, has an excellent prognosis in most cases, although some patients may later present with vomiting and even later episodes of adhesive volvulus in the long term. In stark contrast, the prognosis of a patient presenting emergently with intestinal volvulus will depend on the length of ischemic necrotic bowel resected, irrespective of Ladd's laparotomy and restoration of normal vascular gut flow. In catastrophic cases with irreversible vascular compromise, the whole territory of the SMA is typically affected, with loss of the entire jejunal-ileum and the right colon. As a consequence, death of the patient ("deadly vomit") or short bowel syndrome may require a complex intestinal rehabilitation program with prolonged dependence on parenteral nutrition. Intestinal transplantation is also now available at specialist centers.

HETEROTAXY DISORDERS

Scenario: A full-term newborn baby presents with a prenatal diagnosis of heterotaxy disorder with a single right ventricle, a double outflow tract type complete atrioventricular (AV) channel and severe grade sub-valvular pulmonary stenosis, associated with the liver sited on the left of the abdominal cavity and a single spleen viewed on the right. At 2 months of age, a systemic pulmonary shunt was performed to palliate the underlying heart disease. The plain film X-ray after the cardiac intervention is shown (**Figure 8.11**).

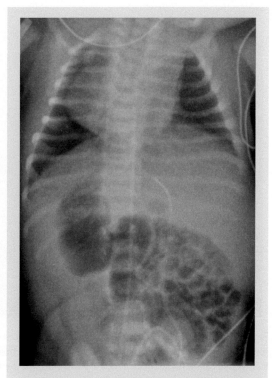

Figure 8.11 X-ray image of a child with heterotaxy syndrome. Note the position of the heart to the right, the liver position to the left and the gastric shadow on the right, with the duodenum lying vertical parallel to the vertebral spine.

Question: What radiographic findings do you note in the patient's X-ray film image?

Answer: Dextroposition of the heart, the liver is located close to the midline and the gastric bubble shadow is on the right, with the duodenum and the rest of the bowel lying in a contralateral position to conventional normal anatomy. All of these radiographic findings are compatible with the prenatal diagnosis of heterotaxy syndrome (HS).

During the postoperative period, the patient presents with an inability to progress, with enteral feeds achieving only a maximum tolerance volume of 5 mL/h.

Question: What imaging studies will you now require to rule out possible causes that may explain this clinical picture?

Answer: In order to rule out possible mechanical cause(s) of intestinal obstruction that explains the patient's current symptoms, an upper GI contrast study can be performed.

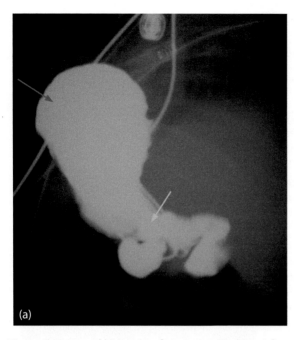 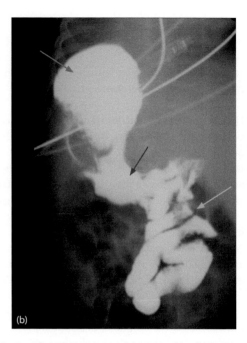

Figure 8.12 (a and b) Image of an upper GI series of a patient with heterotaxy and intestinal malrotation. Note the gastric dextroposition (*blue arrow*) and the presence of a duodenal-jejunal angle to the left of the vertebral spine without crossing the midline (*red arrow*) and a "corkscrew" image associated with intestinal volvulus confirmed (*orange arrow*).

The study shows gastric dextroposition and the DJ flexure apparently not crossing the midline. A "corkscrew" image (associated with intestinal volvulus) is also observed (**Figure 8.12a** and **b**). These findings are thus consistent with intestinal malrotation in a patient with heterotaxy.

Question: What is the relationship(s) between heterotaxy and intestinal malrotation?
Answer: Patients with HS, defined by any arrangement of organs along the left-right body axis that is neither situs solitus nor situs inversus (6), usually have a high rate (%) of associated intestinal malrotation (70%–75%) (7). It is, however, worth mentioning that not all patients with rotation anomalies are "symptomatic" and sometimes the type of associated anomaly cannot clearly be documented. In cases presenting with gastrointestinal symptoms the diagnosis should be established by contrast study, as in the case of our patient.

Question: Once intestinal malrotation is diagnosed in a HS patient, what is the course of action to follow?
Answer: Given that many HS patients have severe congenital heart disease, the decision to perform surgery at the time of detecting a malrotation anomaly in an "asymptomatic" patient and the need to routinely screen for malrotation with a foregut contrast study in all patients with heterotaxy is a highly controversial debate.

Although several surgical centers have reported that the morbidity and mortality associated with a Ladd's procedure in HS patients is not increased when compared to a healthy control population, others have observed worse outcomes with a Ladd's procedure in patients with heterotaxy rotational abnormalities (8). Ladd's procedure is notably associated with a 10%–27% risk of postoperative intestinal obstruction (5, 7).

Langer et al. reported a follow-up study of 152 asymptomatic neonates with HS, of whom only 4 patients developed gastrointestinal symptoms at a median follow-up period of 18 months, and only 1 of these 4 patients had malrotation detected by a contrast study. Of the remaining asymptomatic patients, 43% died of their coexistent heart disease and none developed intestinal symptoms or complications. Therefore, a conservative approach should be adopted in which asymptomatic patients with HS are not routinely screened for intestinal rotational abnormalities unless they become symptomatic (9).

Table 8.1 Characteristics and possible associated malformations in heterotaxy syndromes

	Polysplenia syndrome/Left bilaterality	Asplenia syndrome/ Right bilaterality
Visceroatrial situs ambiguous	Left atrial isomerism	Right atrial isomerism
Atria	Common atrium, atrial septal defects, atrial septal malposition, absence of fossa ovalis	–
AV connection	Single AV valve, common AV channel, accessory pathways	–
AV concordance	Usually normal	Possible mismatch
VA concordance	*Possible discrepancy and/or malformations*: transposition of great vessels, double outlet right ventricle.	
Venous	*Systemic venous anomalies*: IVC interruption, absence of intrahepatic IVC, IVC continuation with azygos system, persistence of the left superior vena cava, bilateral superior vena cava	*Pulmonary venous abnormalities*: partial/ complete anomalous pulmonary venous drainage
Bronchial abnormalities	Left bronchial isomerism	Right bronchial isomerism
Lung abnormalities	Left lung isomerism (two bilobed lungs)	Right lung isomerism (two trilobed lungs)
Extrathoracic visceral abnormalities	Polysplenia, intestinal malrotation, symmetric or inverted liver (left lobe predominance), extrahepatic biliary atresia	Asplenia, intestinal malrotation, stomach in upright position, symmetrical liver
Prognosis	*Survival*: 64% Cardiac malformations present in 90% of cases	*Survival*: 29% Cardiac malformations present in 99% of cases More severe, conotruncal type

Source: Carro Hevia, A; Santamarta Liébana, E; Martín Fernández, M. Síndrome de heterotaxia. Cardiocore [online]. 2011, 46(2), e23–26 [As extracted on March 12, 2022]. ISSN: 1889-898X.

It should be cautiously noted, however, that any symptomatic patient with a documented bowel rotation abnormality should undergo corrective surgery.

Given that our patient did present with symptoms and that a rotation abnormality was found on a contrast study, an operation was indicated.

Question: What other malformations are associated with HS?

Answer: Cardiac malformations vary in complexity (e.g., from atrial septal defects to double outlet right ventricle) and ultimately determine prognosis. The most severe HS patients present with the features of right atrial isomerism. Some notable extracardiac features include the presence of two or three lobes in each lung, absence of the hepatic segment of the vena cava, polysplenia and abnormalities of the cardiac chambers (**Table 8.1**). Systemic and/or pulmonary venous drainage anomalies may also be noted with heterotaxy (10). Heterotaxy syndromes can be associated with asplenia or polysplenia. In these cases, the gastrosplenic ligament is usually poorly developed, predisposing such patients to gastric volvulus. This condition, which usually presents as an acute abdomen similar to midgut volvulus, can result in fatal gastric necrosis if diagnosis and surgical treatment are not established in a timely manner. Gastric volvulus is treated by devolvulation and gastropexy, achieved either by sutures to the abdominal wall or by placement of a gastrostomy tube (11, 12).

BIBLIOGRAPHY

1. Graziano K, Islam S, Dasgupta R, et al. Asymptomatic malrotation: Diagnosis and surgical management: An American Pediatric Surgical Association outcomes and evidence based practice committee systematic review. J PediatrSurg. 2015;50:1783–1790.

2. Torres AM, Ziegler MM. Malrotation of the intestine. World J Surg. 1993;17: 326–331.

3. Ladd WE. Congenital obstruction of the duodenum in children. N Engl J Med. 1932;206:277–283.

4. Ladd WE. Congenital obstruction of the small intestine. J Am Med Assoc. 1933;101: 1453–1458.

5. Abu-Elmagd K, Mazariegos G, Armanyous S, Parekh N, ElSherif A, Khanna A, Kosmach-Park B, D'Amico G, Fujiki M, Osman M, Scalish M, Pruchnicki A, Newhouse E, Abdelshafy AA, Remer E, Costa G, Walsh RM. Five hundred patients with gut malrotation: Thirty years of experience with the introduction of a new surgical procedure. Ann Surg. 2021;274(4):581–596.

6. Langer JC. Intestinal rotation abnormalities and midgut volvulus. Surg Clin. 2017;97: 147–159.

7. Ryerson LM, Pharis S, Pockett C, et al. Heterotaxy syndrome and intestinal rotation abnormalities. Pediatrics. 2018; 142(2):e20174267.

8. Salavitabar A, Anderson BR, Aspelund G, Starc TJ, Lai WW. Heterotaxy syndrome and intestinal rotational anomalies: Impact of the Ladd procedure. J Pediatr Surg. 2015;50(10): 1695–1700. doi: 10.1016/j.jpedsurg.2015.02. 065. Epub 2015 Mar 7. PMID: 25783348.

9. Choi M, Borenstein SH, Hornberger L, et al. Heterotaxy syndrome: The role of screening for intestinal rotation abnormalities. Arch Dis Child. 2005;90: 813–815.

10. Carro Hevia A, Santamarta Liébana E, Martín Fernández M. Síndrome de heterotaxia. Cardiocore [en linea]. 2011;46(2):e23–e26 [fecha de Consulta 12 de Marzo de 2022]. ISSN: 1889-898X.

11. Forenza N, Albuquerque S, Vallejo G, Muzzo G. Síndrome de Ivemark: Vólvulo gástrico asociado con asplenia. Rev. de Cir. Infantil. 2001;11(4):243–245.

12. Miller DL. Gastric volvulus in the pediatric population. Arch Surg. 1991;26(9):1146.

13. Elmo G, Calello S. Intestinal Malrotation. In Fetoneonatología quirúrgica. 1st Edition. M. Martínez Ferro, C. Cannizzaro, G. Chattás Editors. Journal Editors, 2018; Volume 1: pp. 666–676.

9

Hirschsprung's disease

PATRICK CHUNG
Queen Mary's Hospital, University of Hong Kong, Hong Kong

PAUL TAM
Macau University of Science and Technology, Macau
and University of Hong Kong, Hong Kong

Scenario: You are called to assess a 3-day-old Chinese male baby whose abdomen is distended. He was born at term, and the antenatal history was unremarkable. There was a reluctance to feed and a small amount of bilious vomiting noted. The first stool activity was observed some 24 hours from birth with a small amount of meconium allegedly passed.

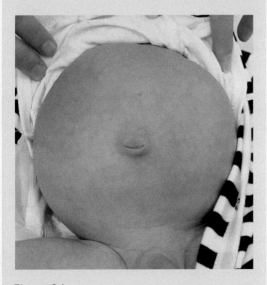

Figure 9.1

On clinical examination, the baby is crying loudly, and no syndromic features are identified. His body height and weight are below the tenth percentile. The abdomen is markedly distended without evident tenderness (**Figure 9.1**). There are no palpable masses evident and a normal-looking anus is seen at the perineum. Digital rectal examination (DRE) resulted in a gush of meconium upon withdrawal of the examiner's finger. Further examination of the back and lower limb neurology is normal.

Question: What are the possible diagnoses for this baby?
Answer: This baby likely has an intestinal obstruction, and from the timing of onset, the diagnosis is linked to a congenital disorder. As the presenting symptom is abdominal distension with minimal vomiting, the level of obstruction is most likely in the lower gastrointestinal tract. Common congenital disorders resulting in distal obstruction include ileal atresia, meconium ileus/plug syndrome and Hirschsprung's disease (HSCR). Nowadays, the broad application of fetal ultrasound allows most small bowel atresia(s) to be detected antenatally. Meconium ileus is more common in Caucasians

and is usually associated with cystic fibrosis. In this case, the most likely diagnosis is HSCR, as the gush of stool expelled after DRE in a baby with abdominal distension is a classical feature of HSCR. Diarrhea suggests HSCR-associated enterocolitis (see next). Not uncommonly, a mild-variant anorectal malformation lesion may also present with constipation, and therefore, the perineum should be examined thoroughly. The lower back of the patient should also be inspected for any stigmata that may suggest underlying spinal anomalies resulting in functional intestinal obstruction.

Question: What investigations would be useful?
Answer: A full blood count with liver and renal function tests should be undertaken as a baseline assessment of the general condition. Thyroid function should be checked also to exclude hypothyroidism as the underlying cause. A plain abdominal X-ray will reveal dilated bowel loops with notably the absence of gas in the rectum, but this is not diagnostic of HSCR (**Figure 9.2**). A contrast enema study may reveal spasticity and narrowing of the rectum, which may extend upward to a more proximal colon (**Figure 9.3**). Increase in the size of the presacral space is consistent also. A transition zone may be observed and is useful to guide the strategy for definitive surgery. However, to ensure the transition zone is best visualized at contrast exam, the DRE should be avoided for 24 hours before the contrast study investigation. To confirm HSCR, a rectal biopsy should be performed. This can be performed using a suction

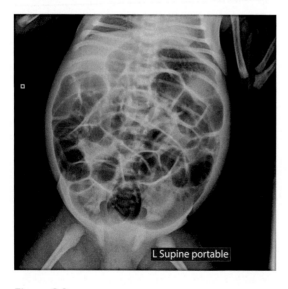

Figure 9.2

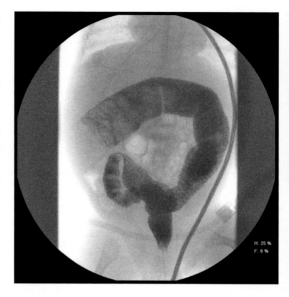

Figure 9.3

device as a bedside procedure. For a proper histology assessment, the specimen should include both the mucosa and submucosa of the area of distal rectum biopsied. The specimen will be examined particularly for the absence of submucosal ganglion cells and the presence of hypertrophic nerve fibers (increased acetylcholinesterase staining) – the two classical pathohistological findings in HSCR. Recently, calretinin immunohistochemistry staining has been added as an adjuvant study analysis to confirm HSCR with a higher sensitivity and specificity.

Question: What is HSCR?
Answer: HSCR is a congenital gastrointestinal disorder with an estimated incidence around 1 in 5,000 live births. A slightly higher incidence is noted in Asian racial groups. This disease is characterized by absence of intrinsic ganglion cells (aganglionosis) in the myenteric and submucosal plexuses of the gastrointestinal tract, starting from the distal rectum with variable extension to the proximal bowel. In more than 80% of the cases, the aganglionosis is limited to the recto-sigmoid colon (i.e., short-segment disease), but a more proximal extension (greater length of colonic involvement) can be found in 10%–15% of index cases. Total colonic aganglionosis (TCA) is a severe form of HSCR and accounts for approximately 5% of all cases. While males are more commonly affected than females in short-segment diseases (ratio = 4:1), the sex ratio appears similar in long-segment HSCR.

Question: How may HSCR present beyond the neonatal period?

Answer: Most HSCR patients will present with intestinal obstruction during the neonatal period, but occasionally, the first symptom manifestations are encountered during infancy and the early childhood period. In such a case, intractable refractory constipation is the usual complaint. In young children, constipation is common and can be due to various self-limiting causes such as inadequate fluid/fiber intake, milk formula diet or poor habit. Sometimes, constipation is a symptom of underlying medical disorders such as hypothyroidism or autoimmune diseases. Occasionally, certain medications can also provoke constipation in infants, but this is usually transient. Children with causes other than HSCR may give a history of fecal soiling, which is unusual with HSCR. On the other hand, HSCR-related constipation tends to be much more severe and may result in malnourishment. In the most severe cases, undiagnosed HSCR may lead to severe bowel inflammation (enterocolitis) resulting in vomiting, diarrhea and life-threatening sepsis, particularly in infants and children.

Question: How do we manage HSCR?

Answer: HSCR is a surgical disease, and until now, the only treatment was elective surgical intervention. While waiting for definitive surgery, patients should receive regular rectal washouts (with or without anal dilatation) by a nurse or caregiver to provide bowel decompression and relieve the obstruction. The first well-described curative surgery for HSCR was a rectosigmoidectomy advocated by Swenson in 1947. Since then, several surgical procedures have been proposed, and they all share the same objective(s) – to resect the aganglionic bowel and reconnect normal bowel to the distal rectum just above the dentate line. While the surgical principle is considered the same, different approaches and techniques are used to achieve this purpose. In recent years, the transanal endorectal pull-through operation (Soave procedure) has become a popular surgical operation for HSCR. The major advantage of this approach is the avoidance of a laparotomy, as most of the dissection is performed via the transanal route. The mobilization of proximal colon can be assisted by laparoscopic surgery (**Figures 9.4** and **9.5**). Excellent functional and cosmetic outcomes have been

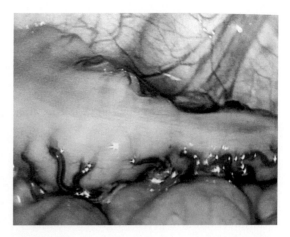

Figure 9.4

consistently reported. The retro-rectal (Duhamel) pull-through is often favored for long-segment disease and 're-do' revisional surgery.

In modern era, there is now a trend to perform one-stage surgery during the neonatal period to avoid the need for a temporary stoma. However, if the patient presents with life-threatening enterocolitis or with long-segment involvement that is often refractory to rectal washouts, initial

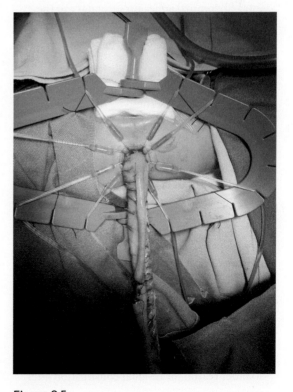

Figure 9.5

defunctioning colostomy will be required. The segment of bowel used for the colostomy (a leveling colostomy) should be fully evaluated for the presence of normal ganglion cells by obtaining a biopsy and frozen section.

Question: What are the potential problems after surgery for HSCR?
Answer:

1. **General complications**
   Surgery for HSCR is a major operation that is subject to the general risks associated with any abdominal or pelvic surgery, including bleeding, intra-abdominal infection, injury to adjacent viscera and anastomotic leak/retraction. Wound complications are potentially minimized by the transanal or laparoscopic approach.
2. **Disease-specific complications**
   Current treatments for HSCR are imperfect, and patients may experience the following long-term problems.

   Obstructive symptoms: Obstructive symptoms can happen in up to 50% of patients. Early obstructive symptoms can be due to intra-abdominal adhesion secondary to the surgery. Patients may present with features of intestinal obstruction. Mild obstruction can be observed for spontaneous resolution, but unrelieved obstruction warrants an adhesiolysis. Constipation that happens after a certain period from surgery could be related to various causes. Mechanical obstruction is most commonly caused by anastomotic stricture and, rarely, by twisting of the pull-through bowel, residual 'spur' (Duhamel procedure) or a long aganglionic muscular cuff (Soave procedure). Not uncommonly, an incomplete resection of the aganglionic bowel during the primary surgery will result in a condition called transitional zone pull-through. When this condition is suspected, the original resected specimen should be fully evaluated and, if necessary, biopsy of the pull-through segment can be carried out to look for the presence of normal ganglion cells. Rarely, dysmotility of the proximal bowel is attributed to intestinal neuronal dysplasia. Internal anal sphincter achalasia is another reason for residual constipation after

surgery. This condition is characterized by high anal sphincteric pressures after exclusion of residual aganglionosis. Botulinum toxin injection or internal sphincterotomy/myectomy can bring symptomatic relief.

Incontinence: Impairment in continence is reported in up to 15% of patients. Genuine incontinence should be differentiated from overflow incontinence, a manifestation of severe constipation. Fecal soiling can be related to sphincter damage during the transanal dissection or pelvic nerve injury with other surgical approaches. Incontinence may be temporary or permanent, and some cases may respond to pelvic floor exercise.

Depending on the etiology, residual bowel dysfunction may or may not be curable.

Nevertheless, an active bowel management program may improve symptoms and minimize distress associated with constipation and incontinence. A stoma or antegrade continence enema (ACE) may be the last resort for intractable cases.

Hirschsprung's disease-associated enterocolitis (HAEC): HAEC can occur in up to 60% of HSCR patients and is potentially life-threatening. This complication occurs more frequently before but is also possible after the pull-through surgery. The typical symptoms of HAEC include abdominal distension, vomiting, fever and the passage of foul-smelling or bloody stool. However, early symptoms can be non-specific, and this condition may be misdiagnosed as an episode of simple gastroenteritis. A high index of suspicion for HAEC is needed for any patients with a history of HSCR presenting with gastrointestinal symptoms. While early HAEC can be managed conservatively with bowel rest, rectal washout irrigations and antibiotics, emergency surgical decompression may be required in severe cases. **Figure 9.6** is an abdominal X ray showing multiple dilated bowel loops in a child with HAEC after Transanal Endorectal Pullthrough operation (TEPT). **Figure 9.7** is the intra-operative photo of the same patient taken during laparotomy. The colon was markedly dilated due to severe inflammation (toxic megacolon), resulting in uncontrolled systemic sepsis.

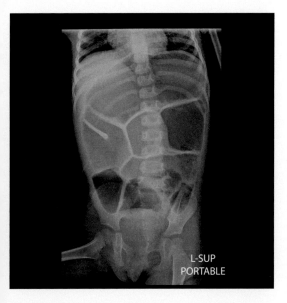

Figure 9.6

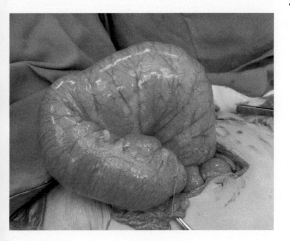

Figure 9.7

Question: How can we prevent HSCR?
Answer: Even though the timing of clinical presentation may be variable, HSCR is a congenital disorder, and the disease is already present at the time the baby is born. Until now, there is no effective way to prevent it. The etiology of HSCR is complex and likely to be multifactorial with a strong genetic basis. 'Damaging'/causative genetic mutations are found in approximately 50% of the rare syndromic, familial and severe HSCR patients and in only 20% of the common isolated short-segment HSCR cases. The majority of HSCR patients thus

carry disease-susceptible genetic variants, some of which are known, while others remain to be fully elucidated. Among 30 or more HSCR-associated genes described to date, the RET proto-oncogene was the first to be discovered. It is the most frequently affected and important HSCR gene, encoding the RET receptor tyrosine kinase protein, a cell-surface molecule that transduces signals. The other major HSCR genes are EDNRB (endothelin receptor B), neuregulin1 (NRG1) (identified in 2009 by the Genome-wide Association Study [GWAS]) and BACE2 (identified in 2018 by whole genome sequencing study), GDNF, GFRA1, NRTN, PHOX2B, SOX10 and SEMA3. Most of these genes are involved in the development of the enteric nervous system. Genetic counseling can be provided to families of HSCR patients who carry the abnormal genes.

BIBLIOGRAPHY

1. Chung PHY, Yu MON, Wong KKY, Tam PKH. Risk factors for the development of postoperative enterocolitis in short segment Hirschsprung's disease. Pediatr Surg Int. 2019; 35(2):187–191.
2. Tam PKH, Chung PHY, St Peter SD, Gayer CP, Ford HR, Tam GCH, Wong KKY, Pakarinen MP, Davenport M. Paediatric Surgery: Advances in paediatric gastroenterology. Lancet. 2017; 390(10099):1072–1082.
3. Neuvonen MI, Kyrklund K, Rintala RJ, Pakarinen MP. Bowel function and quality of life after transanal endorectal pull-through for Hirschsprung Disease: Controlled outcomes up to adulthood. Ann Surg. 2017; 265(3):622–629.
4. Tam PKH. Hirschsprung's disease: A bridge for science and surgery. J Pediatr Surg. 2016; 51(1):18–22.
5. Heuckeroth RO. Hirschsprung disease - Integrating basic science and clinical medicine to improve outcomes. Nat Rev Gastroenterol Hepatol. 2018; 15(3): 152–167.
6. De La Torre L, Langer JC. Transanal endorectal pull-through for Hirschsprung disease: technique, controversies, pearls, pitfalls, and an organized approach to the

management of postoperative obstructive symptoms. Semin Pediatr Surg. 2010; 19(2):96–106.

7. Tang CSM, Li P, Lai FPL, (…), Tam PKH, Garcia-Barcelo MM, Ngan ESW. Identification of genes associated with Hirschsprung disease, based on whole-genome sequence analysis, and potential effects on enteric nervous system development. Gastroenterology. 2018; 155(6):1908–1922.

10

Anorectal malformation

RAGHU SHANKAR AND MARTIN T. CORBALLY
King Hamad University Hospital, Kingdom of Bahrain, Bahrain

Scenario: A full-term male newborn was referred from a regional health center to the neonatal intensive care unit (NICU) with failure to pass meconium after 30 hours of life, abdominal distension and intolerance of feeds.

On clinical examination, the baby is noted to be pink and active, and the abdomen was found to be uniformly distended and non-tender. Loops of intestine were visible. On perineal examination, a dimple was noted in the area of the anus; however, no orifice was clearly visualized. During the examination the baby passed urine and you noticed dark-greenish debris in the infant's urine.

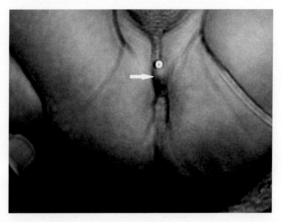

Figure 10.1

Question: What is the likely diagnosis in this baby? What else will you specifically focus your clinical examination on next?

Answer: The newborn would appear to have an 'imperforate anus'. Imperforate anus is not a single index entity, but may be a spectrum of lesion types; hence, anorectal malformation (ARM) is a better term.

Now examine the perineal area carefully for:

1. A meconium or sub-epithelial tract (**Figure 10.1**), which is a tract filled with inspissated meconium or mucus that may extend sometimes into the scrotal raphe, or you may observe a 'meconium pearl', i.e. a singlet droplet of meconium visible along the same line.

2. A skin bridge/tag or ('bucket handle') covering a narrow anal opening (**Figure 10.2**).

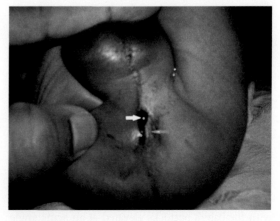

Figure 10.2

DOI: 10.1201/9781003182290-11

These latter findings would suggest that the malformation lesion is termed a 'low' ARM, meaning that the terminal end of the rectum is displaced on the perineum – i.e. rectoperineal fistula. The various forms of ARM will be discussed later at the end of this section.

However, here the infant is passing greenish urine – urine mixed with meconium (meconuria). So, these salient findings indicate that there has to be an abnormal communication (fistula = abnormal connection between two epithelial surfaces) between the rectum/colon and the urinary tract (urethra – 80%, or at the bladder neck – rare). These findings indicate that the malformation likely is a 'high' ARM where the terminal portion of the rectum/colon is not lying on the perineum (has not penetrated the levator muscle/pelvic floor) and has joined and formed an abnormal communication to the lower urinary tract.

RECTO-URETHRAL/RECTO-BLADDER NECK FISTULA

Next the clinician must examine and check the baby's vertebrae and the sacrum in particular. Sacral anomalies such as missing sacral vertebrae, hemi-sacrum or, rarely, sacral agenesis are all associated with ARM anomalies and may have significant bearing on the ultimate and guarded prognosis for attainment of continence of stool following corrective surgery. Spina bifida or neuro-cutaneous markers (i.e. tuft of hair, nevus, hemangioma, lipoma) on the midline of the back should also raise suspicion of an associated spinal cord anomaly, notably a tethered cord.

Question: Do we need any further investigation(s) to fully confirm the diagnosis? If imaging is required, then what is it for and when should it be done?
Answer: We can make the diagnosis of an ARM clinically simply by carefully examining the perineum, but as definitive management will depend on the level of the lesion, i.e. high or low (see variant types of ARM next), we will require additional imaging to help us decide where the distal-most portion of the colon is ending in anatomical terms. **Figure 10.3** shows a cross-table prone lateral (CTPL) plain radiograph. This X-ray examination is undertaken with the baby's buttocks elevated at an acute angle

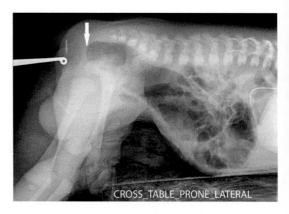

Figure 10.3 Cross Table Prone Lateral X-Ray showing distal level of bowel (white arrow) and radio-opaque marker at level of anus (blue arrow).

to encourage air in the large bowel to travel as far distally as possible – i.e. to the final terminal point of the bowel atresia – and thus allow measurement of the distance between that air shadow on X-ray and the surface perineal skin (note a radio-opaque marker is placed at the perineum).

If the distance between these two points of interest is more than 1 cm, the lesion is considered a 'high' ARM anomaly. Alternatively if the gap distance is less than 1 cm, a 'low' ARM anomaly is suspected. By definition a 'high' ARM anomaly is a malformation that has not penetrated through the levator pelvic muscle complex (i.e. pelvic floor anorectal sphincter).

This evaluation should ideally be best done after some 20–24 hours following birth and delivery, as the air swallowed by the crying infant needs time to travel to the distal terminal colon and rectum. Beware, therefore, that a CTPL imaging study performed too early after birth may give you a false impression of very high ARM anomaly.

Perineal ultrasound with an experienced sonographer can also be utilized to map the perineum to the terminal end of the rectum. This examination is particularly helpful in cases of low ARM anomaly in which a rectoperineal fistula has been missed on a clinical examination and thus saving the infant from undergoing a colostomy.

A plain X-ray of the spine with special focus on the sacrum should also be ordered to look for associated spine abnormalities, as mentioned earlier. Note any newborn with a sacral abnormality suspected on clinical examination or confirmed by plain X-ray must have a spinal ultrasound in the first 6/52 of life to exclude an associated tethered cord lesion.

Question: What are the differences (if any) with an ARM if the baby is female?
Answer: The presence of the female vagina interposed between the terminal large bowel and the urinary tract makes a fistula communicating to the urinary tract much less likely than in males unless the ARM malformation is an extremely high lesion – see **Figures 10.4** and **10.5**.

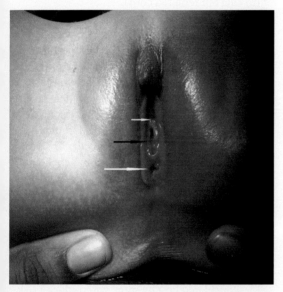

Figure 10.4

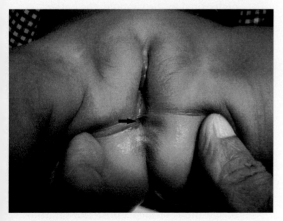

Figure 10.5

Question: Does this female baby have an anorectal malformation (Figure 10.1)? If the female infant has passed meconium stool, where is it coming from?
Answer: By strict definition, an anal opening that is either totally absent or not in an anatomically normal location is an ARM malformation. In the female infant, such ARM lesions are most often found in the posterior regions of the vulva, the vestibule and/or just behind the hymenal ring and vagina orifice. These are best termed **vestibular ARM fistulas**. In newborn females it can be sometimes difficult to be absolutely certain of the exact anatomical location, and it is always wise to seek expert guidance from a pediatric surgeon.

The fistula opening may be of such a reasonable size that meconium can be easily expelled; however, sometimes this may require a gentle probe dilatation with a lubricated cotton bud. In cases of vestibular fistula or a recto-perineal fistula with an anteriorly located anal opening, the female baby may be passing adequate meconium. Corrective surgery to repair the ARM anomaly need not be undertaken emergently in the newborn period. Elective surgery can be scheduled without need for a defunctioning colostomy at 4–6 weeks of life. Definitive ARM surgery in these cases involves an anterior sagittal ano-rectoplasty (ASARP), perhaps best termed a 'mini or modified' posterior sagittal ano-rectoplasty (miniPSARP).

Question: On examination of the external genitalia of a female newborn with an absent anal opening, a single perineal orifice is noted within the labial folds. What kind of ARM is this lesion? (See **Figure 10.6a** and **b**.)
Answer: This is the most severe and complex of ARMs occurring exclusively in the female infant where the distal terminal segments of the rectum, vagina and urinary tract fuse to form a single excretory 'common channel' termed a **cloacal malformation**. This requires complex and very skilled multidisciplinary surgical management over several stages (see next).

The various different classification types of ARM are depicted in **Table 10.1** and **Figure 10.7**.

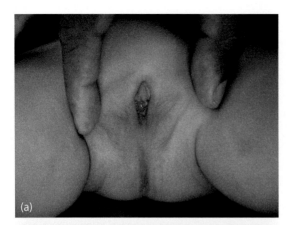

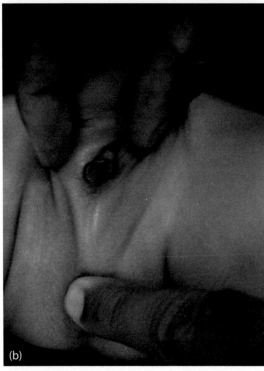

Figure 10.6

Table 10.1

Male	Female
• Rectoperineal fistula	• Vestibular fistula
• Rectourethral fistula-Prostatic, bulbar	• Rectoperineal fistula-anteriorly located, normal location
• Recto bladder neck fistula	• Rectal atresia
• Ano rectal malformation without fistula	• Cloacal malformation
• Rectal atresia	

Question: How do we manage a newborn infant with an ARM?
Answers:

1. **In general:**
   The newborn should first ideally be kept nil by mouth, receive IV fluids, IV antibiotics and an oro/nasogastric tube (O/NGT) for gut decompression. Evaluate the patient for associated defects, notably scheduling a cardiac assessment with echocardiography, urinary tract assessment with ultrasound scan of the renal and bladder anatomy and spine assessment with plain X-rays and spinal ultrasound (to rule out tethered cord).

2. **ARM low anomaly:**
   A primary corrective anoplasty, i.e. definitive surgery to make a new anus, is best performed within 2–3 days of life and without requirement for any covering colostomy. The prognosis for stool and urinary continence is excellent, as there is usually good neural sphincter muscle complex development. A low ARM anomaly does not have a recto-urinary fistula. The position and strength of the anal sphincter should be assessed using a nerve or muscle stimulator.

3. **ARM high anomaly:**
   All high ARM malformations typically require repair in three stages:
   a. *First stage*: Performed shortly after birth, is a diverting colostomy (high sigmoid colostomy); a divided diverting stoma is considered best by some with reduced risk of prolapse. In essence, the more proximally sited in the sigmoid, the better.
   b. *Second stage*: Creation of a new anus by mobilizing and bringing the terminal end of the large bowel colon to the perineum, crucially making sure to place it centrally through whatever anorectal sphincter muscle complex is present. Muscle development here may be poor or absent, and this is the main reason why many of these children have significant lifelong problems with continence of stool. The second operation (i.e. definitive corrective surgery) is usually scheduled at around 2–3 months of age and is termed a posterior sagittal ano-rectoplasty (PSARP). If a high bladder neck fistula is noted, it may difficult to approach the fistula from the posterior sagittal (perineal) route alone, and either

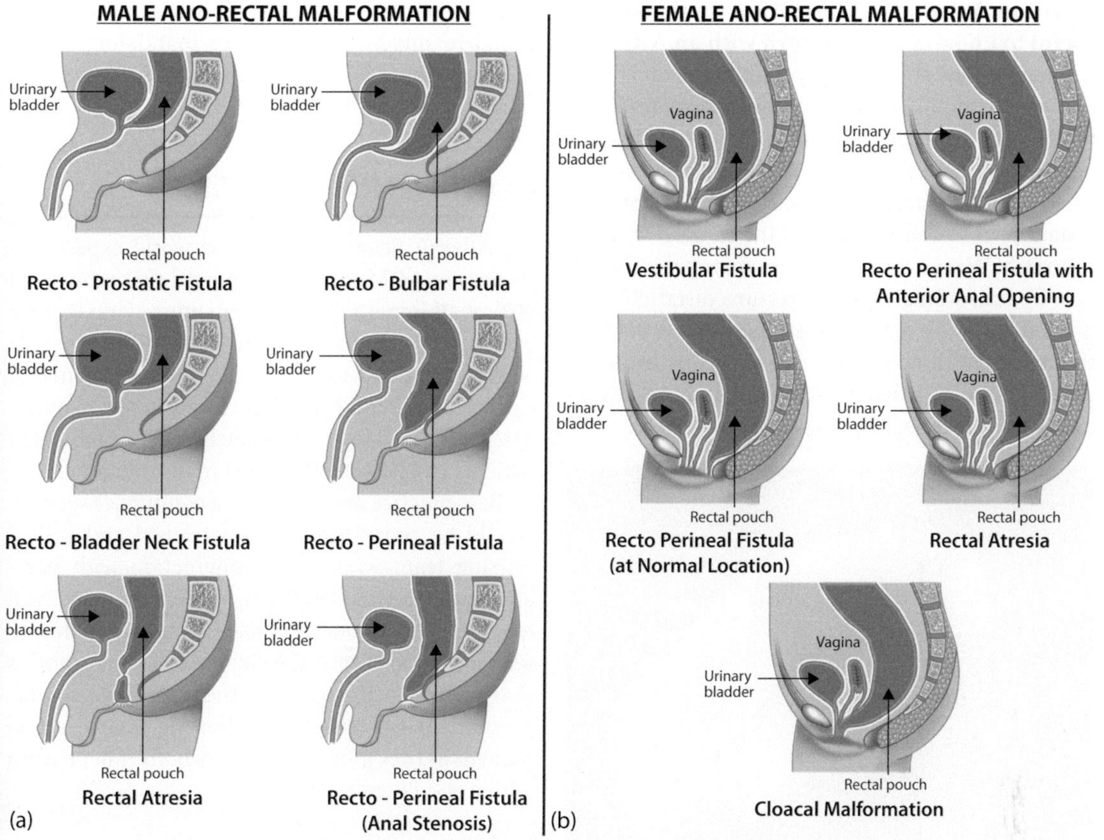

Figure 10.7 (a) Male ano-rectal malformation. (b) Femal ano-rectal malformation.

it is found and dealt with aided by laparoscopy visualization or an additional combined abdominal approach may be deployed in conjunction with PSARP. This strategy is needed in approximately 10% of all high ARMS index cases.

c. *Third stage*: Surgeon schedules to 'take down' and close the diverting covering colostomy, which is generally carried out 3 months or so after the PSARP operation. The parents – after the infant's PSARP operation – are counseled and must be instructed by the care team of doctors and nurses to perform regular anal dilatations using lubricated, graded, sized Hegar dilators to avert neo-anus stenosis. By undertaking infant anal dilatations, the third-stage 'closure of stoma' operation is greatly facilitated and better outcomes anticipated.

4. **Cloaca**

This is a major complex ARM repair, as there is a single common excretory channel into which the large bowel, bladder and vagina terminate and 'open'.

The steps include:

a. Emergent diverting colostomy.
b. Catheterize the common cloaca channel to drain urine.
c. Consider vesicostomy if catheter urine drainage is inadequate, there is renal compromise or subsequent trials of regular bladder emptying are poor.
d. PSARUVP operation (PSARP with uretho- and vaginoplasty) scheduled at 6–12 months to surgically create (1) perineal neo-anus, (2) a neo-urethra orifice opening and (3) vagina. It may not be possible to provide the 'new vagina' at this early stage, and this may require later reconstruction at puberty (with sigmoid colon or other intestinal segment vaginoplasty).
e. Ideal closure of all diverting temporary stomas at 3–6 months' post total reconstruction.

Question: What key information would be very useful to know in any newborn with an ARM?
Answer: If the baby has any possibility of an abnormal fistula communication to the urinary tract, we need to identify its precise anatomical site, as this will need to be corrected at surgery. It would also be helpful to know the exact anatomical site of the terminal distal bowel to define and plan the surgical strategy approach. We can usefully obtain this vital information by scheduling a 'high-pressure distal colostogram study' – i.e. a contrast study instilled through the distal end limb of the stoma mucous fistula to delineate a recto-urinary fistula and, importantly, to assess the rectal pouch anatomy (**Figure 10.8**).

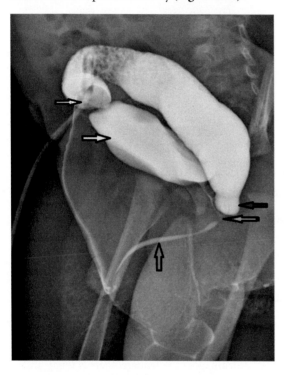

Figure 10.8 Colostogram. Blue arrow shows recto-urethral fistula. White arrow at stoma level. Red arrow is at the tip of the distal rectum. Yellow arrow shows the bladder and the orange arrow the urethra.

LONG-TERM OUTCOMES

All children born with ARM are at increased risk of urinary continence problems with altered physiological bladder compliance/neuropathic bladder, vesico-ureteric reflux (VUR) and symptomatic or 'silent' upper tract urinary infections leading to renal impairment. Regular renal ultrasound surveillance imaging is therefore mandatory in all patients. There is a valid indication for circumcision to promote easy bladder emptying.

CONTINENCE OUTCOMES

Dr. Alberto Pena – a renowned world expert and pioneer in ARM surgery – reported that more than 50% of all imperforate anus patients having PSARP were socially totally continent, while approximately 50% of cases had some degree (%) of incontinence. Constipation requiring adjunct laxative/enema therapies was noted in approximately 18% of high ARM patients vs 43% with low ARM malformations.

Best-practice management of continence services should be coordinated with a trained and skilled nursing team working in conjunction with pediatric surgeons and urology. Modern management together with adjunct medical therapies and neurosensory sacral stimulation/biofeedback programs is now greatly facilitated with the Antegrade colonic enema (ACE) operation, allowing many ARM patients as they grow older to be wholly independent with a good quality of life.

BIBLIOGRAPHY

1. Pena A, Bischoff A, De la Torre L. Anorectal anomalies. Pediatric Surgery Diagnosis And Management Springer Publishers 2023. Eds. P Puri and ME Hollwarth.
2. Narasimharao KL, Prasad GR, Katariya S, Yadav K, Mitra SK, Pathak IC. Prone cross-table lateral view: An alternative to the invertogram in imperforate anus. AJR Am J Roentgenol 1983; 140:227–229.
3. Gross GW, Wolfson PJ, Pena A. Augmented-pressure colostogram in imperforate anus with fistula. Pediatr Radiol 1991; 21:560–562.
4. Malone PS, Ransley PG, Kiely EM. Preliminary report; the antegrade continence enema. Lancet 1990; 336(8725): 1217–1218.
5. Shankar KR, Losty PD, Kenny SE, et al. Functional results following the antegrade continence enema procedure. Br J Surg 1998; 85(7):980–982.

11

Meconium ileus

PIETRO BAGOLAN AND ANDREA CONFORTI
Newborn Surgery Unit, Bambino Gesù Children's Hospital, Rome, Italy
and Department of Systems Medicine, University of Rome "Tor Vergata",
Rome, Italy

FRANCESCO MORINI
Neonatal Surgery Unit, AOU Meyer and University of Florence, Florence, Italy

Question: What is meconium ileus?

Answer: Meconium ileus (MI) is defined as a small bowel obstruction disorder created by inspissated and tenacious meconium occluding a variable length of distal ileum in patients most notably affected by cystic fibrosis (CF). Uniformly poor outcomes are reported if left untreated.

Putty-like green-grey pellets fill a narrowed distal loop of ileum up to the ileo-cecal valve and the colon, leading to marked dilation of the proximal obstructed small bowel, while densely adhesive, dark-green meconium fills the dilated ileum. The distal colon is typically small and unused (micro-colon).

Question: What is cystic fibrosis?

Answer: CF is an autosomal recessive genetic disease that causes a progressive and multisystemic disorder due to mutation of chromosome 7, band q31, coding for the cell membrane protein CF transmembrane regulator (CFTR). To date, there are 2,107 known mutations listed in the CFTR Mutation Database, although the most common mutation (delta-F508) is responsible for approximately 70% of all clinical cases.

The pivotal role of CFTR in the intestine is to modulate secretion of chloride, bicarbonate, and fluid. Gene mutations may result in partial or complete loss of function with abnormally low volume of fluids and aberrant electrolyte composition. All this may lead to MI in up to 20% of affected CF patients. MI is, however, not the only possible gastrointestinal morbid expression of CF, with theoretically all types of congenital intestinal obstruction (isolated intestinal small bowel atresia – 15% of patients may have CF) potentially associated with CF.

The key importance of early diagnosis of CF led the American College of Obstetrics and Gynecology to strongly recommend preconception and prenatal CF carrier screening to all women of reproductive age.

Question: What prenatal findings may be seen (including clinical history)?

Answer: Persistence of hyperechogenic and dilated fetal bowel loops during the second trimester on routine ultrasonography may raise suspicion of uncomplicated MI (**Figure 11.1**). Bowel dilation and polyhydramnios may be variably associated, increasing the chance to diagnose prenatal MI. MI may be suspected on prenatal ultrasound in cases of hyperechoic masses (inspissated meconium in the terminal ileum), dilated and hyperechoic bowel, peritoneal wall calcifications, intra-abdominal cysts, and poor non-visualization of the

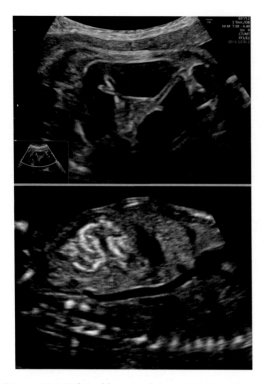

Figure 11.1 Dilated hyperechogenic (*above*) and hyperechogenic bowel contents (*below*) during a second-trimester routine fetal ultrasound scan.

gallbladder. The finding of isolated dilated bowel in association with CF has been reported less frequently than that of hyperechoic bowel.

Although a familial history of CF is commonly reported in MI, all pregnant women with fetal intestinal obstruction should be counselled and advised accordingly to have amniocentesis and genetic counselling. In cases of complicated MI, other possible prenatal findings may include abdominal calcification – a sign of meconium peritonitis often associated with ascites and/or giant pseudocysts, isolated ascites, and, exceptionally, meconium periorchitis in males caused by spillage of meconium into the scrotum via a patent processus vaginalis.

Question: What prenatal management would you advise?
Answer: When MI is suspected, amniocentesis and genetic testing of the fetus and parents may allow a diagnosis of CF. An advantage of prenatal diagnosis is that the fetal medicine team and attending paediatric surgeon can prepare the family's psychological needs before, during, and after delivery. Therefore, with a fetal diagnosis, immediate referral to specialist tertiary centre for multidisciplinary management is recommended. Serial sonographic fetal imaging is advisable on a monthly basis (or earlier based on fetal wellbeing and maternal health) until delivery. These surveillance evaluations allow for early detection of any potential complication as they occur.

Question: How is meconium ileus classified?
Answer: MI is classified as (1) simple or (2) complicated. Each occurs with an equal frequency of approximately 50%. In the simple form, thickened meconium obstructs the distal ileum, as a consequence leading to proximal gut dilatation, bowel wall thickening, and congestion. The unused distal colon is small, described as the 'microcolon' of disuse. Complications of MI include volvulus and intestinal atresia, variably associated with necrosis, perforation, peritonitis, and pseudocyst formation.

Question: What about the postnatal clinical presentation?
Answer: Simple MI usually presents with abdominal distension at birth: Failure or delay to pass meconium with bilious vomiting and intestinal obstruction. Often, dilated loops of bowel become evident at clinical examination when thick and malleable abdominal masses are palpable in the sick newborn. Typically, the rectum and anus are narrowed on careful digital exam/probing – a finding that may be misinterpreted as anal stenosis. In simple MI cases, plain abdominal X-ray will invariably show multiple dilated bowel loops and only a few air-fluid levels (in contrast to atresia not associated with CF). As air mixes with meconium, bubbles of gas may be seen. This classic 'soap bubble' appearance is dependent on the viscosity of the meconium. At contrast enema examination, a small-calibre microcolon with pellets of inspissated meconium is present (**Figure 11.2**). Reflux of contrast media into the distal ileum may reveal dilated bowel loops if and when it bypasses the obstruction.

Complicated MI presents more dramatically. At birth gross distension with abdominal wall erythema and oedema may be present. Abdominal distension may be so severe as to cause marked respiratory distress. Signs of peritonitis and clinically evident signs of sepsis – fever, lethargy, shock – may exist. A palpable mass may indicate pseudocyst formation. The neonate can be critically ill and require urgent resuscitation and emergent laparotomy. Radiographic findings in complicated MI include speckled calcifications, which on a plain abdominal film are highly

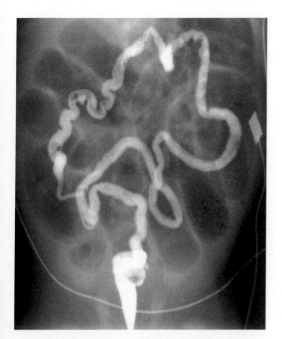

Figure 11.2 Contrast enema. Small-calibre colon (microcolon) with pellets of inspissated meconium.

suggestive of intrauterine intestinal perforation and meconium peritonitis. A pseudocyst should be suspected where there is radiological evidence of a dense mass with a calcification rim, possibly presenting also with an air-fluid level.

Question: What are the other possible differential diagnoses?

Answer: Potential differential diagnoses include meconium obstruction non-CF-related, intestinal atresia, intestinal malrotation and midgut volvulus, Hirschsprung disease, meconium plug syndrome, neonatal small left colon syndrome, and hypothyroidism. Genetic syndromes, prenatal infections, and placental insufficiency should be also considered (**Table 11.1**).

Table 11.1 Meconium ileus – Differential diagnosis

Medical	Surgical
Meconium plug syndrome	Intestinal atresia
Neonatal small left colon syndrome	Malrotation
Congenital hypothyroidism	Midgut volvulus
Prenatal infections	Hirschsprung disease
Placental insufficiency	
Genetic syndromes/ abnormalities	

Question: Which postnatal management strategies will you select and consider?
Answer:

a. *Initial management*: After the diagnosis of MI is confirmed, initial management should include placement of a nasogastric tube and nil by mouth, establishing intravenous access to provide adequate hydration, correction of any electrolyte disorders, and empirical antibiotic coverage. Laboratory test investigations must include electrolytes, haemoglobin, white blood cell count, and lactate to further help determine the clinical status of the infant. Blood should be taken to assess delta-508 before any blood products are given.

b. *Non-operative treatment*: Non-operative management includes the use of therapeutic enemas. It is best reserved for patients with simple MI and has a success rate of over 80%. The most commonly used enema deployed is the hyperosmolar water-soluble contrast agent gastrografin, having an osmolarity of 1900 mOsm/L, as originally proposed by Noblett in 1969. Fluid is osmotically drawn into the obstructed intestinal loops, hydrating and softening the inspissated meconium mass followed by decompressive expulsion of meconium from a resultant osmotic diarrhoea. Late or iatrogenic perforation may be caused from severe bowel distension by osmotically drawn fluid into the intestine or by contrast medium directly injuring bowel wall mucosa; therefore the 'gastrografin enema intervention' should always be performed only in specialist tertiary centres where neonatal surgery is available. The risk of catheter perforation is greatly reduced by the paediatric radiologist carefully placing and guiding the enema catheter tube under fluoroscopy guidance and avoiding inflation of balloon-tipped catheters. Under screening imaging a 25%–50% solution of gastrografin at low hydrostatic pressure is infused through the catheter. The catheter is withdrawn and an abdominal radiograph is taken to rule out perforation. Usually, there is a rapid passage of semi-liquid meconium, which continues over the next 24–48 hours. In the absence of clinical indications, radiographs should be taken every 8–12 hours to confirm relief of obstruction while excluding late perforation. Reflux of the enema agent into the terminal ileum is critical for the bowel obstruction to be relieved. In the absence of reflux or the case of incomplete evacuation, a second enema procedure may be necessary. Serial enemas can be performed at 12- to 24-hour intervals if needed. For further evacuation of meconium, warm saline instilled rectally every 12–24 hours can also be performed. Note that hypertonic enemas may lead to hypovolemic shock; therefore, adequate patient fluid resuscitation (>150 mL/kg per day) with anticipation of fluid losses due to osmotic diarrhoea and diuresis is crucially necessary, usually 10–20 mL/kg as fluid bolus at the time or just before the enema.

Oral N-acetylcysteine solution can be used as an adjuvant agent in conservative management of simple MI. It exhibits a mucolytic action through its free sulfhydryl group, which opens up disulfide chemical bonds in mucoproteins to lower mucus viscosity. It is usually used as a 10% solution that can be given via a nasogastric tube. The dose is typically 1–5 mL tid/qid.

N-acetylcysteine can also be used as a rectal enema at 4% concentrations tid/qid (**Figure 11.3**).

c. *Operative surgical treatments*: Operative treatment is scheduled in simple MI with unsuccessful conservative management or where conservative management is considered not feasible in certain patients or for various logistic reasons and those babies with complicated MI. The key objectives of operative management include the complete evacuation of meconium from the intestine, the establishment of intestinal continuity, and preservation of maximal intestinal length (**Figure 11.3**).

d. *Surgical operations*: The choice of operation depends on the variant form of MI (simple vs complicated) and, to a degree, the surgeon's preference. For uncomplicated disease, an enterotomy can be performed allowing intraoperative irrigation of the bowel to flush out the obstructing meconium, with either primary enterotomy suture closure or creation of a stoma for continued irrigation

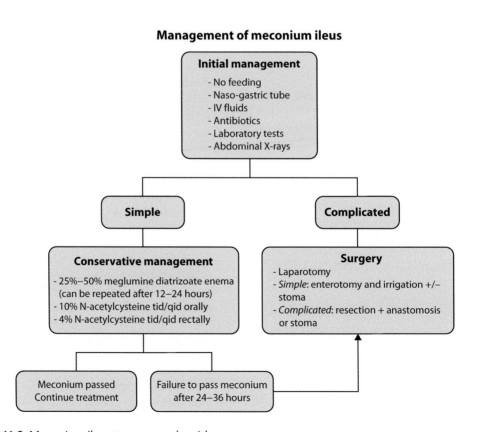

Figure 11.3 Meconium ileus treatment algorithm.

postoperatively. In patients with complicated MI the alternatives are (1) resection with primary anastomosis or (2) resection with enterostomy. Enterostomy options are varied and include creating a Mikulicz double-barrelled enterostomy, distal chimney enterostomy, proximal enterostomy, tube enterostomy, T-tube enterostomy, or appendectomy and inserting a cecostomy catheter through the appendiceal stump for instillation of irrigant and evacuation of impacted meconium (**Figure 11.3**).

Question: What are the desired post-treatment goals?

Answer: The aims and goals are:

1. Restoring continuity and intestinal transit, alleviating symptoms of intestinal obstruction.
2. Preserving as much intestinal length as possible to improve nutrient absorption.
3. Resuming full oral feeding and/or feeding aided by enteral nutrition with adequate volume and caloric intake.
4. Obtaining normal infant weight gain, ideally without parenteral nutrition and with adequate dosage of pancreatic enzyme supplements.
5. Preventing other comorbid problems and complications associated with MI and CF.

Question: Is meconium ileus associated with other gastrointestinal anomalies?

Answer: The pathophysiology of MI is mainly strictly linked to CF and the abnormal chloride and bicarbonate transport due to pathogenic mutations in the *CFTR* located on chromosome 7. At the same time, these gene mutations are responsible for abnormally thickened tenacious mucus and secretions in the lungs, gastrointestinal tract, pancreas, hepatobiliary tree, and vasa deferens ducts. Therefore, the lumen of these varied organ systems becomes obstructed leading to the other clinical findings associated with the disease process.

The most relevant are:

1. *Intestinal atresias*: A fetus with CF is predisposed to segmental intestinal volvulus (complicated MI) due to inspissated meconium, and this may consequently later develop from 'sterile in utero resorption' into a jejunal or ileal gut atresia.

2. *Gastro-oesophageal reflux disease (GERD)*: GERD seems to be more common in CF patients as compared with the healthy general population.
3. Neonatal cholestasis: Cholestatic liver disease in the neonatal period is present in less than 10% of babies with MI and CF. In infancy, cholestasis presents with prolonged conjugated hyperbilirubinemia, which sometimes is so severe as to mimic biliary atresia. Cholestasis tends to regress in early infancy thanks to improved nutrition and appropriate treatment.
4. *Distal intestinal obstruction syndrome (DIOS)*: Formerly termed 'meconium ileus equivalent'. This may occur in any older age group and is frequently associated with pancreatic enzyme deficiency and characterized by acute, complete or incomplete terminal ileal obstruction with inspissated intestinal contents.
5. *Intussusception*: Often typically caused by inspissated bowel contents acting as a 'lead point', with an estimated prevalence of 1% of CF patients.
6. *Rectal prolapse*: Nowadays an uncommon presentation with a typical prevalence 3% of CF patients.
7. Other gastrointestinal problems:
   - Coeliac disease and inflammatory bowel disease (IBD).
   - Small intestine bacterial overgrowth (SIBO).
   - *Pancreatic dysfunction*: This may lead to progressive destruction of pancreatic islet tissue causing abnormal glucose tolerance and CF-related diabetes. Patients with milder variant disease may be considered 'pancreatic-sufficient' though they may later experience pancreatitis.
   - *Liver/Biliary disease*: CF-related liver disease (CFLD) includes a wide range of manifestations ranging from mild elevation of transaminases to liver cirrhosis and portal hypertension. Micro-gallbladder, cholelithiasis, cholecystitis, sclerosing cholangitis, hepatolithiasis, intrahepatic biliary ductular disease, and hepatolithiasis are further concerns associated with CF.
   - *Gastrointestinal cancers*: CF patients have reportedly an increased risk of digestive tract cancers. These include cancers of the small bowel, colon, pancreas, and biliary tract.

BIBLIOGRAPHY

1. Long AM, Jones IH, Knight M, McNally J, BAPS-CASS. Early management of meconium ileus in infants with cystic fibrosis: A prospective population cohort study. J Pediatr Surg. 2021;56(8):1287–1292.
2. Conforti A, Bagolan P. Meconium Ileus In: Rickham's Neonatal Surgery, Springer London 2018. Eds. Losty PD, Flake AW, Rintala RJ, Hutson JM, Iwai N.
3. Casaccia G, Trucchi A, Nahom A, Aite L, Lucidi V, Giorlandino C, Bagolan P. The impact of cystic fibrosis on neonatal intestinal obstruction: The need for prenatal/neonatal screening. Pediatr Surg Int. 2003;19(1–2):75–78.
4. Karem BS, Rommens JM, Buchana JA et al. Identification of the cystic fibrosis gene: Genetic analysis. Science. 1989;245:1073.
5. Cystic Fibrosis Mutation Database Statistics, Dec. 2021: http://www.genet.sickkids.on.ca/Home.html
6. American College of Obstetricians and Gynecologists. Committee Opinion No. 691: Carrier screening for genetic conditions. Obstet Gynecol. 2017;129:e41–e55.
7. Noblett HR. Treatment of uncomplicated meconium ileus by Gastrografin enema: A preliminary report. J Pediatr Surg. 1969;4:190–197.

12

Infantile hypertrophic pyloric stenosis

GERLIN NAIDOO
University of Oxford, UK

PAUL D. LOSTY
Institute of Systems and Molecular Biology, University of Liverpool, Liverpool, UK
and Ramathibodi Hospital, Mahidol University, Bangkok, Thailand

Scenario: A 5-week-old male infant presents to the hospital emergency department of a children's hospital with a 2-week history of progressive vomiting reportedly after feeds that is not green or yellow in colour according to the parents. The infant had an unremarkable antenatal course and delivery. Antireflux therapy has been trialled by the general practitioner (GP) family doctor without success. The parents also describe the vomiting as becoming increasingly forceful in nature, and it is now occurring with almost every feed. Mum and dad have also noted that the baby is wetting nappies less frequently and not stooling with constipation. The infant remains hungry after vomiting.

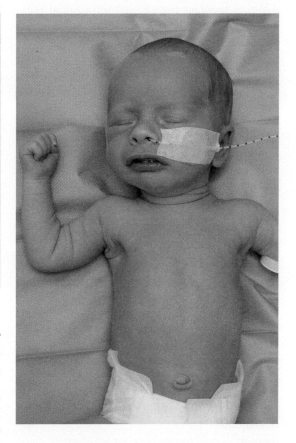

CLINICAL EXAMINATION

The infant appears somewhat thin with poor skin turgor and a sunken anterior fontanelle. You observe on clinical examination that the abdomen appears not distended. A palpable lump possibly is felt in the upper infant's abdomen, and you also notice fluttering movements in the epigastric region (see figure on right).

DOI: 10.1201/9781003182290-13

Question 1: What is your differential diagnosis? What other questions should you elicit in the infant's clinical history to help distinguish and establish a working diagnosis?

Answer: The clinical history appears typical of the classical presentation of infantile hypertrophic pyloric stenosis (IHPS). Other surgical causes of non-bilious vomiting may include a congenital duodenal web anomaly and occasionally intestinal malrotation, which may present with persistent non-bilious vomiting if there is a pre-ampullary obstruction of the duodenum by congenital Ladd's bands.

However, it should always be remembered that the most common causes of non-bilious vomiting in babies tend to be medical in nature. Sepsis is an important differential diagnosis to always consider, as it requires early recognition and emergent intervention. Overfeeding, gastro-oesophageal reflux and lactose feed intolerance are other common medical causes that an expert clinical history should be able to distinguish. Intracranial causes of vomiting resultant from raised intracranial pressure, notably infant brain tumour or hydrocephalus, should always be considered.

A key factor is the timing and nature of the vomiting. Vomiting in IHPS seldom begins before 2 weeks of life. Vomiting that progressively becomes projectile and occurs immediately after feeding is a cardinal symptom of gastric outlet obstruction. IHPS is notably rare after 12 weeks of age. There is a male:female predominance of 4:1. Overall the incidence is estimated at 1–4 per 100 live births in Western Europe.

The family history is also noteworthy, as genetic factors have been implicated in IHPS aetiology. Risk factors include family history (greater transmission risk to offspring if the mother had IHPS as an infant compared with the father), first-born males, formula feeding and a young maternal age. There are rare, though well-documented, co-associations with congenital oesophageal atresia.

The aetiology of IHPS remains poorly understood. Several theories exist, including seasonal viral infections, antibiotic exposure, i.e. erythromycin, or a deficiency in gut nitric oxide synthase (NOS).

Question 2: What next initial investigations would you request?

Answer: A fundamental key aspect of safely managing a vomiting infant is adequate IV fluid resuscitation. When IV access is obtained, a venous blood gas, renal function studies and electrolyte sampling should be obtained. Depending on the clinical scenario, a full blood count, C-reactive protein (CRP) and blood cultures should also be sent to the hospital laboratory to exclude sepsis.

Scenario continued: A venous blood gas is performed, and the results are illustrated in **Table 12.1**.

Table 12.1 Venous blood gas results

Parameter	Result	Normal range
H^+	32 nmol/L	35–45
pCO_2	7.1 kPA	<6
Cl^-	90 mmol/L	95–110
HCO_3^-	39 mmol/L	<28
Na	133 mmol/L	133–146
K^+	3.3 mmol/L	3.4–3.6
Base excess	14 mmol/L	+/–2

Question 3: What does the venous blood gas result show? How can you explain the biochemical abnormalities?

Answer: The venous lab gas result shows a hypokalaemic (low serum K^+), hypochloraemic (low serum Cl^-) metabolic alkalosis. This is the hallmark metabolic derangement seen in infants with IHPS. The extent of alkalosis is dependent on the duration of vomiting. In those babies presenting with vomiting in the first few days after birth, biochemical derangement may not be as marked.

Initially, the vomiting infant loses hydrogen (H^+) and chloride (Cl^-) ions from gastric secretions. This leads to a hypochloraemic state (low Cl^- state), which impairs renal excretion of bicarbonate (HCO_3^-) impacting correction of the alkalosis state. Hypovolaemia causes an increased secretion of aldosterone, which enhances urinary renal sodium (Na^+) retention. The resorption of sodium (Na^+) occurs at the expense of hydrogen (H^+) ions – the sodium/hydrogen pump in the proximal renal tubular system. Therefore, despite the alkalotic state, IHPS infants develop a paradoxical urinary aciduria. Aldosterone also causes an increase in potassium (K^+) excretion, contributing to serum hypokalaemia.

In response to metabolic alkalosis, IHPS infants consequently hypoventilate (reduce central CNS-mediated respiratory drive) in order to retain CO_2. This compensatory respiratory acidosis is demonstrated by a raised pCO_2. Operation, i.e. pyloromyotomy, is never a surgical emergency and is best scheduled when the metabolic biochemical derangement is fully corrected with IV fluid resuscitation in order to avert the significant risks of postoperative respiratory apnoea after general anaesthetic and death.

Question 4: How would you confirm a diagnosis of IHPS?

Answer: IHPS can be readily diagnosed by the surgeon palpating the 'pyloric tumour'. This is aided by undertaking a 'test feed', where the infant is given a feed or clear fluids to help pacify them and relax the abdominal wall. This manoeuvre greatly assists the surgeon's tactile ability to palpate the thickened muscle of pyloric stenosis. The 'test feed 'examination is traditionally best performed from the left side of the infant. Feeding from the bottle may also stimulate vigorous gastric peristalsis readily visible to the observant surgeon examiner.

Ultrasound has largely surpassed the 'test feed' in modern surgical practice. It is now considered the 'gold standard' for the final diagnosis of IHPS. The sensitivity and specificity of ultrasound approach 100% vs the 'test feed' exam where the 'pyloric tumour' may be palpable in only approximately 75% of index cases. Positive ultrasound findings typically correlate with a pyloric muscle

wall thickness >3 mm or a pyloric muscle channel length >15 mm **(Figure 12.1)**.

Question 5: How would you manage this infant before scheduling the operation?

Answer: Overall therapy goals are to improve the infant's fluid volume status to enable correction of the metabolic alkalosis. It is important that the chosen IV crystalloid solution contains adequate supplemental potassium to correct any low dangerous hypokalaemia, which risks cardiac arrhythmias. Often normal saline (0.9%) with potassium and dextrose is used. It is important to recognise if the infant is in fact a neonate, in which case a higher percentage of dextrose is required, notably 10%.

Infants preoperatively are kept 'nil-by-mouth' and have a nasogastric tube inserted. With the infant vomiting, the nasogastric tube should be regularly aspirated and gastric losses replaced millilitre for millilitre with 0.9% saline.

Venous blood gases are repeated daily to monitor correction of the alkalosis. The time to normal metabolic status resolution can vary and may take several days. Operation is never an emergency, and parents should be counselled accordingly.

> **Scenario continued:** The infant is managed with an IV fluid therapy regimen for 48 hours, with 12-hourly blood gases obtained. The most recent blood gas **(Table 12.2)** now shows a restoration of normal serum chloride (Cl^-) and bicarbonate (HCO_3^-) and a reduction in the base excess. The metabolic alkalosis is now considered 'corrected', and the baby may be brought to the operating room.

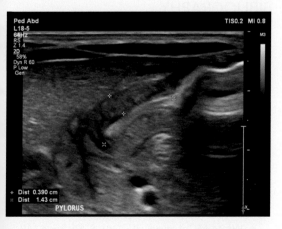

Figure 12.1 Ultrasound image showing IHPS.

Table 12.2 Venous blood gas results

Parameter	Result	Normal range
H^+	43 nmol/L	35–45
pCO_2	5.5 kPA	<6
Cl^-	104 mmol/L	95–110
HCO_3^-	27 mmol/L	<28
Na	134 mmol/L	133–146
K^+	5.8 mmol/L	3.4–3.6
Base excess	1 mmol/L	+/–2

Question 6: What definitive management options are available? What risks (if any) would you inform the parents about as part of the signed consent process?

Answer: Pyloromyotomy is the definitive management of IHPS. The operation was first described by Dufour and Fredet in Paris, France, in 1907. However, it was the German surgeon Conrad von Ramstedt who popularised the classical operation some years later in 1912.

A Ramstedt pyloromyotomy can be performed equally well with classical open surgery or minimally invasive surgery (MIS) techniques. When performed as an open procedure, choices include (i) a right upper quadrant or an (ii) aesthetic umbilical skin fold incision. The pylorus is delivered efficiently via the wound incision. A longitudinal surface myotomy incision is made through the thickened muscle fibres with a scalpel, and it should always extend from the pre-pyloric vein of Mayo pyloric canal region towards the antrum of the stomach. An artery forceps is then used to split the muscle fibres along the length of the myotomy incision down to the level of bulging mucosa. The duodenal fornix is at risk of perforation, and caution should be exercised here with distal myotomy. An air-fluid leak tests the integrity of myotomy, where the surgeon requests air to be insufflated into the stomach via the nasogastric (NG) tube by the anaesthetist whilst keenly observing for the presence (i.e. perforation has occurred) or absence of air-fluid bubbles from saline dripped by the operating surgeon onto the myotomy site.

The MIS operation (Alain et al., 1990) involves securing placement of sub-umbilical optical ports. An atraumatic grasper is then passed through an instrument port. Once the duodenal, i.e. distal end, of the pylorus is controlled with the grasper, a knife device is deployed to make an incision in the pylorus and the hypertrophied muscle split with a spreader. Integrity of the myotomy operation is checked as before by introducing air into the stomach via the NG tube and looking for bubbling.

With both classical and MIS techniques if a duodenal perforation is detected (1–2% of index cases), this should be immediately repaired by the surgeon.

CONSERVATIVE MEDICAL THERAPY FOR IHPS

Use of atropine has been described as a medical therapy, as it is thought to reduce pyloric spasm and thereby ameliorate muscle hypertrophy. Such methods are unpopular and require prolonged administration.

Operative complications of pyloromyotomy may include wound infection (infant skin carriage status typically with *Staphylococcus aureus*), wound dehiscence, incisional hernia, mucosal perforation and incomplete myotomy requiring a 'redo pyloromyotomy'.

Scenario continued: Following the pyloromyotomy operation, the infant recommences feeding and is noted by nursing staff to have several vomiting episodes. The parents are anxious about the vomiting recurring and seek your advice.

Question 8: How would you manage this?

Answer: Transient postoperative vomiting is not uncommon, and varied postoperative pyloric feeding regimens exist with either (i) delayed graded introduction of small incremental feeds or (ii) ad libitum feeding. Gastroesophageal reflux (GER) should also always be considered, and feed thickeners may help the infant, notably Carobel additives. Gaviscon should be avoided because of bezoar formation and risk of gastric outlet obstruction.

If the vomiting is persistent for some days postoperatively, however, then the surgeon must consider and recognise incomplete myotomy (0–2% of cases). A contrast meal may confirm incomplete surgery and support a decision for a 'redo' operation.

BIBLIOGRAPHY

1. Pedersen RN, Garne E, Loane M, Korsholm L, Husby S, A EUROCAT Working Group. Infantile hypertrophic pyloric stenosis: A comparative study of incidence and other epidemiological characteristics in seven European regions. J Matern -Fetal Neonatal Med 2008;21(9):599–604.
2. Murchison L, De Coppi P, Eaton S. Postnatal erythromycin exposure and risk of infantile hypertrophic pyloric stenosis: A systematic review and meta-analysis. Pediatr Surg Int 2016;32(12):1147–1152.
3. White MC, Langer JC, Don S, DeBaun MR. Sensitivity and cost minimization analysis of radiology versus olive palpation for the

diagnosis of hypertrophic pyloric stenosis. J Pediatr Surg 1998;33(6):913–917.

4. Tan KC, Bianchi A. Circumumbilical incision for pyloromyotomy. B J Surg 1986;73:399.

5. Alain JL, Grousseau D, Terrier G. Extramucosal pyloromyotomy by laparoscopy. Chir Pediatr 1990;31(4–5):223–244.

6. Hall NJ, Pacilli M, Eaton S, Reblock K, Gaines BA, Pastor A, Langer JC, Koivusalo AI, Pakarinen MP, Stroedter L, Beyerlein S. Recovery after open versus laparoscopic pyloromyotomy for pyloric stenosis: A double-blind multicentre randomised controlled trial. The Lancet 2009;373(9661):390–398.

7. Meissner PE, Engelmann G, Troeger J, Linderkamp O, Nuetzenadel W. Conservative treatment of infantile hypertrophic pyloric stenosis with intravenous atropine sulfate does not replace pyloromyotomy. Pediatr Surg Int 2006;22(12):1021–1024.

8. Mullassery D, Perry D, Goyal A, Jesudason EC, Losty PD. Surgical practice for infantile hypertrophic pyloric stenosis in the United Kingdom and Ireland – A survey of members of the British Association of Paediatric Surgeons. J Pediatr Surg 2008;43(6):1227–1229.

13

Necrotizing enterocolitis

ELKE RUTTENSTOCK AND AGOSTINO PIERRO
Hospital for Sick Children, Toronto, Canada

AUGUSTO ZANI
University of Toronto, Toronto, Canada

NECROTIZING ENTEROCOLITIS (NEC)

Scenario: A surgical consult is requested for a 3-week-old baby boy, born at 26 weeks of gestation (birth weight: 880 grams) due to lethargy, feeding intolerance, increased oxygen requirements, and passage of a smear of blood per rectum. He was born by emergency caesarean section due to premature rupture of membranes (PROM) from a 26-year-old African American mother. Apgar scores were 1 at 1 minute and 6 at 10 minutes. After intubation, the baby had been admitted to the neonatal intensive care unit and received treatment for respiratory distress syndrome (RDS). The baby had passed meconium on the first day of life and had an otherwise normal physical exam. The infant was starting to receive formula feeds on day 8 of life and reached full enteral feeds within 3 days.

On clinical examination, the baby has a moderately distended but soft and non-tender abdomen. **Figure 13.1** shows a premature baby with distended abdomen.

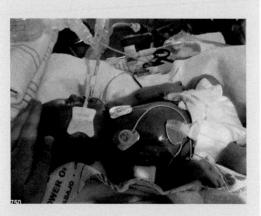

Figure 13.1 A typical preterm infant, incubated and ventilated with a distended abdomen.

NEC RISK FACTORS

Question 1: What risk factors for NEC can you identify in the medical history given?
Answer: Prematurity, low birth weight, Black ethnicity, PROM, low Apgar scores, assisted ventilation/RDS, and formula feeds.

NEC is considered one of the most devastating gastrointestinal emergencies in neonates. Its etiology is multifactorial. Prematurity and low birth weight

DOI: 10.1201/9781003182290-14

are the most consistently identified risk factors for the development of NEC, followed by small for gestational age, assisted ventilation, sepsis, hypotension, PROM, and Black ethnicity (1). Other reported risk factors include low Apgar scores, treatment of patent ductus arteriosus (PDA), erythrocyte blood transfusion, nosocomial infections, and intestinal dysbiosis (2–4). It is important to remember that the more premature the infant, the later NEC may occur after birth (4).

NEC EPIDEMIOLOGY

Question 2: What is the rate of NEC among babies born at <32 weeks of gestation?
Answer: 2%–7%.

The incidence of NEC varies according to the degree of prematurity and the geographic patient location. Overall, NEC incidence varies worldwide from 2% to 7% among babies born <32 weeks' gestation and from 5% to 22% among babies with a birth weight <1000 g. In infants born at <28 weeks of gestation, the lowest reported world incidence of NEC was in Japan (2%) and the highest in Australia, the United States, Canada, and Italy (7–9%) (1). NEC can make up to 9% of the disease burden in neonatal units (2). The wide range in incidence rates between high-income countries suggests that various factors influence the development of NEC, including environment, diet, and genetic predisposition.

NEC PATHOGENESIS

Question: What are the key factors contributing to NEC pathogenesis?
Answer: Gut immaturity, dysbiosis, breakdown of gut barrier function, and overwhelming cytokine-related inflammatory response.

The pathophysiology of NEC is multifactorial and has not been fully elucidated. What we understand so far is that intraluminal bacteria invade the immature intestinal epithelium and subsequently release their endotoxins, leading to a breakdown of the gut barrier and allowing bacteria to translocate. This bacterial invasion provokes an overwhelming cytokine-related inflammatory response. Additionally, vasoactive substances are released and the complement and coagulation systems are activated, thus impairing blood flow in the microvasculature and leading to severe intestinal tissue injury.

Question: What is pneumatosis intestinalis?
Answer: Pneumatosis intestinalis is defined as the presence of gas within the bowel wall. Intramural gas is a by-product of the metabolism of the bacteria that invade the intestine. Pneumatosis intestinalis is probably the most characteristic imaging sign of NEC and can be detected as a typical linear or bubbly pattern on plain abdominal X-ray (**Figure 13.2**) as well as abdominal ultrasound.

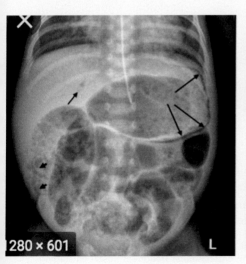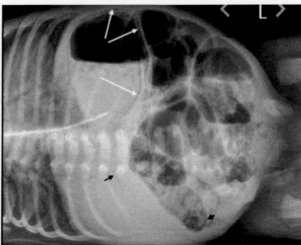

Figure 13.2 X-ray showing abnormal dilated bowel with extensive pneumatosis.

Question: What is portal venous gas?

Answer: Portal venous gas is the presence of gas in the portal vein and its territory branches, and it can be visualized on plain abdominal X-ray and ultrasound. It is hypothesized that it results from the migration of intramural gas produced by bacterial translocation from the intestinal wall to the portal vein. Portal venous gas is typically associated with a worse clinical prognosis.

Question: How can the severity of NEC be categorized?

Answer: Bell's classification and its modifications.

The Bell classification system proposed by the American pediatric surgeon Martin Bell in 1978 (5) remains the most widely used staging system for NEC (1). It categorizes NEC severity based on clinical and radiographic signs into three different stages. A more recent, modified version of Bell's classification is found in **Table 13.1** (2). Neonates with proven (stage II) or advanced (stage III) NEC are at risk of developing peritonitis, sepsis, bowel perforation, and other severe systemic complications including multisystem organ failure. More recently, following a prospective study, Battersby et al. (6, 7) described a novel scoring system based on gestational age.

Question: After physical examination of the patient, plain abdominal X-rays (supine anterior/posterior and left lateral decubitus (left-side-down radiograph) and blood work are initiated. The abdominal X-rays show multiple gas-filled loops of intestine with thickened bowel walls, with no signs of pneumatosis intestinalis or portal venous gas. The laboratory findings on total blood count and blood gas analysis show the combination of neutropenia, thrombocytopenia, and mild metabolic acidosis. Based on these clinical and radiological findings, what stage of NEC is this? Is there an image of this?

Answer: Suspected NEC (Bell stage I).

Given the clinical findings of lethargy, feeding intolerance, and increased oxygen requirements as well as blood per rectum, together with the radiological findings of gas-filled loops with thickened bowel walls without the presence of pneumatosis intestinalis or portal venous gas, your working diagnosis is suspected NEC (Bell stage I).

Question: How would you manage this patient with stage I NEC?

Answer: Conservative management: Nasogastric-tube, nothing by mouth (NPO), parenteral nutrition, broad-spectrum antibiotics, and supportive care.

Table 13.1

Stage	Classification	Clinical signs	Radiologic signs
1	Suspected NEC	Abdominal distention Bloody stools Emesis/gastric residuals Apnea/lethargy	Ileus/dilation
II	Proven NEC	*As in stage 1, plus:* Abdominal tenderness ± Metabolic acidosis Thrombocytopenia	Pneumatosis intestinalis and/or portal venous gas
III	Advanced NEC	*As in stage II, plus:* Hypotension Significant acidosis Thrombocytopenia/disseminated intravascular coagulation Neutropenia	As in stage II, with pneumoperitoneum

Source: Modified from Walsh MC, Kliegman RM: Necrotizing enterocolitis: Treatment based on staging criteria, *Pediatr Clin North Am* 33:179, 1986.

In this early stage of NEC, nasogastric tube decompression, parenteral nutrition, broad-spectrum antibiotics, and supportive care are the widely accepted components of medical conservative management. In case of fungal sepsis (if cultured), empirical antifungal therapy should be considered. The goals of treating NEC are to prevent continued injury to the mucosal epithelium of the gastrointestinal tract, stop disease progression, and treat any infection that may be present.

Question: Over the next 12 hours the patient has continued to deteriorate with more pronounced neutropenia and thrombocytopenia, requiring transfusion of blood products. Blood gas analysis shows severe metabolic acidosis. The patient is hypotensive, and treatment with inotropes has also been initiated. Plain abdominal X-rays are shown in Figure 13.2. An abdominal ultrasound has indicated generalized distension of the intestinal loops, pneumatosis intestinalis, and portal venous gas in the absence of intra-abdominal fluid collections. What stage of NEC has the patient most likely advanced to, and how do you manage the patient at this point?
Answer: The management of the baby at this point is challenging. No evidence of perforation has been found, and it would be too early to consider that medical therapy is failing (antibiotics and bowel rest were started 12 hours ago). Most surgeons would continue with conservative management and supportive care but would consider performing a laparotomy if no improvement or deterioration occurs within the next 12–24 hours.

Question: In the case of a patient who actually improves clinically with medical conservative management, how long will you continue conservative treatment with broad-spectrum antibiotics?
Answer: Traditionally a minimum of 7 days up to 14 days is widely practiced.

While much research has focused on understanding NEC, there are controversies in the care of infants with it. The duration of antibiotic treatment has been mainly based on expert opinion and institutional preferences. In most institutions, the duration of therapy for NEC ranges between 7 and 14 days, and the type of antimicrobial agents can vary. The Infectious Diseases Society of America (IDSA) and World Society of Emergency Surgery (WSES) guidelines recommend treatment

durations of 4–7 days, depending on the NEC severity, for complicated intra-abdominal infection but do not differentiate neonatal intra-abdominal infections (2, 3). The 2017 Surgical Infection Society (SIS) guidelines recommend a course of antibiotic therapy for 7–10 days in neonates (<1 month of age), particularly if affected by NEC (3). Bull et al. (4) have recently established a new NEC severity-guided protocol in which NEC symptom resolution is the determinant for the duration of the antibiotic course. In their study, the median antibiotic duration for patients with mild NEC (normal complete blood count [CBC] or inflammatory markers) was 3 days (range, 1–4), for moderate NEC (abnormal CBC or inflammatory markers but hemodynamically stable) 4 days (range, 1–17), and for severe NEC (hypotension, respiratory failure, severe metabolic acidosis) 9 days (range, 5–21). Interestingly, no difference in NEC recurrence was found based on antibiotic therapy duration (4). This study encourages us to consider a more evidenced-based and patient-specific approach in the future. What remains only partially elucidated is the relationship between antibiotic therapy and the withholding of enteral feeds. Most commonly, feeds are slowly restarted after the antibiotic treatment has been completed.

Continuing Scenario: Twenty-four hours after the start of conservative NEC management, the patient is still not improving. On clinical examination the abdomen is distended and tender with skin discoloration. Abdominal X-ray was performed and shows the following (**Figure 13.3**).

Question: What is the diagnosis and what is the appropriate management?
Answer: Perforated NEC (Bell stage III) – emergent exploratory laparotomy

The finding of a pneumoperitoneum on abdominal X-ray radiography is suggestive of an intestinal perforation and is a definitive indication for surgical intervention. Relative indications include but are not limited to a palpable abdominal mass, fixed intestinal loop, abdominal wall erythema, and clinical deterioration despite maximal medical therapy. The goal of surgical intervention is to remove necrotic bowel while conserving as much intestinal length as possible. Intestinal loops with considerable potential for recovery should not be

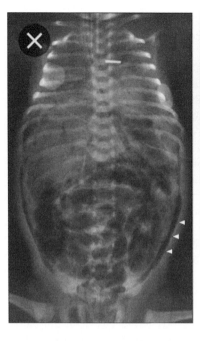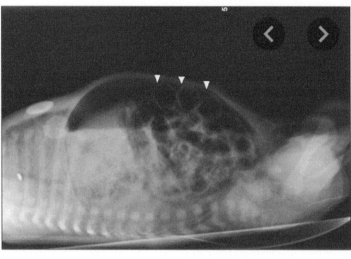

Figure 13.3 X-rays showing extensive pneumoperitoneum.

resected and can be re-evaluated with a second-look laparotomy.

The most common laparotomy approach is via a transverse supraumbilical incision. Utmost caution needs to be used to avoid a potentially fatal liver hemorrhage during retraction or manual dissection.

Question: What are the management options in the case of multisegmental disease?
Answer:

a. Extensive bowel resection + Proximal stoma formation.
b. Bowel resection and anastomosis + Stoma formation.
c. "Clip-and-drop" technique with a second-look laparotomy.

In case of multifocal disease, depending on the patient's perioperative stability, multiple treatment options are available:

a. *Perioperative stable patient and clear delineation between viable and non-viable bowel*: Resection +/– anastomosis of non-viable bowel and formation of a proximal stoma and mucous fistula might be the treatment of choice.

b. *Perioperative unstable patient and/or uncertain bowel viability*: Resection of bowel with full-thickness gangrene. Bowel ends are temporarily sutured or clipped, and a second-look laparotomy will be performed once the patient is stable.

Question: What are your management options in a case of NEC totalis?
Answer: Traditionally managed with comfort care due to high mortality (40%–100%); recent advances in the management of short bowel syndrome have resulted in increasing reports on aggressive surgical therapy.

NEC totalis is defined by the presence of necrotic bowel for 75%–80% of the total length of the small intestine. It is the most aggressive and devastating form of NEC and associated with a high mortality rate. The incidence of NEC totalis is reported to be as high as 10% of all neonates diagnosed with NEC. The management has traditionally been palliative comfort care. However, recently there are increasing reports on aggressive surgical management, especially given the emergence of data demonstrating improved survival in patients requiring long-term total parenteral nutrition (TPN). Surgical management includes diversion of the intestinal stream by high proximal jejunostomy without bowel resection (= fecal diversion) or of extensive bowel resection ("clip-and-drop"). Dukleska et al. recently performed a meta-analysis on NEC totalis, which found that the mortality rate of patients following aggressive surgical treatment was 69%, in contrast to non-aggressive surgical therapy (i.e., exploratory laparotomy only) with a mortality rate of 95% (8).

Question: When is the right time to close the stoma in patients with NEC?

Answer: There are currently no differences in outcomes between early and late stoma closure.

A systematic review and meta-analysis reported no difference in duration of parenteral nutrition, length of hospital stay, and postoperative complications between early (<8 weeks from stoma formation) versus late (after >8 weeks from stoma formation) stoma closure (9).

Question: What are the frequently encountered long-term problems in children with NEC?

Answer: Short bowel syndrome (SBS), failure to thrive, GI problems (strictures, adhesions), and neurodevelopmental impairment.

Common complications of NEC include failure to thrive, gastrointestinal problems including strictures and adhesions, cholestasis, and SBS +/– intestinal failure that can be very challenging to manage. Of note approximately half of all NEC survivors suffer from impairments in cognitive and motor function as well as white matter injury, often resulting in cerebral palsy (10). Close after-care follow-up is essential for NEC patients for early diagnosis, treatment, and monitoring of potential long-term complications.

BIBLIOGRAPHY

1. Solomkin JS, Mazuski JE, Bradley JS, et al. Diagnosis and management of complicated intra-abdominal infection in adults and children: Guidelines by the Surgical Infection Society and the Infectious Diseases Society of America. Clin Infect Dis. 2010;50(2):133–164.

2. Sartelli M, Chichom-Mefire A, Labricciosa FM, et al. The management of intra-abdominal infections from a global perspective: 2017 WSES guidelines for management of intra-abdominal infections. World J Emerg Surg. 2017;12:29. doi:10.1186/s13017-017-0141-6

3. Mazuski JE, Tessier JM, May AK, et al. The Surgical Infection Society revised guidelines on the management of intra-abdominal infection. Surg Infect (Larchmt). 2017;18(1):1–76.

4. Bull KE, Gainey AB, Cox CL, Burch AK, Durkin M, Daniels R. Evaluation of time to resolution of medical necrotizing enterocolitis using severity-guided management in a Neonatal Intensive Care Unit. J Pediatr Pharmacol Ther. 2021;26(2):179–186. doi: 10.5863/1551-6776-26.2.179. Epub 2021 Feb 15. PMID: 33603582; PMCID: PMC7887889.

5. Bell MJ. Neonatal necrotizing enterocolitis. N Engl J Med. 1978:298(5):281–282.

6. Battersby C, Santhalingam T, Costeloe K, Modi N. Incidence of neonatal necrotising enterocolitis in high-income countries: A systematic review. Arch Dis Child Fetal Neonatal Ed. 2018;103(2):F182–F189. doi: 10.1136/archdischild-2017-313880. Epub 2018 Jan 9. PMID: 29317459.

7. Battersby C, Longford N, Costeloe K, Modi N, Group, U. K. N. C. N. E. S. Development of a gestational age-specific case definition for neonatal necrotizing enterocolitis. JAMA Pediatr. 2017;171:256–263. doi:10.1001/jamapediatrics.2016.3633

8. Dukleska K, Devin CL, Martin AE, Miller JM, Sullivan KM, Levy C, Prestowitz S, Flathers K, Vinocur CD, Berman L. Necrotizing enterocolitis totalis: High mortality in the absence of an aggressive surgical approach. Surgery. 2019;165(6):1176–1181. doi: 10.1016/j.surg.2019.03.005. Epub 2019 Apr 27. PMID: 31040040.

9. Zani A, Lauriti G, Li Q, Pierro A. The timing of stoma closure in infants with necrotizing enterocolitis: A systematic review and meta-analysis. Eur J Pediatr Surg. 2017;27(1):7–11. doi: 10.1055/s-0036-1587333. Epub 2016 Aug 14. PMID: 27522125.

10. Rees CM, Pierro A, Eaton S. Neurodevelopmental outcomes of neonates with medically and surgically treated necrotizing enterocolitis. Arch Dis Child Fetal Neonatal Ed. 2007;92:F193–F198. doi:10.1136/adc.2006.099929

11. Samuels N, van de Graaf RA, de Jonge RCJ, Reiss IKM, Vermeulen MJ. Risk factors for necrotizing enterocolitis in neonates: A systematic review of prognostic studies. BMC Pediatr. 2017;17(1):105. doi: 10.1186/s12887-017-0847-3. PMID: 28410573; PMCID: PMC5391569.

12. Alganabi M, Lee C, Bindi E, Li B, Pierro A. Recent advances in understanding necrotizing enterocolitis. F1000Res. 201;8: F1000 Faculty Rev-107. doi: 10.12688/f1000research.17228.1. PMID: 30740215; PMCID: PMC6348433.

13. Berkhout DJC, Klaassen P, Niemarkt HJ, de Boode WP, Cossey V, van Goudoever JB, Hulzebos CV, Andriessen P, van Kaam AH, Kramer BW, van Lingen RA, Vijlbrief DC, van Weissenbruch MM, Benninga M, de Boer NKH, de Meij TGJ. Risk factors for necrotizing enterocolitis: A prospective multicenter case-control study. Neonatology. 2018;114(3):277–284. doi: 10.1159/000489677. Epub 2018 Jul 11. PMID: 29996136.

14. Neu J, Walker WA. Necrotizing enterocolitis. N Engl J Med. 2011;364(3):255–64. doi: 10.1056/NEJMra1005408. PMID: 21247316; PMCID: PMC3628622.

15. Horbar JD, Edwards EM, Greenberg LT, Morrow KA, Soll RF, Buus-Frank ME, Buzas JS. Variation in performance of neonatal intensive care units in the United States. JAMA Pediatr. 2017;171(3):e164396.

16. Gordon PV, Swanson JR, Attridge JT, et al. Emerging trends in acquired neonatal intestinal disease: Is it time to abandon Bell's criteria? J Perinatol. 2007;27(11): 661–671.

14

Intestinal failure

ANNIKA MUTANEN AND MIKKO P. PAKARINEN
The New Children's Hospital, University of Helsinki, Helsinki, Finland

Scenario: In the neonatal intensive care unit, a 1-month-old neonate born at 26 weeks of gestation is diagnosed with sepsis, necrotizing enterocolitis (NEC) and bowel perforation. To remove the necrotic part of the bowel, a laparotomy and an extensive bowel resection with jejunostomy are performed. After operation, the neonate is hemodynamically stabilized but has a high-output stoma and requires long-term parenteral nutrition (PN) support.

Question: What is the working diagnosis of this neonate?

Answer: The neonate has intestinal failure (IF). IF is defined as a reduction of functional gut mass or length below the minimal amount necessary for adequate digestion and absorption to satisfy nutrient and fluid requirements for maintenance of normal growth and development of a child.

In children, the most common etiology of IF is short bowel syndrome (SBS) caused by NEC followed by volvulus, small bowel atresia, gastroschisis and total/near-total intestinal aganglionosis (Hirschsprung disease). Most pediatric SBS cases occur in the neonatal period, while 20% of patients are diagnosed later during childhood with IF caused by volvulus, trauma or, less frequently, by Crohn's disease and malignancies. IF can also be caused by disorders of gastrointestinal motility (e.g. chronic intestinal pseudo-obstruction [CIPO]) and congenital enterocyte disorders (e.g. microvillus inclusion disease, tufting enteropathy and other rare disorders) (**Table 14.1**).

Table 14.1 Etiology of intestinal failure

Short bowel syndrome (70%–80%)	Intestinal motility disorders (5%–20%)	Enteropathies (5%–10%)
• Necrotizing enterocolitis	• Chronic intestinal pseudo-obstruction (CIPO)	• Epithelial dysplasia
• Malrotation midgut volvulus	• Congenital	• Microvillus atrophy
• Adhesive volvulus	• Acquired	• Autoimmune enteropathy
• Small bowel atresia	• Dysmotility in gastroschisis and small bowel atresia	
• Gastroschisis		
• Total/near-total intestinal aganglionosis (Hirschsprung disease)		
• Crohn's disease		
• Trauma		
• Operative complications		
• Malignancy		

DOI: 10.1201/9781003182290-15

Question: How does the remaining bowel anatomy affect the prognosis of IF?

Answer: The probability of weaning off PN depends on the gut length, anatomy, functional state and growth potential of the remaining bowel. IF can be broadly classified based on the remaining visceral anatomy (**Figure 14.1**) to Types 1 (end-jejunostomy), Type 2 (jejuno-colic anastomosis after small bowel and partial colon resection) and Type 3 (jejuno-ileocolic anastomosis after small bowel resection with intact colon and some ileum

preserved). Type 3 anatomy carries the best prognosis, followed by Type 2 and Type 1.

Children with >50% of expected small bowel remaining, regardless of the colon remaining, have a good prognosis, as nearly all will wean off PN support in 1–2 years. In children with <50% of small bowel remaining, the colon has a more important role in improving absorption and ability to reach enteral autonomy. Even patients with <10% of small bowel and remaining colon may be able to wean off PN support in several years' time (1). A preserved ileum, ileocecal valve and colon all improve prognosis and potential for weaning off PN. The remaining ileum is able to absorb water against a concentration gradient, conjugated bile acids, and vitamin B_{12} (**Figure 14.2**). The ileum promotes intestinal adaptation by producing enteroendocrine hormones such as glucagon-like peptide 1 and 2 and peptide YY. The ileum also secretes FGF19, which downregulates bile acid synthesis in the liver, which may protect from liver injury. The colon absorbs water and electrolytes and improves energy salvage by metabolizing carbohydrates to short-chain fatty acids, which are then absorbed. The ileocecal valve slows intestinal transit and prevents colonization of the remaining small bowel by colonic bacteria.

The growth potential of the remaining small intestine affects substantially the prognosis of IF patients, and in addition to absolute gut length, the residual bowel should be evaluated as a percentage of expected bowel length for age (2). The growth potential is greatest in premature neonates. During

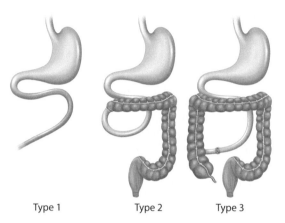

Type 1   Type 2   Type 3

Figure 14.1 IF can be classified based on the remaining visceral anatomy to types 1 (end-jejunostomy), type 2 (jejuno-colic anastomosis after small bowel and partial colon resection) and type 3 (jejuno-ileocolic anastomosis after small bowel resection with intact colon and some ileum preserved).

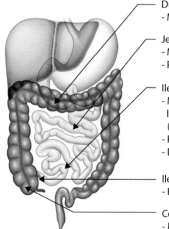

Duodenal resection
- Malabsorption of iron, calcium and B vitamins

Jejunal resection
- Malabsorption of carbohydrates, lipids, amino acids, vitamins and trace elements
- Promotes gastric hypersecretion

Ileal resection
- Malabsorption of conjugated bile acids and B12 vitamin. Bile acid malabsorption leads to impaired micelle formation and promotes malabsorption of lipids (fatty acids and fat-slouble vitamins).
- Fluid and nutrient malabsorption
- Decreased GLP-2 and peptide YY secretion

Ileocaecal resection
- Promotes bacterial overgrowth

Colonic resection
- Malabsorption of electrolytes, water and short chain fatty acids
- Decreased GLP-2 and peptide YY secretion

Figure 14.2 Clinical features associated with different types of intestinal resections.

the last trimester of pregnancy, the small bowel and colon will double in length, making the outcome of a 25-week-gestation neonate very different from a term baby with the same length of residual bowel. The small bowel and colon continue to grow also after birth, since in a term baby the length of the small bowel is approximately 200 cm and the colon 40–50 cm compared to 450 cm of small bowel and 150 cm of colon in an adult.

Question: What is meant by intestinal adaptation?

Answer: After extensive intestinal resection, the remaining bowel starts a compensatory process of adaptation wherein it undergoes structural and functional changes that gradually increase the bowel's absorptive capacity. Histologically, adaptation is seen as increased villus height and crypt depth accompanied by macroscopic bowel lengthening and widening. The adaptation process starts rapidly after bowel resection and continues most actively for the first 2 years and may continue more than 5 years (1). *Enteral nutrition and intestinal continuity are the most important prerequisites for intestinal adaptation.*

Question: What are the surgical treatment options for IF?

Answer: Surgical treatment for IF (i.e. autologous intestinal reconstructive surgery [AIRS]) aims to enhance intestinal adaptation and weaning off PN. By recruiting the entire remaining intestine by closing enterostomies and repairing strictures, blind loops or enteroenteric fistulas, enteral tolerance may be significantly improved. Intestinal motility and function may be improved by performing tapering enteroplasty, longitudinal intestinal lengthening and tailoring (Bianchi) or serial transverse enteroplasty (STEP) of dilated small intestinal loops. Intestinal transit may be slowed down by segmental reversal of small bowel or isoperistaltic colonic interposition, which has been mainly used in adult patients (3).

In the STEP procedure, intestinal tapering and lengthening are accomplished without any loss of surface area and with minimal mesenteric dissection by narrowing the luminal channel with a series of staples from alternating and opposite directions perpendicular to the long axis of the bowel in a zig-zag pattern. After STEP, the length of the operated bowel increases proportionally to the degree of dilatation, even more than 100%. An

SBS patient with imaging-proven bowel dilatation (>3.5–4 cm) with poor peristalsis, symptomatic bacterial overgrowth and inability to wean off PN may be a candidate for this procedure.

In the Bianchi procedure, an avascular plane is opened along the mesenteric border of the dilated bowel. The bowel is split lengthwise, leaving a mesenteric leaf with blood vessels to each side to avoid bowel necrosis and is then tubularized and anastomosed end-to-end in an isoperistaltic fashion. An SBS patient with severe (>5 cm) segmental bowel dilatation, symptomatic bacterial overgrowth and inability to wean off PN could be a candidate for the Bianchi procedure. Patient selection for these operations remains problematic and requires considerable experience and a multidisciplinary care team assessment.

Question: Are there any pharmacological treatment options for IF?

Answer: Adaptation may be promoted with glucagon-like peptide 2 analogues.

Proadaptive medication aims to enhance intestinal adaptation to improve absorption and growth of the bowel. Glucagon-like peptide 2 has been shown to decrease PN requirement and increase villus height in SBS patients. Other medication, such as antisecretory agents (to reduce gastric hypersecretion), antimotility agents (e.g. loperamide to reduce rapid intestinal transit) and cyclic enteral antibiotics (to treat bacterial overgrowth) may be used based on an individualized treatment plan (4).

Question: What are the principles of nutritional therapy in IF?

Answer: The first line of treatment for IF is individually planned nutrition support, including parenterally administered fluid, electrolytes and nutrients together with enteral feeds. In IF, PN is lifesaving and is used to maintain normal fluid and electrolyte balance and growth until intestinal adaptation enables gradual weaning off PN in the majority of patients. PN is administered using a single-lumen, tunneled central venous catheter, preferably as overnight infusions. In principle, neonates with IF are allowed to feed freely as tolerated. Early initiation of enteral feeds, preferentially fresh breast milk, improves oral motor feeding skills, intestinal adaptation and chances of weaning off PN. The amount of enteral feeds is individually adjusted based on the volume of intestinal secretions and stool consistency (4).

Question: What complications are related to IF?
Answer: IF and long-term PN are associated with multiple complications such as intestinal failure–associated liver disease (IFALD), central line–associated bloodstream infections (CLABSIs), mechanical central venous catheter complications (breakage, thrombosis), intestinal bacterial overgrowth, metabolic bone disease, chronic kidney disease and increased mortality (**Table 14.2**).

IFALD results from the combined consequences of PN and compromised intestinal function, bacterial overgrowth, septic episodes and liver immaturity in neonates. Liver disease is initially characterized by histological cholestasis and inflammation combined with variable progression of fibrosis and steatosis over time and increased serum biochemical markers of cholestasis and liver injury. IFALD affects approximately 30–100% of these infants, depending on the definition, while a small proportion of patients develop progressive liver disease, which may lead to biliary cirrhosis. To prevent IFALD, early initiation of oral feeds, choice of modern fish oil–based PN lipids (SMOF), cyclic PN infusions and efficient treatment and prevention of septic episodes and intestinal bacterial overgrowth should all be included in the treatment strategy of IF patients.

CLABSI with symptoms of sepsis, signs of an infected central line site and positive blood culture

Table 14.2 IF-related complications and risk factors

Complication	Risk factors
Intestinal failure–associated liver disease (IFALD)	• Short intestinal remnant • Lack of ileocecal valve • Parenteral nutrition related • Long-term PN dependency • Excess fat, plant sterols, glucose • Lack of PN omega-3 fatty acids • Lack of enteral nutrition • Septic episodes • Bacterial overgrowth • Interrupted enterohepatic circulation • Prematurity and low birth weight
Central line–associated bloodstream infections (CLABSIs)	• Bad central line management, unnecessary line access • No central line lock (taurolidine or ethanol) in use • Bad central line placement (prefer subcutaneous port rather than tunneled catheter)
Central line complications (breakage, thrombosis)	• Bad central line management
Intestinal bacterial overgrowth	• Impaired intestinal motility • Abnormal bowel dilatation • Lack of ileocecal valve
Metabolic bone disease	• Short residual small bowel • Increasing age • Insufficient calcium and vitamin D supplementation
Chronic kidney disease	• Chronic dehydration and electrolyte imbalances due to malabsorptive intestinal losses • Recurrent sepsis • Nephrocalcinosis • Nephrotoxic medications

is a serious complication of IF and PN. The risk of CLABSI may be decreased by standardized aseptic central line management, taurolidine or ethanol catheter locks and by preferably using tunneled single-lumen catheters instead of subcutaneous ports (5).

SBS-related bacterial overgrowth impairing intestinal adaptation and absorptive function is related to defective intestinal motility, abnormal bowel dilatation and lack of the ileocecal valve. Symptoms of bacterial overgrowth include vomiting, increased intestinal secretions, abdominal distension and pain, bacterial translocation–induced septic episodes and D-lactic acidosis. Symptomatic bacterial overgrowth may be treated with empirical cyclic courses of enteral antibiotics and surgically by tapering and lengthening procedures when associated with abnormal small bowel dilatation (4).

IF patients on long-term PN, especially those with a short residual small bowel and insufficient calcium and vitamin D supplementation, have a high risk for metabolic bone disease with incomplete mineralization and consequent disturbances ranging from osteopenia to severe osteoporosis and pathologic fractures. IF-related kidney disease is relatively common and multifactorial from chronic dehydration and electrolyte imbalances due to malabsorptive intestinal losses, recurrent sepsis, nephrocalcinosis and nephrotoxic medications (6).

Question: When is intestinal transplantation indicated?
Answer: IF patients with failed nutritional support due to severe complications, i.e. severe and progressive IFALD, loss of central venous access sites, recurrent catheter-related septic episodes, recurrent and severe dehydration or metabolic abnormalities, may be considered candidates for intestinal transplantation. In case of severe liver disease, a combined liver-intestinal transplant is considered. As current 5-year survival rates after intestinal transplantation (60%) are less than those on long-term PN dependency (90%), poor quality of life alone is not currently considered to justify listing patients for transplantation (5).

BIBLIOGRAPHY

1. Belza C, Fitzgerald K, de Silva N, Avitzur Y, Steinberg K, Courtney-Martin G, et al. Predicting intestinal adaptation in pediatric intestinal failure: A retrospective cohort study. Ann Surg 2019;269:988–993.
2. Struijs MC, Diamond IR, de Silva N, Wales PW. Establishing norms for intestinal length in children. J Pediatr Surg 2009;44:933–938.
3. Pakarinen MP. Autologous intestinal reconstruction surgery as part of comprehensive management of intestinal failure. Pediatr Surg Int 2015;31:453–463.
4. Duggan CP, Jaksic T. Pediatric intestinal failure. N Engl J Med 2017;17:666–675.
5. Wendel D, Cole CR, Cohran VC. Approach to intestinal failure in children. Curr Gastroenterol Rep 2021;23:8.
6. Mutanen A, Wales PW. Etiology and prognosis of pediatric short bowel syndrome. Semin Pediatr Surg 2018;27:209–217.

15

Neonatal abdominal masses

RYO TAMURA AND HANY GABRA
Great North Children's Hospital, Newcastle, UK

Scenario: A 0-day-old newborn baby was referred from a local hospital for a possible intra-abdominal mass. He was born at 39 weeks' gestation via a normal vaginal delivery. His pre-natal fetal ultrasound showed a possible intra-abdominal flank mass.

Question: What information is important at the time of the referral?

Answer: Prenatal ultrasonography is important to evaluate the nature of the intra-abdominal mass. At the same time, details of the pregnancy and delivery history should be noted. Some fetal tumors, including large teratomas or hepatic hemangioendotheliomas, can cause fetal cardiac failure and hydrops fetalis. Oligohydramnios or polyhydramnios can happen together with fetal intraabdominal tumors. From a viewpoint of the newborn baby, the presence of systemic symptoms such as fever, lethargy, and failure to thrive should be reviewed because of its association with neuroblastoma. Symptoms suggesting bowel obstruction, which can be caused by large tumors and can lead to dehydration and electrolyte disturbance, require urgent correction.

In this baby's case, maternal pregnancy and delivery history were unremarkable without problems, and the only concern had been a solid right flank mass, adjacent to the kidney on antenatal ultrasound. No cystic component was noted at this examination. On examination, the baby was alert, active and well perfused. He had fed well and had passed meconium shortly after birth.

Question: What kind of physical findings should be looked for?

Answer: The anatomical location of the mass in the abdomen is an important clue to diagnosis, since it could specify the organ from which the mass originates. At the same time, any qualitative feature of the mass should be recorded such as consistency, size, mobility, and accompanying features like tenderness or surrounding inflammation.

The mass was felt in the right flank and was hard on palpation (**Figure 15.1**). No tenderness and surrounding inflammation were noted. The mass was not mobile and seemed fixed to surrounding tissues.

Question: What is the current suspected differential diagnosis?

Answer: Neonatal intra-abdominal masses have a wide range of differential diagnoses, as described later. In this case, the tumor was noted in the right flank, so the kidney or juxta-renal organs like the adrenal gland could be the organ of origin. From a viewpoint of the kidney, hydronephrosis or multicystic dysplastic kidney should be considered due to their relatively high incidence in newborn babies, but in this case, both are unlikely, as the lesion is solid on prenatal ultrasonography. If a normal kidney is confirmed on previous and postnatal examinations, then neuroblastoma in the adrenal gland

DOI: 10.1201/9781003182290-16

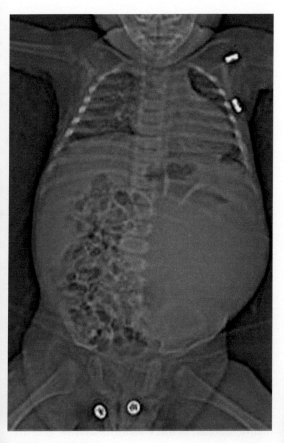

Figure 15.1 MRI scan showing a large left adrenal mass crossing the midline.

is suspected, since it is the most common malignant tumor in neonates. Adrenal hemorrhage is also one of the differential diagnoses of juxta-renal masses, in particular in the right side; however, it is less common than neuroblastoma.

Question: How would you proceed to further make a diagnosis?
Answer: A further imaging study is required. Abdominal ultrasonography is the first modality to be performed, as it is useful to determine further anatomical details (size, location, relationship to adjacent tissues). Furthermore, it can show whether the mass is solid or cystic and provide more information on vascularity. In addition to ultrasonography, cross-sectional imaging with computed tomography (CT) or magnetic resonance imaging (MRI) is employed, in particular when malignant tumors are suspected. MRI is often superior in terms of showing the qualitative characterization of the mass. However, MRI is not

always available, and CT may have an advantage of short examination time and being able to be performed without sedation, even in infants, compared to MRI, while its main disadvantage of ionizing radiation should be always considered. Blood or urinary tumor markers are also assessed in a case of suspected malignancy.

In this case, abdominal ultrasound and then MRI were both performed (**Figure 15.2**). A solid right adrenal mass was evident, and neuroblastoma is now the most likely diagnosis. There was no apparent invasion into adjacent tissues, but it crossed the midline of the abdomen. No distant metastasis was observed on MRI. According to an institutional treatment protocol, tumor biopsy was initially performed and the diagnosis was confirmed. The mass didn't seem amenable for primary resection, and the patient underwent neoadjuvant chemotherapy and had radical resection of the tumor several months later. No recurrence emerged, and the patient remained completely free from disease recurrence.

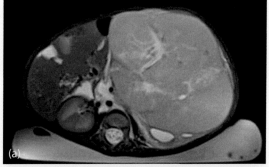

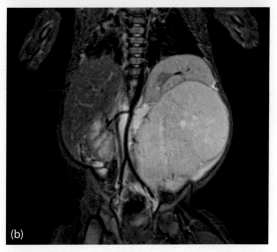

Figure 15.2 (a) Transverse section view. (b) Coronal section view.

GENERAL DISCUSSION

Neonatal abdominal masses include a wide variety of pathologies ranging from benign simple cysts to solid malignant tumors and can arise from various organs in the abdomen including intraperitoneal and retroperitoneal organs and tissues. Although malignant tumors should always be considered in the differential diagnosis, it seems worthwhile to note that the most common abdominal masses in infancy and childhood are non-pathological, including a normal liver, feces, and full bladder (1). At the same time, the three most common pathological abdominal masses are abdominal neuroblastoma, Wilms tumor, and neonatal hydronephrosis. An annual incidence of neonatal solid tumors was reported as 36.6 cases per million live births in a population study in France and accounted for 2% of all childhood malignancies (2). In the United States, the prevalence of cancer in the first month of newborn babies was reported as 36.5 cases per million live births (3). Neuroblastoma is the most common neonatal abdominal malignant tumor, which accounts for roughly 40%–50% and is followed by Wilm's tumor and liver tumors (4).

Clinical presentation

Most neonatal abdominal masses are usually asymptomatic and are noticed by family members incidentally (when not diagnosed on antenatal ultrasound). One exception is neuroblastoma, which may cause systemic symptoms such as fever, failure to thrive, and general malaise. Apart from the systemic symptoms, a large tumor may cause obstructive symptoms of the gastrointestinal tract like vomiting and early satiety. Urinary retention may be noticed by decreased numbers of wet nappies or a weak urine stream.

Differential diagnosis

A wide range of pathologies is included in a differential diagnosis of neonatal abdominal masses, and they can be divided based on the location where they arise (**Table 15.1**). Each organ or tissue included in the location where the mass emerges can be an organ of origin. Initially, the abdomen is divided into five locations including left and right upper quadrant, flank abdomen, mid-abdomen, and pelvis. Each location has several organs, and then the origin of the mass can be narrowed according to the organ in the location.

Diagnostic work-ups

A comprehensive history ought to be obtained first. As described earlier, systemic symptoms such as failure to thrive, irritability, or being unwell may indicate the presence of neuroblastoma. GI symptoms like vomiting may be induced by a large tumor itself, and hematochezia may be caused by GI hemorrhage due to ectopic gastric mucosa occurring with intestinal duplications or direct invasion of malignant tumors into the GI tract. A history of multiple urinary tract infections or decreased number of wet nappies may indicate a congenital issue relating to the urinary tract or the kidney. Antenatal ultrasound is extremely useful to raise suspicion of congenital hydronephrosis, multicystic dysplastic kidney, ovarian cysts/teratoma, neuroblastoma, and hepatoblastoma (5).

Plain abdominal X-ray is the first imaging study which ought to be performed. Calcification within the mass is suggestive of neuroblastoma or teratoma.

Laboratory blood examination is useful to detect any ongoing inflammatory process and electrolyte disturbance. It is also important to check for tumor markers, which could be raised in germ cell tumors, neuroblastoma, and hepatoblastoma. In a case of neuroblastoma, urinary vanillylmandelic acid and homovanillic acid are important clues for diagnosis.

Distribution of blood vessels in the mass can be also depicted with Doppler ultrasound. It can be performed bedside and so is an appropriate initial and sequential modality to document any chronological change in the tumor. At the same time, CT or MRI is preferred in a case of suspected malignant tumor as a second survey to evaluate cross-sectional, sagittal, and coronal views of the tumor; metastasis; and direct invasion into adjacent tissues. In case of a mass arising in the kidney or causing urological obstruction, nuclear scans like MAG3 renograms or DMSA scintigram (after 3/12 of age) may be employed to examine renal parenchymal and excretory function, but these examinations are not routinely performed in neonates since their renal function is not sufficient to draw out a valid diagnosis.

GENERAL MANAGEMENT

Management is usually based on the initial presentation, imaging, discussion by the multidisciplinary team (MDT) (if malignancy suspected), and pathology. Initial tissue diagnosis via image-guided biopsy may be required to determine the

Table 15.1 Differential diagnosis of neonatal abdominal masses classified by the location and the organ

Location	Organs	Differential
Flank		
	Kidney	Hydronephrosis
		MCDK
		Solid tumors of the kidney
	Juxta-renal	Adrenal hemorrhage
		Neuroblastoma
		Pulmonary sequestration
Right upper quadrant		
	Liver	Hemangioendothelioma
		Hamartoma
		Hepatoblastoma
	Biliary tree	Choledochal cyst
Left upper quadrant		
	Spleen	Splenic cysts
Mid-abdomen		
	Pylorus	Hypertrophic pyloric stenosis
	Intestine	Intestinal duplications
		Lymphatic malformations
		Meconium disease
		Constipation
	Abdominal wall	Mid-abdominal wall defects
		Omphalomesenteric remnants
Lower abdomen/Pelvis		
	Uterus	
	Ovary	Ovarian cysts
	Urachus	Urachal cyst
	Sacral	Sacrococcygeal teratoma

Source: Reference 6.

nature of the mass and hence the subsequent management. However, up-front surgical resection in the form of excision biopsy could also be considered or required for diagnostic and treatment purposes. This may require a nephrectomy or oophorectomy for a renal or ovarian solid mass, respectively. In other scenarios, such as a neonatal neuroblastoma, a conservative approach is justified based on the risk stratification and the histology of the tumor. A decision to watch and wait must always be based on the conclusion of an MDT discussion.

BIBLIOGRAPHY

1. Hutson JM, O'Brien M, Beasley SW, Teague WJ, King SK. Jones' Clinical Paediatric Surgery: John Wiley & Sons; 2015.

2. Desandes E, Guissou S, Ducassou S, Lacour B. Neonatal solid tumors: Incidence and survival in France. Pediatr Blood Cancer. 2016;63(8):1375–80.

3. Bader JL, Miller RW. US cancer incidence and mortality in the first year of life. Am. J. Dis. Child. 1979;133(2):157–9.

4. Campbell A, Chan H, O'brien A, Smith C, Becker L. Malignant tumours in the neonate. Arch Dis Child. 1987;62(1): 19–23.

5. Lee TC, Olutoye OO. Evaluation of the prenatally diagnosed mass. Semin Fetal Neonatal Med. 2012;17(4):185–91.

6. Chandler JC, Gauderer MW. The neonate with an abdominal mass. Pediatr Clin North Am. 2004;51(4):979–97, ix.

16

Cardiac surgery

DAVID VONDRYS AND MARK REDMOND
Children's Health Ireland, Crumlin, Dublin, Ireland

The surgery of congenital cardiac disease is at times quite complex. In this chapter the most common anomalies will be discussed under the four headings of:

Oxygen
Blood flow
Blood return
Airways

OXYGEN

Scenario: You are called to see a Caucasian, full-term, male newborn with a birth weight 5.2 kg, Apgar score 9-9-8 who seems to be pale, or rather purple in colour and is struggling to breathe on room air. His parents are concerned that after an initial period of lively crying he became rather lethargic. He is now 48 hours old.

Question: What is the first and best simple investigation required?
Answer: Pulse oximetry. Pulse oximetry measures the saturation of blood with oxygen. Normal saturation in a healthy newborn depends on the quality, quantity and separation of pulmonary and systemic blood circulations and should be higher than 90% on any extremity.

A pulse oximetry screen exam is considered positive if the measured oxygen saturation is lower than 90%. Any infant with a positive pulse oximetry screen should have a diagnostic echocardiogram (1).

Question: This child has saturation of 80–85% on all extremities. While you are waiting for the echocardiography study to be performed, what should you next do as an initial treatment of choice?
Answer: Schedule an infusion of prostaglandin. The most likely diagnosis will be:

1. Transposition of the great arteries (TGA).
2. Pulmonary atresia.
3. Tetralogy of Fallot.
4. Total anomalous pulmonary venous return (TAPVR).
5. Hypoplastic left heart syndrome.
6. Truncus arteriosus

These are so-called 'ductus-dependent malformations', and the prostaglandin infusion will usually re-open the fetally open but postnatally closed arterial duct (PDA). As the duct opens, more blood will flow into the lungs via the pulmonary artery (P), and the oxygen saturation in peripheral blood will improve. This will give us time to stabilize the patient, and after the echocardiography confirms the diagnosis, the patient should be transferred to an appropriate specialist facility for cardiac surgery (**Figure 16.1**).

Question: Describe the principles of the most common cardiac surgery operations for congenital malformations.
Answer:

1. *TGA:* The aorta and pulmonary artery are transected just above the valves and the coronary arteries are liberated. Both arteries are

DOI: 10.1201/9781003182290-17

Normal Heart

Transposition of great arteries

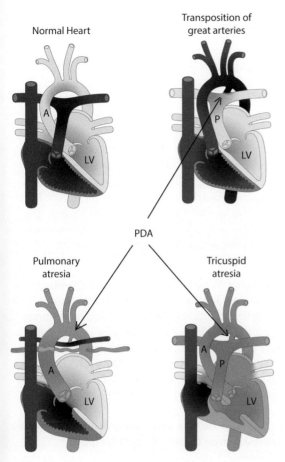

PDA

Pulmonary atresia

Tricuspid atresia

Figure 16.1 *Abbreviations:* Aorta (A); left ventricle (LV).

then moved above the correct ventricle (the aorta is connected with the left ventricle and the pulmonary artery is connected with the right ventricle), and the coronary arteries are reimplanted into the root of the neoaorta. The arterial septal defect is closed.

2. *Pulmonary atresia, tetralogy of Fallot*: A Blalock Taussig (BT) shunt (3–3.5 mm in diameter created with a PTFE [Gore-Tex] tube) is anastomosed between the innominate and pulmonary artery. This allows the blood to flow into the lungs until the full repair. This is performed later, and the shunt is removed. The ventral septal defect (VSD) is closed and the right ventricle to the pulmonary artery (PA) connection is created (either a valved conduit or valveless connection – direct anastomosis called a transannular patch). This will require further interventions, most likely percutaneous

implantation of a larger sized right ventricle (RV)-PA conduit or surgical replacement.

3. *TAPVR*: The confluence of pulmonary veins needs to be identified and ligated. A new direct connection is then created between the confluence and the posterior wall of the left atrium. This is mostly done in so-called 'deep hypothermic circulatory arrest', where the circulation is stopped after the patient is cooled down to 16 degrees Celsius with the help of a heart-lung machine to allow surgical anastomosis. This has an obvious negative impact on the perfusion of all organs and can lead to multiorgan failure.

4. *Hypoplastic left heart syndrome*:

   First stage: Norwood operation in the newborn period. The small ascending aorta is connected with the large pulmonary artery (Daymus Key Stensel procedure), and the blood flow is maintained via a BT shunt. A common atrium is created via atrial septectomy.

   Second stage: Glenn operation at the age of 3–6 months. The BT shunt is taken down and the superior vena cava is transected and directly anastomosed into the right PA.

   Third stage: Fontan operation at the age 3–5 years. The inferior vena cava is separated from the common atrium and is connected directly into the pulmonary artery with the help of a PTFE (Gore-Tex) graft conduit with a diameter of 18–20 mm.

5. *Truncus arteriosus*: The anomalously originating PA is explanted from the ascending aorta, the VSD is closed with a patch and a new conduit is implanted between an incision in the RV and an incision in the PA.

BLOOD FLOW

Scenario: A female patient of Asian origin is born at term, birth weight 3.5 kg and now 4 days old. She was originally discharged from hospital but has now come back with a fever, vomiting and a very low urine output. During physical examination she moves her lower extremities less, which are also very cold compared to her arms, body and head. You measured the saturation and there is 100% on the right hand and 90% on the left hand and both legs.

Question: What is the most appropriate investigation now?

Answer: Non-invasive blood pressure measurement of all four limbs. Palpation of femoral pulses shows reduced pressure waves on both sides. The blood pressure measured will be as follows: right arm 80/40, left arm 60/30, right leg 50/25 and left leg 50/25 mm Hg. This represents restriction of blood flow from the left ventricle into the descending aorta and hence into the kidneys and gastrointestinal tract.

The most likely diagnosis will be coarctation of the aorta or hypoplastic or interrupted aortic arch.

Question: What is the solution?

Answer: Echocardiography should confirm the diagnosis. Prostaglandin and catecholamine infusion and volume resuscitation should be initiated to increase the peripheral blood pressure and improve the lower body blood supply. The patient is in urgent need of an emergency operation or stenting **(Figure 16.2)**.

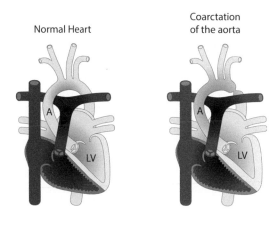

Normal Heart

Coarctation of the aorta

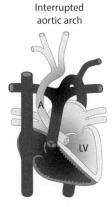

Interrupted aortic arch

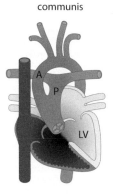

Truncus arteriosus communis

Figure 16.2 *Abbreviations:* Aorta (A); pulmonary artery (P); left ventricle (LV).

BLOOD RETURN

Scenario: A patient in the ICU requires your attention. It is a mildly preterm baby boy, birth weight 2.8 kg, who was admitted on the fifth day of life with the preliminary diagnosis of sepsis. He is now 7 days old, intubated on 40% FiO_2, saturation 90% on all extremities, catecholamine support and requiring IV diuretics. He has good urine output and signs of sepsis: white blood cells (WBC) 18, C-reactive protein (CRP) 125. Nurses report that there are copious amounts of rose-coloured foamy secretions suctioned from the airways during the last 24 hours.

Question: What is the first and simple investigation?

Answer: Chest X-ray. This shows whiteout of both lung fields. This is most likely caused by pulmonary oedema, which could be caused by impaired drainage of blood from the lungs via the pulmonary veins. The most likely diagnosis is TAPVR with obstruction. This is often not seen on fetal echocardiography, as the lungs are not perfused before the birth.

Question: In this case, what is a more specific investigation than echocardiography?

Answer 2: Contrast angiography. The contrast study investigation can better delineate the exact anatomy of venous return and help to establish the urgency of an operation. The pulmonary veins do not enter straight into the left atrium, but they create a confluence which can be connected to the heart from above, from below or from behind (supracardiac, infracardiac or a retrocardiac type of TAPVR, respectively) **(Figure 16.3)**.

AIRWAYS

Scenario: A 3-year-old boy presents in the emergency department with a peri-arrest situation. He has had a respiratory infection for the last 2 weeks and was treated with antibiotics by his general practitioner (GP). He has a history of a repaired trachea-oesophageal fistula as a baby. Now he is hyperventilating and unsettled, and you can already hear a very loud stridor from a distance. His oxygen saturation is 95% on 2 litres of oxygen, and he has normal blood pressure with mild tachycardia.

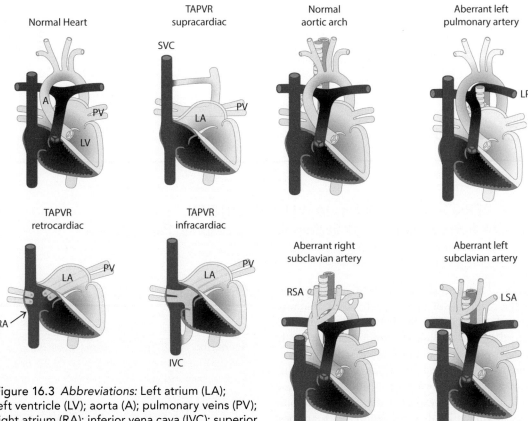

Figure 16.3 *Abbreviations:* Left atrium (LA); left ventricle (LV); aorta (A); pulmonary veins (PV); right atrium (RA); inferior vena cava (IVC); superior vena cava (SVC).

Question: What investigation should be performed?
Answer: Contrast CT scan of the chest. It is very likely that his stridor is caused by an external compression of his airways. Tracheoesophageal fistulas are associated with co-existent congenital cardiovascular anomalies (VACTERL). A CT angiogram will probably show some vascular malformation. For example, a double aortic arch, a right-sided aortic arch or just a malposition of great arteries, all which can cause a compression of the airways.

Question: What should the initial management be?
Answer: The patient should be admitted to hospital and further investigations should be performed. These include (1) bronchoscopy, (2) echocardiography and (3) contrast bronchography to establish the exact anatomy and give enough information for further treatment. The most common procedures undertaken would be aortopexy (i.e. fixation

Figure 16.4 *Abbreviations*: Left pulmonary artery (LPA); left subclavian artery (LSA); right subclavian artery (RSA).

of the aorta and brachiocephalic artery away from the airways), division of a double aortic arch or aberrant great arteries. In recent years some hospitals have used metallic or biodegradable stents for stenting of the airways **(Figure 16.4)**.

BIBLIOGRAPHY

1. Harold JG. Screening for Critical Congenital Heart Disease in Newborns. Circulation. 2014;130:e79–e81
2. Illustration taken from http://www.chd-diagrams.com. Illustrations are licensed under Creative Commons NonCommercial NoDerivatives 4.0 International License by the New Media Center of the University of Basel.

17

Fetal surgery

CARA BERKOWITZ AND WILLIAM H. PERANTEAU

The Children's Hospital of Philadelphia, Philadelphia, Pennsylvania

Advances in prenatal care with fetal imaging allow for the diagnosis of most structural or anatomical birth defects prior to birth. The benefits of in utero diagnosis include the ability for families to consider pregnancy options, increased health provider fetal well-being surveillance and planning ahead for the newborn patient to include site and mode of delivery at expert centers. Although most surgical anomalies detected before birth are best managed after birth, some structural birth defects result in progressive damage and even fetal mortality before birth. In these select cases, and when there are no maternal contraindications, fetal surgical interventions may be an option at specialized medical centers after multidisciplinary, nondirectional counseling is provided to the expectant parents. The more commonly prenatally diagnosed structural birth defects, including those which, in select cases, may be amenable to fetal intervention, are listed in **Table 17.1**. It should be noted that fetal surgery for structural birth defects involves a large, multidisciplinary, highly specialized team of skilled practitioners including but not limited to pediatric/fetal surgeons, maternal-fetal medicine specialists, fetal cardiologists, anesthetists with expertise in fetal surgery, genetic counselors, neonatologists, psychologists, social workers and a dedicated team of operating room nurses. In this chapter we will seek to highlight three common structural birth defects managed at fetal diagnosis and treatment centers, including the rationale for prenatal interventions for these anomalies.

CONGENITAL LUNG LESIONS

Scenario: A 28-year-old female carrying a 22-week-gestation fetus underwent a 20-week fetal ultrasound scan during which a hyperlucent lesion is noted in the left lung. No other anatomic abnormalities were seen. The mum is referred to your fetal care center for further management.

Question: What is the likely fetal diagnosis, and what further studies should be performed?
Answer: The initial ultrasound findings are consistent with a congenital pulmonary airway malformation (CPAM). CPAMs consist of a spectrum of diagnoses including microcystic and macrocystic congenital cystic adenomatoid malformations (CCAMs); intralobar and extralobar bronchopulmonary sequestrations (BPSs); hybrid lesions (have characteristics of both a CCAM and a BPS); and mainstem, lobar or peripheral bronchial atresia. Although the different CPAM lesions have different pathologic findings, the prenatal and postnatal management for most of these lesions is similar. Additional workup should include a repeat fetal ultrasound scan with particular attention to the vascular supply and drainage of the lung lesion, size (cm) and presence of additional findings. For large lesions or those in which the diagnosis is in question, an ultrafast fetal MRI is recommended.

DOI: 10.1201/9781003182290-18

Table 17.1 Prenatally diagnosed structural anomalies including the possible prenatal intervention and rationale for that intervention in select cases for certain diagnoses

Structural anomaly	Possible prenatal intervention	Rationale for prenatal treatment/Delivery via EXIT
Cervical masses (teratoma, lymphatic malformation)	EXIT procedure	To secure an airway
Congenital lung lesions	Open fetal surgery (OFS) or EXIT to resect involved lung lobe	Alleviate mass affect and fetal heart failure, minimize pulmonary hypoplasia and respiratory failure at birth
Congenital diaphragmatic hernia	Fetoscopic tracheal occlusion	Minimize pulmonary hypoplasia
Renal anhydramnios	Serial amnioinfusions	Minimize pulmonary hypoplasia
Lower urinary tract obstruction	Vesicoamniotic shunt; ablation of valves	Prevent renal failure and pulmonary hypoplasia
Pericardial teratoma	OFS or EXIT and resection of teratoma	Prevent cardiac failure
Sacrococcygeal teratoma	OFS and debulking	Prevent death from high-output cardiac failure
Myelomeningocele/ Myeloschisis	OFS and repair of vertebral defect	Minimize need for postnatal ventriculoperitoneal shunt and improve hindbrain herniation and motor function
Twin-twin transfusion syndrome	Fetoscopic ablation of communicating vessels	Prevent vascular steal

Structural anomalies diagnosed prenatally but without prenatal intervention options/lack of rationale for a fetal intervention

Abdominal wall defects (gastroschisis, omphalocele, OEIS)	Pure esophageal atresia	Duodenal atresia
Jejunoileal atresia	Anorectal malformations	Enteric duplication cysts
Cleft lip/Palate	Conjoined twins	Ovarian cysts
Biliary cysts	Limb/Skeletal anomalies	Lymphatic malformations (noncervical)
Ventriculomegaly/ Hydrocephalus	Renal mass/hemorrhage	

Question: What findings on ultrasound differentiate a BPS from other CPAMs?

Answer: BPSs are characterized by the presence of an abnormal systemic arterial blood vessel (often arising from the aorta) supplying the BPS. The venous drainage can be either directly into the systemic system or into the pulmonary venous system. A BPS with systemic venous drainage is an extralobar lesion, while one with pulmonary venous drainage is an intralobar sequestration.

Question: What ultrasound findings are critical for evaluating the prognosis of the fetus with a CPAM and determining the appropriateness of a prenatal intervention?

Answer: Findings on prenatal ultrasound scan that inform the prognosis and prenatal management include the CPAM-volume ratio (CVR), the presence of signs suggestive of hydrops fetalis and whether the lesion is a microcystic or macrocystic lesion. The CVR is the ratio of the volume of the lung lesion (height × length × width × 0.52) to the fetal head circumference. The lower the CVR, the better the prognosis with lesions, with a CVR >1.6 portending a poor prognosis without intervention. Most lung lesions grow in absolute and relative (CVR) size until 26–28 weeks' gestation after which they plateau or even reduce in size. Nonimmune hydrops fetalis is traditionally defined as the accumulation of serous fluid in at least two body cavities (pericardial effusion, pleural effusion, skin/scalp edema, ascites and placentomegaly) and is indicative of fetal heart failure. In cases of large lung lesions, heart failure is believed to be related to compression. Finally, the characteristic of the lung lesion, microcystic versus macrocystic, will inform potential prenatal treatment options if indicated.

Question: Repeat fetal ultrasound at the clinic demonstrated a left lower lobe lung lesion without a systemic arterial feeding vessel, no evidence of hydrops and a microcystic lesion with a CVR of 0.4. What are the next steps in the management of this patient?

Answer: This fetus has a small lung lesion that is not compromising the fetal cardiac function. No prenatal intervention is therefore required. The fetus should be monitored with serial maternal ultrasounds to monitor for the growth of the lesion and the presence of hydrops fetalis (**Figure 17.1**). Of note, the vast majority of lung lesions present like the lesion discussed in the current scenario. *Note*: A small lung lesion usually never requires

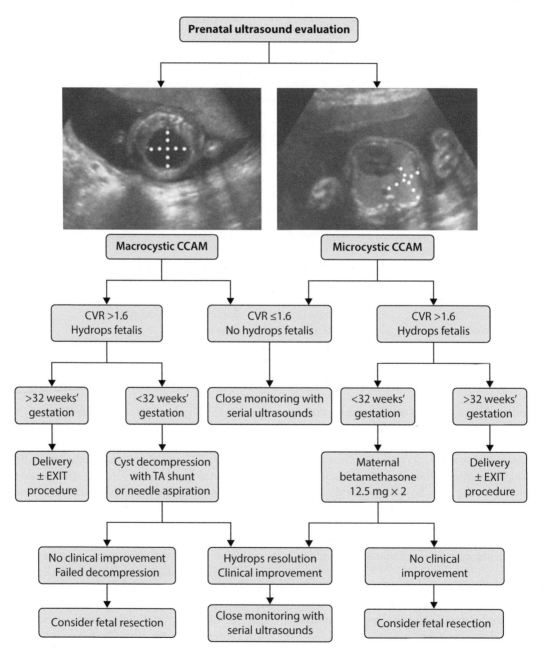

Figure 17.1

prenatal intervention and can be managed expectantly after birth.

Question: Another mum presented with a fetus at 23 weeks' gestation with a macrocystic lung lesion with a CVR = 2.1 and trace evidence of pericardial effusion and ascites. What would your initial management of this patient be? How would management differ if the lung lesion was a macrocystic lung lesion?

Answer: This fetus has a large lung lesion (CVR >1.6) and signs of early hydrops fetalis. Assuming there are no maternal complications, the option of ultrasound-guided CPAM macrocyst drainage with subsequent placement of a thoracoamniotic shunt if there is reaccumulation of the cyst fluid should be offered to the family. This approach has been shown to reduce the size of the lesion, be associated with resolution of hydrops fetalis and improve outcomes (**Figure 17.2**). One known complication of thoracoamniotic shunt placement is an increased incidence (%) of thoracic rib deformities on the side of the shunt when the shunt is placed early in gestation. If the lesion was a microcystic lesion, providing single or multiple courses of maternal betamethasone has been shown to decrease the size of the lesion, encourage resolution of hydrops and improve outcome/survival in fetuses with large lung lesions without drainable macrocyst(s) (**Figure 17.1**).

Question: Despite placement of a thoracoamniotic shunt or administering three courses of maternal betamethasone, the fetal lung lesion in the patient discussed continued to grow and there was an increase in pericardial fluid and ascites. What would the management of the fetus be at this point? How does the gestational age of the fetus affect your management decision?

Answer: Fetuses with large lung lesions that do not respond to cyst drainage or maternal betamethasone would be candidates for open fetal surgery or an ex utero intrapartum treatment (EXIT) procedure to remove the offending lung lesion depending on the gestational age (fetuses <30 weeks' gestation = open fetal surgery; fetuses >30 weeks' gestation = EXIT procedure) (**Figure 17.2**). Open fetal surgery requires maternal general anesthesia, a maternal laparotomy and hysterotomy with exposure of the fetal chest. Fetal thoracotomy and resection of the involved lung lobe is performed

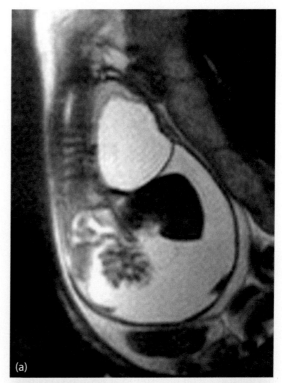

(a)

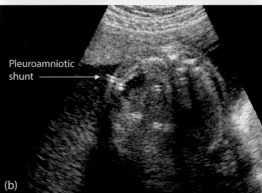

Pleuroamniotic shunt →

(b)

Figure 17.2

and the hysterotomy closed with the goal of maintaining the pregnancy and minimizing preterm labor. An EXIT procedure involves a maternal laparotomy under general anesthesia with a hysterotomy and resection of the fetal lung lobe involved in which the lung lesion is located while the fetus is maintained on placental support. After resection, the baby is then delivered. Both procedures involve a multidisciplinary skilled team at specialized fetal treatment centers and requires nondirective multidisciplinary counseling of the family prior to the surgery (**Figure 17.1**).

Question: What is the postnatal management of CPAMs?

Answer: As indicated earlier, most CPAMs do not require fetal intervention, and many babies are asymptomatic at birth. Furthermore, many CPAMs can be difficult to visualize on late gestation fetal ultrasound, giving the false impression that they have fully resolved. It is highly unlikely that a prenatally diagnosed CPAM will resolve, and thus we always recommend a low-dose irradiation CT scan at ~1 month of age after birth for infants prenatally diagnosed with a CPAM. With the exception of small extralobar BPSs, we generally recommend surgical resection either via a thoracotomy or a thoracoscopic approach of the involved lung lobe after birth for symptomatic and asymptomatic lesions to remove the risks of infection and the low risk of cancer.

SACROCOCCYGEAL TERATOMA

A 30-year-old mother presents with a 23-week fetus to your multidisciplinary fetal care center after having had a fetal ultrasound at her OB/GYN physician's hospital which demonstrates a large mass in the area of the fetal coccyx.

Question: What is the likely diagnosis, and what imaging studies are recommended?

Answer: The most likely diagnosis in this scenario is a sacrococcygeal teratoma (SCT). SCTs are typically benign extragonadal germ cell tumors that involve the coccyx. They are believed to originate from the Hensen's node region. Although many are considered benign, 11%–35% of SCT tumors may contain malignant elements such as yolk sac or embryonal carcinoma. Further workup for the fetus should include a detailed fetal ultrasound, an ultrafast fetal MRI and a fetal echocardiogram.

Question: What are different ways of classifying SCTs based on fetal imaging, and what are the implications for outcomes?

Answer: SCTs can be classified into four distinct categories according to the location and extent of the tumor according to the Altman Classification Scheme (**Figure 17.3**):

Type I: Primarily external with a small presacral component.
Type II: External with intrapelvic extension.

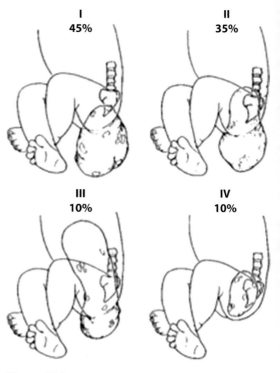

Figure 17.3

Type III: Primarily pelvic and intra-abdominal with external component.
Type IV: Completely intrapelvic with no external component.

Additionally, SCTs can be classified based on the amount of solid and cystic components they contain. Solid tumors tend to be much more vascular and, if large, can be associated with an increased risk of high-output cardiac failure, hydrops fetalis, tumor rupture/hemorrhage and fetal demise. Furthermore, SCTs with large intra-abdominal/pelvic components have an increased risk (%) for long-term urologic and anorectal complications even after surgical resection.

Question: What is the treatment for SCTs?

Answer: Surgical resection is the definitive treatment for SCTs. Complete resection of the tumor and coccyx is required. Most SCTs are resected within days of birth.

Question: What are the indications for fetal resection or caesarean delivery with immediate resection of an SCT?

Answer: Large, predominantly solid SCTs portend an increased risk of fetal heart failure, hydrops fetalis and fetal demise. If the solid component is predominantly external, then debulking the external component either at open fetal surgery (fetuses <28 weeks' gestation) or immediately following caesarean section delivery (fetuses >28 weeks' gestation) is an option in 'high-risk' fetuses with progressive fetal cardiac strain and/or early signs of hydrops. Thus, serial ultrasound evaluation and echocardiograms (sometimes twice weekly) to assess the size of the SCT, presence of hydrops, inferior vena cava diameter and the combined cardiac output (CCO) are required. In fact, for fetuses with large, predominantly solid external tumors at significant risk for hydrops fetalis, elective C-section delivery at 28–30 weeks' gestation with immediate neonatal debulking of the external component is often planned, as unexpected fetal demise has occurred in attempts to delay delivery until later in gestation. Importantly, a second surgery to complete the resection of any remaining external components, the coccyx and internal components of the tumor is required after the infant is stabilized and recovered from surgical debulking (often 2–3 months later around the 40-week-gestation date).

MYELOMENINGOCELE

Scenario: A 27-year-old mother with a body mass index (BMI) of 30 presents with a 23-week fetus noted to have a myelomeningocele (MMC) located at the first lumbar vertebrae and hindbrain herniation reported on ultrafast fetal MRI and ultrasound. The fetus has a normal karyotype and no other anomalies. The mother has no other comorbidities and a good psychosocial support network.

Question: Are this mother and fetus candidates for fetal MMC repair? Is there a benefit to fetal MMC repair compared to postnatal MMC repair? Answer: Yes – the mother and fetus are eligible candidates for fetal MMC repair. MMC is the most common form of spina bifida neural tube defect and is characterized by the extrusion of the spinal cord/meninges into a cerebrospinal fluid (CSF)–filled sac through a defect in the vertebral arches. The postnatal standard of care is early surgical closure of the birth defect within the first 24–48 hours of life. After compelling animal laboratory studies

demonstrating the safety and feasibility of fetal MMC repair and the growing clinical experience with open fetal surgery for MMC repair, the Management of Myelomeningocele Study (MOMS) multicenter trial showed that evidence is overwhelmingly favorable for prenatal repair. MOMS demonstrated that, for select patients, fetal MMC repair resulted in a significant reduction (%) of ventriculoperitoneal (VP) shunt placement at 1 year following surgery (40% vs. 82%, $P < 0.001$), improved infant neuromotor function including the ability to walk independently (42% vs. 21%, $P < 0.01$), and amelioration of hindbrain herniation. Although clinically beneficial, prenatal MMC repair is associated with an increased risk of maternal spontaneous rupture of membranes (46% vs. 8%, $P < 0.001$), oligohydramnios (21% vs. 4%, $P = 0.001$) and preterm labor (79% vs. 15%, $P < 0.001$). The inclusion and exclusion criteria for fetal MMC repair based on the MOMS trial are listed in **Table 17.2**.

Table 17.2 Inclusion and exclusion criteria for MOMS trial

Inclusion
• Maternal age ≥18 years
• GA from 19.0 to 25.6 weeks
• Normal karyotype
• Vertebral defect at S1 level or higher
• Hindbrain herniation noted on prenatal ultrasound and MRI

Exclusion
• Multiple gestation pregnancy
• Insulin-dependent pregestational diabetes
• Additional fetal anomalies
• Fetal kyphosis ≥30°
• History of incompetent cervix or cervix <20 mm on ultrasound
• Placenta previa
• Coexisting serious maternal comorbidities
• BMI ≥35
• Previous spontaneous singleton delivery at <37 weeks GA
• Maternal-fetal Rh isoimmunization
• Maternal HIV+, Hepatitis B+ or Hepatitis C+
• Inadequate maternal psychosocial support or maternal psychosocial limitations
• Uterine anomaly
• Unable to travel and follow-up

Abbreviations: BMI: Body mass index, GA: Gestational age.

Question: What is the rationale for fetal MMC repair?

Answer: The pathology related to MMC results from a 'two-hit process'. Failure of the neural tube to close early in gestation results in exposure of neural elements to trauma and the neurotoxic effects of amniotic fluid. Additionally, the open neural tube defect allows CSF to leak externally, predisposing the fetus to developing hindbrain herniation termed Arnold-Chari II malformation. The rationale for fetal MMC repair is therefore to (1) close the neural tube defect prenatally with a watertight seal, preventing exposure of the neural elements to additional trauma and the toxic elements in amniotic fluid, and (2) stopping the CSF leak, thus facilitating resolution of hindbrain herniation.

BIBLIOGRAPHY

1. Adzick NS, Thom EA, Spong CY, et al. A randomized trial of prenatal versus postnatal repair of myelomeningocele. N Engl J Med 2011;364:993–1004.
2. Crombleholme TM, Coleman B, Hedrick H, Liechty K, Howell L, Flake AW, et al. Cystic adenomatoid malformation volume ratio predicts outcome in prenatally diagnosed cystic adenomatoid malformation of the lung. J Pediatr Surg 2002;37(3):331–8.
3. Cass DL, Olutoye OO, Cassady CI, Zamora IJ, Ivey RT, Ayres NA, et al. EXIT-to-resection for fetuses with large lung masses and persistent mediastinal compression near birth. J Pediatr Surg 2013;48(1):138–44.
4. Tsao K, Hawgood S, Vu L, Hirose S, Sydorak R, Albanese CT, et al. Resolution of hydrops fetalis in congenital cystic adenomatoid malformation after prenatal steroid therapy. J Pediatr Surg 2003;38(3):508–10.
5. Peranteau WH, Boelig MM, Khalek N, et al. Effect of single and multiple courses of maternal betamethasone on prenatal congenital lung lesion growth and fetal survival. J Pediatr Surg 2016;51(1):28–32.
6. Peranteau WH, Adzick NS, Boelig MM, Flake AW, Hedrick HL, Howell LJ, Moldenhauer JS, Khalek N, Martinez-Poyer J, Johnson MP. Thoracoamniotic shunts for the management of fetal lung lesions and pleural effusions: A single-institution review and predictors of survival in 75 cases. J Pediatr Surg 2015;50:301–5.
7. Baumgarten HD, Gebb JS, Khalek N, Moldenhauer JS, Johnson MP, Peranteau WH, Hedrick HL, Adzick NS, Flake AW. Preemptive delivery and immediate resection for fetuses with high-risk sacrococcygeal teratomas. Fetal Diagn Ther 2019;45:137–44.
8. Partridge EA, Canning D, Long C, Peranteau WH, Hedrick HL, Adzick NS, Flake AW. Urologic and anorectal complications of sacrococcygeal teratomas: Prenatal and postnatal predictors. J Pediatr Surg 2014;49:139–42.
9. Hedrick HL, Flake AW, Crombleholme TM, Howell LJ, Johnson MP, Wilson RD, Adzick NS. Sacroccygeal teratoma: Prenatal assessment, fetal intervention, and outcome. J Pediatr Surg 2004;39:430–8.

PART 2

Surgical Disorders of Infancy

18

Inguinal hernia and hydrocele

NABEEL ASHEERI
Salmanya Hospital, Kingdom of Bahrain, Bahrain

Scenario: A 25-day-old male infant is brought to the pediatric surgery clinic by his parents with a history of a swelling in the right groin and scrotum noted by the mother while changing diapers the day before. The swelling appears mostly during infant crying or straining and disappears when the child is at rest or asleep.

On clinical exam there is an obvious swelling noted in the right inguinal region. On palpation the swelling is smooth, soft, non-tender, and with gentle pressure was easily reduced.

Question: What is the most likely diagnosis? What particular findings will confirm your diagnosis?
Answer: The most likely diagnosis is a right inguinal hernia. The history of an intermittent inguinal swelling is a classical presentation for inguinal hernia. Physical exam showing a reducible groin swelling would also provide confirmatory diagnosis.

Question: How would you confirm a diagnosis of inguinal hernia if there was no visible swelling in the groin during the clinic examination?
Answer: Demonstrating the 'silk glove sign' – palpation of the hernia sac over the cord structures while rolling the spermatic cord gives a sensation similar to rubbing two layers of silk together and is highly suggestive of an inguinal hernia.

Bedside maneuvers to increase intra-abdominal pressure may be attempted to demonstrate a groin swelling. Depending on the patient's age, these may include lifting the infant to an upright standing position on the exam couch to allow gravity to accentuate a groin swelling. In the older child, asking them to stand up, jump up and down several times or cough or try inflating a balloon (Valsalva) may also be attempted. A cord that is palpably thicker and more easily palpated is also evidence of a hernia.

Question: What else might you wish to examine at the clinic visit?
Answer: Examining the contralateral groin is important to detect the presence of a synchronous hernia, as inguinal hernias may be bilateral. Inguinal hernias are notably twice as common

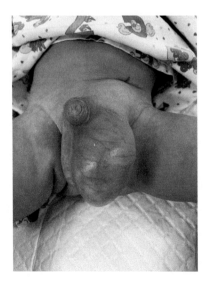

Figure 18.1 Inguinal hernia and hydrocoele

DOI: 10.1201/9781003182290-20

on the right side than the left and are bilateral in some 10% of all patients. Check also the testes and genitalia. Undescended testes, retractile testicles and hypospadias can be encountered in patients with inguinal hernias.

Question: Do we need further investigations to confirm the diagnosis of inguinal hernia?
Answer: No further investigations are required. The diagnosis of an inguinal hernia can be confidently made on history and clinical examination in most cases.

Question: What is the cause of an inguinal hernia in a child?
Answer: Inguinal hernias arise due to failure of the processus vaginalis to obliterate during fetal life. So they are always indirect inguinal hernias. In males, the processus vaginalis normally obliterates once descent of the testis is complete. In females, the anlage of the processus vaginalis is known as the 'canal of Nuck' which leads to the labia majora; typically obliterates by the seventh month of fetal life following descent of the ovaries to the pelvis. Factors that drive the patent processus vaginalis to obliterate are not fully understood; however, pediatric disorders associated with increased intraabdominal pressure such as ascites, ambulatory peritoneal dialysis or chronic cough increase the incidence of indirect inguinal hernias. The overall incidence of inguinal hernias is around 5% in males. The incidence is typically 5–10 times more common in males than in females. There are additional several risk factors for the development of inguinal hernias which also include prematurity, cystic fibrosis, the presence of a ventriculoperitoneal shunt (VP shunt) and certain connective tissue disorders.

Question: What is the treatment for this infant?
Answer: Inguinal hernia requires operative repair. The basic principles involve careful skeletonization of the spermatic cord structures, avoiding injury to the vas and vessels, with isolation and high transfixion ligation of the hernia sac (ensuring sac contents are empty), most often undertaken by a classic open approach. Premature infants will often require an overnight hospital stay with postoperative observation for apnea. In healthy newborns and older infants, surgery can be safely done as an ambulatory day case procedure. Laparoscopic or minimally invasive surgery (MIS) involving purse string closure of the internal ring is now increasingly popular. MIS has the practical advantage of the surgeon operator having direct visualization of the contralateral internal ring for the ready detection of a contralateral inguinal hernia, which will undergo synchronous repair.

> **Scenario:** A male child is brought to the hospital emergency department by his parents with a similar history of groin swelling in the inguinal region, which is now present all the time. In addition the patient is irritable and has been vomiting since morning.
>
> On examination the baby is irritable and continuously crying with the abdomen distended and non-tender. On abdominal exam percussion, it appears somewhat tympanic. The right inguinal region has a swelling which is tender on palpation with no obvious skin color changes noted.

Question: What is the diagnosis in this child?
Answer: This child also has a right inguinal hernia, *but* the presence of irritability and painful swelling indicates the presence of incarceration. Vomiting and abdominal distention are indicative of bowel obstruction. The diagnosis is therefore incarcerated and obstructed right inguinal hernia.

Question: How would you manage this child?
Answer: The patient has an incarcerated and obstructed right inguinal hernia. As there are no current findings to indicate peritonitis, manual reduction or 'taxis' should be attempted after ensuring adequate resuscitation in the stable child. In the presence of hemodynamic instability, septic shock or peritonitis, manual reduction *must not* be undertaken and the patient scheduled for *an urgent* operation.

Manual reduction is best achieved by sedating the infant and applying gentle pressure on the hernia to encourage the contents to return to the peritoneal cavity. A 'gurgle' often signifies successful hernia reduction. Taxis is successful in approximately 90% of patients undertaken by pediatric surgeons. It is a skill quickly acquired in the early training years. A 24- to 48-hour recovery period is then practiced by most surgeons for resolution of spermatic cord edema followed by semi-elective repair with hospital discharge.

Question: What will your management strategy be in a patient if the hernia is not reducible or only partially reduced?
Answer: Urgent surgical exploration is indicated if the taxis hernia reduction exam is unsuccessful to avert bowel gangrene, necrosis and perforation.

Scenario: A 5-month-old healthy male infant is brought to the outpatient hospital clinic with a history of a right scrotal swelling since birth. The swelling is noted to be present all the time by the parents, and the patient is well with no other symptoms. On clinical examination a uniform swelling of the right scrotum is observed. On palpation the swelling seems confined to the scrotum, is non-tender and is not reducible. You cannot readily palpate the ipsilateral right-sided testis. The left testis is felt in the scrotum.

Question: What is the most likely diagnosis?
Answer: Hydrocele is the most likely diagnosis in this scenario, as the swelling was reportedly present since birth. On examination it is confined to the scrotum and not reducible in an otherwise well infant, which all support a working diagnosis of a hydrocele.

Question: What is the cause of a hydrocele? How do you confirm a diagnosis?
Answer: A hydrocele is collection of fluid typically within the processus vaginalis surrounding the testis. It develops due to failure of the processus vaginalis to obliterate, allowing fluid to pass easily from the peritoneal cavity to the scrotum. The diagnosis may be further confirmed by demonstrating the ready identification of the presence of fluid within the scrotum by a transillumination test performed by placing a torch behind the scrotum, which will illuminate or 'light it up' (aka Chinese lantern sign), which is diagnostic for a hydrocele.

Question: How are hydroceles classified?
Answer: (1) Communicating hydrocele and (2) non-communicating hydrocele. An encysted hydrocele of the cord develops when the proximal and distal portions of the processus vaginalis obliterate, thereby entrapping a fluid-filled sac within the spermatic cord. In females, a failure of obliteration of the processus vaginalis will lead to fluid accumulation within the processus termed 'hydrocele of the canal of Nuck'.

Question: How would you then manage a child with a hydrocele?
Answer: Most hydroceles resolve spontaneously within 1–2 years after birth. Hydroceles can be observed safely ('active observation') in the early years. Surgical treatment is traditionally indicated for hydrocoeles that typically are persistent beyond the age of 2–3 years. Operation entails a day care groin procedure with isolation and transfixion suture of the processus vaginalis. Don't forget to empty the distal hydrocele sac at operation, as retained fluid can otherwise take some weeks to resolve!

Surgical practice and debate prevail with regard to age at operation (3, 4, 5 years, etc.) and the controversy of pediatric hydrocele operation being 'non-essential' in public health–funded services.

BIBLIOGRAPHY

Marte A, Caldamone AA, Aguiar LM. The history of the pediatric inguinal hernia repair. J Pediatr Urol. 2021;17(4):485–491.

Othersen Jr HB. The pediatric inguinal hernia. Surg Clin North Am. 1993;73(4):853–859.

Esposito C, Escolino M, Turra F, et al. Current concepts in the management of inguinal hernia and hydrocele in pediatric patients in the laparoscopic era. Semin Pediatr Surg. 2016;25(4):232–240.

Jobson M, Hall NJ. Current practice regarding timing of patent processus vaginalis ligation for idiopathic hydrocele in young boys; a survey of UK surgeons. Pediatr Surg Int. 2017;33(6):667–681.

Farrelly PJ, Losty PD. Essential and non-essential paediatric surgery: Implications for the future delivery of state health care in the UK. Pediatr Surg Int. 2015;31(9):879–883.

19

Umbilical hernia, epigastric hernia and allied conditions

STEVE DONNELL
Alder Hey Children's Hospital, Liverpool, UK

Scenario: A 4-month-old infant is referred with an enlarging umbilical hernia. The parents have been advised to attend accident and emergency (A&E) urgently if they think the hernia has become obstructed.

Question: What information is relevant in the history?
Answer:

1. *Ethnicity*: For reasons that are unclear but which may include social inequality, umbilical hernias are more common in black than in white infants. Studies from the United States indicate an 8- to 10-fold increase in incidence (25%–58% versus 2%–18% in the first year of life), but this is much less marked in South Africa (23% versus 19%). Overall, 15%–23% of young infants will have an umbilical hernia. There is no gender difference.
2. *Gestational age at birth*: The more premature the child, the more likely an umbilical hernia. Infants with a birth weight below 1,500 g have a 75%–84% incidence compared to 20% in those with a birth weight over 2,000 g.
3. *Timing*: Although childhood umbilical hernias occur through an unclosed, congenital umbilical ring, they are rarely apparent until the umbilical cord separates, at 5–8 days of age.

4. *Symptoms*: In the absence of incarceration or obstruction, childhood umbilical hernias are best considered to be asymptomatic. Any reported symptoms are likely to have another cause – colic, reflux, constipation, etc. – and should be managed accordingly.
5. *Medical history*: Rarely, an umbilical hernia will be the initial presentation of an underlying condition. These may include autosomal trisomy (21 and 18), metabolic disorders (hypothyroidism and mucopolysaccharidoses) and certain dysmorphic syndromes (Beckwith-Wiedemann and Marfan).
   A review of the antenatal and postnatal history may alert the clinician further. The presence of a ventriculoperitoneal shunt or peritoneal dialysis catheter may influence the natural history, and hence management of an umbilical hernia.

Question: What should you focus on in your clinical examination?
Answer:

1. *General appearance*: Does anything suggests an associated condition? Is the child healthy and interacting as expected?
2. *Abdominal examination*: Is there any distension, discolouration or tenderness?
   Exclude other abnormalities, including organomegaly, masses and ascites.

DOI: 10.1201/9781003182290-21

3. *Umbilical examination*: Is there a hernia, and is it reducible? What size is the open umbilical ring? Umbilical hernias can be classified as small (ring diameter <0.5 cm), medium (0.5–1.5 cm) and large (>1.5 cm).

4. *Linea alba*: Is there divarication of the recti? This is often visible as an infant strains or moves and manifests in an older child by aiding them or asking them to sit up and lie down.

Other discrete swellings may also be noted in the midline (see later – supraumbilical and epigastric hernia).

Question: Are any investigations indicated?
Answer: In the absence of symptoms and signs of incarceration or obstruction, no investigation should be necessary, unless the diagnosis of a hernia is in doubt or there appears to be another lesion. In those instances, an ultrasound scan may be appropriate. Possible alternative diagnoses include a supraumbilical hernia, lymphovenous malformations and, in older children, lipomatous lesions, implantation dermoid cysts within the umbilical cicatrix and prominent umbilical skin after a hernia has resolved.

Question: What should you tell the parents?
Answer:

1. *Natural history*: Although most umbilical hernias typically appear to enlarge at first, the umbilical ring does not. As an infant grows, its muscles become stronger and more intestine can be pushed into the peritoneal sac, making the swelling enlarge. As the umbilical ring contracts, the hernia stops getting visibly bigger before typically resolving. The stretched skin of the hernia may take months or years to fully contract but seldom merits treatment. Whilst more than 50% of umbilical hernias have resolved by 2 years of age and 80–95% by age 6 years, half of those still present will resolve by 11–13 years of age. It has been stated that the large hernia (>1.5 cm) is unlikely to resolve, but not all surgeons agree.

2. *Risk of complications*: Despite the sometimes alarming size and appearance of an umbilical hernia when an infant is crying or straining, the risk of incarceration is very small (0.07 %–0.3%). The medium-sized (0.5–1.5 cm) hernias may be most at risk. Thirty percent occur in the first 6

months of life, and the median age is 2.5 years. Perforation is even less common.

The relationship between a persistent childhood umbilical hernia and a symptomatic adult umbilical hernia is unknown. Most adult umbilical hernias occur through a defect in the linea alba adjacent to the true umbilicus and are more common with pregnancy, obesity and liver disease, with a female predominance.

The risk of complications from surgical repair is low, but there is a 2% recurrence rate, and the risk of an adverse respiratory event with general anaesthesia reduces 8% for each added year of age in childhood.

As a hernia reduces in size, the stretched skin contracts, but surgical intervention impairs this natural contraction. Generally, the younger the patient, the greater the need for umbilicoplasty.

3. *Non-surgical treatment*: Although there are proponents of hernia strapping or taping, this is probably of little benefit and carries risks of skin injury.

Question: When would you recommend surgical repair?
Answer:

1. There is no consensus for the timing of umbilical hernia repair, with minimum age recommendations varying from 2 to 12 years.

2. In the UK, best practice guidelines recommend waiting until at least 3 years of age, while the American College of Surgeons recommends 5 years of age. The author's personal practice is to wait until 7 years of age to allow the patient to more actively participate in decision making and for the resolution of any associated divarication (see later).

3. Complications aside, the indications for surgery are vague, but notably include cosmetic and social issues. Related ventriculoperitoneal shunt or peritoneal dialysis catheter problems may mandate hernia repair.

Question: How would you repair the hernia?
Answer:

1. In the absence of comorbidity, umbilical herniorrhaphy is a day case procedure, performed

under general anaesthesia, usually with muscle relaxation to reduce the risks of bowel injury. Laparoscopic repair is not commonplace in paediatric surgery.

2. An infraumbilical skin crease incision is made.
3. The peritoneal sac is adherent to the overlying dermis, and there is no need to separate the two – rather, the sac is divided by direct vision or transected after circumscription, leaving the distal sac adherent to the skin.
4. Secure fascial closure is obtained by interrupted absorbable or non-absorbable sutures, taking care not to injure the bowel. A Mayo double-breasting technique is suitable, but simple sutures are equally effective.
5. The peritoneum fused to the dermis can be attached to the repaired fascia with absorbable sutures, or a formal umbilicoplasty can be performed.
6. Absorbable subcuticular sutures oppose the skin edges.
7. The application of a pressure dressing for 48 hours to reduce the risk of haematoma is still practised, but may not be necessary.
8. A return to normal activities may be delayed for a week or two, dependent on the surgeon's preference.
9. Clinic review follow-up is optional.

Scenario: A 4-year-old patient presents with a reducible swelling just above the umbilicus.

Question: What is the diagnosis?
Answer: A supraumbilical hernia.

Question: What is the anatomy?
Answer: Usually a crescentic defect in the linea alba, concave inferiorly, with extraperitoneal fat protruding into the subcutaneous tissues.

Question: What is the natural history?
Answer: Usually asymptomatic, but unlikely to resolve spontaneously unless developing in infancy, when resolution may occur as the linea alba matures. Reminiscent of the defect described in adult umbilical hernia, surgery is usually appropriate.

Question: When should surgery be performed?
Answer: Any abdominal symptoms are likely to have another cause and should be investigated accordingly. An associated umbilical hernia should take precedence and be given time to resolve.

Question: How is the hernia repaired?
Answer:

1. Day case repair under general anaesthesia. Muscle relaxation is optional, as the peritoneum is not opened.
2. A supraumbilical skin crease incision is made.
3. The herniated extraperitoneal fat is dissected free from the fascial defect and either reduced or excised.
4. The defect is closed with simple, interrupted, absorbable or non-absorbable sutures.
5. Subcutaneous fat is optionally opposed with absorbable sutures.
6. Skin is closed with a subcuticular, absorbable suture. A dressing is optional.
7. Return to activities is the same as for umbilical herniorrhaphy.

Scenario: A 6-year-old patient is referred with a painless, irreducible swelling midway between the xiphisternum and the umbilicus.

Question: What is the likely diagnosis?
Answer: An epigastric hernia.

Question: What is the anatomy?
Answer: Through a 1- to 2-mm transverse defect in the linea alba, usually to one side of the midline, extraperitoneal fat has mushroomed into the subcutaneous fat. These hernias vary greatly in position between the xiphisternum and umbilicus and may be multiple in 10% of cases.

Question: Are investigations necessary?
Answer: There is usually little doubt in the clinical diagnosis, but an ultrasound will exclude other lesions, such as lipomatous or vascular lesions.

Question: What is the natural history?
Answer: If reducible, resolution is possible, particularly in infancy, but most will not resolve. Although symptoms from pinching during exercise are reported, many remain asymptomatic. They often become invisible, or much less obvious, with increase in the subcutaneous fat layer and pubertal changes in the midline abdominal tissues.

Question: When should surgery be offered?
Answer:

1. If there are symptoms and other causes have been excluded.
2. For cosmetic considerations. It is important that the patient and parents understand the natural tendency for cosmetic improvement with time, that a scar will be permanent with operation and can lengthen with growth and that there are potential surgical complications, including recurrence (more likely to be an iatrogenic hernia above or below the original due to splitting of the fibres of the linea alba).

Question: How is the hernia repaired?
Answer:

1. It is essential to carefully mark the site of the hernia while the child is still awake, as it may be impossible to find once the patient is anaesthetised!
2. Day case under general anaesthesia.
3. Occasionally a natural skin crease can be used to optimise the future cosmetic appearance of the scar, but generally a 1.5- to 2.5-cm vertical midline incision is made, centred on the hernia.
4. The hernia is identified as a rounded swelling of slightly different colour to the subcutaneous fat and carefully dissected down to its origin on the linea alba.
5. It is frequently helpful to gently widen the fascial defect with tissue forceps before excising or reducing the herniated fat.
6. One or two simple, interrupted, absorbable sutures close the defect, taking care to avoid splitting the fibres above or below by inserting the needle at slightly different levels.
7. Absorbable sutures to the subcutaneous fat and subcuticular layer close the wound.
8. Normal activities can resume after 48 hours, given the very small fascial defect that requires closure.

Scenario: A 2-year-old child is referred with a ventral hernia. Examination reveals an elliptical protrusion, akin to the upturned hull of a rowing boat, between the xiphisternum and the umbilicus.

Question: What is the diagnosis?
Answer: Divarication of the recti (rectus muscles).

Question: How common is it?
Answer: Extremely. Almost all infants will have evidence of divarication if actively looked for.

Question: What is the natural history?
Answer: Most divarications have resolved by the age of 10 years.

Question: What is the significance?
Answer: Although needing no treatment, a divarication indicates immaturity and lack of strength of the linea alba. Outcome studies for umbilical, supraumbilical and epigastric hernia in children lack information with regard to the coexistence of divarication, but adult studies show increased recurrence rates for sutured repair of these hernias when there is a divarication. Given the natural history of these hernias in childhood, delaying repair until the divarication has resolved may be beneficial.

SUMMARY

Umbilical hernia: Repair urgently for complications and electively for persistence, if patient wishes.
Supraumbilical hernia: Repair electively for persistence.
Epigastric hernia: Repair electively for symptoms or at patient request.
Divarication of the recti: Do not repair but consider when planning elective repair of midline hernias.

BIBLIOGRAPHY

1. MacKinnon AE. Herniae and hydrocoeles IN Burge DM, Griffiths DM, Steinbrecher HA and Wheeler RA eds. Paediatric Surgery (second edition). Hodder Arnold 2005:308
2. Weber TR. Umbilical and other abdominal wall hernias IN Holcomb III GW, Murphy JP and Ostlie DJ eds. Holcomb Ashcraft's Pediatric Surgery (sixth edition). Elsevier Saunders 2014:673–5
3. Bowling K, Hart N, Cox P and Srinivas G. Management of paediatric hernia. BMJ. 2017:359–64

4. Tulloh B and Nixon SJ. Abdominal wall, hernia and umbilicus IN Williams NS, O'Connell PR and McCuskie AW eds. Bailey and Love's Short Practice of Surgery (twenty seventh edition). CRC Press 2018:1036–9

5. Yoshida S, Yanai T, Tei E, Sueyoshi R, Koga H and Yamataka A. Incarceration of umbilical hernia in infants. J Pediatr Surg Case Rep. 2018;34:27–9

6. Zens TJ, Cartmill R, Muldowney BL, Fernandes-Taylor S, Nichol P and Kohler JE. Practice variation in umbilical hernia repair demonstrates a need for best practice guidelines. J Pediatr. 2019;206:172–7

20

Vitello-intestinal duct disorders

NICK LANSDALE
Royal Manchester Children's Hospital, Manchester, UK

Scenario: A 4-week-old infant born at term was referred to the specialist paediatric surgery clinic by their community midwife. There were concerns that the baby's umbilicus looked abnormal, and the abnormality had persisted despite application of silver nitrate cautery on a number of occasions.

On examination, the baby was noted to be well and the abdomen soft, flat and not tender. There was a prominent pink-coloured, fleshy polyp like a lesion at the umbilicus.

Question: What are the differential diagnoses that could explain this presentation?

Answer:

- Umbilical 'granuloma' due to incomplete epithelialisation of the umbilicus and the overgrowth of granulation tissue.
- *Vitello-intestinal (omphalomesenteric) duct remnant*: There are a spectrum of abnormalities that can result here from failure of involution of the vitello-intestinal duct, a process that is usually complete by the eighth or nine week of gestation (**Figure 20.1**). These abnormalities include a patent vitello-intestinal duct, a Meckel's diverticulum, a vitelline cyst, an umbilical polyp and a fibrous band.

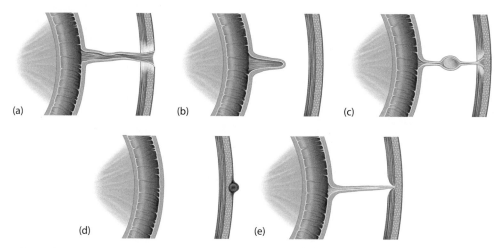

Figure 20.1 The variant types of vitello-intestinal duct abnormalities: (a) Patent vitello-intestinal duct, (b) Meckel's diverticulum, (c) vitelline cyst, (d) umbilical polyp and (e) fibrous band.

DOI: 10.1201/9781003182290-22

- *Urachal remnant*: Whilst these usually present as a suprapubic or infraumbilical mass due to a urachal cyst (which can become infected), they can occasionally cause an abnormality at the umbilicus itself. Urachal remnants result from a failure of involution of the urachus in fetal life.

Question: What might the polyp discharge?
Answer:

- Clear fluid, which may include gastric acid from the presence of ectopic mucosa. This can irritate the surrounding skin.
- Enteral tract fluid contents.
- Blood.
- Urine (persistent urachus).

Question: What investigation might be helpful, and what will this look for?
Answer: Ultrasound scan of abdomen. This will help look for a urachal remnant with connection from the bladder to the umbilicus or a vitelline cyst.

Question: What is the management of this condition?
Answer: Surgical exploration of the umbilicus and excision of the lesion are clearly indicated given that silver nitrate therapy has failed. This can be achieved using a mini-laparotomy with a curved skin fold crease incision just below the umbilicus. The umbilicus can be inspected and any connections to the bowel or bladder ascertained. Laparoscopy can also be useful, particularly in cases of urachal remnants that have been demonstrated at ultrasound.

Scenario: A 7-year-old child presented to the emergency department with bilious vomiting and abdominal distension.

On examination there were signs of volume dehydration. The abdomen was distended and mildly tender. There was no history of previous surgery and no surgical scars.

An abdominal radiograph was carried out (**Figure 20.2**).

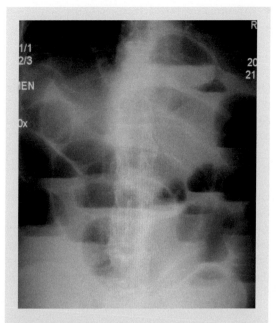

Figure 20.2 Abdominal radiograph demonstrating dilated intestinal small bowel loops with air/fluid levels. (From James Heilman, MD, CC BY-SA 3.0 https://creativecommons.org/licenses/by-sa/3.0, via Wikimedia Commons. No changes have been made to the image.)

Question: What is the diagnosis?
Answer: Small bowel obstruction.

Question: What are the possible causes of this condition in a child of this age?
Answer: The following are possible causes:

- Congenital obstructing band, e.g. mesodiverticular band ('Meckel's band'). The mesodiverticular band is an embryologic remnant of the vitelline circulation, which carries the arterial supply to Meckel's diverticulum.
- Adhesions from a previous inflammatory process, e.g. unrecognised or partially treated appendicitis.
- *Intussusception*: Whilst not the typical age group for idiopathic intussusception, there could be a small bowel intussusception due to a pathological lead point such as a tumour, polyp or Meckel's diverticulum.
- Obstructed hernia, e.g. inguinal hernia with an incarcerated bowel loop.

- Inflammatory bowel disease (IBD).
- *Midgut volvulus*: This could occur due to an unrecognised predisposition to volvulus such as a malrotation anomaly or congenital band.

Question: What is the initial management of this problem?

Answer: Intravenous fluid resuscitation should be commenced promptly.

A nasogastric tube should be inserted, aspirated regularly and left on free drainage.

Question: What is the surgical management of this problem?

Answer: An exploratory laparotomy or laparoscopy should be performed to diagnose the cause of these symptoms. The surgical treatment will depend on the actual findings at operation but may include division of bands/adhesions and/or bowel resection.

Scenario: A 5-year-old child presented to the hospital emergency department with a single episode of painless, profuse bleeding per rectum. The blood was brick-red in colour and not mixed with stool. The child was haemodynamically stable, and on examination, the abdomen was noted to be soft and not tender with no palpable mass or signs of distension.

Question: What are the potential causes of painless rectal bleeding in this case?

Answer:

- Meckel's diverticulum
- Bleeding intestinal polyp
- Inflammatory bowel disease
- Intestinal duplication
- Gastroenteritis/infective colitis
- Milk protein allergy
- Intussusception
- Ischaemic bowel
- Angiodysplasia

Question: What is the initial treatment for this child?

Answer: Intravenous access should be secured, and blood taken for a full blood count, clotting screen and blood cross-match to transfuse if required. Intravenous fluid and blood volume therapy should be tailored to the child's clinical state condition and haemoglobin level.

Question: What investigations should be carried out?

Answer: In addition to the blood tests listed earlier, renal status and liver function should be assessed. Initial imaging may include an ultrasound scan, as this can usually be arranged quickly and may yield an obvious source for the bleeding. Otherwise, the choice of investigation should be tailored to the clinical case; for example, if there is a history consistent with IBD, then early GI endoscopy may be needed: Biomarker tests such as faecal calprotectin may also be particularly helpful when judging the likelihood of IBD.

If a Meckel's diverticulum is suspected, then a technetium-99 m pertechnetate scan (Meckel's scan) can be done in the haemodynamically stable child. This investigation has a sensitivity of around 90% and specificity of >95% in children with rectal bleeding. In the more unstable child or in the event of a negative Meckel's scan with ongoing suspicion of Meckel's diverticulum, diagnostic laparoscopy will need to be undertaken to confirm or exclude the diagnosis

In cases when an obvious cause for bleeding cannot be found, a number of other key investigations can be undertaken. Cross-sectional imaging, usually computed tomography (CT), can be helpful and may demonstrate a mass or inflammation responsible for the bleeding. Mesenteric CT angiography can detect the presence of active bleeding, for example, due rarely to angiodysplasia. More advanced endoscopy techniques such as video capsule endoscopy and double balloon enteroscopy may also be employed in cases of occult bleeding. Combined endoscopy and laparotomy techniques (including the option of using a surgical enterotomy for endoscopy access) may be very helpful to diagnose the exact source of bleeding when initial external inspection of the bowel surface wall has not yielded the abnormality.

Question: If the bleeding is due to a vitello-intestinal duct disorder, what is the mechanism for the bleeding and how should it be treated?

Answer: Meckel's diverticulum frequently contains ectopic gastric mucosa. This mucosa can secrete acid and thus result in ulceration of the adjacent ileum, which then bleeds. This is important to consider when definitively treating Meckel's diverticulum, as surgical excision should best incorporate the adjacent ileum with a bowel resection and anastomosis.

BIBLIOGRAPHY

Snyder CL. Current management of umbilical abnormalities and related anomalies. Semin Pediatr Surg. 2007;16(1):41–9. doi: 10.1053/j.sempedsurg.2006.10.006. PMID: 17210482.

O'Donnell KA, Glick PL, Caty MG. Pediatric umbilical problems. Pediatr Clin North Am. 1998;45(4):791–9. doi: 10.1016/s0031-3955(05)70045-6. PMID: 9728186.

Lane VA, Sugarman ID. Investigation of rectal bleeding in children. Paediatr Child Health. 2010; 20(10):465–72. doi: 10.1016/j.paed.2010.06.008.

Moore TC. Omphalomesenteric duct malformations. Semin Pediatr Surg. 1996;5(2):116–23. PMID: 9138710.

Boonthai A, Mullassery D, Losty PD. Omphalomesenteric duct remnants. Pediatric Surgery Diagnosis and Management. Springer Publishers 2023 (Second Edition). Eds. Puri P and Hollwarth ME.

21

Undescended testes

SPENCER W. BEASLEY

Christchurch Hospital, Christchurch, New Zealand

Undescended testes (UDT) represent one of the most common disorders seen by paediatric surgeons and occurs in approximately 1%–2% of boys. The major clinical significance of UDT is that if orchidopexy is performed, i.e. an operation to bring the testis into the scrotum before the age of 2 years, this will likely maximize male fertility potential and also potentially reduce the risk of subsequent late malignancy of the maldeveloped testis.

The following clinical scenarios cover most of the key clinical decisions that need to be made by the clinician when confronted with a boy with suspected UDT.

Question: You are asked to see a 26-week-gestation infant boy with UDT. What guidance can you provide on how to manage the testes?

Answer: Testes are not normally fully descended at 26 weeks gestation age. Inguinoscrotal descent usually commences at around 26 weeks in the fetus and continues throughout development until term delivery at 37 weeks (and sometimes beyond term). Typically, in this scenario the baby should be subject to surveillance follow-up at clinic visits, where the natural history in this case may well be that the testes will eventually descend spontaneously into the scrotum with advancing months of age. Most testes in males are descended at birth, but further descent is recognised to occur particularly in the 3 months after term delivery.

The best advice, therefore, is to re-examine the baby after 3 months post-term. In everyday practice this is often at 6–9 months of age. If the testes at that stage are confirmed to be descended to the scrotum, no further action – other than reassurance – is required. If they are shown to be undescended at this follow-up clinic visit, an orchidopexy is scheduled to be performed, which in many hospital centres is now typically between 9 and 18 months of age.

Question: Just prior to discharge from the neonatal intensive care unit (NICU) it is noticed that a male infant has a right-sided inguinal hernia. The testes are undescended. What management would you advise?

Answer: The challenge in this scenario is to balance the risks of leaving an inguinal hernia that may incarcerate with all the consequences of strangulation versus anaesthetic and surgical aspects of a potentially 'difficult operation' where the hernia will need to be simultaneously repaired and the undescended testis brought down into the scrotum at the same procedure. There is an emerging expert consensus that the best approach involves a single operation, i.e. inguinal herniotomy and orchidopexy concurrently, which is superior to first repairing the hernia at one operation (i.e. leaving the testis undescended) and coming back later at a second operation to undertake orchidopexy. Adhesions from the first groin hernia operation make the second procedure, i.e. orchidopexy, more demanding and notably associated with a higher complication risk, mainly from damage to the vascular pedicle or vas deferens leading to testicular atrophy or infertility.

DOI: 10.1201/9781003182290-23

The contralateral undescended testis – if present in this male patient – can be brought down following normal guidelines as referred to earlier (9–18 months) at the usual time.

Question: A 6-month-old boy is referred to you with an absent testis on one side but also a small hard lump is palpable within the scrotum. What are the possible explanations for this condition? How is the boy best managed?

Answer: The most likely explanation for these findings is that a perinatal torsion event has occurred and the affected testis has subsequently involuted and atrophied. On taking a full history, both testes may have been documented at some point as having been in the scrotum at birth. It may also have been noticed that one hemiscrotum is larger than the other, either from a reactive hydrocele or from inflammation/induration around a recently torted testis. On examination, it may be noted here that the contralateral scrotal testis is larger than expected from compensatory hypertrophy.

In this scenario there is an ongoing risk of torsion affecting the contralateral healthy scrotal testis, so the normal testis in this situation should be fixed ('pexy') surgically and ideally soon. It is not necessary to remove the atrophic testis 'lump' as it poses no long-term risks to the child, but many surgeons do so, mostly to have confirmatory histological diagnosis of the involuted 'perinatal torted' testis.

Question: You see an 18-month-old boy in clinic who has been referred by the family general practitioner (GP) because the testes have become increasingly difficult to find and allegedly appear to be undescended. What key information will you now ask from the parents? What clinical findings do you expect to find?

Answer: Clinical assessment is directed at distinguishing whether the testes are retractile or undescended. Retractile testes occur during childhood when androgen levels are low and the cremasteric muscle reflex is prominent. It is a normal occurrence in young boys but can vary in intensity. The key questions to ask the mother are whether the testes were 'down' at birth (if so, it makes retractile testes as a diagnosis much more likely) and whether the mum or dad have ever observed the child's testes in the scrotum particularly after a warm bath.

On clinical examination a retractile testis is best defined as one that can be easily manipulated into the scrotum without excessive tension on the cord structures and then may later spontaneously retract from the scrotum to the groin region. The affected testis is generally considered of normal size to the other contralateral scrotal testis. The scrotum in boys often appears well developed and symmetrical.

In contrast, a true undescended testis cannot either be delivered easily into the scrotum or, if it can be, with difficulty; once it is released, it disappears immediately into the groin. The spermatic cord in such boys feels tight with no redundancy. In males, the maldeveloped testis is sometimes often smaller than a normally descended contralateral testis. This discrepancy in size tends to become much more evident as boys get older.

Question: You examine a 9-month-old boy and are unable to palpate one testis. What are the possible explanations for this? What specific findings do you seek on clinical examination? What is your approach to case management?

Answer: The possible explanations include:

1. Intra-abdominal testis (i.e. the testis is proximal to the internal inguinal ring and cannot therefore be palpated in the groin).
2. Intracanalicular testis (the testis here resides within the inguinal canal and cannot be felt; it is located proximal to the external inguinal ring though distal to the internal ring).
3. Absent testis on one side (testis has never developed).
4. An atrophic testis, as after perinatal torsion, with consequent ischaemia and resorption.
5. Simple failure to palpate an otherwise palpable testis. This is something much more likely to occur in boys with adiposity or obesity, an undeveloped hypoplastic scrotum, an ectopic testis (e.g. located in the perineum region or femoral in location) or lack of clinician experience and familiarity with the UDT examination technique. Many family practitioners/ community health care professionals often have difficulty palpating markedly retractile testes.

Assuming it is one of the first four explanations, examination of the scrotum can provide additional valuable information. Note whether there is scrotal asymmetry, as where there is, for example, a poorly developed hemiscrotum – this now suggests that no testis has ever resided in it. Palpate the contralateral testis because if it is larger in size than expected, as occurs with compensatory hypertrophy, it implies either that there is no testis on the 'empty' side or that any testis may be intra-abdominal and/or hypoplastic. A small, hard, 'pea-size' lump felt within the scrotum is highly suggestive of perinatal torsion with subsequent atrophy of the involved testis. The only residual evidence of the testis is a small, hard, hemosiderin-stained nodule or nubbin.

If no testis is palpable and clinical assessment confirms an impalpable testis, the next key step is to schedule laparoscopy. This will clarify the diagnosis. On entering the pelvic peritoneal cavity at endoscopy, the course of the vas and testicular vessels is followed by the surgeon. This manoeuvre will permit the position of any intra-abdominal testis to be established. If the vessels and vas are seen to continue entering through the internal ring, the diagnosis is either (1) an intra-canalicular testis or an (2) atrophic (previously descended) testis.

Where an intra-abdominal testis is confirmed, the operative decision that needs to be made by the surgeon is whether to proceed with a standard laparoscopic-assisted orchidopexy or to consider performing a staged orchidopexy in which the testicular vessels are ligated or clipped laparoscopically at the same procedure. Later, usually 6–9 months later, once a good blood supply nourishing the testis has been established through the artery accompanying the vas deferens, the second-stage operation is undertaken. The second-stage operation involves division of the testicular pedicle distal to the previous clips/ligation and mobilization of the testis into the scrotum that is efficiently now nourished by the artery of the vas.

If at initial laparoscopy, vessels and vas are shown running through the internal ring into the inguinal canal, most surgeons will proceed to exploration of the groin in the expectation that they will find either (1) an intra-canalicular testis (which is then brought down into the scrotum) or (2) a hemosiderin-stained nubbin remnant of testis from previous torsion. In this latter case, consideration should always be given to fixation ('pexy') of the contralateral healthy side to protect the boy from a potential later torsion event – true life risk rate undefined and catastrophic male anorchia.

Strictly speaking, as mentioned earlier in the chapter, it is not necessary to always remove an atrophic testicular remnant, although most surgeons do so for histological confirmation of what has occurred perinatally.

Question: You are requested to see a newborn baby with impalpable gonads and a bifid scrotum. What other clinical findings do you seek and why?
Answer: The major concern here is that the infant may have a disorder of sexual differentiation (DSD). The combination of a bifid scrotum (in this situation, more appropriately termed labioscrotal folds) and UDT (until established with certainty, it is best to use the term gonads) and an abnormal phallus (is it a penis or enlarged clitoris?) is particularly suggestive of a DSD. In effect, the genitalia should be considered ambiguous, and the protocol of investigations should follow the lines outlined in Chapter 73.

Question: You performed an orchidopexy operation on a boy 2 years ago. You are asked to see him at clinic because the parents do not believe the testis is now in the scrotum. What are the possible clinical findings? And what should you do for each?
Answer: Occasionally, a testis can move out of the scrotum following an orchidopexy. This is uncommon but much more likely if the undescended testis was very high to start with (being farther to bring down into the scrotum) and had a shortened tight spermatic cord despite its full mobilisation. Clinical review will either reveal that everything in fact is fine, with the testis fully descended in the scrotum and of good size; alternatively the parents' suspicions may prove correct and the testis is now found sitting 'high' proximal to the scrotum. In this later instance a 'redo' orchidopexy revision operation is indicated. The parents should be advised here that it may be more difficult than the first original procedure because of adhesions with scarring and that the success rate may be lower than hitherto previously There is a paucity of 'real-world' data on the actual success rates of surgery in this latter situation that are considered lower than for initial primary orchidopexy. Redo orchidopexy should be scheduled therefore as an elective procedure best undertaken by an experienced surgeon, as risks to the vessel, vas and testis with subsequent loss of the gonad are notably greater.

BIBLIOGRAPHY

1. Hutson JM, Thorup JM, Beasley SW Eds. Descent of the Testis. 2015 Springer Publishers (2nd edition).
2. Gates RI, Shelton J, Diefenbach KA, et al. Management of the undescended testis in children: An American Pediatric Surgical Association Outcomes and Evidence Based Practice Committee Systematic Review. J Pediatr Surg 2022;57(7):1293–1308.
3. Lip Lin Zhao S, Murchison Denheen LE, Cullis PS, Govan L, Carachi R. A meta-analysis of the risk of boys with isolated cryptorchidism developing testicular cancer in later life. Arch Dis Child 2013; 98(1):20–26.
4. Driver CP, Losty PD. Neonatal testicular torsion. Br J Urol 1998;82(6):855–888.
5. Rhodes HL, Corbett HJ, Horwood JF, Losty PD. Neonatal testicular torsion: A survey of current practice amongst paediatric surgeons and urologists in the United Kingdom and Ireland. J Pediatr Surg 2011;46(11):2157–2160.
6. Corbally MT, Quinn FJ, Guiney EJ. The effect of two-stage orchidopexy on testicular growth. Br J Urol 1993;72(3):376–378.

22

Intussusception

EMMA SIDEBOTHAM
Leeds Teaching Hospitals NHS Trust, Leeds, UK

Scenario: A 9-month old baby presents with an 18-hour history of vomiting which has become bile stained. The parents report the child has been crying and difficult to settle; there are episodes when they appear to fall asleep then within minutes become distressed again. The infant had a normal bowel action earlier in the day.

On examination the infant is lying on its front with its knees drawn up to the chest. Placing the child supine, you note they have cool peripheries and are tachycardic with a heart rate of 160/min and a capillary refill time of 4 seconds. Examining the abdomen, it appears full and distended. It is soft, but tenderness and guarding are noted in the right upper quadrant, where examination rouses the infant and they become distressed. Rectal exam reveals pinkish fluid on the fingertip of the glove.

Question: What are your working differential diagnoses?

Answer: This is a classic and typical age for children presenting with intussusception: 6–18 months for primary idiopathic intussusception, the triad of diagnostic symptoms being vomiting, which becomes bilious, cyclical abdominal pain and red currant jelly stools. The bloody stools tend to occur later in the course of the illness and are thus often not reported in the history; if they are, the parents or referring doctors tend to describe blood passed per rectum. Occasionally children do not appear to have pain, which is the most classic defining symptom: Cycles of pain when patients cry and draw their knees to their chest last about 10 minutes (older children will turn prone with their knees to their chest and their bottom raised in the air) after which they will have a similar short period of being very quiet, typically bradycardic if on cardiac monitoring, which is a vagal response to stimulation of the bowel.

Sometimes the intussusception is palpable as a sausage-shaped mass, most commonly in the right upper quadrant. More often the child is tender in the region of the intussusception with guarding; this combined with its position adjacent to the liver often makes the mass difficult to feel.

Important differential diagnoses are malrotation volvulus for any child with bilious vomiting. This presents most commonly in infants in the first week of life but can occur at any age, and it is vital it is promptly recognised and treated. If the child has had previous abdominal surgery, this could be the presentation of an adhesional obstruction; this can also occur more rarely with congenital bands such as a Meckel's band. Infectious gastroenteritis, especially if associated with foreign travel (Salmonellae Typhi), needs to be explored in the history. This child is quite young for obstruction due to an ingested foreign body, e.g. magnets.

Regardless of the diagnosis, the child requires intravenous access, baseline blood tests should be sent including a group and save, and fluid resuscitation given with a 10 mL/kg fluid bolus repeated as necessary. A nasogastric (NG) tube should be sited and placed on free drainage. Analgesia should be administered.

DOI: 10.1201/9781003182290-24

Question: What is intussusception, and why does it happen?

Answer: Intussusception is where one segment of the intestine, the intussusceptum, is drawn into the downstream intestine, the intussuscipiens.

In the classic infant/toddler age group, enlargement of Peyer's patches (anti-mesenteric lymphoid aggregates) in the ileum results in them protruding

Table 22.1 Pathological lead points in intussusception (most common in bold); small bowel tumours are rare but most commonly present with intussusception

Structural

- **Meckel's diverticulum**
- Ectopic gastric mucosa
- Ectopic pancreas
- Appendix (normal, appendicitis or mucocele or appendiceal stump)
- Enteric duplication cyst
- Anastomotic suture line

Vascular/Haematological

- **Henoch-Schoenlein purpura**
- Haemophilia
- Abdominal trauma – haematoma
- Leukaemia
- Idiopathic thrombocytopenic purpura
- Haemolytic – uraemic syndrome

Neoplastic

- **Polyps (adenomas, hamartomas, Peutz-Jeghers, juvenile)**
- **Lymphoma**/Lymphosarcoma
- Small bowel carcinoid tumours
- Haemangioma
- Lymphangioma
- Lipoma
- Adenomyoma, mesenchymoma
- Leiomyoma
- Fibrosarcoma
- Metastatic tumours
- Colonic adenocarcinoma

Other

- **Foreign bodies, e.g. trichobezoars**
- Granulomas (amoebic, eosinophilic, Crohn's)
- Ascaris lumbricoides
- Cystic fibrosis – 1% of 9- to 12-year-olds – presumably linked to viscid bowel contents

into the bowel lumen, then being caught by a peristaltic wave and dragged into the downstream bowel causing ileocolic intussusception. Reasons for this enlargement may be systemic viral infections and weaning from milk formula to solids; the loss of maternal transferred immunity may also be significant. This is primary idiopathic intussusception, which has a peak incidence at 5–9 months of age. Intussusception has an incidence of 7 in 10,000 and is more common in males (2:1) at all ages.

The rotavirus vaccine (Rotarix, RotaTeq) is associated with an increased incidence of intussusception: 1–2 excess cases per 100,000 infants vaccinated. In the UK this vaccine is given at 8 and 12 weeks of age, and it is thus important to obtain a full vaccination history in a younger infant presenting with suggestive symptoms.

The older patients become, the more likely it is that there will be a pathological lead point – a persistent abnormality protruding into the bowel lumen rather than the transient enlargement of Peyer's patches. Ten to twenty-five percent of cases of intussusception occur in patients older than 2 years. (**Table 22.1**)

Question: What investigations are needed to establish the diagnosis?

Answer: A plain abdominal X-ray is simple to perform but often fails to be very instructive. It may show evidence of small bowel obstruction and absence of the normal caecal shadow in the right iliac fossa (RIF). There may be a paucity of gas in the area of the intussusception, typically in the right upper quadrant, consistent with a soft tissue mass (**Figure 22.1**).

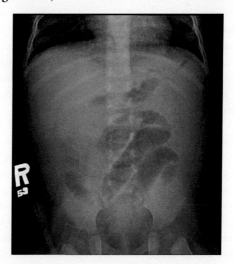

Figure 22.1 Plain X-ray showing dilated central small bowel loops and the impression of a soft tissue mass in the right upper quadrant.

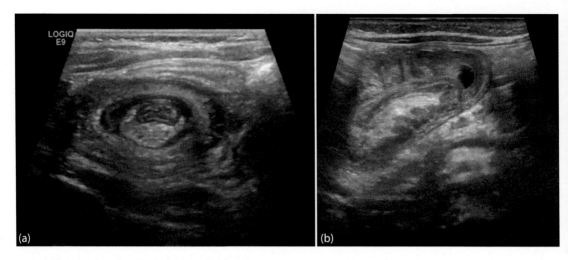

Figure 22.2 Ultrasound scan images of intussusception. (a) Target sign in transverse section. (b) False kidney in longitudinal section.

Ultrasound is diagnostic. The intussusception appears as a "target" sign in transverse section and a "false kidney" in longitudinal section. Proving the absence of intussusception can be difficult for the inexperienced sonographer, especially in the presence of a lot of dilated gas-filled small bowel loops (**Figure 22.2**). Intermittent self-resolving ileoileal intussusception is sometimes seen. These occur with disordered bowel motility, most commonly with gastroenteritis, but testing for coeliac disease should be considered if the history is suggestive. In one study 25% of children diagnosed with coeliac disease were demonstrated to have an ileoileal intussusception on ultrasound prior to commencing a gluten-free diet.

Question: How is intussusception treated?
Answer: Once the diagnosis is confirmed, enema reduction is first-line treatment. In the UK this is typically an X-ray–guided air enema reduction, but ultrasound-guided fluid enema reduction or contrast enema can also be utilized.

A catheter is placed into the anal canal and the balloon inflated. Typically the buttocks need to be held together manually or with tape to achieve an adequate seal. Filtered air is then pumped in, with pressure monitoring, typically aiming to achieve sustained pressures of 80–100 mmHg over 1–2 minutes. The reduction is monitored fluoroscopically. The soft tissue mass of the intussusceptum is seen to reduce proximally as the air column progresses, with a rush

of air up the small bowel signifying complete reduction. Antibiotics and opiate analgesia are typically administered to cover the procedure.

If the small bowel is very gas filled on the initial film or the ileocaecal valve has become very oedematous, giving the appearance of a soft tissue mass protruding into the caecum, it can be difficult to be sure if the intussusception has fully reduced. Ultrasound or a contrast enema may help to confirm this or a period of observation in which the patient should recover rapidly if the reduction is complete. Enema reduction is successful in ≥70% of cases. If the intussusception has not reduced after two to three good attempts, then enema reduction is unlikely to be successful.

There is a risk of perforation of the bowel. In reported series this risk is similar for air and fluid enema reduction at around 0.3%–0.5%. With air reduction perforation may result in a tension pneumoperitoneum compromising respiration, requiring a cannula to be placed urgently through the abdominal wall to help release the air. Failure of reduction or perforation requires surgical management of the intussusception, but enema reduction will avoid the need for surgery in the majority of patients.

Classically a laparotomy is performed through a right infraumbilical transverse incision or a midline laparotomy in older patients. Reduction of the intussusception should be attempted by pressure on the bowel in the region of the tip of the intussusception, aiming to progressively reduce the intussusceptum proximally until it reduces fully. If the bowel does not reduce relatively easily with sustained pressure, the segment of the bowel involved in the intussusception should be resected. Reduction of ischaemic bowel can result in release of endotoxins into the circulation and circulatory collapse/shock.

Traditional teaching was that reduction should not be attempted by traction on the bowel proximal to the intussusception, but if a laparoscopic reduction is attempted, then this technique tends to be cautiously utilized.

If the bowel reduces, it should be palpated for a pathological lead point and an enterotomy considered if there is concern, as oedema may make this assessment difficult. An intussusception due to a pathological lead point is less likely to reduce.

Question: Should all patients with intussusception undergo an air enema?

Answer: Not all cases of intussusception are suitable for enema reduction. Intussusception not only causes obstruction of the lumen of the bowel by the intussusceptum but also compromises blood supply to that segment of bowel. Initially venous return is impaired resulting in oedema, mucus production and transudation of blood breakdown products through the bowel wall, producing the red currant jelly stool. If the intussusception persists, arterial inflow is also compromised resulting in ischaemia and necrosis of the intussusceptum.

Enema reduction should not be attempted in a patient who is shocked and not responding rapidly to fluid resuscitation or a patient who has peritonitis. The length of the history/duration of the intussusception is not an absolute contraindication but needs to be considered.

Age is a further contraindication, with both older patients and rare cases presenting in very young infants, due to the likelihood of there being a pathological lead point. However, two-thirds of childhood intussusception cases presenting in children over 2 years of age will still have idiopathic intussusception. Nonetheless, as a child gets older and stronger, an enema reduction is increasingly difficult to attempt without requiring general anaesthesia.

Question: How quickly will the patient recover?

Answer: Infants typically recover quickly once the intussusception is successfully reduced. They often sleep for a period after the enema procedure as a result of relief of the preceding symptoms and the opiate analgesia administered, then typically awaken and are keen to feed. A child may have ongoing symptoms due to the underlying cause of the intussusception, but failure of complete reduction of the intussusception needs to be carefully considered. Older children after surgical management for a pathological lead point will make a slower recovery, and in any child bowel resection and anastomosis will require a delay in reintroduction of oral intake.

Question: Can the intussusception recur?

Answer: The highest risk of recurrence is in the first few days after air enema reduction when the Peyer's patches remain enlarged. Recurrence of symptoms within the first 24 hours is suspicious of incomplete reduction, as general oedema of the bowel tends to prevent very early recurrence. Occasionally patients present with a further completely separate episode of intussusception; in older patients a pathological lead point should always be considered.

Question: Can patients die from intussusception?

Answer: Deaths do occur with intussusception, as the affected bowel will eventually become ischaemic and perforate. Thirty-three childhood deaths were identified in England and Wales in a 6-year period from 1984 to 1989. Delayed diagnosis was a factor, but inadequate fluid resuscitation, sepsis and aspiration due to failure to adequately decompress the stomach were also highlighted, with some 20 of the 33 patients felt to have had avoidable deaths. Forty years on, these basic tenets of timely diagnosis and good patient resuscitation still apply.

BIBLIOGRAPHY

Jiang J, Jiang B, Parashar U, Nguyen T, Bines J, Patel MM. Childhood intussusception: A literature review. PLoS ONE 2013;8(7):e68482.

Gluckman S, Karpelowsky J. Management of intussusception in children. Cochrane Database Syst Rev 2017;2017(6):CD006476.

Guo W, Hu Z, Tan Y, Sheng M, Wang J. Risk factors for recurrent intussusception in children: A retrospective cohort study. BMJ Open 2017;7(11):e018604.

Stringer MD, Pledger G, Drake DP. Childhood deaths from intussusception in England and Wales, 1984–9. BMJ 1992;304:737–739.

Ondhia MN, Al-Mutawa Y, Harave S, Losty PD. Intussusception: A 14 year experience at a UK tertiary referral centre. J Pediatr Surg 2020;55(8):1570–1573.

Yen C, Healy K, Tate JE, Parashar UD, Bines J, Neuzil K, Santosham M, Steele AD. Rotavirus vaccination and intussusception – science, surveillance and safety: A review of evidence and recommendations for future research priorities in low and middle income countries. Hum Vaccin Immunother 2016;12(10):2580–2589.

23

Intestinal foreign bodies and corrosive esophagitis

PRINCE RAJ, ABEER FARHAN, AND MARTIN T. CORBALLY
King Hamad University Hospital, Kingdom of Bahrain, Bahrain

PAUL D. LOSTY
Institute of Systems and Molecular Biology, University of Liverpool, UK
and Ramathibodi Hospital, Mahidol University, Bangkok, Thailand

It is normal for children to inspect objects with their mouths. Occasionally these are accidently swallowed. Often this is not a cause for concern, but certain items do pose a problem and indicate the need for urgent removal. This chapter will describe these.

FOREIGN BODIES

Scenario: A 4-year-old girl is brought to hospital by her mother with a 2-hour history of having swallowed a foreign body associated with a single episode of vomiting. There is no history of coughing or cyanosis. On clinical examination she is well hydrated, and vital signs are stable with a soft, non-tender abdomen.

The emergency department physician requested an X-ray **(Figure 23.1)**.

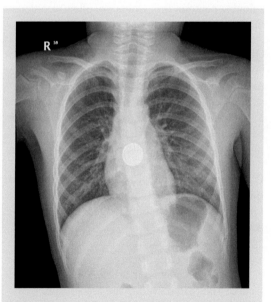

Figure 23.1 Plain chest X-ray showing an oesophageal foreign body lodged at junction of mid and lower oesophagus.

Question: Can you interpret the X-ray findings?
Answer: This is a chest radiograph showing a rounded foreign body in the distal oesophagus suggestive of a button battery.

Question: What is your next differential diagnosis?
Answer: Foreign body ingestion: A coin, magnet or a battery.

Question: What is the mechanism of injury for button batteries?
Answer: Externally the button battery is composed of two metallic discs. The larger is the cathode and the smaller surface the anode. Electrolytic production of an alkaline fluid via formation of a local circuit from the ingested battery creates oesophageal tissue contact with both the anode and cathode, which causes direct mucosal damage.

Question: How would you differentiate between a battery and a coin on plain film X-ray?
Answer: Button batteries will appear as a round, smooth object on plain radiographs and are often misdiagnosed as coins. However, on closer inspection, some larger button batteries will demonstrate a double contour rim. Coins are often of different shapes and size and do not have a double rim.

Question: What are the most common foreign bodies accidentally ingested by children?
Answer: The majority of foreign body ingestions occur in children between the ages of 6 months and 3 years. Commonly ingested objects include coins, button batteries, small toys, toy parts, magnets, safety pins, screws, marbles, bones, and food boluses.

Question: Name and list the anatomical locations within the gastrointestinal tract where a foreign body may become lodged.
Answer:

1. Cricopharyngeus
2. Mid-oesophagus, in the region where the aortic arch and carina overlap the oesophagus
3. Gastroesophageal junction
4. Pylorus
5. Ileocecal junction

Question: A battery is in the oesophagus. Is this an emergency scenario?
Answer: Oesophageal batteries are associated with increased morbidity due to the profound tissue injury that can occur through pressure necrosis with release of a low-voltage electric current or leakage of an alkali solution causing liquefaction necrosis. The mucosal injury may occur in as little as under 15 minutes of contact time and may continue to progress even after battery removal. Therefore, in any suspected case of oesophageal battery impaction, *immediate* removal is mandatory.

Question: Why are lithium cells more dangerous as compared to traditional battery cells?
Answer: The chemical composition of batteries has trended toward larger-diameter lithium batteries, and these are now ubiquitous in working devices within the household. Lithium cells are typically 3.0 V, as compared with the 1.5 V of traditional alkaline button batteries. The increased voltage is a major factor in the type and degree of injury transmitted by these newer-age batteries, as according to Ohm's law, the higher voltage will drive an increase in current. Most major paediatric button battery injuries are caused by

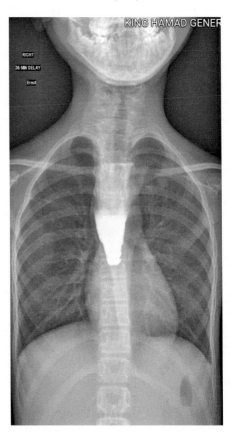

Figure 23.2 (a) Contrast study showing complete obstruction of oesophagus.

lithium batteries >20 mm. These batteries cause injury through several mechanisms, most notable being via caustic injury. Mucosal surfaces in contact with the positive and negative battery terminals complete a circuit allowing battery current to flow. This process generates hydroxide radicals, which begin to cause necrosis of tissue within 15 minutes of contact. Severe oesophageal damage and perforation can occur within only a few hours (**Figure 23.2**).

Question: How would you manage this patient?

Answer: Management depends on the general condition of the patient, type of foreign body ingested and its anatomical location. Age of the patient, size of the battery and timing of ingestion are equally important, as the site location of the battery will help predict the severity of the injury. Ensure adequate resuscitation with urgent scheduling of upper GI endoscopy undertaken by a paediatric gastroenterologist or paediatric surgeon. Liquefactive necrosis of the oesophagus may occur due to the electrical current, leading to ulceration within only a few hours of ingestion and perforation as early as 8 hours post ingestion.

Question: What are the possible complications from battery ingestion?

Answer: Button batteries warrant special attention due to their potential for severe complications including oesophageal perforation, trachea-oesophageal fistula, vocal cord paralysis and, rarely, fatal death from an aorto-oesophageal vascular fistula (AEF) due to massive exsanguinating upper GI haemorrhage.

Question: What are the complications of foreign body magnet ingestion?

Answer: Based on the North American Society of Pediatric Gastroenterology, Hepatology and Nutrition (NASPGHAN), urgent endoscopic removal is recommended in the presence of more than one magnet device even in asymptomatic patients. If the swallowed magnets have been present for more than 12 hours, then paediatric surgery consultation is advisable. Once the magnets pass beyond the pylorus, surgical intervention is strongly recommended, as they are unlikely to pass spontaneously and become inaccessible.

Multiple magnet ingestion or co-ingestion of a single magnet with another metal object must be

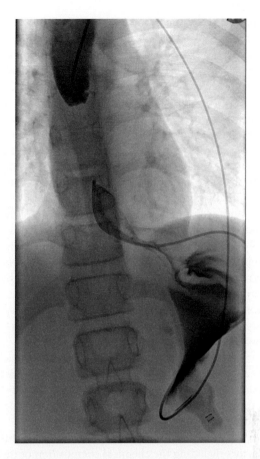

Figure 23.2 (b) Pain X-ray under fluoroscopy in attempt to pass guide wires from above and via gastrostomy.

treated urgently. Complications in this scenario are due to pressure necrosis with subsequent fistulisation across adjacent intestinal gut segments. Other complications may include ulceration, oesophageal perforation and gastroenteric fistulae.

CORROSIVE ESOPHAGITIS

Scenario: A 12-year-old girl is brought to hospital by her mother with an inability to swallow and recurrent vomiting associated with weight loss. The patient has a history of previous admission with aspiration pneumonia. Upon further questioning it is learned that the patient ingested detergent cleaner 4 months ago. On examination weight is 13 kg and the abdomen is soft and non-tender (**Figure 23.2b**).

Question: Define what is meant by the term corrosive substances.

Answer: Corrosive substances are chemical agents capable of causing direct tissue injury due to their strong acid or alkaline properties. The physical form of the substance ingested and its pH play a substantial role in the site and type of post-ingestion oesophageal injury, with a substance pH greater than 12 or less than 1.5 being associated with severe corrosive organ injury. Acidic ingestions most commonly cause gastric injury. Alkali ingestion more commonly results in an oesophageal injury.

With acid ingestion, coagulation necrosis of the mucosa occurs with eschar formation and usually a limitation of acid penetration through the injured mucosa. With alkali ingestion, tissue penetration with liquefactive necrosis is followed by severe destruction of the epithelium and submucosa, which may extend through all the muscle layers. Ischemia and thrombosis are dominant early events in the injury process.

The most common causes of caustic oesophageal burns are alkali household cleaning products containing sodium, potassium hydroxides and other cleaning agents with sodium phosphate, sodium carbonate and ammonia.

The extent of injury is dependent on several factors including the chemical composition of the substance, volume ingested, concentration and duration of organ contact.

Question: Interpret the following X-ray studies.

Type of study – Upper GI contrast swallow
Answer: The study shown (**Figure 23.2**) is a contrast esophagogram showing a complete 'cutoff' at the distal region of the oesophagus with proximal dilatation of the oesophagus. The additional study shown is taken under fluoroscopy imaging screening, and the contrast is instilled via the oral route and the gastrostomy device. The image shows a 'long gap' between the proximal and the distal oesophagus suggestive of a complete long-segment stricture of the distal oesophagus.

Question: What is the best initial management?
Answer: History and examination.

1. *ABCDE approach*: Initial emergent management is directed at maintaining an adequate airway and patient oxygenation and ensuring cardiovascular stability with ingestion.

2. *Endoscopic examination*: Fibre-optic endoscopy examination is both accurate and safe, especially when done carefully within 24–48 hours after accidental ingestion.

3. *Indirect fibre-optic laryngoscopy*: In the presence of visual evidence of a pharyngeal burn in those patients having stridor, early oesophagostomy is contraindicated because of the risks of aggravating major airway obstruction; hence, indirect fibre-optic laryngoscopy is useful and timely to assess the upper airway.

Question: When will you consider performing an upper GI endoscopy?
Answer: When signs of airway compromise are present or when there is strong evidence of significant burn.

Evidence of oesophageal obstruction: Patients will often have hyper-salivation and have an inability to swallow liquids. They will have a high risk for aspiration and require an emergent (preferably within 2 hours, but at the latest within 6 hours) endoscopic intervention.

Question: What is the role (if any) of inducing vomiting?
Answer: In cases of caustic ingestion, inducing vomiting or encouraging the ingestion of any neutralizing liquids is contraindicated. Moreover, vomiting or reflux regurgitation may cause further secondary injury. Inhaled or aspirated vomitus will introduce corrosive injury into the upper major airway leading to inflammation and oedema with airway obstruction.

Question: Is there a role for scheduling a technetium-labelled sucralfate scan?
Answer: Technetium-labelled sucralfate radioisotope scanning of the oesophagus has been deployed by some surgeons as a screening study, with poor sucralfate adherence indicating the absence of significant organ injury.

Question: When would you then undertake a contrast esophagogram examination?
Answer:

1. If fever, systemic sepsis and upper abdominal signs/symptoms are present, organ perforation may have occurred, and a water-soluble contrast esophagogram may be useful to provide evidence of perforation.

2. A contrast esophagogram examination is usually scheduled approximately 10–14 days after accidental ingestion, when an assessment of the entire oesophagus and upper GI tract can identify the extent of injury and may help in choosing the best appropriate therapy programme.

Question: The patient later had an upper GI endoscopy exam. List the grading system used for oesophageal injury.
Answer:

Grade 0 – Normal mucosa.
Grade 1 (superficial) – Mucosal oedema and hyperaemia.
Grade 2 (transmucosal) – Friability, haemorrhage(s), erosions, blisters, whitish membranes and superficial ulcerations.
  Grade 2A – No deep focal or circumferential ulcers.
  Grade 2B – With deep focal or circumferential ulcers.
Grade 3 – Areas of multiple ulceration and areas of brown-black or greyish discoloration suggesting necrosis.
  Grade 3A – Small scattered areas of focal necrosis.
  Grade 3B – Extensive necrosis.

Question: What is the management protocol for a caustic stricture?
Answer: If a stricture is demonstrated on contrast radiography taken 10–14 days after the injury, a program of oesophageal dilatation therapy should be scheduled. Various methods can be used:

- Mercury-filled boogies – not common today.
- Flexible-graded boogie dilatation.
- Guidewire-directed metal olives (Eder-Puestow system).
- Balloon dilators (Boston Scientific Manufacturers).

If several strictures are encountered and visualization is difficult, it is then much safer to secure placement of a transoesophageal string, which is then used to guide the passage of the dilators either in a retrograde manner through the gastrostomy or antegrade via the mouth.

Dilatations should be initially undertaken at least once per week, commencing with catheters that are one or two French sizes smaller than the estimated diameter of the stricture.
Factors indicating poor prognosis are:

- Delay in presentation.
- Extensive grade III injury.
- Ongoing oesophageal ulceration.
- Densely fibrotic stricture that cracks on dilatation.
- A stricture length greater than 5 cm.
- Inadequate lumen patency despite repeated dilatations over a 9- to 12-month period.

During recovery from caustic ingestion, it is essential to provide adequate patient nutrition with access through either (1) nasogastric tube or by (2) placement of a feeding gastrostomy or (3) jejunostomy tube.

If dilatation fails and a dense stricture develops, it requires aggressive treatment. Local injection of steroids into short strictures has had some limited success when combined with dilatation but has not been assessed prospectively. Likewise, application of mitomycin C has also been used with some reported success.

Some surgeons advocate oesophageal stenting by means of an indwelling NG tube. However, for many patients these tubes are not well tolerated and they promote gastroesophageal reflux. With extensive injury stents must be in place for a much longer duration to be of any useful effect. Stents have been deployed in the management of oesophageal fistulae resultant from caustic injury or dilatation therapy, mainly as a temporizing measure before later operative repair or oesophageal bypass operations.

Question: What are the possible complications?
Answer:

1. Gastroesophageal reflux disease (GERD).
2. Oesophageal stricture.
3. Oesophageal perforation.
4. Residual motility dysfunction.

Carcinoma of the injured caustic oesophagus is a real risk in later adult life, usually with a latency period of approximately 15–40 years. If the injury is extensive and transmural, necrosis may involve the surrounding mediastinum, leading to mediastinitis, or in an anterior direction migrate to the trachea resulting in acquired tracheoesophageal fistula or even fatal aorto-oesophageal vascular injury.

If a dilatation therapy programme fails or if the oesophagus cannot be salvaged, oesophageal replacement is then indicated. Colon interposition, gastric tube esophagoplasty, and jejunal grafts are the options available and best undertaken by an experienced surgeon.

BIBLIOGRAPHY

1. Mubarek A, Benninga MA, Broekaert I, et al. Diagnosis, management and prevention of button battery ingestion in childhood: A European Society for Paediatric Gastroenterology Hepatology and Nutrition Position Paper. J Pediatr Gastroenterol Nutr 2021;73(1):129–36.
2. Gibbs H, Jatana KR. Pediatric button battery injuries – current state and what's next? JAMA Otolaryngol Head Neck Surg 2022;148(7):683–5.
3. Houston R, Powell S, Jaffray B, Ball S. Clinical guidelines for retained button batteries. Arch Dis Child 2021;106(2):193–4.
4. Paediatric Surgery Trainee Research Network. Magnet and button battery ingestion in children: Multicentre observational study of management and outcomes. BJS Open 2022;6(3):zrac056.
5. Reddy SM, Lander AD, Stumper O, Botha P, Khan O, Pachl M. Esophago-vascular fistulae in children: Five survivors, literature review and proposal for management. J Pediatr Surg Oct 2023;58(10):1969–75.
6. Spitz L, Lakhoo K. Caustic ingestion. Arch Dis Child. 1993;68(2):157–8.
7. Hammond P, Jaffray B. Hamilton L. Tracheosophageal fistula secondary to disk battery ingestion: A case report of gastric interposition and tracheal patch. J Pediatr Surg 2007;42(7):E39–41.
8. Millar AJ, Numanoglu A, Mann M, et al. Detection of caustic oesophageal injury with technetium 99m-labelled sucralfate. J Pediatr Surg 2001;36(2):262–5.
9. Panieri E, Rode H, Millar AJ, Cywes S. Oesophageal replacement in the management of corrosive strictures: When is surgery indicated? Pediatr Surg Int 1998;13(5–6):336–40.
10. Spitz L, Ruangtrakool R. Esophageal substitution. Sem Pediatr Surg 1998;7:130–3.

24

Gastro-oesophageal reflux

NATALIE DURKIN AND PAOLO DE COPPI
Zayed Centre for Research, Great Ormond Street Institute of Child Health, London, UK

Question: What are the anatomical and physiological anti-reflux mechanisms which normally contribute to prevention of gastro-oesophageal reflux?

Answer: Many mechanisms contribute to the presence of the anti-reflux barrier. The first of these to consider is the presence of the highly specialised *lower oesophageal sphincter* (LOS), a physiological area of high intrinsic tone near the gastro-oesophageal junction (GOJ). Thickened circular muscle fibres superior to the GOJ generate a continuous tonic pressure of 15–30 mmHg, although this pressure typically varies throughout the day; the basal LOS tone is notably higher when supine and fasting, for example.[1] This high-pressure zone is sufficiently higher than the intra-gastric pressure (~5 mmHg), thus preventing reflux of caustic gastric contents into the oesophagus.

Periodic increases in intra-gastric pressure (e.g. secondary to inspiration or straining) which may surpass that of the LOS require additional mechanisms to be protective against reflux. The sling-shaped oesophageal hiatus in the right crus region of the diaphragm encloses the proximal LOS and acts as a *pinchcock*: an external sphincter mechanism reinforcing the LOS. In addition, the hiatus marks the transition between the intra-thoracic and intra-abdominal oesophagus which is anchored to the crural diaphragm by the phreno-oesophageal ligament. The presence of a sufficient length of *intra-abdominal oesophagus* is also key; this is compressed when intra-abdominal pressure increases, again reinforcing the anti-reflux mechanism. As such, maintenance of the intrabdominal oesophagus and repair of the crura during fundoplication is key to success of this operation. The *angle of His* is an added anti-reflux mechanism. Its location between the intra-abdominal oesophagus and the greater curvature of the stomach should be acute, therefore acting as a secondary protective valve; intra-luminal mucosal folds further create a *mucosal rosette* at the GOJ, which are squeezed together when an increase in intrabdominal pressure occurs, acting as an additional weak anti-reflux valve mechanism. Finally, reflux is also prevented by *oesophageal peristalsis* which promotes oesophageal clearance and promotes oesophageal clearance and limits exposure of the oeosphageal epithelium to acidic luminal contents.

Question: Why does reflux occur?

Answer: The role of the LOS and transient lower oesophageal relaxation (TLOSR) in gastro-oesophageal reflux (GOR) appears to be key. During swallowing, relaxation of the LOS is co-ordinated by activation of afferent sensory neurones in the pharynx and oesophagus as part of the sequence of primary peristalsis. Subsequent stimulation of inhibitory

DOI: 10.1201/9781003182290-26

efferent neurones in the myenteric plexus leads to a brief relaxation of tone and of the LOS, allowing the passage of food or, conversely, the retrograde passage of swallowed air or vomit.[2] However, TLOSR also occurs independent of peristalsis or swallowing due to stimulation of stretch receptors within the fundus secondary to gastric distension from air or food. Whilst this is a normal phenomenon allowing, for example, belching, it is also the dominant mechanism of pathological reflux; a higher incidence of TLOSR is notably seen in patients with GORD vs. healthy controls.[3] In addition to TLOSR, anything which interferes with other anti-reflux mechanisms can also increase the incidence of GOR. Disruption of the phreno-oesophageal ligament, as with a hiatus hernia, results in separation of the internal and external LOS mechanisms leading to a lower basal LOS pressure and a higher incidence of GOR. Reduction of the angle of His has also been shown to increase reflux (e.g. by gastrostomy creation pulling the stomach inferiorly). Obesity increases risks secondary to rises in intra-abdominal and subsequently intra-gastric pressure. Finally, impaired peristalsis, abnormal hiatal compliance and delayed gastric emptying have also been shown to play a role.[4]

Question: When assessing an infant presenting with regurgitation, how will you differentiate between GOR and GORD? What information in the patient's history is relevant to aid discrimination between the two conditions?
Answer: GOR is considered a normal physiological event marked by a tendency to effortlessly regurgitate milk due to the relative immaturity of the LOS, consumption of large quantities of liquid feeds, supine positioning and a shallower angle of His in children under the age of 1 year. GOR is thus very common in infants, affecting up to approximately 40% at 4 months and resolving in 95% of infants by aged 14 months.[5] Where it occurs with no other symptoms, it does not require further investigation or treatment other than parental reassurance. In contrast, a diagnosis of gastro-oesophageal reflux disease (GORD), is typically associated with clinical symptoms or complications of GOR.

Key questions to differentiate between the two states include the presence of worsening symptoms of GOR or evidence of sequelae of GORD including distress/crying, choking/gagging, coughing, feed refusal, back arching, abnormal posturing, apnoea spells, faltering weight, recurrent pneumonia and otitis media infection, all of which have been associated with GORD.[6] A maternal history of GORD and passive smoking in the household have also been shown to increase the incidence of GORD in infants. Additionally, many medical disorders are known to independently predispose children to GORD including prematurity, neurological disability, oesophageal atresia, congenital diaphragmatic hernia, Down's syndrome and cystic fibrosis.[7] Finally, a thorough history with food diary and assessment of the onset and pattern of regurgitation helps exclude potential differential diagnoses. Regurgitation associated with GOR is more likely to occur before 8 post-natal weeks, but rarely before 1 week old or after 1 year. As such, onset before or after these timepoints may indicate alternative diagnoses. Regurgitated contents must be milky in nature; the presence of bilious or bloody vomit warrant further investigation. Finally, a history of atopy in the family, chronic diarrhoea or straining at stool may indicate the alternative diagnosis of non-IgE-mediated cow's milk protein allergy.

Question: Which investigations may help confirm a diagnosis of GORD in an infant or child?
Answer: The presence of GOR with symptoms such as apnoea and vomiting refractory to medical treatment requires further investigation for consideration of surgical treatment. The diagnosis of GORD is largely based on clinical suspicions, but the importance of corroboration by the use of targeted diagnostic tests is key, particularly where the history may not be clear-cut as in infants and young children. Commonly used tests with relative advantages and disadvantages are discussed later. There is, however, no absolute gold-standard tool for the diagnosis of reflux in infants and children; no test has been recommended in isolation for the diagnosis of GORD by the NASPGHAN/ESPGHAN guidelines, which recommend that one or more diagnostic tests are used as an adjunct to aid diagnosis on an individual patient basis after consideration of symptoms, age and likelihood of differential diagnoses.[8]

1. **Oesophago-gastro-duodenoscopy (OGD) +/– biopsy**
   The role of OGD in the diagnosis of symptomatic children with GOR is threefold. It can diagnose erosive reflux oesophagitis by

visualisation of inflammation and erosions/ulceration in the oesophageal mucosa, which is particularly useful where haematemesis is suggested in the clinical history. Biopsy can readily indicate the presence of microscopic oesophagitis by evidence of eosinophils and basal cell hyperplasia, and finally, OGD can exclude other oesophageal pathologies mimicking reflux, particularly in the presence of dysphagia, including eosinophilic oesophagitis. Whilst endoscopy alone has a low sensitivity for oesophagitis, biopsy is highly sensitive and specific. Additionally, OGD can readily identify hiatus hernia, Barrett's oesophagus and strictures and provides an opportunity for gastric biopsy to exclude *Helicobacter pylori.*

2. **pH and pH/impedance monitoring (pH-MII)**
   In pH-metry, a transnasal probe continuously measures the frequency and duration of the reflux index, episodes where the lower oesophageal pH is <4, indicating the presence of acidic gastric contents in the oesophagus. This is then assessed in conjunction with a diary of activities and symptoms. Stand-alone pH-metry has limitations for several reasons; firstly, a reflux index of <4 was determined in adults with no determination of true normative values in children. In addition, although it has been shown to have a high sensitivity and specificity for *acid* reflux, it is unable to identify *non-acid* reflux, which is common in infants and estimated to account for 45–89% of GOR episodes in this population.[9] Additionally, usefulness will be limited if patients are unable to stop acid suppressant medication for the test because of symptom severity.

   The development of multichannel intraluminal impedance and pH monitoring (pH-MII) has significant advantages over standard pH-metry. It accurately detects pH < and >4 and correlates this with the amount and type of refluxate in the oesophagus (liquid or gas). Additionally, it can differentiate between low pH due to swallow vs. reflux episodes. As such, pH-MII has a much higher sensitivity compared to pH-metry, particularly when non-acid reflux is present. pH-MII is endorsed in:
   i. Patients with persistent typical symptoms despite appropriate acid suppression to clarify between different types of GOR: Patients with non-erosive reflux disease (pathological reflux regardless of symptoms), hypersensitive oesophagus (positive symptom correlation with acid or non-acid events but no pathological reflux) and functional heartburn disorders (negative symptom correlation and no pathological reflux) to tailor medical treatments accordingly.
   ii. Understanding of the efficacy of acid suppression: The mean sensitivity of pH-MII was 80% in patients taking acid suppression, whereas this dropped to 47% in pH-metry alone in one study.[10]
   iii. The presence of extra-oesophageal (respiratory) symptoms: Seven impedance sensors along the probe allow for accurate detection of full-column reflux events, which can help understand their role in patients with allied respiratory symptoms.

3. **Upper gastrointestinal contrast study**
   Upper gastrointestinal contrast studies are insensitive and non-specific for the diagnosis of GORD; however, they offer the best definition of foregut anatomy and are therefore useful in evaluation of children with refractory symptoms to exclude other conditions which contribute to or mimic GORD. These include hiatal hernia, malrotation, pyloric stenosis, duodenal stenosis or web, oesophageal narrowing secondary to strictures or external compression and achalasia. In addition, comment can be made on oesophageal motility, helping to understand the risk of aspiration. Supplementary videofluoroscopic swallow studies can aid exclusion of oropharyngeal dysphagia with reflux aspiration, which can mimic GORD. Finally, contrast imaging is very useful for assessment of children with recurrence of symptoms post anti-reflux surgery to assess for obstructing or a slipped fundoplication.

4. **Oesophageal manometry**
   High-resolution oesophageal manometry is used to measure the contractility of the oesophagus and LOS pressure. It was the key technique used to identify TLOSR and its role in reflux and can identify other causes of reflux including hypotonic LOS or a hiatus hernia. In combination with impedance, it is able to quantify the proportion of TLOSRs associated with bolus movement of gastrointestinal contents in the oesophagus but is not specifically predictive of GORD. The measurement of oesophageal motility can be helpful in detecting motility

abnormalities which may increase the risk of aspiration such as dysmotility or outlet obstruction. Newer uses of manometry pre- and post-fundoplication include the development of a dysphagia risk index, assessing parameters of oesophageal motility that are associated with a higher risk of postoperative complications such as dysphagia,[11] but it is not used routinely in clinical practice.

Question: You are asked to see an 18-month-old neurologically normal child in clinic presenting with a year-long history of regurgitation and a new presentation with apnoea spells. Symptoms persist despite 8 weeks of treatment with full-dose proton pump inhibitor (PPI), and symptoms were ongoing once the PPI was weaned. What are your next steps?

Answer: Assessment of treatment compliance with PPI therapy and consideration of differential diagnoses are the most likely causes of treatment failure in this scenario. In the absence of lack of compliance, recurrence or no improvement in symptoms post weaning, the PPI agent indicates either an alternative diagnosis or the presence of non-acid reflux. Investigations should include pH-MII to assess for the presence of non-erosive reflux disease and the extent of full-column reflux contributing to apneoas; an OGD with biopsy to identify the presence of oesophagitis and aid exclusion of contributing factors such as a hiatus hernia; and an upper gastrointestinal imaging study to exclude potential differential diagnoses, comment on oesophageal motility and assess gastric emptying.

Question: What surgical treatment options exist for a child with GORD? What are the relative advantages and disadvantages?

Answer: Anti-reflux surgery is recommended in children in whom optimal medical management has failed, chronic pharmacotherapy for control of symptoms is required, a chronic condition means here the risk of GORD-associated complications are high (e.g. neurological impairment) or life-threatening symptoms exist after optimal medical management (e.g. apneoas, bradycardia or aspiration pneumonia).

Minimally invasive surgery (MIS) or open classical Nissen's fundoplication is considered the gold-standard surgical option for severe GORD refractory to medical treatment. Fundoplication has been shown to reduce reflux symptoms, total acid exposure time and number of non-acidic reflux episodes. This is achieved through many mechanisms; fundoplication has been shown to increase the length of the intra-abdominal oesophagus, thereby increasing the angle of His and the baseline LOS pressure and thus decreasing the incidence of TLOSRs by 50% due to changes in compliance of the cardiac region.[12] Overall, operative success is considered high; a systematic review of the paediatric literature involving over 1,200 patients reported complete relief of GORD symptoms in as many as 86% of patients.[13] However, risks include gas bloat, dysphagia, retching, dumping syndrome, worsening aspiration from oesophageal stasis and wrap migration. Many studies, though, demonstrate poorest outcomes in those patients where fundoplication is primarily used to treat extra-oesophageal symptoms of GORD, e.g. aspiration pneumonia. Re-do fundoplication rates range from 4.6% to 12.2%, and this risk is notably associated with retching, younger age at operation, extensive hiatal dissection and neurological impairment.[8] Survival is variable and difficult to assess as it is considerably influenced by the underlying status of the patient; a 5-year prospective, observational study of 255 patients undergoing fundoplication by a single surgeon showed 100% survival in those with no underlying medical history, but only 59% in those with neurological impairment and a gastrostomy.[14] As such, patient selection is critical, and only those with clearly proven GORD should undergo surgery.

The use of transpyloric feeding with surgically inserted gastro-jejunal tubes (GJTs), either by open/laparoscopic GJT placement or by percutaneous endoscopic techniques (PEG-J), can be used in those patients requiring enteral feeding but are wholly unable to tolerate gastric feeding because of reflux. This is most commonly used in infants with failure to thrive secondary to reflux, which may improve over time, e.g. neonates or those with significant extra-oesophageal complications of GOR such as aspiration, apnoea and bradycardias. Studies appear to suggest lower numbers of reflux events recorded by pH-MII compared to fundoplication with comparable rates of GORD complications.[11,15] However, one retrospective study of over 100 matched patients also showed higher rates of failure to thrive, repeat of initial intervention(s) and crossover intervention(s) in the GJT arm.[16] The reasonably high incidence of tube-related complications (including displacement, kinking, blocking, intussusception and, rarely, jejunal perforation) and the requirement for periodic tube replacement mean that fundoplication is still currently the preferred definitive surgical option for GORD.

Total oesophago-gastric disassociation (TOGD), described by Bianchi in 1997, is most often used as a rescue procedure when previous fundoplications have failed. It completely eliminates the possibility of reflux by transecting the GOJ, re-anastomosing the oesophagus to the distal jejunum, anastomosing the biliopancreatic segment loop 30 cm distal to the oesophagojejunal anastomosis and creating a gastrostomy for intra-gastric feeding. A recent systematic review (discussed later) has shown TOGD in neurologically impaired patients to be as effective as fundoplication – if not more – at reducing reflux with equivalent complication rates.[17] As such, it is increasingly being advocated by some surgeons as a potential primary treatment in a 'select risk group' of patients who are severely neurologically impaired and completely dependent on tube feeding, although this view is not endorsed by ESPGHAN/NASPGHAN.

Question: In clinic, you are asked to see a 3-year-old with neurological impairment, vomiting and failure to thrive. What impact does neurological impairment have on the incidence of reflux and why? How may symptoms or presentation of GORD be different in a child with a neuro-disability compared to a patient with no medical history? What implications does neuro-disability have on surgical strategy?

Answer: The incidence of feeding difficulties in neurologically impaired children is significantly higher than in those without. Whereas older children with reflux symptoms may self-report symptoms such as heartburn, acid reflux, epigastric or abdominal pain,[7] the diagnosis is more challenging in neurologically impaired children due to deficits in verbal communication and a high incidence of general feeding difficulties including feed refusal and vomiting. As such, the true prevalence is largely unknown but is estimated to be 20–30%. Symptoms warranting investigation include vomiting, rumination, haematemesis, anaemia, behavioural problems and dental erosion. However, several patients may not display symptoms and present with significant complications; a large study in the Netherlands of 1,500 neurologically impaired patients showed a pathological pH test in 48% with reflux oesophagitis in 96% of these, Barrett's oesophagus in 14%

and peptic strictures in approximately 4%, in the absence of obvious GORD symptomatology.[18] This increased incidence is due to a combination of factors; central nervous system dysfunction results in foregut dysmotility leading to delayed gastric emptying; a lower LOS pressure with increased incidence of TLOSRs; and spasticity, scoliosis and seizures, all resulting in a higher intra-abdominal pressure often exacerbated by a non-ambulatory position.

In addition to significantly more complications from GOR, these vulnerable patients are more likely to fail medical management therapies mandating a surgical procedure.[7] Additionally, this 'at risk' population has higher rates of surgical complications and symptom disease recurrence after surgery. The success rate of fundoplication appears to be highly dependent on severity of neurological status of each individual patient. Wrap migration into the chest is the most common cause of surgical failure, likely due to spasticity, scoliosis and seizure convulsions. A recent meta-analysis study showed a higher recurrence rate of symptoms of GOR, a higher incidence of re-do fundoplication and a higher risk of failure of re-do in the neurologically impaired population compared to the neurologically normal patient. Comparison between fundoplication and TOGD in this patient group showed similar intensive care unit length of stay and time to achieve full postoperative feeds with significantly higher recurrence rates of symptoms in the fundoplication treated group (25% vs. 1%), with no statistical differences in complication rates apparent between the two procedures.[17] Interestingly, two further meta-analyses have shown that the placement of a GJT compared to fundoplication as treatment of GORD in this population was associated with similar incidence of recurrence of symptoms but a lower incidence of complications.[19] When deciding on a surgical strategy for these special vulnerable patients, all of this must be taken fully into account and the family best counselled appropriately by a specialist multidisciplinary team (MDT).

BIBLIOGRAPHY

1. Schoeman et al. Gastroenterology (1995). PMID: 7806066
2. Boeckxstaens. Neurogastroenterology Motility (2005). PMID: 15836451

3. Schneider et al. Journal of Surgical Research (2010). PMID: 19577763
4. Falk. Gastroenterology (2010). PMID: 20600061
5. Martin et al. Pediatrics (2002). PMID: 12042543.
6. Curien-Chotard et al. BMC Paediatrics (2020). PMID: 9446923.
7. Sherman et al. American Journal of Gastroenterology (2009) PMID: 19352345
8. Rosen et al. Journal of Pediatric Gastroenterology and Nutrition (2018). PMID: 29470322
9. Vandenplas et al. Journal of Paediatrics (2007). PMID: 17498193
10. Rosen et al. Clinical Gastroenterology and Hepatology (2006) PMID: 16469676.
11. Loots et al. Journal of Pediatrics (2013). PMID: 23102795
12. Ireland et al. Gut (1993). PMID: 8472975
13. Mauritz et al. Journal of Gastrointesintal Surgery (2011). PMID: 21800225
14. Stone. Pediatrics (2009). PMID: 28159744.
15. Srivastava et al. Pediatrics (2009). PMID:19117901
16. Wockenforth et al. British Journal of Surgery (2011). PMID: 21351077
17. Lauriti et al. Pediatric Surgery International (2018). PMID: 30105496
18. Böhmer et al. The Netherlands Journal of Medicine (1997). PMID: 9446923.
19. Livingston et al. Journal of Pediatric Surgery (2015). PMID: 25783384

25

Necrotizing pneumonia

PRINCE RAJ, MOHAMMED AMIN AL AWADHI, AND MARTIN T. CORBALLY
King Hamad University Hospital, Kingdom of Bahrain, Bahrain

Scenario: A 3-year-old girl presented to the hospital emergency department with a 5-day history of cough, sore throat, high-grade fever and difficulty in breathing. There was no significant prior medical history. On examination, she was febrile, tachycardic and tachypnoeic. Respiratory examination revealed chest in-drawing, reduced air entry on the right side and dullness to percussion over the right lower lung zone.

Question: What is your diagnosis?
Answer: The most common cause for this acute presentation in a child with symptoms typical of lower respiratory tract infection in this age group is a community-acquired pneumonia (CAP). It is a potentially serious infection affecting children globally, accounting for almost 20% of childhood death worldwide. Diagnosis is best made from the patient's history and clinical examination.

Question: How will you next investigate the patient?
Answer: History: Workup should begin with reviewing the child's history to identify any underlying medical diseases. History should be elicited for any possible foreign object aspiration or ingestion of toxic substances. There should be a note made on other findings unrelated to the respiratory tract such as abdominal pain, loose stools, vomiting, lethargy, poor feeding, irritability and/or signs of dehydration.

Physical examination: Careful note should be made of the overall appearance of the child and identification of any obvious signs of toxaemia, hypoxia and dehydration. The child should next be assessed for tachypnoea, elevated temperature, chest wall retraction, grunting and use of accessory respiratory muscles. The upper respiratory tract should be closely examined for evidence of ear, nose or throat infection. Older children like the index case listed are more likely to have findings such as lung rales, dullness to percussion, bronchial breath sounds, tactile vocal fremitus and a pleural rub. Chest auscultation with a stethoscope may reveal localized rales and wheezing in younger children.

Diagnostic workup: This is required for all patients with severe pneumonia or complicated pneumonia.

Question: The child has developed hypoxia and increased respiratory distress, and chest radiology imaging shows an extensive right-sided thorax consolidation with effusion.
Answer: The clinical picture of tachypnoea with hypoxia and imaging showing extensive right lung consolidation with a parapneumonic effusion (PPE) points towards a severe pneumonia. This child requires emergent hospital in-patient admission, preferably to the intensive care unit.

1. Supplemental oxygen (O_2) therapy should be started to maintain saturations.

2. Parenteral IV ampicillin (or penicillin) and gentamicin is a recommended first-line treatment.
3. Hydration status should be maintained with a crystalloid infusion.

Question: The patient further deteriorates with progression of the right-sided pleural effusion and an opaque right hemithorax with mediastinal shift (Figure 25.1). Chest ultrasound reveals a PPE (Figure 25.2). What are the next steps?
Answer: In view of the deteriorating condition and increased oxygen requirements and a chest X-ray (CXR) showing mediastinal shift, it is pertinent to consider placing an intercostal drain (ICD). Drain insertion will help relieve respiratory distress and also improve ventilation and blood gas status.

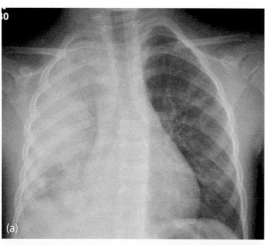

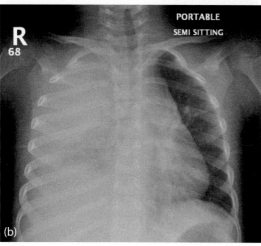

Figure 25.1 Chest X-ray AP view showing extensive right-sided pulmonary consolidation with ipsilateral parapneumonic effusion and mediastinal shift to the left side.

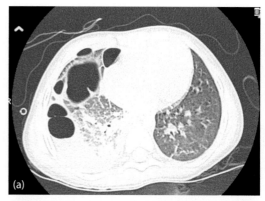

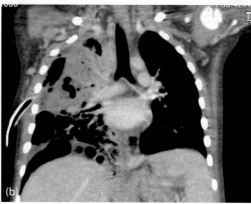

Figure 25.2 CT thorax showing total consolidation of the right lung upper lobe containing an air bronchogram, hypodense multiple necrotic centres and air loculi, suggestive of necrotizing pneumonia. Compression atelectasis is also seen affecting the right middle lobe. Atelectasis-consolidation of the right lower lobe is also evident.

Question: The IV antibiotic therapy is continued for 7 days, but the patient has developed recurrent spikes of fever, and the pleural fluid analysis showed gram-positive cocci. What are the next steps to progress patient management?
Answer: As the patient is still spiking temperatures with an ICD in situ, there is now the distinct possibility of a lung abscess, empyema and/or necrotizing pneumonia. The next steps should be to organize a computed tomography (CT) thorax scan for better delineation of the underlying pathology.

Question: A chest CT scan (Figure 25.3) shows signs of parenchymal necrosis, pleural air loculations, parapneumonic hydropneumothorax and right lung atelectasis. What is your diagnosis now?
Answer: The patient's condition has progressed with a protracted clinical course despite IV

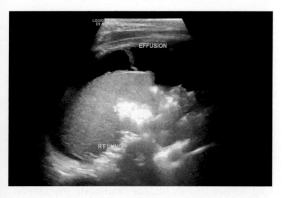

Figure 25.3 Ultrasound scan showing a parapneumonic effusion with underlying consolidation of the lung parenchyma.

antibiotic therapy and adequate intercostal drainage. The clinical scenario now fits a working diagnosis of complicated necrotizing pneumonia (NP). CT thorax findings further clinch the diagnosis.

Question: What is the pathogenesis of NP?
Answer: NP is an uncommon and severe complication of CAP. It is also known as a cavitary pneumonia and involves massive parenchymal lung damage despite early and appropriate antibiotic therapy in an otherwise previously healthy child.

MICROBIOLOGY

The most common organisms associated with NP are *Streptococcus pneumoniae* and *Staphylococcus aureus*.

Though pneumococci possess numerous virulence factors, the most important one is the bacteria polysaccharide capsule, which helps in evading the immune system. Serotypes most commonly involved with NP are types 3 and 19A. *S. aureus* also has multiple virulence factors to help evade the immune response and cause tissue invasion leading to NP, but recently strains expressing Panton-Valentine Leucocidin (PVL) – a pore-forming exotoxin – has been found to be associated with severe forms of the disease in previously healthy children and adults.

Other bacteria implicated with NP include *Streptococcus mitis, Streptococcus pyogenes, Mycoplasma pneumoniae, Pseudomonas* and *Fusobacterium*. Viruses like influenza, adenovirus and cytomegalovirus (CMV) have also been implicated

in occasional reports. Fungi (e.g. *Aspergillus*) causing NP are extremely rare but should always be kept in mind in those with immunodeficiency syndromes and oncology patients.

PATHOLOGY

NP is characterized by necrosis of lung parenchyma from a combined coagulative and liquefactive necrosis and leads to formation of thin-walled cavities. It typically lies somewhere between the spectrum of lung abscess and pulmonary gangrene. PPE and empyema result when the necrotic disease regions involve pleura. A possible mechanism is infection leading to a vasculitis and activation of the coagulation cascade, which then predisposes to thrombotic events and occlusion of intrapulmonary vessels. This along with the bacterial toxin induces a profound cytokine and interleukin 8–mediated inflammatory response, which releases proteolytic enzymes, which cause tissue destruction and cavity formation.

Question: What are the major clinical features of NP, and how will you investigate a patient?
Answer: NP most commonly involves toddlers and preschool-age children. Generally, the child is healthy and has no prior medical history. Symptoms are similar to uncomplicated pneumonia to start with initially, but then the illness runs a protracted course. The patient invariably presents with fever, cough, sore throat, chest pain and difficulty in breathing. On clinical examination they have tachycardia and tachypnoea. Chest examination may be stony dull to percussion, and on auscultation there will be decreased breath sounds, bronchial breathing and signs of mediastinal shift. The affected child usually fails to respond adequately to IV antibiotic therapy and may well have persistent fever, cough, tachypnoea and hypoxia. Rarely a patient with NP may show a sudden deterioration and develop sepsis, shock and respiratory failure.

A diagnosis of NP should therefore always be kept in mind while dealing with a child with a pneumonia when they become more ill and don't respond to broad-spectrum antibiotics and where there is evidence of PPE, empyema or bronchopleural fistula (BPF) despite adequate chest tube drainage not showing improvement.

Investigations:

1. Blood.
   a. *Complete blood count (CBC)*: Anaemia – mild to moderate leucocytosis
   b. Antistreptolysin titre (ASO)
   c. Blood cultures
   d. Electrolytes – Hyponatremia is not uncommon
   e. C-reactive protein (CRP) – Highly raised >100 mg/L
   f. Protein – Hypoalbuminemia
2. Pleural fluid
   a. Gram staining
   b. Leukocyte counts – Raised and neutrophilic
   c. pH – Acidic < 7.20
   d. Glucose – < 2.2 mmol/L
   e. Lactate dehydrogenase (LDH) – >1000 U/L
   f. Proteins – > 30 g/L

RADIOLOGY INVESTIGATIONS

Chest X-ray

Initial investigation ordered in all suspected cases of pneumonia. The sensitivity to detect NP is poor. Findings on CXR will show consolidation, effusion and mediastinal shift (**Figure 25.1**). Pneumatoceles or small-pattern lucencies may be missed on the initial CXR film.

CT thorax: This is the investigation of choice to diagnose NP. It is more sensitive than CXR for parenchymal lung disease, and moreover it rules out any other underlying congenital lung malformations. Findings suggestive of NP on CT imaging are multiple small gas- or fluid-filled, thin-walled, non-enhancing cavities; loss of lung parenchymal architecture; and poor perfusion (**Figure 25.3**). Gas-filled pneumatoceles may be noted in the later disease stages.

Ultrasound: A good imaging modality to evaluate the pleural space in children with complicated pneumonia (**Figure 25.3**). In the hands of a skilled paediatric radiologist and when combined with colour Doppler, lung consolidation along with areas of hypoperfusion can be readily discerned.

Question: What are the differential diagnoses to consider?
Answer: There are many causes of cavitary lung lesions, but differentiating NP from a lung abscess is important, as the underlying pathology and management differ. Generally, a child with a lung abscess runs an indolent course for weeks, and radiologically the inflamed cavities are thick walled and enhancing on CT scan. Other potential cavitary lung lesions include tuberculosis, actinomycosis, fungal infections like *Aspergillosis* and mucormycosis including helminthic infections like *Echinococcus*. Congenital lesions which can be secondarily infected include congenital pulmonary airway malformation (CPAM), which should always be considered in the appropriate clinical setting. Other causes include traumatic pseudocyst, vasculitis syndromes and immunodeficiency states, which can all occur rarely as cavitary lesions.

Question: How would you best manage a case of NP?
Answer: There are no standard guidelines for management of NP, and most of the treatment protocols are largely based on expert opinions and single-centre published reports. So practice management will best require a multidisciplinary team approach. Therapy goals are to control the infection and reverse the pathological events in the affected lung to near normal by providing prolonged antibiotic therapy. Primary objectives are also to prevent hypoxia by providing supplemental oxygen therapy and relieve pleuritic chest pain in order to improve ventilation by giving adequate analgesia. Secondary objectives are to drain intrapleural fluid collection by ICD, correcting any serum fluid and electrolyte abnormality and supporting adequate nutrition.

Medical management:

1. Supplemental O_2.
2. Analgesia.
3. *Antibiotic therapy*: Prolonged IV antibiotic therapy is a key aspect of medical management. Ampicillin or IV penicillins should be the first line of treatment. Vancomycin should be added to therapy regimens when there is suspicion of methicillin-resistant *S. aureus* (MRSA) or if the pleural fluid culture is confirmatory. Addition of clindamycin, linezolid or rifampicin have all been shown to improve outcomes.

The duration of antibiotic treatment is not well defined, though some reports suggest a median duration of approximately 28 days. Switching to oral antibiotics from parenteral therapy should be considered once the patient is improving and clinically stable, tolerating feeds with inflammatory markers (CRP) on a decreasing profile trend. Oral antibiotics should ideally be continued for another 2 weeks (10–14 days).

SURGERY

Surgical intervention should be considered only in those patients with loculated empyema, pneumothorax or pyo-pneumothorax leading to mass effect and compromising ventilation. BPF is one of the complications linked to operative intervention, though spontaneous BPF may also occur in advanced cases of NP.

ICD: Chest tube drainage (as in the index case illustrated) may alone suffice in moderate to large PPE and pyo-pneumothorax, but for a loculated empyema, instillation of fibrinolytic agents is considered very useful.

Video-assisted thoracoscopic surgery (VATS)/ mini-thoracotomy with debridement/decortication: Required when symptoms and signs persist despite ICD and on serial chest imaging there is an increasing or persistent collection.

Management of BPF: If a BPF is persistent despite adequate and prolonged ICD drainage, further surgery may be later required to seal the troublesome air leak. Fibrin glue or muscle flaps may be used to seal a persistent leak.

Lobectomy/Pneumonectomy: Rarely required in the paediatric population.

Indications are:

a. Progressive parenchymal lung necrosis
b. Massive haemoptysis
c. Multiple tension pneumatoceles
d. Pulmonary gangrene involving >50% of involved lobes

Question: What follow-up after-care practice would you undertake?
Answer: NP has a favourable outcome generally in children compared to adult sufferers, where the mortality rate may be high, in the range of 40–50%. Most paediatric patients have a full recovery within 2 months of index hospital admission. CXR and CT imaging tend to normalize or improve 5–6 months from the primary illness (**Figure 25.4**).

After-care outpatient clinic: Ideally three outpatient visits at 2 weeks, 3 months and 6 months after the first hospital discharge for clinical

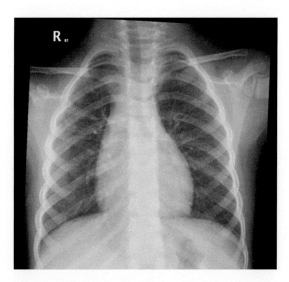

Figure 25.4 Follow-up chest X-ray taken 3 months after primary hospitalization.

health assessment and CXR radiology evaluation. Spirometry for those children who can adequately perform the test should ideally be done at hospital discharge and at 6 months.

BIBLIOGRAPHY

1. Kerem E, Bar Ziv Y, Rudenski B, Katz S, Kleid D, Branski D. Bacteremic necrotizing pneumococcal pneumonia in children. Am J Respir Crit Care Med. 1994;149:242–4.
2. Gillet Y, Vanhems P, Lina G, et al. Factors predicting mortality in necrotizing community-acquired pneumonia caused by *Staphylococcus aureus* containing Panton-Valentine Leucocidin. Clin Infect Dis. 2007;45:315–21.
3. Hodina M, Hanquinet S, Cotting J, Schnyder P, Gudinchet E. Imaging of cavitary necrosis in complicated childhood pneumonia. Eur Radiol. 2002;12:391–6.
4. Wheeler JG, Jacobs RF. Complications of pneumonia. In: Cherry JD, Harrison GJ, Kaplan SL, Steinbach WJ, Hotez PJ, editors. Feigin and Cherry's textbook of Pediatric infectious diseases. 7th ed. Philadelphia: Elsevier Saunders; 2014. pp. 306–22.
5. Bradley JS, Byington CL, Shah SS, et al. The management of community acquired pneumonia in infants and children older than 3 months of age: Clinical practice guidelines by the Pediatric Infectious Diseases Society

and the Infectious Diseases Society of America. Clin Infect Dis. 2011;53:e25–76.

6. Lai JY, Yang W, Ming YC. Surgical management of complicated necrotizing pneumonia in children. Pediatric Neonatol 2016 Oct 28. doi: 10.1016/j.pedneo.2016.06.002

7. Grimwood K, Chang AB. Long-term effects of pneumonia in young children. Pneumonia. 2015;6:101–14.

8. Long AM, Smith Williams J, Mayell S, Couriel J, Jones MO, Losty PD. 'Less may be best '- Pediatric parapneumonic effusion and empyema management: Lessons from a UK center. J Pediatr Surgery. 2016;51(4):588–91.

9. Islam A, Calkins CM, Goldin AB, et al. The diagnosis and management of empyema in children: A comprehensive review from the APSA Outcomes and Clinical Trials Committee. J Pediatr Surg. 2012;47(11):2101–10.

10. Balfour-Lynn IM, Abrahamson E, Cohen G, et al. BTS guidelines for the management of pleural infection in children. Thorax. 2005;60(Suppl 1):i1–21.

PART 3

Surgical Conditions in Childhood and Adolescence

26

Acute and recurrent abdominal pain of childhood

HIND ZAIDAN AND MARTIN T. CORBALLY
King Hamad University Hospital, Kingdom of Bahrain, Bahrain

Scenario: A 12-year-old boy presents to the hospital emergency department with a 1-day history of abdominal pain, which was initially periumbilical in onset but is now localised to the right iliac fossa. The patient has had one episode of vomiting and reports he's had very little to eat over the last 2 days.

Question: What are the potential differential working diagnoses?
Answer:

- Acute appendicitis
- Acute non-specific abdominal pain (ANSAP)
- Mesenteric adenitis
- Gastroenteritis
- Gastritis
- Renal/Ureteric stones
- Pyelonephritis
- Henoch-Schoenlein purpura

It is important to remember that 60–70% of cases of abdominal pain in childhood are caused by ANSAP. The aetiology is frequently idiopathic and the course self-limiting. ANSAP and mesenteric lymphadenitis may present with a preceding history of upper respiratory tract infection (URTI) in the past 2 weeks and may or may not be associated with GI symptoms such as nausea or vomiting.

Yersinia/viral/bacterial gastroenteritis will present predominantly with diarrhoea and vomiting and a history of likely affected family members. Renal stones present as colicky flank pain in a crescendo-decrescendo manner and manifest with severe episodes of sharp stabbing pain radiating from the loin to the right iliac fossa (RIF) and groin.

This short history may appear confusing at times, as the symptoms of appendicitis classically present over a 2- to 3-day period. An accurate history is therefore key in diagnosing the condition, and the Alvarado Score is useful. This scoring system is a set of clinical prediction rules to enhance the clinical diagnosis of appendicitis. The 10-point score adds up each symptom of MANTRELS (migration of pain, anorexia, nausea, tenderness in right lower quadrant, rebound pain, elevated temperature, leucocytosis, shift of white blood cell count to the left) to a total yielding one of three groups: A score of 1–4 is least likely to be appendicitis, and the management is discharge with instructions; 5–6 suggests a possibility of appendicitis, and the patient is to be admitted and actively observed; and a score of 7–10 suggests the diagnosis is most likely appendicitis, and the treatment is to operate. Ninety-three percent of patients who fall into the last category score are successfully predicted to have appendicitis. However, the Alvarado Score accuracy in correctly diagnosing women and children is much lower (1). All or none of these signs may be present. Children below the age of 5 years and those who are non-verbal

148

DOI: 10.1201/9781003182290-29

are especially challenging and typically present with an appendix perforation rate as high as 50%.

Question: What tests will to help establish a correct diagnosis?

Answer: Diagnosing appendicitis may involve utilising a combination of laboratory and radiological investigations, but most importantly, the history and serial clinical examination are key (2). A full blood count will indicate a bacterial infection (increased white blood cells [WBC], left neutrophil shift), increased inflammatory markers (C-reactive protein/erythrocyte sedimentation rate [ESR]). Radiological tools in the paediatric population are considerate of radiation risks; therefore, ultrasound is the first-line investigation. Sensitivity ranges between 40% and 50% (2) due to multiple factors such as the sonographer, body habitus, location of the appendix, presence or absence of a fecalith or overlying bowel gas obscuring an accurate view. CT scans are also deployed in patients with a higher body mass index (BMI), but hospital policies may vary from centre to centre.

PRESENTATION OF APPENDICITIS

The clinical presentation of appendicitis varies with age and anatomical position of the appendix. The most common mode of presentation in children under 5 years is diarrhoea and fever, which may therefore lead to the highest rates of misdiagnosis in this vulnerable age group. Up to 50% of preschool children with appendicitis are misdiagnosed as having gastroenteritis. Perforation rate and rapidly evolving peritonitis are higher because of the small appendicular lumen requiring less pressure to breech the thin appendicular wall, compounded with an underdeveloped omentum acting as a poor protective barrier in limiting the spread of infection. Other uncommon presentations include symptoms of small bowel obstruction associated with fever. The greatest negative predictor of appendicitis is a low WBC count and lack of neutrophil shift, amongst other negative clinical signs, which include absent Rovsing's sign, percussion tenderness and little evidence of nausea and vomiting. Becker et al. reported that 44% of children (a series of 750 cases) may present with six or more atypical clinical signs (3). Rebound tenderness is assessed by the 'jump test' which is up to 87% sensitive in diagnosing appendicitis combined with raised inflammatory markers. Asking the child to 'jump up and down' to reach a hanging toy will result in grimace or refusal to jump and is considered a positive test.

Older children may present with referred pain to the loin, groin and leg, and some boys may even present with testicular pain. By contrast, in cases of testicular torsion, the initial clinical presentation may only be abdominal pain; therefore, testicular examination is crucially an important part of the surgeon's abdominal examination.

McBurney's point is located approximately two-thirds of the distance from the umbilicus to the right anterior superior iliac spine – a point of maximum abdominal wall tenderness encountered in acute appendicitis. The tip of the inflamed appendix, though, can vary greatly in its anatomical site location – anterior, retro-caecal, pelvic, ileal and, rarely, sub-hepatic. Pelvic appendicitis causing local inflammation of the bladder can present with typical urinary symptoms such as dysuria, urgency and frequency. Diarrhoea is common if the tip of the appendix lies in the pararectal space, and similarly, symptoms of colitis are common with ileal-sited appendicitis. In menarchal girls, an inflamed appendix adherent to the uterus or fallopian tube may simulate early menstrual cycle pain. Retro-caecal and sub-hepatic appendicitis often present with the highest perforation rates because of atypical symptoms. Retro-caecal appendicitis may give rise to referred leg pain, and clinical examination will then often confirm a positive psoas sign. Sub-hepatic appendicitis can mimic renal colic or acute cholecystitis with renal angle tenderness or focal tenderness in the right upper quadrant and a positive Murphy's sign. Ultrasound is therefore especially useful in atypical clinical presentation and can help aid in diagnosing appendicitis and excluding other variant pathologies **(Figure 26.1)**.

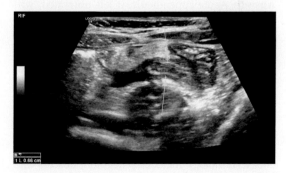

Figure 26.1 Ultrasound scan in acute appendicitis. Ultrasound showing inflamed appendix; measurements >6 mm are indicative of acute appendicitis. Yellow arrows depict the walls of an inflamed appendix measuring 6.6 mm.

Question: What are your clinical management plans?

Answer: Some patients may present with a short history and inconclusive clinical examination or normal laboratory tests; therefore, diagnosing appendicitis at an early stage is not always clear-cut. If early appendicitis is therefore suspected, the patient should be admitted to hospital and actively observed for a minimum of 24 hours. Through serial bedside examination, an inflammatory process will eventually manifest with peritoneal signs, pyrexia or other signs indicative of appendicitis. Active observation is a useful tool deployed by paediatric surgeons to help accurately diagnose appendicitis, and in many cases, it remains a firm clinical diagnosis rather than a radiological one.

Treatment of acute appendicitis involves antibiotic therapy and appendectomy with laparoscopic or open classical operation. Recent studies have also explored non-operative medical management of appendicitis as first-line therapy. A recent meta-analysis showed a 92% efficacy rate in the initial management of uncomplicated appendicitis. On the other hand, an increased number of repeat hospital emergency department visits and recurrent symptoms of abdominal pain were also a common finding in those children treated non-operatively. Sixteen percent of patients thus went on to have an appendectomy because of reported disturbed quality of life (QoL) (4). Outcomes also were observed to vary with the presence of an appendicolith. Some studies have thus reported a higher failure rate, while others found no statistical differences.

Question: What are the complications of appendicitis?

Answer: Acute appendicitis, if left untreated, will progress to complicated appendicitis whereby the omentum and surrounding viscera (small and large bowel) form a phlegmon around the focus of inflammation to shield the neighbouring peritoneal organs from spreading infection. This phlegmon can further progress to liquefy at its centre, forming an appendicular abscess. Generalised peritonitis is a consequence of a ruptured appendicular abscess and secondary perforation. Complicated appendicitis terminology includes phlegmon, abscess and perforated appendicitis. Uncomplicated appendicitis is defined as an inflamed or suppurative appendicitis without the aforementioned complications.

Question: How do you treat complicated appendicitis?

Answer: Diffuse peritonitis secondary to perforated appendicitis with significant sepsis (tachycardia, fever) despite resuscitation efforts and antimicrobial therapy is one of the few indications for timely urgent 'middle of the night' appendectomy. In uncomplicated appendicitis appendectomy may be routinely scheduled during normal hospital working hours (7:30 a.m. to 6:00 pm), i.e. the following morning, so long as IV antibiotics have been commenced promptly in line with UK National Confidential Enquiry into Patient Outcome and Death (NCEPOD) recommendations. This incentive was designed to help minimise operative risk and intraoperative complications during the late hours of the night caused by lack of experienced staff and resource shortages compounded with human error (5). There is now a growing trend of carefully timed operative intervention in acute or complicated appendicitis to help minimise postoperative complications. Time for resuscitation and overnight antibiotic therapy have proved to significantly reduce the risk of intrabdominal collections (6).

Complicated appendicitis presenting as appendicular phlegmon/appendix mass or appendix abscess is typically managed conservatively with 1–2 weeks of antibiotics followed by elective interval appendectomy scheduled 8–12 weeks after the initial infection. Interval appendectomy ('non-essential surgery') is also an optional decision-making process for patients/family carers, as a significant number of children will never develop recurrent appendicitis (7–9).

Appendicular abscess is best managed with percutaneous image-guided drainage or, rarely, open methods followed by conservative antibiotic therapy and interval appendectomy 8–12 weeks later (7–9).

Question: What are the complications of appendectomy?

Answer: The most common postoperative complications in order of frequency are wound infection, postperative intrabdominal collections, lung atelectasis, adhesive bowel obstruction, stump appendicitis, 'stump blowout' and retained fecalith. Soft tissue infection (SSI) rates vary from 0.76% to 16.6%, with intrabdominal collection reportedly occurring in 0.55% to 32.3% of patients (7). Wound infection and intrabdominal collections typically represent 60–70% of all postoperative complications.

> **Scenario:** A 13-year-old female presents to your hospital clinic with a history of abdominal pain for the past 6 months. It is intermittent in nature, not exacerbated by identifiable factors, severe in onset and lasts for approximately 10–25 minutes. There are no obvious precipitating or relieving factors, and she has visited the emergency department a number of times for this pain.

Question: How will you manage this patient?
Answer: The first and most important steps are to obtain a detailed patient clinical history using the SOCRATES approach (site, onset, characteristic, radiation, associated symptoms, time course, exacerbating and relieving factors, severity). Recurrent abdominal pain of childhood may be diagnosed along with the appropriate patient work-up once 'red flag' symptoms are ruled out.

Question: What are the red flag symptoms?
Answer: Fever, vomiting, blood in the stool, diarrhoea, failure to thrive or poor weight gain, jaundice, recurrent urinary tract infections (UTIs) and unexplained lymphadenopathy.

Question: What is your working differential diagnosis list?
Answer:

- Recurrent abdominal pain of childhood
- Biliary colic
- Renal colic
- Constipation
- Malrotation
- Gastritis/*Helicobacter pylori*/duodenitis
- Chronic pancreatitis
- Inflammatory bowel disease
- Coeliac disease
- Biliary dyskinesia
- Gynaecological disorders

It is important to recognise that significant and/or invasive investigation is rarely indicated in the child confidently suspected by the experienced paediatric surgeon as having recurrent abdominal pain (RAP). However, many patients will or may have already undergone extensive investigations at other hospitals before they first attend your paediatric surgery service. The yield from CT scans, barium enema and colonoscopy is typically very low, and these investigative studies are only of value when red flag symptoms are apparent. In general, laboratory tests such as a full blood count and renal and liver profiles are sufficient in addition to scheduling an abdominal and pelvic ultrasound exam.

Once all tests are negative – and they generally are – treatment is best directed at managing the family and patient's perception of the condition and considering using a combination of patient-centred behavioural therapy and reassurance.

The value of an abdominal ultrasound exam is to reassure the patient and parents that 'all appears normal' and that the pain will in due course resolve. Occasionally a laxative or stool softener may be prescribed, e.g. lactulose, if constipation seems a major feature. It is finally important to emphasise that any prolonged pain or pain unusual in character or site should prompt a visit to the family doctor or hospital emergency department. Studies show the majority of patients with idiopathic recurrent abdominal pain improve over time (10, 11).

BIBLIOGRAPHY

1. Ohle R, O'Reilly F, O'Brien KK, Fahey T, Dimitrov BD. The Alvarado score for predicting acute appendicitis: A systematic review. BMC Medicine. 2011;9(1):139.
2. Zaidan H, Alkhalfan F, Ahmed H, Corbally M. Positive and negative rates in children with acute appendicitis. Bahrain Medical Bulletin. 2018;40:82–5.
3. Becker T, Kharbanda A, Bachur R. Atypical clinical features of pediatric appendicitis. Academic Emergency Medicine. 2007; 14(2):124–9.
4. Maita S, Andersson B, Svensson JF, Wester T. Nonoperative treatment for nonperforated appendicitis in children: A systematic review and meta-analysis. Pediatr Surg Int. 2020;36(3):261–9.
5. Campling E. Who operates when? London: National Confidential Enquiry into Perioperative Deaths; 1997.

6. Burjonrappa S, Rachel D. Pediatric appendectomy: Optimal surgical timing and risk assessment. The American Surgeon. 2014;80(5):496–9.

7. Degrate L, Chiappetta MF, Nigro A, Fattori L, Perrone S, Garancini M, et al. The uncharted severity of complications after appendectomy for acute appendicitis in children: Results from 348 consecutive patients. Updates in Surgery. 2021.

8. Okoye BO, Rampersad B, Marantos A, Abernethy LJ, Losty PD, et al. Abscess after appendicectomy in children: The role of conservative management. British Journal of Surgery. 1998;85(8): 1111–3.

9. Fawkner-Corbett D, Jawaid WB, Mc Partland J, Losty PD. Interval appendectomy in children clinical outcomes, financial costs and patient benefits. Pediatric Surgery International. 2014;30(7):743–6.

10. O'Donnell B. Abdominal pain in children. Blackwell Scientific Publications Ltd. 1985.

11. Reust CE, Williams A. Recurrent abdominal pain in children. American Family Physician. 2018;97(12):785–93.

27

Disorders of the spleen

RICCARDO COLETTA
Department of Paediatric Surgery, Meyer Children's Hospital
Department of Neurosciences, Drug Research and Child Health, University of Florence, Florence, Italy; and School of Heath and Society, University of Salford, Manchester, UK

BICI KEJD
Department of Paediatric Surgery and Transplantation Pediatric Unit, IRCCS-ISMETT, UPMC (University of Pittsburgh Medical Center), Palermo, Italy

ANTONINO MORABITO
Department of Paediatric Surgery, Meyer Children's Hospital
Department of Neurosciences, Drug Research and Child Health, University of Florence, Florence, Italy and School of Heath and Society, University of Salford, Salford, UK

Scenario: The case report describes a 1-year-old girl who presented with symptoms of abdominal pain, fever, nausea, and vomiting lasting 24 hours. Her physical examination revealed poor overall condition and diffuse tenderness upon abdominal palpation. The blood tests indicated a slight increase in white blood cell count and neutrophils. An abdominal ultrasound revealed a non-vascularized, undefined mass in the pelvic area, measuring 6 cm × 8 cm × 9 cm (**Figure 27.1**).

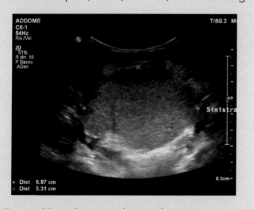

Figure 27.1 Ultrasound scan showing homogenous mass in pelvis.

A 5-mm optical camera was introduced via umbilical access, and an ectopic necrotic spleen was identified in the left iliac fossa and pelvic area. The hilum of the spleen was characterised by multiple torsions along its main axis, presenting a whirled appearance (**Figure 27.2**). A midline periumbilical surgical incision was performed to provide access for prompt de-rotation of the splenic hilum, but

DOI: 10.1201/9781003182290-30

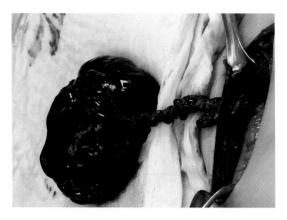

Figure 27.2 Operative picture showing splenic torsion and necrotic spleen.

no improvement in colour or vascularisation was noted. Hence, vessels were tracked up to their origins, ligated and the spleen excised.

The postoperative course was uneventful. Serial blood exams did not show any major variations. The patient had vaccination against capsulated pathogens 4 days after the splenectomy and was discharged home on postoperative day 6. Haematological follow-up at 3, 6 and 12 months showed no complications, and the patient is living a normal life.

This case is illustrative of a complicated wandering spleen (WS). The first description of the condition was attributed to Van Horne, who confirmed a diagnosis of WS in an autopsy exam in 1667. It has an incidence rate of 0.2% and mainly affects children aged <10 years. In paediatric patients, most WS cases are typically seen in children <1 year old, and it is 2.5 times more common in boys than in girls. After the first decade, WS predominantly occurs among females compared to males, with a ratio of 7:1.

WS is a consequence of congenital anomalies in the development of the dorsal mesogastrium that induce an absence or hyperlaxity of the peritoneal ligaments. In paediatric patients, prune-belly syndrome, renal agenesis, gastric volvulus, diaphragmatic eventration and congenital diaphragmatic hernia may be notably associated. Depending on the torsion degree, splenic infarction, gangrene, abscess formation, peritonitis, gastrointestinal obstruction or splenic rupture are possible events.

The clinical presentation of patients with WS varies from asymptomatic to an emergent acute abdomen. Fifteen percent of paediatric patients are totally asymptomatic, while a majority present with abdominal pain (55%) or a palpable mass (90%) related to its complications. Torsion has been described in 64% of children with WS. Laboratory tests are usually non-specific; for this reason diagnosis of WS and its complications relies on imaging techniques. On colour Doppler, there is absence of flow in the parenchyma (in the presence of torsion) and in the splenic hilum. The twisted pedicle can show the well-known characteristic whirled appearance. Computed tomography (CT) scan is an accurate study to diagnose WS and its potential complications in most cases. Absence of the spleen in its usual anatomical location and splenomegaly typically define the existence of this condition. Low signal intensity on T1- and T2-weighted MRI images are signs of acute infarction, while evolutive images are characterised by homogeneous high signal intensity on T2-weighted images and a peripheral hyperintense rim surrounding a hypointense central area on T1-weighted images.

In cases of acute complications and infarction of the spleen, surgery is mandatory and splenectomy commonly performed if non-viable tissue is present. For patients who have milder symptoms and present with no complications, a conservative non-operative management plan may be considered as a standard of care. Increasing knowledge of the spleen's vital role in the hematopoietic reticuloendothelial system makes unnecessary removal of the spleen unwarranted. Thus, when no signs of splenic infarction arc confirmed, open or laparoscopic splenopexy is best recommended to preserve splenic function.

Question: What is the surgical anatomy of the spleen?

Answer: The spleen is composed of three main sections: The body, the central pole and the lower pole. The main venous drainage of the upper pole of the spleen goes through the short gastric vessels. The peritoneal attachments are fixed to the diaphragm and the lateral abdominal wall (**Figure 27.3a** and **b**). It lies along the axis of the left ninth rib.

The main splenic artery is a branch of the celiac artery, and the main splenic vein joins the superior mesenteric vein to form the portal vein, which then drains into the liver. The spleen is fixed to the diaphragm and to the lateral abdominal wall by the peritoneal attachments, which normally prevent torsion or volvulus of the spleen.

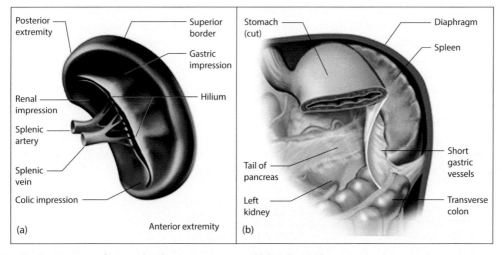

Figure 27.3 Diagram of normal splenic anatomy and blood supply.

Question: What are the indications for splenectomy?

Answer: When the spleen is involved in various disease states, splenectomy may be performed to either alter the clinical course of disease or provide symptomatic relief. Currently, indications for splenectomy have expanded to a broad spectrum of benign and malignant diseases.

The most common indications for paediatric splenectomy are:

Hematologic conditions:
- Autoimmune thrombocytopenia and haemolytic anaemia
- Felty's syndrome
- Idiopathic thrombocytopenic purpura (ITP)
- Erythrocyte membrane disorders
- Erythrocyte enzyme deficiencies
- Hemoglobinopathies
- Primary hypersplenism

Neoplastic conditions:
- Hodgkin's disease
- Non-Hodgkin's lymphoma
- Chronic myelogenous leukaemia
- Chronic lymphocytic leukaemia
- Hairy cell leukaemia
- Metastatic tumours

Benign vascular tumours:
- Haemangioma
- Hamartoma
- Lymphangioma

Uncertain behaviour vascular tumours:
- Littoral cell angioma
- Haemangioendothelioma
- Haemangiopericytoma

Malignant vascular tumours:
- Angiosarcoma

Other benign conditions:
- Gaucher's disease
- Wiskott–Aldrich syndrome
- Chediak–Higashi syndrome
- Splenic cysts
- Splenic abscesses
- WS and splenic torsion
- Trauma

Iatrogenic injuries

Question: What is considered the best management strategy for splenic trauma?

Answer: The spleen is one of the most common solid organs injured in trauma due to its high vascularity and vulnerable anatomical location. Suspicion of splenic injury without signs of haemodynamic instability should be followed by CT imaging, which is up to 98% sensitive in detecting active bleeding and is the imaging modality of choice for grading the severity of splenic trauma.

Paediatric surgeons introduced the concept of non-operative treatment of children with blunt spleen injury more than 50 years ago. In the 20th century, immediate splenectomy for major organ injury trauma was often advocated by surgeons, as misconceptions were portrayed that the spleen was an expendable organ.

The importance of preservation in children sustaining splenic injury is now increasingly widely recognised; however, published reports do continue to show practice variation in treatment depending on where children are managed and by whom, i.e. adult vs paediatric surgeon. There is robust evidence that the rate of non-operative management is higher when children are treated in paediatric trauma centres and that young patients treated in adult trauma centres are more likely to undergo splenectomy. It has now been accepted that the haemodynamic physiological status of the 'stable patient' is pivotal rather than the injury grade of the spleen, which should lead therapeutic decision making towards splenic preservation.

In 2000, the American Pediatric Surgical Association (APSA) Trauma Committee developed evidence-based guidelines introducing the concept that the grade of injury should determine treatment and resource utilisation in stable children. Paediatric surgeons can now witness with some pride that clinical protocols for adult patients sustaining splenic injury more closely mirror paediatric trauma protocols. Despite all these medical advances, teenagers with spleen injuries may still undergo angiography and splenectomy at a higher rates when treated by adult trauma surgeons (**Figure 27.4**).

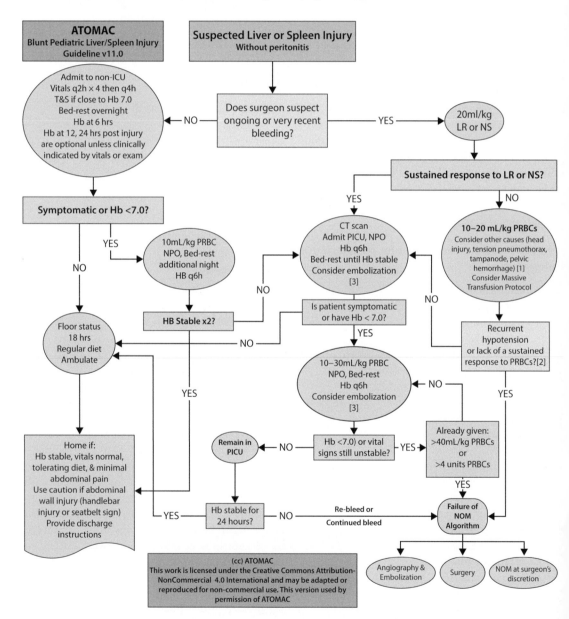

Figure 27.4 Algorithm of management of blunt liver and splenic injury.

Question: How should splenic cysts be managed?
Answer: Non-parasitic splenic cysts (NPSCs) are rare in children and are usually asymptomatic until they compress adjacent organs. Other symptoms and signs may include a palpable mass, thrombocytopenia, early satiety or abdominal swelling and distension. NPSCs can be congenital (also referred to as primary) with an inner epithelial lining or acquired. Ultrasonography can help distinguish cysts from solid lesions, and MRI with CT imaging can provide valuable information regarding the size and location of the cyst in relation to other abdominal structures. Ultimately, the final diagnosis of the specific category of splenic cyst can only be confirmed by immunohistochemistry examination and histopathology.

Asymptomatic smaller splenic cysts (<5 cm in diameter) are often treated conservatively with observation and imaging follow-up. If the cysts increase in size or become symptomatic, intervention should be considered due to the risk of complications. These complications include rupture, haemorrhage, peritonitis, renal compression, hypersplenism or infection. Options for intervention include cystectomy, partial or total splenectomy and, more recently, percutaneous aspiration with or without sclerotherapy.

Question: How should solid splenic mass lesions be managed?
Answer: Splenic tumours may be classified as lymphoid tumours, non-hemato-lymphoid tumours or tumour-like lesions. Lymphoma is the most common malignancy in children to involve the spleen. Splenic involvement is evident in approximately 33% of children with Hodgkin's disease and 15% of children with non-Hodgkin's disease. Yet primary involvement of the spleen by lymphoma is much less common than secondary involvement and usually here it represents non-Hodgkin's lymphoma of B-cell origin. Secondary disease involvement of the spleen is much more common and is seen typically in association with enlarged lymph nodes. Splenic lymphoma in children presents with splenomegaly associated with a solitary mass or multiple mass lesions. The appearance of splenic lymphoma on CT scan also broadly reflects the spectrum of pathology ranging from splenomegaly, only to miliary multifocal lesions, to a solitary mass. On MRI scan, areas of lymphoma appear as hypointense foci on MRI T1-weighted images and as hyperintense foci on T2-weighted images. However, MR cannot reliably depict infiltrative lymphoma because both the normal spleen and lymphomatous infiltrated tissues may have similar T1 and T2 weight values.

Primary angiosarcoma of the spleen is the most common malignant tumour. Its prevalence in the paediatric population varies from 0.14 to 0.25 per million, making this the rarest form of cancer. Paediatric primary angiosarcoma is an aggressive tumour that always presents with splenomegaly associated with palpable mass in the upper left abdominal quadrant. Other symptoms may include abdominal pain, with or without fever, fatigue and weight loss. The histologic features show disorganised anastomosing vascular channels, atypical endothelial cells with large, irregular, hyperchromatic nuclei and a high mitotic rate. These tumours may be so extensive as to replace almost the entire splenic parenchyma. Ultrasound will show multiple complex heterogeneous masses involving the spleen. On contrast-enhanced CT scan, hypervascular lesions are evident that present a heterogeneous appearance. On MRI, areas of mixed high and low signal on T1- and T2-weighted images are seen. In all suspected cases of splenic angiosarcoma, percutaneous needle biopsy should be best avoided, as it is associated with risks of massive haemorrhage. Angiosarcoma may be chemotherapy responsive in some cases; however, an aggressive multidisciplinary approach including chemotherapy and a surgical excision of the primary tumour and all metastases is vital to achieve cure and remission.

Haemangioma is one of the most common primary spleen vascular malformations. Prevalence ranges from 0.3% to 14%, with the highest incidence seen in those at ages 30–50. It is characterised by a proliferation of vascular channels of variable size that are lined with a single layer of endothelium and filled with red blood cells. Most haemangiomas are small lesions (<2 cm), totally asymptomatic and usually found incidentally occasionally associated with skin lesions. However, in rare cases splenic lesions may be multiple and diffuse or part of a systemic disorder such as Kasabach–Merritt and Klippel–Trenaunay syndromes. This condition is usually managed conservatively, though splenectomy is recommended for very large haemangiomas due to the inherent risk of life-threatening bleeding. Recently, propranolol has been successfully used as primary therapy for infantile haemangiomas.

On ultrasound imaging, haemangiomas appear as well-defined, intrasplenic or pedunculated, echogenic, solid or complex cystic masses with abundant colour flow. On CT scan, cavernous haemangiomas appear heterogeneous and show mottled enhancement with contrast at the lesion periphery, whereas capillary haemangiomas tend to be more homogeneous. MRI scan will show haemangiomas are hypointense or isointense on T1 weighting and hyperintense on T2 weighting.

Splenic hamartoma is a rare benign lesion composed of malformed splenic red pulp elements without organised lymphoid follicles. Hamartoma is a rare tumour, but it is considered one of the most common primary non-lymphopoietic neoplasms of the spleen in children. Usually a splenic hamartoma is asymptomatic, while larger lesions may manifest with a palpable mass, splenomegaly or rupture. Moreover, thrombocytopenia and anaemia may occur from sequestration of hematopoietic cell elements.

Considering its derivation from the red pulp of the spleen, hamartomatous lesions will be characterized on ultrasound colour Doppler imaging as exhibiting increased vascularity, in contrast to the typically hypoechoic appearance of the normal splenic tissue. Radiology imaging or percutaneous biopsy may not be enough to reach a definitive diagnosis, and more often, splenectomy is thus undertaken to achieve diagnosis.

Question: What is post-splenectomy sepsis and how can it be prevented?
Answer: Overwhelming post-splenectomy infection (OPI) is a noteworthy complication of splenectomy with an associated mortality of 50–70%. The pathogenic bacteria most often involved in OPI are *Streptococcus pneumoniae*, *Neisseria meningitides* and *Haemophilus influenzae*, with the excess risk of bacteraemia greatest in the first 90 days after splenectomy and occurring in approximately 10% of all patients. The incidence is notably higher after splenectomy for hematologic or malignant disease.

OPI manifests with a short prodromal phase with fevers, chills, malaise and GI complaints without an obvious source of infection. A rapid deterioration with hypotension, disseminated intravascular coagulation (DIC), respiratory distress, coma and death may occur within a few hours. Risk factors linked to OPI mortality include children younger than 4 years of age, thrombocytopenic purpura and spherocytosis. Vaccination against encapsulated pathogens 2 weeks prior to elective splenectomy or 2 weeks after emergency splenectomy is the treatment of choice, and a booster vaccine must be administered every 5 years.

Question: What are the risks of thrombosis events after splenectomy?
Answer: Following splenectomy, platelet counts usually increase by 30–100%, reaching the highest levels between 10 and 20 days postoperatively. Post-splenectomy reactive thrombocytosis (RT) is a very common event, and it is estimated to affect 75–90% of patients undergoing splenectomy. Commonly, thrombocytosis persists over the subsequent 2–3 months, but RT persists indefinitely in a few patients. Portal, splenic and mesenteric vein thrombosis have occurred after splenectomy, with a reported incidence of 1.6–11%. In children affected with haemolytic disorders, the incidence of symptomatic portal vein thrombosis is low but not entirely negligible. Large spleens, long operating times and higher postoperative platelet counts have all been demonstrated to be risk factors for thrombotic events after splenectomy.

Symptoms include fever, vomiting and/or abdominal pain as early as 2 days postoperatively, and urgent abdominal imaging is therefore needed to exclude complications. In asymptomatic individuals with no associated risk factors, routine Doppler ultrasound scan is advisable 1 week postoperatively. Routine administration of antiplatelet prophylaxis after splenectomy is not generally advised in children, including in those who may develop postoperative thrombocytosis.

28

Inflammatory bowel disease

BRUCE JAFFRAY
The Great North Children's Hospital, Newcastle upon Tyne, UK

Scenario: A 13-year-old girl presents with a 6-month history of abdominal pain aggravated by eating. Upon further questioning, she has ceased menstruation, having previously been menstruating regularly. Inspection of her medical records shows that her height and weight were on the 50th percentile 2 years ago, but her weight is now on the 25th percentile. There is no history of diarrhoea. She has a maternal aunt with a history of bowel surgery in early adulthood. Both parents smoke.

Examination reveals a thin girl with erythema ab igne on her abdomen and a fullness in the right iliac fossa. A rectal examination is not performed, but multiple anal skin tags are noted.

Question: What is the differential diagnosis?

Answer: This history is strongly suggestive of Crohn's disease. Small intestinal Crohn's disease is a common cause for a previously well adolescent to exhibit growth failure. While an abdominal mass may be felt in advanced cases, a fullness or no palpable anomaly is more typical. Either a prior history of perianal sepsis or a local perianal anomaly such as skin tags are often seen. A first-degree relative with inflammatory bowel disease may be apparent from history taking. Smoking within the household aggravates a genetic predisposition.

The differential diagnosis is functional pain, followed by pain of ovarian origin in a girl, typically a simple ovarian cyst. In both sexes chronic appendicular pain is often considered but seldom substantiated. Meckel's diverticulum may cause bleeding or an acute perforation but is seldom a cause of chronic pain.

Question: What investigations are indicated?

Answer: The screening investigations should include measurement of faecal calprotectin and an ultrasound scan of the terminal ileum (**Figure 28.1**).

If both of these tests are normal, inflammatory bowel disease is excluded. If these tests are confirmatory, then biopsy proof of the terminal ileum is required by ileo-colonoscopy.

Question: Which imaging modality is preferred?

Answer: Although contrast radiology was traditionally employed to aid diagnosis, this has now been superseded by ultrasound and magnetic resonance enterography (**Figures 28.2–28.5**).

Question: Should the patient be offered surgical resection?

Answer: Diagnosis and management of paediatric Crohn's disease should be under the care and direction of a paediatric gastroenterologist with suitable experience of the condition. Modern management is directed at mucosal healing guided by endoscopic assessment rather than simply

DOI: 10.1201/9781003182290-31

Faecal calprotectin

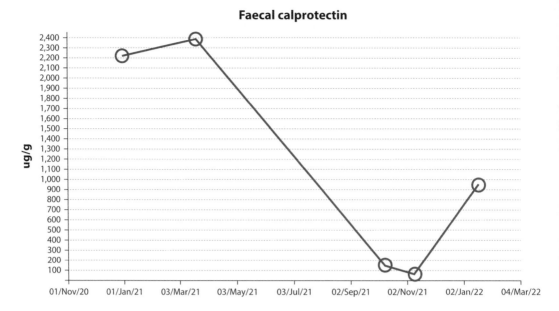

Figure 28.1 Monitoring disease activity with faecal calprotectin. The level falls following resection but then starts to rise again as disease activity flares.

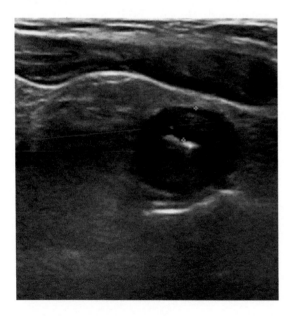

Figure 28.2 Cross-sectional ultrasound image of thickened terminal ileum.

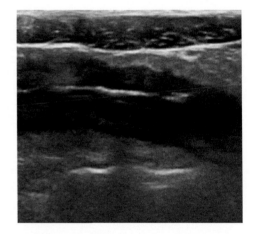

Figure 28.3 Longitudinal ultrasound view of thickened terminal ileum.

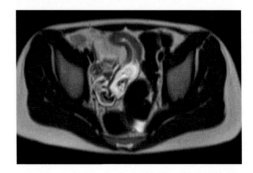

Figure 28.4 MRI scan image of thickened terminal ileum.

symptomatic improvement. However, the LIRIC trial emphasised that for selected phenotypes, surgical resection offers comparable outcomes to medical therapy [1]. In the example listed, if the disease is confined to the terminal ileum, then consideration should be made for surgical resection as a primary therapy.

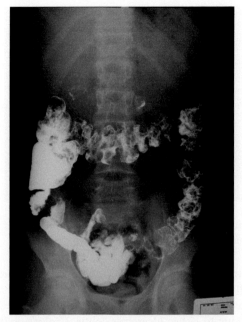

Figure 28.5 Contrast follow-through study showing an ileal stricture. This is a historical image for illustrative purposes only.

The response of children to ileal resection can be dramatic, as seen in this growth chart of a child who underwent resection (**Figure 28.6**).

Complications of Crohn's disease include obstruction, internal fistulation and perforation. These all mandate resection, and it is important to recognise this when you are confronted by complex Crohn's disease (**Figure 28.7**).

Question: What are the potential surgical options?

Answer: The typical patient will have short-segment terminal ileal disease. Macroscopically, the diseased segment is recognised by creeping 'fat wrapping'. When attempting to manipulate the diseased segment with a laparoscopic grasper, it is often difficult to hold because of the increased thickness of the bowel wall. The usual operative procedure undertaken is resection of the terminal ileum and adjacent caecum and appendix. The procedure is completed by anastomosis of the ileum to the ascending or transverse colon. It is usually necessary to mobilise the hepatic flexure to

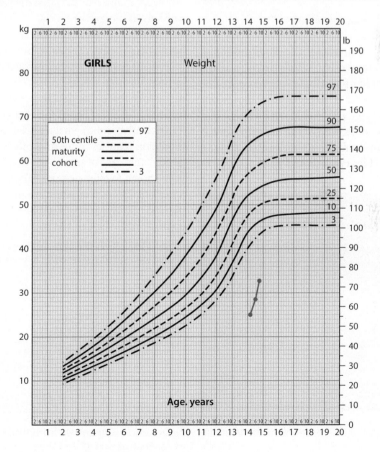

Figure 28.6 Growth chart of a child following ileal resection.

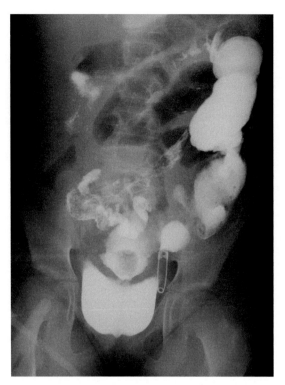

Figure 28.7 Entero-vesical fistula.

allow a tension-free anastomosis. Anastomosis is typically stapled side to side, which can be accomplished either intracorporeally or extracorporeally. Intracorporeal intestinal stapling is a significant laparoscopic challenge and should not be attempted by occasional operators, who would be better served by an extracorporal anastomosis through a small midline incision (**Figures 28.8** and **28.9**).

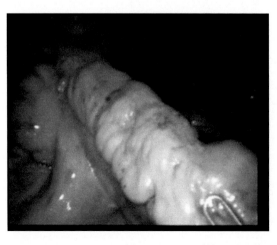

Figure 28.8 'Creeping fat' wrapping of the terminal ileum.

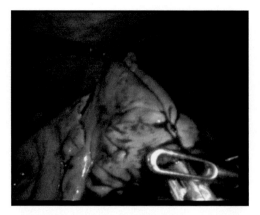

Figure 28.9 Side-to-side intracorporeal stapled anastomosis following Crohn's resection.

Question: Does the absence of diarrhoea exclude inflammatory bowel disease?
Answer: Diarrhoea signifies colitis, which may be due to either ulcerative colitis, Crohn's colitis or indeterminate colitis. Infectious causes should always be excluded. Severe Crohn's colitis is usually accompanied by perianal disease, which is very unlikely in ulcerative colitis.

There is uncertainty about the best surgical management of Crohn's colitis. While the disease distribution suggests segmental resection as a reasonable option, the high disease recurrence rates often lead to further resection. Severe perianal disease often leads to a final end ileostomy after colonic resection.

Ulcerative colitis that cannot be brought into remission requires restorative proctocolectomy. Ileal pouch anal anastomosis (IPAA) has consistently been shown to offer superior functional outcomes to a straight ileo-anal anastomosis. In a Canadian comparison of IPAA and straight ileo-anal anastomoses, approximately half of the straight ileo-anal anastomoses never achieved anal defaecation and 30% were excised or converted to an IPAA (**Figure 28.10**) [2].

Type of anastomosis	Number in follow-up	Mean follow-up (yr)	Total (%) with transanal defecation restored by original IAA	Total (%) with IAA/pouch taken down
J-pouch	41	5.5 ± 3.4	36 (88%)	3 (7%)
S-pouch	13	6.8 ± 3.0	8 (62%)	4 (32%)
Straight	19	5.8 ± 3.3	10 (53%)	6 (32%)[b]
Total	73[a]	5.8 ± 3.3	54 (74%)	13 (18%)

Figure 28.10 Outcomes from three different types of reconstruction. (From Durno et al. [2].)

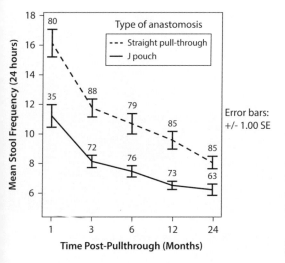

Error bars:
+/- 1.00 SE

Figure 28.11 Stool frequency following IPAA and straight ileo-anal anastomosis. (From Seetharamaiah et al. [3].)

In a comparison of functional outcomes, a combined American and Finnish study emphasised that at every time point following resection, children with IPAA had significantly fewer stools per day than straight ileo-anal anastomosis (**Figure 28.11**) [3].

Stages in restorative proctocolectomy:

The distinction between ulcerative colitis and Crohn's disease is crucially important to avoid constructing an ileal pouch in a patient with Crohn's disease. However, in a patient requiring emergency surgery for either perforation or toxic dilatation, the procedure required is sub-total colectomy with the top of the rectum stapled off and an end ileostomy, so the distinction is immaterial in the acute emergent scenario.

Question: How should perianal disease be managed?

Answer: Perianal sepsis is a frequent and distressing component of Crohn's disease. Significant pain is strongly suggestive of an abscess. While there is a temptation to proceed immediately to exploration, a preliminary urgent MRI can be very helpful. The author has encountered suppurative collections which can be neither seen nor felt but can be drained when guided by preoperative MRI.

Surgery should be minimal. Drain collections by simple incision, either over the perianal skin or the adjacent rectal wall. Do not use wide drainage,

which will simply become a large non-healing ulcer. Do not pack cavities, which is painful to the patient and adds nothing to the treatment.

Fistulae are very common. Probing a collection will usually lead to a point where there is only the thinnest mucosa between the cavity and a finger in the rectum. Pass a Seton suture through this point and tie it loosely with non-absorbable silk; I find vascular sloops ideal for this purpose. It is a mistake to think that you may create a fistula; the fistula is already present but is masked by tissue oedema. The object of the Seton is to allow drainage while medical therapy works.

Severe perianal disease may require temporary diversion in the form of an end sigmoid colostomy. This may allow healing and is certainly a relief for the patient.

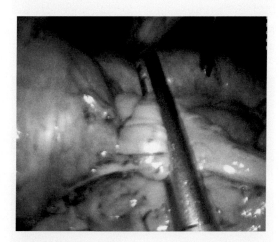

Figure 28.12 Laparoscopic ileal division from devascularised colon.

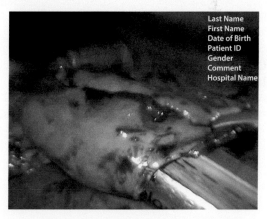

Figure 28.13 Intracorporeal laparoscopic ileal J pouch formation.

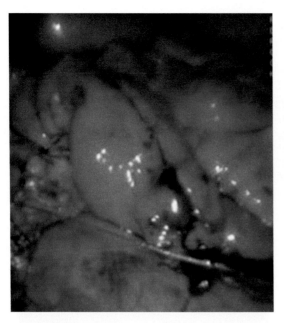

Figure 28.14 Completed ileal J pouch prior to anal anastomosis.

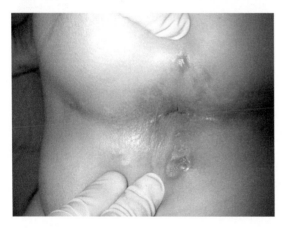

Figure 28.15 External openings of perianal fistulae at three and nine o'clock.

Question: What are the outcomes of paediatric inflammatory bowel disease?

Answer: Around 20% of cases come to surgical resection. Historically, 20% of cases of Crohn's

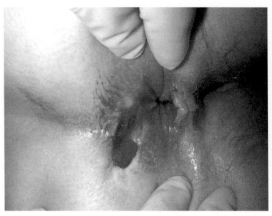

Figure 28.16 A large Crohn's ulcer.

disease then relapse to require further resection, but this may be lesser now in the modern era. Ulcerative colitis cases should receive IPAA, either as a single stage if well or staged if in poor condition. There should be zero mortality for both conditions in advanced health care systems.

BIBLIOGRAPHY

1. Stevens TW, Haasnoot ML, D'Haens GR, Buskens CJ, de Groof EJ, Eshuis EJ, et al. Laparoscopic ileocaecal resection versus infliximab for terminal ileitis in Crohn's disease: retrospective long-term follow-up of the LIR!C trial. Lancet Gastroenterol Hepatol 2020;5(10):900–7.
2. Durno C, Sherman P, Harris K, Smith C, Dupuis A, Shandling B, et al. Outcome after ileoanal anastomosis in pediatric patients with ulcerative colitis. J Pediatr Gastroenterol Nutr 1998;27(5):501–7.
3. Seetharamaiah R, West BT, Ignash SJ, Pakarinen MP, Koivusalo A, Rintala RJ, et al. Outcomes in pediatric patients undergoing straight vs J pouch ileoanal anastomosis: A multicenter analysis. J Pediatr Surg 2009;44(7):1410–7.

29

Lower gastrointestinal bleeding and polyps in children

OLUGBENGA AWOLARAN AND BRUCE OKOYE
Department of Paediatric Surgery, St George's University Hospitals NHS Trust, London, UK

INTRODUCTION

Lower gastrointestinal bleeding (LGIB) is defined as bleeding originating from the intestine distal to the ligament of Treitz. LGIB is uncommon in children and is responsible for 0.3% of emergency presentations. The median age at presentation is 8–10 years. About 80% of presentations are self-limiting. Bleeding from the colon, rectum and anal region is usually bright red. From the small bowel the blood is darker, while melaena is seen in proximal gastrointestinal (GI) lesions.

AETIOLOGY

The most common causes of LGIB by age groups are:

- *Infants*: Allergic colitis, anal fissures
- *2–5 years*: Polyp, anal fissure, infectious enterocolitis
- *Older children*: Anal fissure, infectious enterocolitis, polyp, inflammatory bowel disease (IBD) (**Table 29.1**)

CLINICAL PRESENTATION

Commonly, bleeding is painless and detected on wiping after defaecation or may be seen in the pan. The blood may coat the outside of the stool or be

Table 29.1 Common differential diagnoses of LGIB

Perianal lesions: Anal fissure, haemorrhoids
Colitis: Infectious, allergic, IBD
Polyps
Vascular disorders: Arteriovenous malformation, Dieulafoy lesion, angiodysplasia
Congenital malformations/obstructive causes: Meckel's diverticulum, duplication cyst, malrotation with volvulus, intussusception
Systemic disorders: Henoch-Schoenlein purpura, haemolytic uraemic syndrome, bleeding disorders
Upper GI causes
Non-GI causes: Haematuria, menstruation, ingested substances (red – beets, candies, ampicillin; black – iron supplements, blueberries)

separate from the stool in the pan. Bright red blood suggests a distal source in the anal region, rectum or colon. Less commonly, patients present with a severe and large rectal bleed requiring emergency admission. Occasionally, patients may present with intermittent moderate bleeds. Maroon-coloured blood suggests a source within the small bowel. Melaena is rarer in children.

DOI: 10.1201/9781003182290-32

INVESTIGATIONS

Depending on the clinical presentation, the following investigations will be appropriate:

- Blood tests – routine tests including full blood count, electrolytes, liver function tests, clotting profile and cross-match (rarely needed unless bleeding is massive).
- Stool sample for faecal calprotectin, microscopy and culture.
- Ultrasound may identify GI malformations including Meckel's diverticulum, polyps, duplication cyst and intussusception.
- Rectosigmoidoscopy and colonoscopy.
- Meckel scan (technetium-99 pertechnetate scintigraphy).
- Red blood cell scan (technetium-99 labelled).
- Angiography.
- Video capsular endoscopy (VCE).
- Small bowel enteroscopy.
- Diagnostic laparoscopy.

MANAGEMENT

When a child presents with mild rectal bleeding, they are usually seen in an outpatient setting. Careful history taking and physical examination will often reveal the cause of the bleeding. An association with painful defaecation usually suggests an anal fissure, although this is not always the case. Bright red blood suggests a distal source. A history of constipation should be sought, as this may be the underlying cause. There may be a history of a lesion prolapsing from the anus suggesting a polyp.

Physical examination should be thorough assessing the overall condition of the child, including nutritional state, signs of anaemia or cutaneous vascular lesions. Examination of the abdomen should be performed mainly to assess for faecal masses. Perineal examination is essential. Examination should look for the presence of anal skin tags suggesting anal fissure. Gentle stretching of the anus may reveal an obvious fissure. Digital rectal examination may be performed during which a polyp may be detected. However, if this is considered necessary, it may be more appropriate to perform an examination under general anaesthetic when a proctosigmoidoscopy can also be performed. Any polyp detected at this examination can be excised at the same time. Should findings all be negative

at this point, it is appropriate to observe and perform no further investigations, as sinister aetiology is extremely rare in children. If symptoms persist, then a colonoscopy should be performed to investigate further.

For acute rectal bleeding, the priority is to assess the severity of bleeding and haemodynamic status of the child and resuscitate as necessary. Following resuscitation, subsequent management depends on the clinical course. If the child stabilises and there is no further bleeding, then investigations can be carried out electively.

MECKEL'S DIVERTICULUM AND BOWEL DUPLICATIONS

Meckel's diverticulum occurs due to failure of regression of the vitelline duct. It is a true diverticulum present on the antimesenteric border of the ileum. It is found in about 2% of the general population, and it is symptomatic in about 2–4%. Duplication cysts can occur anywhere along the GI tract. Bleeding occurs due to the presence of ectopic gastric mucosa within the diverticulum or duplication cyst. Ultrasonography may detect a duplication cyst or, rarely, a Meckel's diverticulum. Technetium-99 pertechnetate scintigraphy (Meckel's scan) has a 60–80% sensitivity for detecting Meckel's diverticulum. The ectopic gastric mucosa within the Meckel's diverticulum takes up the technetium selectively, thereby allowing detection (**Figure 29.1**). Premedication with a histamine H2-receptor antagonist or proton pump inhibitor increases diagnostic yield. A negative scan, however, does not rule out Meckel's diverticulum. This investigation could also pick up ectopic gastric mucosa within a duplication cyst. If these lesions are detected, they can be excised surgically.

Should these lesions not be detected by ultrasound or Meckel's scan following a large bleed, a laparoscopic investigation of the bowel is indicated, and this may be carried out in conjunction with colonoscopy if needed.

MANAGEMENT OF ACUTE PERSISTENT RECTAL BLEEDING

Occasionally there is persistent rectal bleeding which is unresolving, requiring ongoing resuscitation. In this scenario, the aim of management is to locate the source of bleeding and stop it.

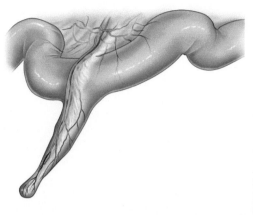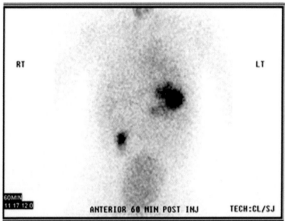

Figure 29.1 Schematic diagram of Meckel's diverticulum and appearance on Meckel's scan.

CT angiography and/or occlusion of bleeding vessels by interventional radiologists may be a feasible option where these services are available. However, these may not always reveal the source of the bleeding if the rate and volume of blood loss are not significant (<0.5 mL/min). Likewise, red blood cell scans are only helpful if there is active bleeding in excess of 0.1 mL/min.

If it is not possible to identify the source of bleeding, then laparoscopy (with or without laparotomy) is indicated, along with upper and lower GI endoscopy (**Figure 29.2**). Sequential clamping of the small bowel may help identify the source of the bleeding, and segmental bowel resection may be required.

GASTROINTESTINAL POLYPS

GI polyps are one of the most common causes of rectal bleeding in children. The incidence is 1–2% of the paediatric population. Polyps are found in 20% of children undergoing colonoscopy for rectal bleeding; 80% present with painless rectal bleeding, 10% with prolapsing polyp and the remaining 10% with complex symptoms (including anaemia, intussusception, diarrhoea and oedema from hypoalbuminaemia). Eighty percent are located in the colon and rectum, of which 80% are solitary.

CLASSIFICATION

Simple juvenile polyp

This is the most common type of polyp found in children, responsible for over 80% of cases. They commonly present between age 2 and 5 years. They can be solitary or multiple (two to four). Histologically, they are benign hamartomas. Some present as a prolapsing polyp, which can be expelled spontaneously. Polyps in the distal colon may be excised during proctosigmoidoscopy. Of importance, full colonoscopic evaluation is recommended when polyps are detected, as there may be multiple polyps. There is a 5–10% risk of polyp recurrence. Surveillance colonoscopy is not required in solitary cases. However, repeat colonoscopy after 5 years is recommended where there are multiple polyps.

Polyposis syndromes

These are multiple polyps in children that are commonly associated with genetic mutations and present with extraintestinal manifestations.

JUVENILE POLYPOSIS SYNDROME (JPC)

Diagnosis is made if there are five or more juvenile polyps in the colon/rectum in a lifetime or any number of juvenile polyps with a positive family history. They are hamartomas histologically. About 50% will have germline mutation (*SMAD4* or *BMPR1A* genes. Genetic testing should be carried out in all diagnosed cases.

JPC confers about a 50% lifetime risk of later GI malignancy. Management is by endoscopic removal of polyps >10 mm followed by annual surveillance until no polyp >10 mm is identified, then 1- to 5-yearly surveillance colonoscopy. Asymptomatic

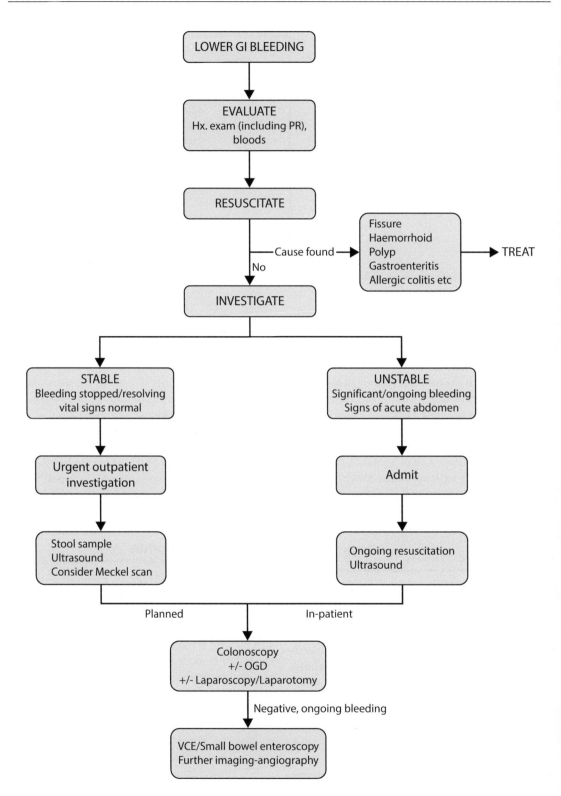

Figure 29.2 Suggested management approach for LGIB in children. *Abbreviations*: OGD: Oesophago-gastroduodenoscopy, VCE: Video capsular endoscopy.

family members should have genetic testing from age 12 and 1- to 5-yearly surveillance colonoscopy. Colectomy is recommended in those with high polyp burden or dysplasia on histology.

PEUTZ–JEGHERS SYNDROME (PJS)

This is diagnosed if two or more histologically confirmed PJS polyps are found or any number of polyps in a child with characteristic mucocutaneous pigmentation or positive family history. A germline mutation is found in 95% of cases (*STK11* gene). They are histologically hamartomas but distinct from juvenile polyps. More than 80% of polyps are located in the stomach and small bowel. Intussusception is the most common complication experienced, found in about 50% of cases.

Sixty percent will develop cancer (GI and extraintestinal) by age 60. Endoscopic polypectomy is performed for polyps >1.5 cm. Asymptomatic family members should have genetic testing from age 3 and 3-yearly oesophagogastroduodenoscopy (OGD), colonoscopy and VCE from age 8 years. These investigations should be performed every 3 years in asymptomatic children diagnosed with PJS and earlier in symptomatic cases.

FAMILIAL ADENOMATOUS POLYPOSIS (FAP)

Diagnosis is made if there are >100 adenomatous polyps. The *APC* gene mutation is responsible for this condition, and there is a 100% GI cancer risk by age 50.

Polypectomy is recommended for polyps >10 mm or that show signs of malignancy. Asymptomatic family members should undergo genetic testing from age 12 and 1–3-yearly surveillance colonoscopy if the gene is confirmed. Colectomy is recommended for all cases, which is usually performed in early adulthood. The two main surgical options are colectomy with ileorectal anastomosis (IRA) and proctocolectomy with ilea-pouch anal anastomosis (IPAA). IPAA is recommended in those with significant rectal burden of adenomas (>20 rectal polyps).

CONCLUSION

Surgeons are frequently involved in the diagnosis and management of children with LGIB. The clinical stability and severity of bleed should the direct management approach. Simple diagnostic tools like focused and systemic examination, laboratory tests and ultrasound scan could provide diagnosis in a significant number of cases. These should be employed first before more invasive investigations. A logical algorithm is provided. Colonoscopy plays a major role in the diagnosis and management of LGIB. While most polyps are simple and solitary, some will be multiple and syndromic, needing genetic testing and long-term surveillance. Prompt involvement of the paediatric gastroenterologist is crucial.

BIBLIOGRAPHY

1. Kawada PS, O'Loughlin EV, Stormon MO, Dutt S, Lee, CH, Gaskin KJ. Are we overdoing pediatric lower gastrointestinal endoscopy? J Pediatr Gastroenterol Nutr. 2017, 64(6), 898–902.
2. Kay M, Eng K, Wyllie R. Colonic polyps and polyposis syndromes in pediatric patients. Curr Opin Pediatr. 2015;27(5):634–41
3. Thakkar K, Fishman DS, Gilger MA. Colorectal polyps in childhood. Curr Opin Pediatr. 2012; 24(5):632–7.
4. Sahn B, Bitton S. Lower Gastrointestinal Bleeding in Children. Gastrointest Endosc Clin N Am. 2016;26(1):75–98.
5. Romano C, Oliva S, Martellossi S, Miele E, Arrigo S, Graziani MG, Cardile S, Gaiani F, de'Angelis GL, Torroni F. Pediatric gastrointestinal bleeding: Perspectives from the Italian Society of Pediatric Gastroenterology. World J Gastroenterol. 2017;23(8):1328–1337.
6. de Ridder L, van Lingen AV, Taminiau JA, Benninga MA. Rectal bleeding in children: endoscopic evaluation revisited. Eur J Gastroenterol Hepatol. 2007;19(4): 317–320.
7. Hu Y, Wang X, Jia L, Wang Y, Xin Y. Diagnostic accuracy of high-frequency ultrasound in bleeding Meckel diverticulum in children. Pediatr Radiol. 2020;50(6):833–839.
8. Qu NN, Liu RH, Shi L, Cao XL, Yang YJ, Li J. Sonographic diagnosis of colorectal polyps in children: Diagnostic accuracy and multifactor combination evaluation. Medicine (Baltimore). 2018;97(39):e12562.

9. Cohen S, Hyer W, Mas E, Auth M, Attard TM, Spalinger J, Latchford A, Durno C. Management of juvenile polyposis syndrome in children and adolescents: A position paper from the ESPGHAN polyposis working group. J Pediatr Gastroenterol Nutr. 2019;68(3):453–462.

10. Hyer W, Cohen S, Attard T, Vila-Miravet V, Pienar C, Auth M, Septer S, Hawkins J, Durno C, Latchford A. Management of familial adenomatous polyposis in children and adolescents: Position paper from the ESPGHAN polyposis working group. J Pediatr Gastroenterol Nutr. 2019;68(3):428–441.

11. Latchford A, Cohen S, Auth M, Scaillon M, Viala J, Daniels R, Talbotec C, Attard T, Durno C, Hyer W. Management of Peutz-Jeghers syndrome in children and adolescents: A position paper from the ESPGHAN polyposis working group. J Pediatr Gastroenterol Nutr. 2019;68(3):442–452.

30

Constipation and fecal incontinence

PAYAM SAADAI
University of California, Davis and Shriners Hospitals for Children-
Northern California, Sacramento, USA

MARC A. LEVITT
Children's National Hospital, Washington, DC, USA

Severe chronic refractory constipation is a substantial health and emotional burden for affected children and their families. Chronic constipation with or without fecal soiling may be secondary to a variety of conditions treated by pediatric surgeons, including anorectal malformations, Hirschsprung disease, spinal cord problems, and colonic dysmotility. True (anatomic) fecal incontinence must be distinguished from soiling related to constipation, sometimes referred to as encopresis. Understanding this major differentiation is key to determining the correct bowel treatment plan. Various medical and surgical interventions are reviewed. Manometric and motility evaluation, both anorectal and colonic, can be helpful in the workup of children with constipation and can guide therapy including several key surgical options.

> **Scenario:** A 4-year-old girl is referred to a surgeon by their pediatric gastroenterologist for fecal incontinence, stool withholding, and pain with defecation despite daily therapy with polyethylene glycol. The child's parents are concerned because these symptoms started at 6 months of age and seem to have worsened in the last year.

Question: What is the definition of constipation for pediatric patients? Does the patient's developmental age affect the defining criteria?

Answer: Severe chronic refractory constipation results in a significant burden on the affected child and their family. Functional (sometimes referred to as idiopathic) constipation is a diagnosis of exclusion when no anatomic, physiologic, or histologic etiology for constipation can be identified. The Rome IV criteria have been created to help standardize the definition of functional constipation (https://theromefoundation.org/rome-iv/rome-iv-criteria/). Definitions exist for children less than 4 years of age and those over the age of 4 years. For infants and toddlers up to 4 years old, two or more of the following symptoms must be present for at least 1 month: A maximum of two stools per week, a history of excessive stool retention, painful bowel movements, large-diameter stools, or a large fecal mass in the rectum. For a child with a developmental age of at least 4 years, two or more of the following symptoms must be present each week for at least 1 month: A maximum of two stools per week, an episode of incontinence, volitional stool retention, painful bowel movements, large-diameter stools, or a large fecal mass in the rectum. Difficult and painful bowel movements often

DOI: 10.1201/9781003182290-33

promote withholding behavior and stool accumulation, perpetuating the cycle of constipation.

In addition to physical symptoms, constipation can lead to school absence, multiple medical consultations, exclusion from social activities, and embarrassment, especially if the patient has fecal soiling. These children and their caregivers often suffer from emotional distress, including anxiety, depression, and low self-esteem, and they may suffer from a decrease in their quality of life (QoL), necessitating a behavioral component to their therapy.

In the scenario described, the child is exhibiting typical stool-withholding behavior. The history of constipation beginning at age 6 months, when solid foods are typically introduced, and worsening during the toilet-training years is common for functional constipation. Intervention should begin by identifying psychosocial stressors contributing to stool withholding, an assessment of dietary behaviors with a focus on increasing water and fiber intake, and initiation of medical therapy if needed to break the cycle of stool-withholding behavior.

Question: How is fecal continence achieved in a normal child and how does this differ from children with anorectal malformations?

Answer: Fecal continence depends on three factors: Anal sphincter muscles (internal and external), anal canal sensation, and reliable appropriate colonic motility. In the typical patient, the voluntary muscle structures (skeletal) are represented by the levator muscles, the sphincter muscle complex, and the parasagittal muscle fibers. For patients with anorectal malformations (ARMs), these voluntary striated muscles have different degrees of hypodevelopment. The involuntary (smooth) muscles, the internal sphincter, are often absent, as they exist in the wall of the distal rectum, which is usually fistulous tissue that is resected at the time of the anoplasty. In a patient without ARM, these structures are intact. However, they may be dysfunctional in that they do not relax at the appropriate time thus leading to constipation.

Voluntary muscles are used only when the patient has an intact anal sensory mechanism that triggers activation. Most patients with ARMs, excluding those with rectal atresia, are born without an anal canal. Therefore, sensation does not exist or is rudimentary. Another group of patients who may lack anal canal sensation are those with spinal cord abnormalities. In contrast, children with Hirschsprung disease are born with a normal anal canal, but this can be injured at the time of their pull-through operation, leading to a dysfunctional anal sensory mechanism. Patients with perineal trauma may likewise have an injured anal canal. Unlike these groups of patients, children with functional constipation have normal anal sensation.

Most individuals can perceive distention of the rectum. This point is important for patients undergoing repair of an ARM. The distal rectum and anus must be placed within the sphincter mechanism for patients to sense stretching of the voluntary muscles. These children might not feel liquid or soft fecal material because the rectum is not adequately distended. Thus, to achieve some degree of bowel control, a patient must have the capacity to form solid stool.

The internal sphincter maintains a closed anus most of the time. When stool is present in the rectum, the stool is detected, and the internal sphincter relaxes secondary to the presence of a recto-anal inhibitory reflex (RAIR). It is at this time that the voluntary muscles take over the role of closing the anus, holding in the stool until the appropriate time, when these muscles are allowed to relax. Various disturbances in the internal sphincter – uncoordinated relaxation – can lead to constipation.

Most patients with an ARM suffer from some disturbance of bowel motility. Constipation is the main clinical manifestation of this disturbance and seems to be more severe in patients with lower defects. Constipation that is not aggressively treated eventually results in an ectatic, distended colon with or without rectosigmoid dilation. This causes more severe constipation and soiling. For patients without an ARM, poor motility can exist (colonic dysmotility). Poor colonic function can be diffuse throughout the entire colon or be limited to one segment of the colon (the sigmoid, most commonly).

Question: How do you define true (anatomic) incontinence vs constipation with soiling?

Answer: Severe constipation with or without fecal soiling may be secondary to a variety of conditions that are treated by pediatric surgeons. True (anatomic) fecal incontinence must be distinguished from overflow soiling (also called encopresis). Children with true fecal incontinence are unable to be clean for stool because of a physiological or anatomic abnormality. These patients can include some surgical patients with ARM, Hirschsprung disease, and congenital or acquired spinal cord problems. Patients with overflow soiling have the potential for bowel control, but they soil because of severe constipation with rectal fecal impaction.

Question: Are all patients with ARM or Hirschsprung disease born with the ability to achieve voluntary fecal continence?

Answer: Most patients who have undergone repair of an ARM have some level of deficiency in their fecal continence mechanism. Some patients with Hirschsprung disease suffer from fecal incontinence because of surgical damage to their anal canal or sphincters or due to dysmotility of their otherwise ganglionated colon. Hirschsprung patients may also need to "learn" how to overcome their nonrelaxing internal sphincters before they can achieve bowel control. Botulinum toxin may help with this sphincter dysfunction.

Patients with a poorly developed or a damaged anal canal or sphincters may not have the ability to achieve fecal continence and will need a mechanical means to stop fecal soiling. This mechanical means involves a high-volume enema program which can be administered either retrograde or anterograde.

Patients with constipation and overflow soiling, on the other hand, are born with the ability to achieve voluntary continence. They have this potential for continence unless they sustain long-term damage that chronic encopresis may cause over many years. Patients with overflow soiling require optimal medical treatment of constipation as the first and often definitive management. This major difference between these two groups of patients – does the patient have potential to achieve voluntary bowel movements or are they anatomically unable to do so – is the key to determining the correct bowel management program that is effective.

Scenario: A 2-month-old is referred by their pediatrician for constipation. The child's parents say that the infant is on formula feeds and will not stool without rectal stimulation.

Question: What are the causes of constipation in a newborn or infant?

Answer: The first stool is passed within 24 hours of birth in about 90% of newborns, and nearly 98% will have passed their first meconium stool within 48 hours. A newborn who fails to pass stool within the first 48 hours of life should be closely monitored and evaluated. A careful exam of the perineum should be performed to rule out an ARM (such as a rectoperineal or rectovestibular fistula anal stenosis). Plain abdominal radiographs will sometimes suggest a particular diagnosis, such as a hemisacrum associated with a presacral mass, or simply reveal evidence of distal intestinal obstruction. Unless the patient has evidence of peritonitis, a water-soluble contrast enema should be performed to evaluate for small left colon syndrome, meconium ileus, meconium plug syndrome, or Hirschsprung disease. A suction rectal biopsy should be performed if there is clinical or radiographic concern for Hirschsprung disease. In patients older than 6 months, a full-thickness biopsy is often necessary to obtain an adequate specimen. It is important to note that premature infants may have a delayed passage of meconium without an underlying problem.

There are several key medical conditions that lead to colonic distension (**Table 30.1**). Organic etiologies such as cystic fibrosis, neuromuscular, metabolic, or endocrine disease are other possible causes of constipation. However, constipation in infants is more likely to be of a functional nature. The typical onset of functional constipation in this age group is around the time of transition from breast milk to formula or to the introduction of solid foods. The infant may have hard stools that are difficult and painful to pass. This traumatic stooling experience may result in voluntary withholding of stool. This behavior is characterized by grunting, arching of the back, and stiffening of the legs and the body.

Infants with functional constipation may respond to the addition of fruit juices to their intake, such as

Table 30.1 Common causes of newborn colonic obstruction

- Hirschsprung disease
- Distal small bowel atresia
- Anorectal malformation
- Meconium plug
- Meconium ileus (associated with cystic fibrosis)
- Allergic proctocolitis (milk protein allergy)
- History of magnesium sulfate intrapartum
- History of diabetic mother (leading to small left colon syndrome)
- History of opioids
- Hypothyroidism

prune juice. Changing formula, especially if the current formula contains iron, may be helpful. Some solid foods that are introduced to the infant's diet such as rice cereal may also be constipating.

Question: What medical therapies should be considered for an infant with constipation?

Answer: If dietary modification is unsuccessful, then a stool softener or a stimulant laxative should be added to the regimen. In patients with mild constipation, a trial of polyethylene glycol, milk of magnesia, lactulose, or sorbitol should be considered. More effective treatment can usually be achieved by a stimulant laxative, but the parent must be taught to adjust the dosage with the goal to achieve a soft and easy-to-pass daily bowel movement. In children with more severe functional constipation, a history of ARM repair, or those who have had prior surgery for Hirschsprung disease, a stimulant laxative by itself or in addition to a stool softener should be used. Adding a water-soluble fiber also helps, as it makes the laxative more effective by providing a little bulk to the stool, so a more formed, yet soft, bowel movement can be passed.

It is important to be aware of a small group of infants who are exclusively breastfed who may not have a daily bowel movement. These patients may have a bowel movement once every 2–14 days (average of 5 days). They do not exhibit any discomfort, and their stools are soft to loose in consistency. These infants do not require further workup. Infant dyschezia is another entity often mistaken as constipation. These infants will typically present in the first few months of life with excessive discomfort and straining during bowel movements and eventually pass soft or loose stool. This is due to the lack of coordination between the increased intra-abdominal pressure and pelvic floor muscle relaxation. In this scenario, parental reassurance is all that is needed, as the problem is self-limited. In the most severe of cases, botulinum toxin of the anal canal can help by relaxing the sphincter complex which allows for the passage of stool.

Scenario: A 3-year-old is having new-onset constipation. Their parents report that they are working on toilet training for both urine and stool. Their older child had no issues with toilet training at all, and they are wondering what they can do.

Question: How is the management of new-onset constipation in a toddler different from the newborn or infant?

Answer: A new onset of constipation in the toddler age group is often related to toilet training. It is still prudent to closely review the stooling history of the patient, as organic etiologies, in the appropriate clinical setting, may be the cause of constipation. If the history, physical exam, and contrast enema do not reveal an anatomical reason for the constipation and medical therapy is not effective, then motility studies may be indicated. Some of these studies may not be readily available at all institutions, requiring referral to specialty centers. However, transit studies such as sitz markers, radionuclear scintigraphy, or a plain X-ray timed for the day after a contrast enema should be available in most places. Anorectal and colonic manometries, when indicated clinically, can play a key role in the therapeutic decision making. If a child is having incontinence for both urine and school or is having lower extremity neuromuscular symptoms, then imaging of the spinal cord with MRI is warranted.

Treatment in this age group generally includes dietary modifications, teaching good toileting habits, and use of stool softeners with or without stimulant laxatives. ARM patients at this stage usually require a more aggressive bowel management program, often with the initiation of rectal enemas.

Scenario: A 10-year-old is referred by the pediatric gastroenterologist for new-onset constipation. She has been having difficulty due to frequent accidents and no longer wants to go to school.

Question:

Answer: New onset of constipation in this age group is uncommon. It must be determined if the constipation is really a new issue or if it is a chronic one that has never been investigated or treated effectively. If it is truly a new problem, then one must consider the possibility of a behavioral cause, psychosocial components, or physical and/or sexual abuse. The start of a new school may be associated with new-onset constipation. Constipation-predominant irritable bowel syndrome (IBS) is another common diagnosis to be considered. Other potential etiologies include tethered spinal cord or occult spina bifida, which should be considered especially if there are persistent urinary symptoms in the absence of a rectal impaction. The evaluation of these children should include at least a contrast enema and possibly the addition of motility studies.

Question: What motility test can be particularly helpful in the workup of an older child with functional constipation?

Answer: Anorectal manometry is useful in that it can provide real-time functional data such as squeeze pressure and the presence of dyssynergia. In addition, an intact RAIR can be documented, which effectively will rule out Hirschsprung disease. Anorectal manometry can also help determine if internal anal sphincter achalasia (IASA) is the cause of severe constipation in an older child. The diagnosis is made when manometry demonstrates an absence of the RAIR in a child who has normal ganglion cells on rectal biopsy. While not common, IASA may be identified in approximately 4% of chronically constipated children. These patients present with severe constipation that is refractory to medical therapy. Intrasphincteric injection of botulinum toxin has been used to treat this condition. It is safe but has variable success. Typically, 100 IU of botulinum toxin diluted in 1 mL of saline is injected equally into the four quadrants of the anal sphincter. The advantage of botulinum toxin injection is that it can be both diagnostic and therapeutic and lasts no more than a few months. Correct diagnosis of this condition and appropriate treatment with botulinum toxin may preclude unnecessary high-dose use of laxatives and unneeded colon resections.

Older children with constipation will occasionally present with recurrent fecal impaction. An initial attempt at disimpaction with retrograde high-volume enemas is reasonable, but manual disimpaction in the operating room under general anesthesia may be required. It is critical to ensure that the patient does not have stool impacted in the rectum prior to initiating oral cathartics, as this clinical scenario represents a distal bowel obstruction, and the medications will lead to severe cramping or even stercoral perforation.

RADIOGRAPHIC AND MOTILITY EVALUATION

Question: What imaging and motility studies can be helpful in a patient with constipation refractory to medical management?
Answer: Please see the following sections.

Contrast enema

A contrast enema provides information regarding the diameter, length, and redundancy of the colon, stool burden, and provides catharsis (disimpaction). An anal or colonic stricture or a transition zone may also be assessed for patients who have had prior anorectal or Hirschsprung surgery. A plain abdominal radiograph the following day provides useful information regarding the motility of the colon. If much of the contrast remains on plain X-ray, then it can be concluded that the child has a slow-moving (hypomotile) colon. If the colon is empty the day after the contrast enema, this is an ideal time to initiate stimulate laxative therapy. Colonic hypermotility is suspected if the patient has fecal incontinence with a tendency toward diarrhea, a normal-caliber colon, and no contrast on the follow-up X-ray.

Sitz marker study

A Sitz marker study is an efficient, inexpensive, and readily available colonic transit study. It involves having the patient swallow radiopaque rings (markers) and subsequently have plain abdominal X-rays performed over the course of several days. A child with normal motility will have passed most of the markers on day four and all of them on day seven (**Figure 30.1**). In a patient with total colonic inertia and diffuse dysmotility, these markers accumulate in the right colon. In patients with more of an outlet obstruction and normal colonic motility, the markers will be located predominately in the rectosigmoid colon. Other patients with segmental colonic dysmotility may have markers retained in the affected segment.

Colonic nuclear transit study (colonic transit scintigraphy)

A colonic nuclear transit study using scintigraphy has the advantage of being a more senstive measure of colonic motility than a Sitz marker study while remaining noninvasive. In this study, a radioactive isotope is ingested and its progression through the colon followed. Several measurements, including overall colonic transit as well as transit through several anatomic areas of interest, can be obtained. The scintigraphic technique uses minimal radiation, but like the Sitz marker study, can take a few days to complete.

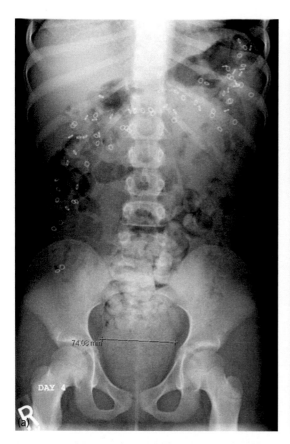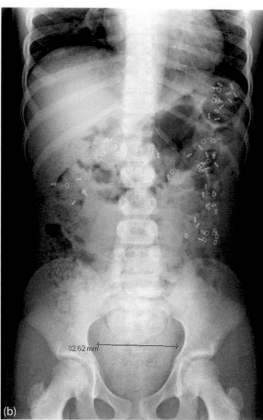

Figure 30.1 Sitz marker study demonstrating distal dysmotility. Abdominal radiograph day 4 (a) and day 7 (b) after the patient swallowed 24 marker capsules.

Manometric evaluation

Children with chronic constipation with or without encopresis who have failed aggressive medical therapy should undergo additional testing and are good candidates for colonic manometry. It is important to evaluate colonic motility prior to surgical intervention such as a diverting stoma, antegrade enema procedure, or segmental colonic or rectosigmoid resection. This evaluation entails functional and anatomic mapping of the colon and is enhanced by performing anorectal manometry to assess the function of pelvic floor musculature and the anal sphincters.

Colonic manometry requires an adequate bowel prep. The study begins with placement of a manometry catheter with equally spaced recording sites either endoscopically or using fluoroscopic guidance. Typically, the study is performed over 6 hours.

The patient's motility is observed for the first 2 hours while still fasting, and then the patient is given an age-appropriate meal. This is followed by a postprandial observation period. The colonic motility index is expected to increase following a meal due to the gastrocolic reflex mechanism. An abdominal X-ray is typically done following the postprandial observation period to document the location and course of the catheter as well as the position of the pressure sensors. A colonic stimulant such as liquid bisacodyl or glycerin is then infused through the catheter to induce high-amplitude propagating contractions (HAPCs). If, and when, the patient has a response to the stimulant medication, one can accurately localize the origin of each HAPC, the duration, and the distance traveled. A normal HAPC is defined as contractions with a pressure amplitude greater than 60 mmHg, lasting at least 10 seconds and propagating 30 cm or more.

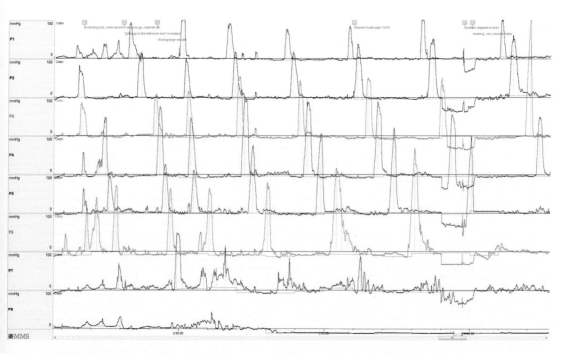

Figure 30.2 Normal colonic manometry tracing. An eight-sensor water-perfused catheter tracing with sensors spaced 10 cm apart is shown. The top tracing is from the most proximal sensor. A normal high amplitude propagating contraction is defined as contractions with a pressure amplitude greater than 60 mmHg, lasting at least 10 seconds and propagating 30 cm or more.

The information obtained from a colonic manometry study may demonstrate that a patient has one of the following scenarios:

1. *Normal motility*: Normal or mildly slow motility with strong HAPCs that propagate fully to the rectosigmoid junction, where they are normally expected to stop (**Figure 30.2**).
2. *Diffuse dysmotility*: Absent motility without any HAPC in the entire colon despite repeated and escalating doses of a stimulant laxative.
3. *Segmental dysmotility*: Normal motility in the proximal colon with HAPCs that terminate at some point prior to reaching the rectosigmoid junction. Identifying the affected segment of colon is helpful prior to therapeutic intervention (**Figure 30.3**).

The SmartPill motility system (Medtronic) is a newer method of noninvasive testing that can provide information not just from the colon but the entirety of the gastrointestinal tract. It is especially helpful if a motility disorder that is not confined to the colonic area is suspected. The child ingests a capsule that measures pressure, pH, transit time, and temperature as it passes through the gastrointestinal tract. The sensor is sensitive enough to capture gastric emptying time, whole gut transit time, colonic transit time, and pressure patterns from the antrum and duodenum.

MEDICAL TREATMENT

Scenario: A 7-year-old boy has suffered with constipation for several years. He has been to the emergency room three times in the past 12 months for disimpactions and admissions for cleanouts. During these admissions, he has required enemas, but he has never had a maintenance treatment after these episodes.

Question: What are the initial medical therapies for chronic constipation, and what screening laboratory tests should be obtained?
Answer: Please see the following section.

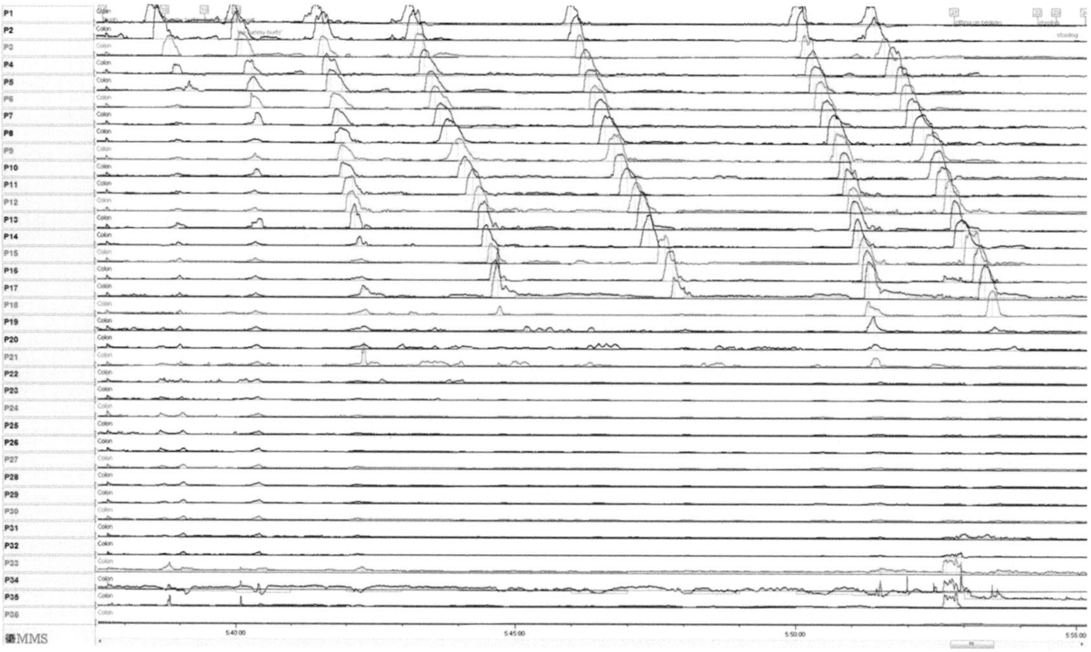

Figure 30.3 Colonic manometry tracing with distal dysmotility. High-resolution solid-state colonic manometry catheter with sensors spaced 3 cm apart is shown. The top tracing is from the most proximal sensor. Normal motility is seen in the proximal colon with high amplitude propagating contractions that terminate prior to reaching the rectosigmoid junction.

Dietary modification and medical laboratory screening

The first step in any bowel management program must include a thorough assessment of the patient's diet. The vast majority of children in Western societies would benefit from increased water and fiber intake, and a registered dietitian can be invaluable in identifying deficiencies in nutrient intake and making recommendations for dietary modifications. For some children, changes in nutritional intake, such as removing lactose from the diet, can completely resolve constipation symptoms if initiated early in the onset of symptoms. Routinely screening children with significant constipation symptoms after the age of potty training for celiac disease, food allergies, and hypothyroidism is recommended.

Question: How does the treatment for a child who is soiling due to loose stools differ from one who has constipation from hard stools?
Answer: Children with loose stools have an overactive colon. First, a cause for hypermotility

must be checked for, such as inflammatory bowel disease, infectious diarrheas, and IBS, diarrheal type. In patients with fast motility, a constipating diet, bulking agents (e.g., water-soluble fibers), and/or medications (e.g., loperamide) to slow down the colon are used. Constipating and laxative foods are shown in **Table 30.2**. If the patient has a foreshortened colon related to prior surgery (such as in an ARM patient who has had an abdominal perineal pull-through with loss of the rectum, a Hirschsprung disease patient with loss of a significant amount of their colon for the pull-through, or a patient with ulcerative colitis who has had an ileoanal pull-through), a daily small-volume enema may also be required. To determine the right combination, treatment is initiated with enemas, a very strict diet, loperamide, and a water-soluble fiber. Most children respond to this aggressive management within 1–2 weeks. The child should remain on a strict diet until clean for 24 hours for 2–3 days consecutively. This diet includes three scheduled meals and no snacks. They can then choose one new food every 2–3 days, and the effect of this new food on the child's

Table 30.2 Food products and stool consistency

Constipating foods	Laxative foods
Refined Foods	*Whole Grain Foods*
White bread	Whole wheat bread
White rice	Whole grain pasta
Pasta	Brown rice
Sweets (chocolate)	Bran cereal
Fruits	*Fruits and Vegetables*
Banana	Apples with skin
Apple without skin	Berries, dried figs
Apple sauce	Carrots, peas,
Foods High in Fat	broccoli
French fries	Pears, peaches,
Fast food	prunes
Fried foods	Fruit juices
Meats	*Beans*
Red meat	Black beans
Boiled, broiled, baked	Kidney beans
chicken or fish	Pinto beans
Dairy	*Dairy*
Cheese	Yogurt
Milk	

colonic activity is observed. If the child soils after eating a newly introduced food, that food must be eliminated from the diet. Over several months, the most liberal diet possible should be sought. If the child remains clean with a liberal diet, the dose of the medication can gradually be reduced to the lowest effective dose to keep the child clean for 24 hours.

Some children with hypermotility, especially those patients with total colonic Hirschsprung disease, may develop a severe and painful buttock rash. The management of this excoriation requires diligent local and systemic care. We recommend the addition of the following in an escalating fashion depending on the severity of the rash and treatment response: Constipating diet, fiber supplementation, small-volume enemas, loperamide, cholestyramine, hyoscyamine, diphenoxylate/atropine, and clonidine (see Bibliography). Involvement of a pediatric gastroenterologist with experience in motility disorders is recommended for patients who require multimodal pharmacological therapy. The buttocks should also be covered with zinc oxide–based barriers, skin emollients, and/or liquid skin protectants with each diaper change.

Question: How should medical management be escalated in a child who does not respond to the initial steps of treating constipation?
Answer: Please see the following sections.

Fiber

Both water-soluble and water-insoluble fibers are mainstays in fiber treatment for the management of constipation. When mixed with a liquid, soluble fibers dissolve to form a gel-like substance, as opposed to insoluble fibers which pass through the gastrointestinal tract relatively unaltered. Both can provide bulk to stools, but we often recommend water-soluble fiber (e.g., psyllium, pectin, methylcellulose, guar gum [Table 30.3]) to maximize the bulking effect and maintain a good balance between stool frequency and consistency. This bulking of the stool is important, as it allows the child to be more aware of the stool in the rectum and can help provide feedback as to when it is time to have a bowel movement. There are many kinds of fiber that are available over the counter in stores, but it is important to get the sugar-free versions of these. Foods and supplements high in sugar can make stools looser and cause a reverse effect.

Stimulant laxatives

A more aggressive management regimen is required when dietary measures fail. Medications that are designed to increase the colon's motility are much more effective than stool softeners. One common misconception is that softening of the stool without a stimulant medication is all that is needed to produce effective bowel movements. This approach, however, may be self-defeating, because loose stool may not result in adequate rectal distention that triggers an urge to defecate. Therefore, the softer stool is not felt in the rectum (no rectal distension), and this leads to more soiling.

High-dose stimulant laxatives and bulking agents such as pectin or water-soluble fiber such as psyllium are initiated once the patient has been disimpacted. The disimpaction process is a vital and often neglected step. This includes the administration of enemas three times a day until the patient is disimpacted (confirmed radiographically). If the patient remains impacted after 3 days, despite saline enemas, then an oral bowel prep is

Table 30.3 Commercially available soluble fiber options

Type	Dosage and use	Where to find it
Pectin (Sure-Jell©)	1 Tablespoon = 2 grams of fiber	Found in the grocery store in the jelly/canning section or online at www.pacificpectin.com Get the sugar-free version.
Citrucel©	Powder 1 Tablespoon = 2 grams of fiber Capsule 2 capsules = 1 gram of fiber	Found in the pharmacy section of the store. or online at www.citrucel.com You can use the generic or the brand name. Get the sugar-free version.
Metamucil© (psyllium husk)	Powder 1 Teaspoon = 2 grams of fiber Capsule 5 capsules = 2 grams of fiber Wafer 1 packet (2 wafers) = 3 grams of fiber	Found in the pharmacy section of the store or online at www.metamucil.com Get the sugar-free version.
Nutrisource© (guar gum)	1 Tablespoon (scoop) = 3 grams of fiber *Can be sprinkled on food or mixed in drinks.*	Found in the pharmacy section of the store, online, or through homecare companies.

needed, sometimes via nasogastric tube, and if this is not successful, then manual disimpaction under anesthesia should be considered.

Stimulant laxative therapy includes senna-based products. The starting dose of senna is variable depending on the child's age and history, but typically begins with 15–30 mg and is titrated according to response. Bisacodyl is another stimulant that has been very effective in inducing colonic contractions and stool evacuation. If the child does not have a bowel movement within 24 hours, a bowel cleanout with polyethylene glycol is often needed to evacuate the distal stool, and the laxative dose is increased once the rectum is confirmed to be clean on abdominal X-ray. Sometimes a rectal enema is helpful. Water-soluble fiber administered to patients receiving stimulant laxatives will add bulk and increase the efficacy of the laxative. This is usually dosed at 1 tablespoon three times a day.

It is important to remember that patients may have laxative requirements that are much greater than the manufacturer's recommendation. Occasionally, in the process of increasing the amount of laxatives, patients may experience severe abdominal cramping, nausea, or vomiting before reaching the desired effect. In these patients, a different medication can be tried, but some patients may not tolerate any of these laxatives at a dose that allows for the colon to empty effectively. These patients are considered to have an intractable

condition and may need to be switched to enemas or considered for surgical intervention. Segmental colon resection is rarely needed. Only if there is a dysmotile segment on motility testing and the patient cannot empty medically with medicines or retrograde or antegrade enemas is surgery indicated. The dysmotile segment usually corresponds with a significantly redundant and dilated segment of colon, usually the sigmoid, but sometimes the left or transverse colon can be dysmotile as well.

Question: What is a typical enema program, and which patients should begin the treatment of their constipation with enemas?
Answer: Please see the following section.

Enemas

Patients with true (anatomic) fecal incontinence who have a tendency toward constipation (*hypomotility*) should not be treated with laxatives; instead, these patients need a mechanical emptying program. The patient and their caregivers are taught how to clean the colon once daily with a retrograde or antegrade enema, so the child stays completely clean for 24 hours until the next enema. A plain radiograph performed shortly after the enema will confirm that the enema led to an empty rectosigmoid colon. If passage of stool happens many hours after the enema and the X-ray shows persistent stool in the rectosigmoid colon, then the enema provided inadequate cleaning and the patient needs a larger-volume enema, a stronger irritating enema, or both. If stool passes quickly after the enema and the X-ray is clean, then the enema may be too irritating. and the enema itself may be the cause of the "accidents."

In contrast, children with true fecal incontinence who have loose stools (*hypermotility*) make up a very small percentage of those with fecal incontinence. This scenario is generally the result of resection of the rectum and sigmoid colon. Rapid transit of stool results in frequent episodes of diarrhea even when an enema effectively cleans their colon. To treat this situation, laxative-type foods are eliminated and a constipating diet with or without medications (loperamide and water-soluble fiber), as described earlier, to slow down the colon are necessary.

Large-volume enema therapy includes a saline solution (0.9% saline can be made by adding 2 teaspoons of salt to 1000 mL of water) and often requires the addition of stimulants. The initial enema volume is generally 20 mL/kg of normal saline. It is rare to use a volume greater than 750 mL. Most enema cocktails start with 400 or 500 mL of saline. In children over 5 years of age plain water is also fine, but is slightly less provocative in emptying of stool. We have not found the volume of contrast used on the contrast enema to be predictive of the therapeutic volume of saline. If normal saline alone is ineffective, glycerin (10–30 mL) or another unscented soap (Castile or a baby soap or shampoo; 1–3 packets, 9–27 mL) is added. To make an enema even stronger, bisacodyl liquid can be added, particularly in patients in whom the motility testing showed a response to this medication. It should be noted that colitis has rarely been reported with enemas containing soap, and this possibility should always be considered in a patient doing well with an enema routine for a while who suddenly starts having diarrhea, which may be mucus laden or blood tinged.

Patients are taught to hold the retrograde enema for 10 minutes and then sit on the toilet for 30–45 minutes. The solution is adjusted until the child effectively empties their colon with the enema and has no accidents between enemas. Bowel management may be performed in a similar way in children with a colostomy who are being considered for definitive repair but who have a cloacal

exstrophy malformation, for example, and an end stoma. If the patient can form solid stool and if the stoma bag remains empty of stool for 24 hours after the enema, then the child can potentially undergo a pull-through of that colon and be expected to remain clean thereafter with anterograde enemas.

During the initial week of bowel management, a daily outpatient abdominal X-ray is obtained, and the patients/parents are contacted by phone/email/video call to evaluate treatment. Treatment regimens are adjusted based on the child's clinical and radiographic response. The treatment plan is considered successful when the abdominal radiograph is empty of stool in the rectum and left colon and the child has no soiling.

Question: What is a typical bowel management program or "bootcamp"?
Answer: Please see the following sections.

Bowel management program

Children with severe constipation or fecal incontinence may go through an intensive week of tailored bowel management at specialized centers that have bowel management programs. Most of these therapy programs are undertaken as outpatients, although some centers prefer inpatient bowel management to limit the number of extraneous variables affecting care. Details vary from center to center, but typically the week begins with a water-soluble contrast enema the day before the visit and an abdominal X-ray the day of the clinic evaluation. The provider can determine the diameter and length of the colon and the stool burden. This also provides catharsis and allows for the patient to start the program with an empty colon. Motility may be roughly assessed based on the X-ray then obtained the day after the contrast enema. A treatment plan is designed based on the patient's history and imaging results. The therapeutic goal is determined in collaboration with the patient and caregivers at the outset, but most often the objective for most patients is to empty the colon regularly and to be free of soiling or abdominal pain between the emptying maneuver (either medicines or enemas). Other specialists including a nutritionist, social worker, psychologist, and child life therapist can be invaluable in the initial assessment of the child and for determining an appropriate treatment plan for each individual patient.

If the contrast enema has not adequately evacuated the colon, then a mechanical cleanout with polyethylene glycol or enemas should be initiated so as to begin the program with an empty colon.

Once there is minimal stool burden in the colon as confirmed by radiograph, management plans generally consist of either high-dose senna-based stimulant laxatives or a daily large-volume enema. However, there is a small group of patients with a foreshortened colon and a tendency toward diarrhea who are managed with small-volume enemas, a constipating diet, a bulking agent such as psyllium, and antimotility agents such as loperamide.

In older patients who have been toilet trained in the past but have soiling from encopresis or have severe constipation without soiling but with other significant symptoms (abdominal pain, bloating, poor appetite), high-dose laxatives are initiated following stool disimpaction. In patients who have never been toilet trained and have a history of soiling or in those patients with a megarectum, daily large-volume enemas are initiated. It is important for a child to have been toilet trained or have had a period of being clean, wearing normal underwear, prior to initiating a laxative program. This may be more easily accomplished with the initial use of enemas. For children who do not tolerate retrograde enemas or oral laxatives, such as those with severe autism, severe anxiety disorder, or a history of abuse, a manual disimpaction is scheduled under general anesthesia followed by behavioral and aggressive medical therapy. If a trip to the operating room for disimpaction is necessary, the surgeon should consider whether anorectal manometry with rectal biopsy to rule out Hirschsprung disease and/or injection of botulinum toxin to treat a high pressure external sphincter or internal anal achalasia may be of benefit. An antegrade continence enema procedure (ACE stoma) is the next therapy resort if this strategy fails.

Follow-up

After a successful regimen has been initiated, children should be followed closely, as this is the key to preventing relapse of soiling or severe constipation. When a child has been successful on enemas for 3–6 months, a laxative trial can be attempted if the child is felt to have the potential for adequate bowel control. The laxative trial is performed as previously described. Patients who are repeatedly unsuccessful with laxatives are given the option to continue retrograde enemas and try laxatives again in 6–12 months or undergo an ACE procedure. A Malone appendicostomy or cecostomy tube may be used for antegrade continence enemas. Patients are also encouraged to undergo laxative trials periodically following the ACE procedure, if appropriate. The antegrade flushes are a valuable aid tool for "potty training" as the child can practice holding in the flush and releasing it, which simulates bowel control.

SURGICAL TREATMENT

Scenario: A 3-year-old boy is having new-onset constipation. His parents report that they are working on toilet training for both urine and stool. Their older child had no issues with toilet training at all, and they are wondering what they can do.

Question: What is the role of a pediatric surgeon in the management of functional constipation?
Answer: Pediatric surgeons are often consulted by pediatricians, emergency physicians, or pediatric gastroenterologists to assist in children with severe cases of fecal impaction. If a child is to undergo general anesthesia for disimpaction, that is a prime opportunity to obtain valuable diagnostic information in select patients. In a child with a suspicious history for Hirschsprung disease but in whom the diagnosis has not been ruled out, a rectal biopsy may be warranted. If an anorectal manometry has not been done by the gastroenterologists, this is an ideal time for that study to be scheduled as well. Botulinum toxin injection into the anal canal can be given under the same anesthetic if the anorectal manometry shows either an absent RAIR (which requires a biopsy to rule out Hirschsprung disease) or high sphincter resting pressure.

Antegrade enemas

For children in whom bowel management with retrograde enemas has been successful and in whom a long-term enema program is indicated, or for children who are resistant to rectal maneuvers but would benefit from mechanical emptying, the pediatric surgeon may offer a surgical antegrade continence operation such as appendicostomy, neo-appendicostomy, or cecostomy.

Malone appendicostomy

In the laparoscopic ACE procedure, also known as a Malone procedure, an appendicostomy is created. The appendix is connected to the umbilicus or in the right lower quadrant. The orifice site matures to be intermittently catheterized, or a skin-level tube can be left in place. This operation allows enemas to be given in an antegrade fashion using the patient's native appendix as a catheterizable channel. The cecum is plicated around the base of the appendix to create a valve mechanism that prevents stool from leaking back through the umbilicus (**Figure 30.4**). The operation is usually recommended when patients want to become more independent, as it allows administration of enema without parental assistance. For children who are "anally defensive" and cannot tolerate rectal enemas, an appendicostomy is highly beneficial as a "bridge to continence".

Some children with spina bifida or other urologic problems either may already have a Mitrofanoff stoma accessing the bladder for self-catheterizations at the umbilicus or they will need one. If the child needs both a Mitrofanoff and an ACE, a preoperative discussion with the pediatric urology team is necessary to determine for which procedure the appendix will be best used or if splitting of the appendix is an option (**Figure 30.5**).

In patients with a thicker abdominal wall, the appendix may not reach the body surface without compromising its blood supply. This point should be carefully considered preoperatively. A nice option in this case is to bring the appendiceal tip to the skin and not perform a plication.

The most frequent complication of appendicostomy is stomal stricture. The V-V advancement technique for the umbilical-appendiceal anastomosis has been shown to decrease the incidence of this complication. A broad V-shaped skin incision is made with the apex of the V at the base of the umbilicus (**Figure 30.6a**). The incision is extended inferiorly through the skin and fascia to externalize the appendicocecal junction for cecal plication. The tip of the appendix is spatulated away from the mesentery, and the circumferential anastomosis is begun by approximating the apex of the skin flap to the spatulated portion of the appendix (**Figure 30.6b**). The completed anastomosis is partially lined with epithelium, which reduces the risk of stricture. Occasionally patients or parents will elect to have

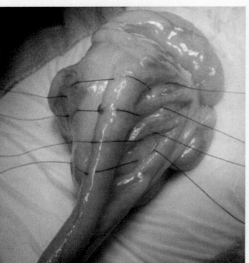
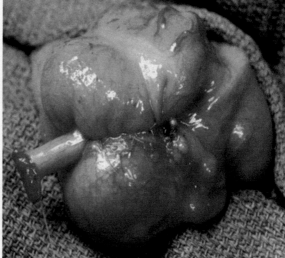

Figure 30.4 Creation of a Malone appendicostomy. After creation of mesenteric windows, a plication is performed using several nonabsorbable sutures to prevent fecal reflux.

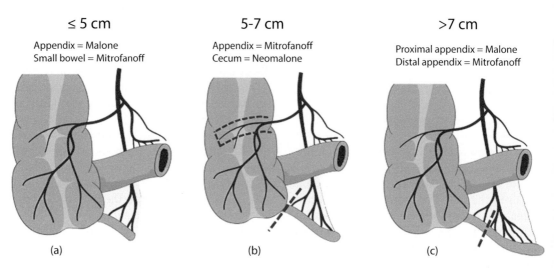

≤ 5 cm

Appendix = Malone
Small bowel = Mitrofanoff

5-7 cm

Appendix = Mitrofanoff
Cecum = Neomalone

>7 cm

Proximal appendix = Malone
Distal appendix = Mitrofanoff

(a)　　　　　　　　(b)　　　　　　　　(c)

Figure 30.5 In patients in whom both a Malone and a Mitrofanoff are indicated, there are various strategies that may be employed depending on whether the appendix is less than 5 cm in length (a), between 5 and 7 cm in length (b), or greater than 7 cm in length (c).

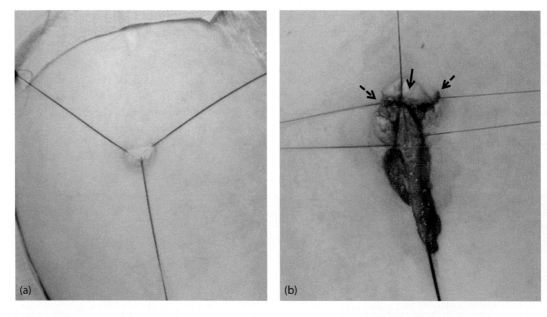

(a)　　　　　　　　(b)

Figure 30.6 The V-V advancement technique for the umbilical-appendiceal anastomosis. The broad V-shaped skin incision is shown with the apex of the V at the base of the umbilicus oriented toward the bottom of the photograph (a). The tip of the appendix is spatulated away from the mesentery and the circumferential anastomosis created by approximating the apex of the skin flap to the spatulated portion of the appendix (b). Dashed arrows represent the corners, and solid arrow represents the apex.

an indwelling silicone device placed through the appendicostomy in order to avoid daily catheterization. An algorithm pathway for initiation of postoperative antegrade enemas is outlined in **Table 30.4**.

Neo-appendicostomy

If there is no appendix or if the appendix is needed for a Mitrofanoff, creating a tube from a flap of cecum (continent neo-appendicostomy) is an option. A triangular skin flap is created at the umbilicus as in

Table 30.4 Postoperative antegrade enema protocol

Appendicostomy (native appendix)

Begin antegrade enema postoperative day 1:

Postoperative day 1: ½ volume (pre-op enema solution) × 1

Postoperative day 2: Full-volume flush, daily

Follow up: Indwelling tube stays in place 4–6 weeks

Neo-Appendicostomy

Begin antegrade enema when starting solid food

Day 1 (of solid foods): ½ volume (pre-op enema solution) × 1

Day 2 (of solid foods): ½ volume (pre-op enema solution) twice a day

Discharge enema: ½ volume (pre-op enema solution) twice a day × 4 weeks

Follow up: Indwelling tube stays in place for 4–6 weeks

the Malone procedure. The right colon is mobilized. A site located on the ascending colon away from the ileocecal valve is selected for creation of the flap. A feeding vessel from the mesentery is identified and the transverse flap created (**Figure 30.7**). The flap must be large enough to tubularize over an 8 Fr feeding tube. The colonic wall is then plicated around the neo-appendix, taking care to avoid apposition of the two suture lines. The umbilical-appendiceal anastomosis is then performed as in the Malone in a V-V fashion.

Cecostomy

An alternative to an appendicostomy for antegrade enemas is a skin-level device such as a Chait trapdoor cecostomy or a low-profile gastrostomy feeding tube.

These tubes may be placed through the abdominal wall in the right lower quadrant directly into the cecum using laparoscopic or percutaneous techniques. The benefits of a skin-level device include the avoidance of daily catheterization and elimination of the risk of stomal stricture. This option is ideal for children with sensory processing disorders in whom intermittent catheterization is impractical. However, issues such as abscess, granulation tissue, leakage, parastomal cutaneous fecal fistula, and inadvertent tube dislodgement are common.

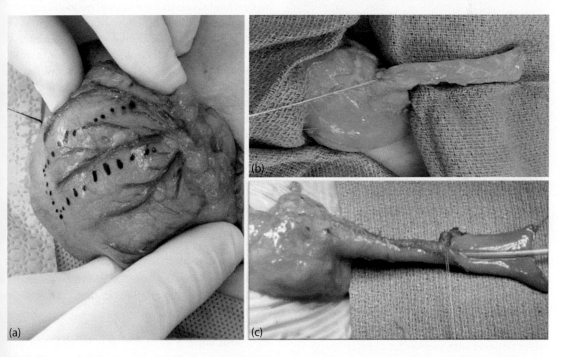

Figure 30.7 Technique for a neo-appendicostomy. A feeding vessel is identified and preserved (a). The colonic wall is plicated around the neo-appendix, taking care to avoid apposition of the two suture lines (b). A transverse flap large enough to tubularize over an 8 Fr feeding tube is created (c). The umbilical-appendiceal anastomosis is then performed as in the Malone in a V-V fashion.

COLONIC RESECTION

Question: Is there a role for colon resection in pediatric functional constipation?

Answer: In children with a megarectosigmoid or very redundant sigmoid colon who require long-term bowel management, segmental bowel resection will reduce their daily laxative requirement or required daily enema volume. The rectum is generally divided at the level of the peritoneal reflection, removing the redundant sigmoid (**Figure 30.8**). We recommend segmental colectomy in children only after they have had a thorough motility assessment, and who have failed antegrade flushes.

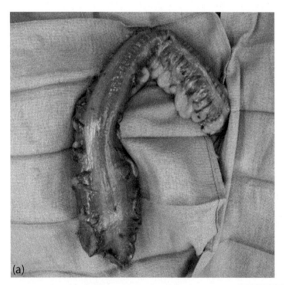

(a)

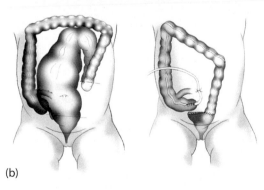

(b)

Figure 30.8 Partial colectomy may be useful in select patients with segmental dysmotility (a). This is often performed in conjunction with an antegrade enema program (b). Recently, we have found that performing an ACE prior to colectomy may help obviate the need for partial colectomy.

A colectomy does not cure their constipation, but rather will assist in subsequent bowel management, making it an easier colon to empty, either by laxatives or flushes. A staged approach beginning with a trial of an antegrade enema program with an ACE or cecostomy and progressing to a sigmoidectomy only if that fails is best to avoid the morbidity of colon resection. These patients must be followed closely afterward because the remaining colon and rectum are most likely abnormal and there may be recurrence of their severe symptoms long-term.

In patients with an ARM, the rectum should remain intact because the patient needs it for continence, as discussed earlier. From a technical point of view, if the sigmoid colon ever needs to be resected in an ARM patient, the surgeon must take great care to preserve the sigmoid vessels to the distal rectum. Because these patients often have had a colostomy, the marginal vessel to the distal rectum may have been interrupted. In addition, the rectum was likely fully dissected to perform the anoplasty; thus, the inferior and middle hemorrhoidal arcades have likely also been ligated. In these patients, the rectum depends on the superior hemorrhoidal vessels for its nutritive blood supply.

For patients with functional constipation who have not undergone any rectal surgery and have a normal anal canal and sphincters, the upper rectum and sigmoid can be resected with preservation of fecal continence (i.e. a low anterior resection). The very distal rectum (6 cm) should be preserved so as to not interfere with the continence mechanism. It is good to remember that resection of the rectosigmoid down to the dentate line is what is performed for patients with Hirschsprung disease, and these patients can maintain their continence provided the anal canal and sphincters are preserved.

OUTCOMES

Question: What are the outcomes of bowel management for functional constipation, and how is success defined?

Answer: Bowel management can be considered successful when a patient is able to wear normal underwear and stay totally clean for 24 hours. This is achievable in approximately 85%–95% of children with ARMs, Hirschsprung disease, spinal disorders or severe intractable idiopathic constipation.

Regardless of the underlying disorder, bowel management plans often require tailored modification over time. Thus, careful patient follow-up is a key component to a successful program.

Surgical complications

Stomal stricture is the most common indication for appendicostomy revision. This complication ranges from 13% to 50% and is often used to support placement of a cecostomy tube by many surgeons. By creating the stoma using the V-to-V technique described earlier and using an indwelling tube for a longer period of time, this complication may be reduced. Leakage accounts for approximately one quarter of stoma revisions, occurring in 6–35% of patients. The cause of leakage is likely multifactorial. Leakage will often occur when the patient is not effectively emptying the colon with the antegrade enema and becoming progressively impacted. Once a successful enema is found, the leakage will improve or resolve. In some patients, leakage may be related to breakdown of the cecal plication. The need for cecal plication is debated, as the appendix has a normal antireflux valve in many patients, and no consensus or large prospective series exists evaluating this technical aspect of the procedure. Interestingly, the incompetence of the ileocecal valve may play a role in "failure" of antegrade flushes, as the flush goes into the terminal ileum causing nausea and cramping and obviously not cleaning the colon. Interventional radiology can fashion a longer tube that sits in the right colon to solve this problem. Stomal prolapse occurs in less than 5% of patients but will require a skin-level revision to prevent mucus from constantly soiling clothing. In children who undergo partial colectomy, anastomotic stricture is a rare but possible complication. This can usually be managed endoscopically with dilations.

FUTURE CONSIDERATIONS

Sacral nerve stimulation

The effect of sacral nerve stimulation (SNS) on bowel function was initially appreciated in early studies evaluating its effect on voiding dysfunction. The exact mechanism of action is unknown, but some evidence suggests that SNS normalizes intestinal transit by modulation of the enteric nervous system or its reflex pathways at the spinal cord level. Studies in children are limited, with variable outcomes reported. However, data suggests that when used in carefully selected patients, SNS results in an increased frequency of defecation and decrease in abdominal pain in many cases.

Summary Points

- A variety of organic, functional, and anatomical problems can lead to constipation and fecal incontinence. These must be thoroughly evaluated and addressed before the symptom of constipation can be effectively treated.
- Contrast studies are indicated in most patients for diagnosis, treatment, and predictive purposes.
- Evaluation of challenging patients can be greatly enhanced by motility studies.
- The management of patients with ARMs or Hirschsprung disease must be proactive in order to avoid progressive dilation and dysfunction of the bowel.
- The ACE procedure can be very effective in medically refractive cases or patients with neurological problems.
- Practitioners caring for children with severe constipation or fecal incontinence must be committed to finding the best therapy program that works for the individual patient. This program will often require modification over time.

BIBLIOGRAPHY

1. Wood R, et al. One-year impact of a bowel management program in treating fecal incontinence in patients with anorectal malformations. J Pediatr Surg, published online: May 8, 2021;56(10):1689–93.
2. Chatoorgoon K, et al. Neoappendicostomy in the management of pediatric fecal incontinence. J Pediatr Surg. 2011;46(6):1243–9.
3. Eradi B, et al. The role of a colon resection in combination with a Malone appendicostomy as part of a bowel management program for the treatment of fecal incontinence. J Pediatr Surg. 2013;48(11):2296–300.
4. Khan WU, et al. The percutaneous cecostomy tube in the management of fecal incontinence in children. J Vasc Interv Radiol. 2015;26(2):189–95.

5. Lawal TA, et al. Laparoscopic-assisted Malone appendicostomy in the management of fecal incontinence in children. J Laparoendosc Adv Surg Tech A. 2011;21(5):455–9.

6. Levitt MA, Kant A, Pena A. The morbidity of constipation in patients with anorectal malformations. J Pediatr Surg. 2010;45(6):1228–33.

7. Rangel SJ, et al. The appendix as a conduit for antegrade continence enemas in patients with anorectal malformations: Lessons learned from 163 cases treated over 18 years. J Pediatr Surg. 2011;46(6):1236–42.

8. Russell KW, Barnhart DC, Zobell S, Scaife ER, Rollins MD. Effectiveness of an organized bowel management program in the management of severe chronic constipation in children. J Pediatr Surg. Published online: December 5, 2014. doi: 10.1016/j.jpedsurg.2014.08.006

9. Clarke MC, et al., Quality of life in children with slow transit constipation. J Pediatr Surg. 2008;43(2):320–4.

10. Athanasakos EP, et al. Clinical and psychosocial functioning in adolescents and young adults with anorectal malformations and chronic idiopathic constipation. Br J Surg. 2013;100(6):832–9.

11. Loening-Baucke V. Prevalence, symptoms and outcome of constipation in infants and toddlers. J Pediatr. 2005;146(3):359–63.

12. Vilanova-Sanchez A, et al. Total colonic Hirschsprung's disease: The hypermotility and skin rash protocol. Eur J Pediatr Surg. 2020;30(4):309–16. doi: 10.1055/s-0039-1694744. Epub 2019 Aug 20. PMID: 31430765.

13. Lu PL, Mousa HM. Constipation: Beyond the old paradigms. Gastroenterol Clin North Am. 2018;47(4):845–62. doi: 10.1016/j.gtc.2018.07.009. Epub 2018 Sep 28. PMID: 30337036.

14. Tabbers MM, DiLorenzo C, Berger MY, Faure C, Langendam MW, Nurko S, Staiano A, Vandenplas Y, Benninga MA. Evaluation and treatment of functional constipation in infants and children. J Pediatr Gastroenterol Nutr. 2014;58(2):258–74.

15. Rodriguez L, Sood M, Di Lorenzo C, Saps M. An ANMS-NASPGHAN consensus document on anorectal and colonic manometry in children. Neurogastroenterol Motil. 2017;29(1). doi: 10.1111/nmo.12944. Epub 2016 Oct 9. PMID: 27723185.

16. Siminas S, Losty PD. Current surgical management of pediatric idiopathic constipation – a systematic review of published studies. Ann Surg. 2015;262(6):925–33.

31

Chest wall deformities

ELIZABETH O'CONNOR AND HANY GABRA
Great North Children's Hospital, Newcastle, UK

Scenario: A 15-year-old male attends outpatient clinic stating his chest has "caved in". He had noticed a depression in his chest for a few years, but it has gotten a lot worse over the last 6 months.

Question: What is the diagnosis (Figure 31.1)?

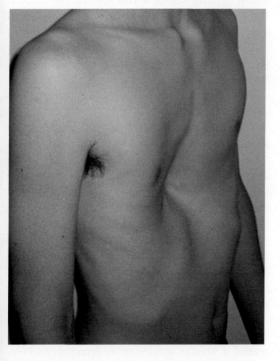

Figure 31.1 Photograph of a post pubertal male with significant pectus deformity.

Answer: Pectus excavatum.

This is the most common type of chest wall deformity, characterised by a posterior depression of the anterior chest wall, usually affecting the lower sternum. The defect can be mild, moderate or severe.

In a third of patients the pectus deformity may be noted in infancy, but it typically presents at puberty, when the defect rapidly worsens with the pubertal growth spurt. The incidence of pectus excavatum ranges from 1/400 to 1/1000 population, although there may be geographical variations. There is typically a male predominance (M>F 4:1).[1,2]

Question: What symptoms would you ask this boy about?

Answer: Chest pain, palpitations, shortness of breath and reduced exercise tolerance. Any psychological effects of the condition impacting on his self-esteem or daily lifestyle? Any associated conditions?

Although the defect may present notably earlier in young children, pectus deformities tend to be asymptomatic because of significant pulmonary and cardiac reserve and a pliable chest wall. At puberty, symptoms then develop as the deformity becomes more severe and the chest wall more rigid.

Patients may complain of reduced exercise tolerance and difficulty keeping up with their peers at sports. Males often become embarrassed by the appearance of their chest and seek to avoid sporting physical activities at school. Patients often adopt a typical "pectus posture" with a thoracic kyphosis, forward-sloping rounded shoulders and a protuberant abdomen appearance.[1]

DOI: 10.1201/9781003182290-34

Question: Is there a genetic component to pectus excavatum?

Answer: Yes – there is a genetic predisposition, with the condition being inherited in an autosomal dominant, autosomal recessive, X-linked and multifactorial fashion. Pectus excavatum is associated with Marfan's syndrome (2.7% of patients), Ehlers-Danlos syndrome (0.7%) and idiopathic scoliosis (20%).

Twenty medical genetic disorders have been shown to be associated with pectus excavatum, and genetics referral is thus recommended if patients fulfil certain criteria (**Figure 31.2**).[3]

Question: What examination features will you specifically look for?

Answer: It is important to examine the patient both in the erect standing and supine positions, as posture can affect the appearance of the defect.[2]

The pectus deformity can have a focal or cup-shaped appearance or be a diffuse/saucer-shaped depression. Next assess the deepest point of the deformity. If this is not in the midline, then it is considered an asymmetric defect. Look for the typical pectus posture plus any associated scoliosis. Any rib flaring should be recorded, and carefully examine for any phenotype features associated with Marfan's syndrome – very tall thin patients with a wide arm span, which can also be noted with Ehlers-Danlos syndrome.

Question: What is Marfan's syndrome?

Answer: Marfan's syndrome is an autosomal dominant inherited connective tissue disorder characterised by tall stature and hypermobile joints with dislocation of the lens of the eye. Patients can also present with spontaneous recurring pneumothorax, dissecting aortic aneurysm and mitral valve prolapse.

Question: Are there cardiac and pulmonary effects as a result of having pectus excavatum?

Answer: This is a much-debated controversial topic with some surgeons believing that pectus excavatum is mainly a cosmetic problem. As more patients come forward seeking minimally invasive pectus repair, preoperative and postoperative investigations do show improvements in exercise tolerance and striking evidence of preoperative cardiac and pulmonary restriction (ACTS, Sigalet D et al, Maagard et al - Normalised CP exercise function in patients with PE 3 years after operation).

The severity of the defect, the status fitness level of the patient and any associated conditions will influence the extent of the cardiopulmonary effects of pectus excavatum. Additionally respiratory function tests taken at rest or during exercise may show impairment. Patients may often keep up with peer groups at rest, with reduced exercise tolerance becoming apparent when they are challenged with sporting physical activity.

Cardiac effects include decreased cardiac output, mitral valve prolapse and arrhythmias, which have all been shown to be associated with pectus excavatum. Significant compression of the heart leads to reduced cardiac filling, reductions in stroke volume and therefore impaired cardiac output. Compression of the heart can also interfere with normal heart valve function. Mitral valve prolapse is recorded in up to 65% of patients with pectus excavatum compared to only 1% in the normal healthy paediatric population. Dysrhythmias such as Wolf-Parkinson-White syndrome are seen in 16% of affected patients.

Pulmonary effects result from restricted movement of the depressed part of the thoracic cage. Lung function tests show a reduction in forced vital capacity (FVC) and forced expiratory volume (FEV).

Question: What investigations would you schedule for this patient?

Answer: After taking a full history and clinical examination, several investigations can help plan treatment.

Clinical photography is important to document the deformity and will be used to monitor progress during treatment.

Some clinicians will rely on a chest X-ray (CXR) alone.[4]

CT scan: Very helpful study to show the degree of cardiac compression and displacement with the deformity and pulmonary compression with atelectasis. CT can be used to calculate the Haller index (transverse diameter divided by the antero-posterior [AP] diameter of the chest). MRI does not give adequate bone images.

Echocardiography: Important to document heart compression, reduced chamber filling and reduced cardiac output. It is important to document a structurally normal heart before embarking on corrective pectus surgery.

Lung function studies and cardiopulmonary exercise testing: Cardiorespiratory workup is essential if Marfan syndrome is detected. As mentioned earlier, with severe pectus deformity, these parameters will be notably affected, and the cardiorespiratory exercise index often returns back

Scoring list referral of patient with pectus excavatum for genetic counseling

Patient with pectus excavatum

≥1 Major criteria or ≥2 Minor criteria*

Major criteria

Family
- First degree family member with PE and/or a congenital anomaly (for example congenital heart defect).

Growth
- Height< 2SDS or >2SDS
- Micro- of macrocephaly

Neurology and senses
- Intellectual disability or developmental delay or autism
- Muscular hypotonia
- Hearing loss

Congenital anomalies and dysmorphisms
- Craniosynostosis
- Dysmorphic facial features, score 1 for each (Low set ears, Downslanting palpebral features, long facies, Short webbed neck, Arachnodactyly or brachydactyly)
- Cleft palate or high arched palate
- Increased span and/or limited elbow extension
- Cardiovascular anomalies
- Diaphragmatic hernia
- Anomalies of thumb and/or halluces
- Loose redundant skin and/or three or more café-au-lait spots or lentigines
- Cryptorchidism

Other medical problems
- History of pneumothorax
- Malignancy

Minor criteria

Congenital anomalies and dysmorphisms
- Dysmorphic facial features, score 1 for each (dysplastic ears or hypertelorism or malar hypoplasia or retrognathia and/or micrognathia or widow's peak or coarse facial features)
- Joint hypermobility and/or dislocations
- Rib and spinal deformities
- Pes planus
- Shawl scrotum
- Hypoplasia of the pectoralis major and/or Anomalies of thumb/halluces
- Kidney anomalies
- Limb joint contractu res and/or Limb defects

Neurology and senses
- Movement disorder
- Seizures

Other medical problems
- Lung emphysema in childhood

Referral for genetic counseling

Our advice is to refer to a clinical geneticist those patients with pectus excavatum who have at least 1 major criterium or at least 2 minor criteria.

*Some features of the identified genetic disorders have not been added to the major and minor criteria as they are not easily recognizable in a surgical consultation setting. These features however may be important in recognizing an underlying molecular defect. Examples are dural ectasia, lisch noduli of the eye , hormonal deficiencies, bleeding diathesis and Multiple jaw keratocysts.

Figure 31.2 Criteria for referral for genetic counselling for patients with pectus excavatum.

towards normal expected values with corrective surgery.

Psychological assessment: Is crucial, as patients may have low self-esteem because of perceived distorted body image, and the Pediatric Quality of Life evaluation (PDQL) is an invaluable baseline before and after the operation.

Question: What is the Haller index for the patient shown in the Figure 31.3?

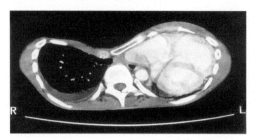

Figure 31.3 CT of severe pectus excavatum patient showing dept of sternal depression.

Answer: The Haller index (HI) is the number obtained by dividing the transverse diameter of the chest by its AP diameter.

In healthy patients without a pectus deformity, this index would be typically <2. If the HI is >3.2, the patient is deemed to have a significant pectus defect, and surgical correction is traditionally warranted based on these criteria.

Question: How will you manage this patient?
Answer: Consider non-surgical options first (bracing).

He does not complain of chest pain, palpitations or shortness of breath. He does not like to go swimming any more, however, as he is very embarrassed by the appearance of his chest. He also states difficulty keeping up with his peers while running or playing football at school.

The following flow chart shown in **Figure 31.4** is used to guide management.[5]

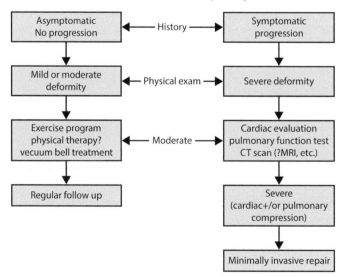

Figure 31.4 Algorithm of suggested evaluation and treatment.

In the UK, National Health Service (NHS) funding for corrective surgery has been discontinued. UK paediatric surgeons are now mainly deploying bracing.

Question: What is meant by pectus bracing?
Answer: The vacuum bell therapy (VBT).

This is a suction device used to create a vacuum and lift forward the chest wall designed by Dr Eckart Klobe in 2005. It is a safe therapy for treating pectus excavatum non-operatively. VBT has been shown to have higher success rates in those younger patients who present earlier, with milder deformities (pectus excavatum depth <3 cm), have a symmetric pectus excavatum or have a more compliant chest wall with lack of costal flaring. The recommendation is to use the vacuum bell for a minimum of 30-minute sessions twice daily. More recent literature now suggests VBT can be extended for a maximum of several hours per day. Around 79% of pectus patients will have a sternal elevation of more than 1 cm after only 3 months of VBT therapy. The sternum is lifted to a normal level in 13.5% of index patients after approximately 18 months. Outcomes are reportedly best in patients with mild and symmetrical pectus.

The vacuum bell has also been useful for elevating the sternum during operative pectus repair (see next).

Question: What are the current surgical procedures described to treat pectus excavatum?
Answer: See the following sections for more information.

RAVITCH OPERATION

Ravitch introduced and popularised this pectus operation in 1949.[5] It is an open procedure, involving an anterior chest wall incision. Skin and muscle flaps are then elevated, exposing the underlying costal cartilages. The rib perichondrium is incised longitudinally and the deformed cartilages partially/completely excised. An anterior wedge-shaped sternal osteotomy is then performed at the site of the defect. The sternum is subsequently elevated with this operation and the osteotomy closed. One of the main significant complications that may develop after a Ravitch operation is acquired asphyxiating thoracic chondrodystrophy (ACT), so various modifications have been subsequently introduced to provide more stability to the chest wall in an effort to reduce ACT risk.

A much less aggressive approach detailed next is employed by many surgeons nowadays, and the open Ravitch approach is now best reserved for older patients with significant asymmetrical and/or recurrent pectus after a Nuss operation, discussed later.

NUSS PROCEDURE – MINIMALLY INVASIVE REPAIR OF PECTUS EXCAVATUM (MIRPE)

In 1997 Nuss et al. pioneered and reported a 10-year experience with a new minimally invasive technique. Later in 1998 thoracoscopy was added to the key operation steps to make the procedure safer to avoid iatrogenic cardiac injury.

Steps: The chest is marked with a circle using an ink pen at the site of the deepest depression, then two crosses are made on either side of the sternal defect. Metal bar(s) used to correct the deformity are custom measured for the patient and bent into shape using a bar bender.

Incisions are made on the skin surface on either side of the chest wall. A subcutaneous tunnel is created and then bilateral thoracotomy incisions are made. An introducer device is inserted into the chest cavity guided under thoracoscopic vision. The pleura and pericardium are carefully dissected off the under-surface of the sternum. The introducer device is then slowly advanced across the mediastinum and exteriorised through the thoracostomy incision on the opposite side. When the introducer is secure in place, the sternum is lifted out of its depressed position by the introducer.

An umbilical tape is then attached to the introducer and the device slowly withdrawn. The pectus support bar (or bars) are then attached to the umbilical tape and slowly guided into place via the substernal tunnel. The bar convexity faces posteriorly until it emerges on the patient's contralateral side.

Once the bar is positioned in the chest with the convexity facing posteriorly, it is 'flipped over' with bar flippers. This manoeuvre corrects the pectus excavatum defect like 'sucking out a motorcar dent'. The bar is safely secured into position using bar stabilisers and peri-costal sutures. Occasionally an additional correction bar may be needed.

More recently a 'pectus up' procedure has also been described – a new minimally invasive surgical technique with an implant placed on top of the sternum, at the subpectoral level in the most sunken depressed area of the chest. Then by means of a smart elevation system, the sternum is lifted to the desired corrective position and fixed with the implant.

Question: What complications may occur during the operative procedure(s)?
Answer: Damage to the important mediastinal and thoracic structures, leading to pneumothorax, haemothorax and cardiac injury. These complications have reduced significantly with the introduction of thoracoscopy, allowing direct visualisation of the thoracic cavity, and now with the deployment of the screw-crane system for pre-lifting the sternal depression intraoperatively, which allows for safer repair.[6]

Question: What complications would you discuss when taking informed consent for the operation from the patient and family when you are planning to undertake the Nuss procedure?

Answer: Please see the following table.

Early	Late
Haemothorax	Bar displacement
Pneumothorax	Failure to adequately correct the defect
Cardiac injury	Infection
Pain	Recurrence of the deformity
Complications associated with the epidural site	Metal allergy

Question: When would you remove the pectus bar?

Answer: The bars are not required permanently to correct the pectus defect. They can be removed after approximately 2–3 years when their in situ support has successfully recontoured the pectus defect.

Scenario: Case 2

Question: What is this anomaly in Figure 31.5?

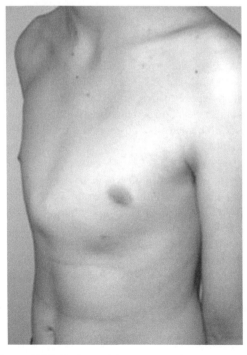

Figure 31.5 Patient with pectus carinatum.

Answer: Pectus carinatum ('Pigeon chest').

A protrusion deformity of the anterior chest wall. It is 10 times less common than pectus excavatum. This defect is not normally apparent until the pubertal growth spurt. It is thought to be due to an abnormal overgrowth of the costal cartilages, resulting in protruberance of the sternum and adjacent costal cartilages.

There are two main types – (1) chondro-manubrial, where the protruberance is maximal at the upper portion of the sternum, and the more common (2) chondro-gladiolar type, where the protruberance is maximal at the xiphi-sternum. The current management is mainly via non-surgical orthotic bracing. Surgery can be considered if bracing fails with either a modified Ravitch procedure or, more recently, an operation involving the insertion of anterior Nuss bar – the Abramson technique.

BIBLIOGRAPHY

1. Holcomb GW, et al (eds). Ashcraft's Pediatric Surgery sixth ed. (2014).
2. Parikh DH, Crabbe DC, et al (eds). Pediatric Thoracic Surgery. Springer Publishers (2009).
3. Billar RJ, Manoubi W, Kant SG, et al. Association between pectus excavatum and congenital genetic disorders: A systematic review and practical guide for the treating physician. J Pediatr Surg. 56, 2239–2252 (2021).
4. Mueller C, et al. Chest X-ray as a primary modality for preoperative imaging of pectus excavatum. J Pediatr Surg. 43, 71–73 (2008).
5. Nuss D, et al. Nuss bar procedure: Past, present and future. Ann Cardiothorac Surg. 5, 422–433 (2016).
6. Park HJ, Rim G. Development of a screw-crane system for pre-lifting the sternal depression in pectus excavatum repair: A test of mechanical properties for the feasibility of a new concept. J Chest Surg. 54, 186–190 (2021).
7. Obermeyer RJ, et al. Nonoperative management of pectus excavatum with vacuum bell therapy: A single center study. J Pediatr Surg. 53, 1221–1225 (2018).

8. Haje DDP, et al. Localized pectus excavatum treated with brace and exercise: Long term results of a Brazilian technique. Acta Ortop Bras. 29, 143–148 (2021).

9. Emil S. Current options for the treatment of pectus carinatum: When to brace and when to operate? Eur J Pediatr Surg. 28, 347–354 (2018).

10. Pilegaard H, Licht PB. Minimal invasive repair of pectus excavatum and carinatum. Thorac Surg Clin. 27, 123–131 (2017).

11. Nuss D, Kelly RE, Croitoru DP, Katz ME. A 10-year review of a minimally invasive technique for the correction of pectus excavatum. J Pediatr Surg. 33, 545–552 (1998).

32

Acute disorders of the ovary

SARAH BRAUNGART
Leeds Teaching Hospitals NHS Trust, Leeds, UK

PAUL D. LOSTY
Institute of Systems and Molecular Biology, University of Liverpool, UK;
and Ramathibodi Hospital, Mahidol University, Bangkok, Thailand

Scenario: A 14-year-old female presents to the hospital emergency department with acute-onset lower abdominal pain. She is pale and clearly in pain. The patient reports the pain started acutely 48 hours ago and was so severe at the onset that she vomited several times. On examination tenderness is noted in the lower abdomen. Vital signs show no fever evident, and blood tests are normal apart from a raised white cell count.

Question: What is your differential working diagnosis?

Answer: The differential list of diagnoses is wide ranging in a 14-year-old girl with lower abdominal pain. These include functional abdominal pain, acute appendicitis, inflamed Meckel's diverticulum, menstrual cycle–related pain such as Mittelschmerz, and acute ovarian pathology – most importantly, acute ovarian torsion and ruptured ovarian cyst. Tubo-ovarian abscess and ectopic pregnancy are less common in this teenage age group, but must not be forgotten. It is important to establish her pubertal status and undertake a full detailed report including gynaecological history. One must not forget to establish if the patient is sexually active and obtain a urine pregnancy test. Bear in mind your professional responsibility in terms of safeguarding. The patient reports that she has had a regular menstrual cycle for 2 years and generally does not suffer from pain. She has never been sexually active. You are very concerned she may have ovarian torsion.

Question: How do you proceed?

Answer: If there is a high suspicion of ovarian torsion, emergency diagnostic laparoscopy should be performed, as this is the only way to reliably diagnose or rule out ovarian torsion. The threshold to proceed to diagnostic laparoscopy should be low, as missing an ovarian torsion will invariably result in ovarian necrosis. There is no imaging investigation that can reliably rule out ovarian torsion, even if Doppler ultrasound is obtained. However, ultrasound may be helpful in establishing an alternative diagnosis such as acute appendicitis.

Question: You proceed to theatre. Intraoperatively you find the right ovary is torted. It is macroscopically dark blue in colour and enlarged even following detorsion. What is your intraoperative management?

Answer: Laparoscopic detorsion of the ovary is the recommended procedure. Even if the ovary appears macroscopically necrotic (dark blue or black in colour), it should not be resected.

DOI: 10.1201/9781003182290-35

Macroscopic findings in ovarian torsion are unreliable to predict viability of an ovarian follicular mass, even if the history is prolonged. Very rarely is resection unavoidable, for example, when the ovary spontaneously disintegrates due to advanced-stage necrosis.

Question: What will be your postoperative management and follow-up?
Answer: The patient can be discharged home once recovered from the operation. A follow-up ultrasound scan and outpatient clinic visit following discharge are useful to assess the sonographic appearance of the ovary after a period of recovery and for patient counselling. A multidisciplinary team (MDT) should be organised to define best practice after-care management and follow-up.

> **Scenario:** You have a 10-year-old girl in outpatient clinic. She has been referred by her family doctor because an abdominal ultrasound (which was obtained because of a urinary tract infection) has identified a 3-cm cyst likely arising from the left ovary. The family is concerned the child will need an operation to remove it.

Question: What information do you require before you can firmly establish a diagnosis?
Answer: In most cases ovarian cysts are asymptomatic and an incidental finding on ultrasound scan. In order to decide on the most appropriate management, it is important to know if the cyst is simple or complex, how large it is (in centimetres) and if the patient displays any clinical signs suggestive of malignancy or precocious puberty.

A simple cyst is typically unilocular, thin-walled and fluid filled, without any solid parts, calcifications or septations. In peri-pubertal and postpubertal females, they are frequently a physiological finding during the menstrual cycle. They may occur when no egg is released from a developing follicle (and so the fluid remains in the cyst) or when the corpus luteum forms a cyst rather than naturally involuting. Simple cysts are not always ovarian in origin; they may also be parafimbrial, paratubal or arise from the broad ligament.

Question: The ultrasound scan shows a simple cyst 3 cm in size, and the patient is otherwise well, prepubertal, with no clinical features suggestive of precocious puberty or malignancy. What is your management plan now?
Answer: As the cyst is small and simple, no intervention is required, and the patient and family can be reassured. A follow-up ultrasound scan should however be obtained in 3 months' time to ensure the cyst is resolving and not growing in size.

Question: When would you recommend intervention for a simple ovarian cyst?
Answer: Cyst removal by minimally invasive ovarian-sparing cystectomy is generally recommended for cysts >5 cm, for two reasons: Large cysts are more likely to act as a lead-point for triggering ovarian torsion and also are more likely to be neoplastic in origin.

Question: Do you know any of other non-neoplastic ovarian cysts?
Answer:

- *Haemorrhagic cysts*: These usually result from haemorrhage into a simple or corpus luteum cyst. Most resolve spontaneously. A follow-up ultrasound scan 2–3 months later will confirm resolution.
- *Endometrioma*: Growth of ectopic endometrial tissue within the ovary may cause an endometrioma or a "chocolate cyst". These usually cause cyclical pain and may be associated with dysmenorrhea and dyspareunia. These do not normally resolve without treatment.

> **Scenario:** A 15-year-old girl presents to the hospital emergency department. She is mid-cycle and experienced a sharp lower abdominal pain this morning. The pain has now improved. On examination her lower abdomen is mildly tender. Blood tests and pregnancy test are unremarkable. An ultrasound scan shows some free fluid in the pelvis; the ovaries otherwise appear normal.

Question: What is the most likely diagnosis?
Answer: The most likely diagnosis is that of a ruptured functional ovarian cyst. This occurs most commonly mid-cycle and is associated with a sharp pain when the follicle ruptures, followed by a dull pain in the lower abdomen, which is caused by peritoneal irritation from the haemorrhagic fluid.

Question: What is your management of this patient?

Answer: The management plan is conservative with simple analgesia and reassurance. The patient should be advised that the pain will resolve spontaneously over the next couple of days. Follow-up is generally not required.

> **Scenario:** A healthy baby girl is delivered. The neonatal doctor calls you for advice as the fetal antenatal ultrasound scan identified a 2.5-cm intra-abdominal cyst, which was thought to be arising from the left ovary.

Question: What are your recommendations on management?

Answer: Antenatal detection of an intra-abdominal cyst is a relatively common scenario in paediatric surgery. The majority of these cysts are ovarian in nature; however, it is never possible to fully make the diagnosis solely based on the antenatal scan. Therefore, the ultrasound scan should be repeated following delivery in order to (1) establish the nature of the cyst, i.e. the organ it is originating from; (2) determine the current size of the cyst; and (3) assess if it is causing any compression or obstruction.

If the baby is clinically well a repeat ultrasound scan may be performed on an outpatient clinic basis at 2–3 weeks of age. If there are any concerning features such as significant abdominal distension, abdominal pain, signs of bowel obstruction or jaundice, further investigations should be obtained on an urgent basis before contemplating hospital discharge.

Question: The baby is well and discharged. The parents return to your clinic following a repeat ultrasound scan with the baby now 6 weeks of age. The repeat ultrasound was not able to clearly identify the cyst, but both ovaries are visualised and normal. What do you now tell the parents?

Answer: Most neonatal ovarian cysts resolve spontaneously. It is believed these cysts originate from fetal stimulation by maternal oestrogens and placental beta-human chorionic gonadotropin (HCG).

They are most often diagnosed in the third trimester, are usually unilateral and are simple in appearance. As the baby is well and no abnormalities were visualised on ultrasound scan, no further follow-up is required.

Question: You have a medical student in clinic with you. He wants to know what your management would have been if the cyst had persisted.

Answer: Most neonatal ovarian cysts resolve spontaneously. In general, it is recommended to perform surgical intervention for cysts larger than 5 cm in diameter, because such large cysts increase the risk for torsion of the ovary. Intervention may also be necessary if the baby appears symptomatic or the cyst causes compression of other structures. Furthermore, if the ultrasound shows a complex cyst or if the origin of the cyst remains unclear, intervention may be necessary.

A diagnostic laparoscopy may be required to establish the nature of the cyst. Treatment options for large simple cysts include ultrasound-guided needle aspiration or minimally invasive or open ovarian-sparing cystectomy. Needle aspiration is regarded as the less preferable option due to a higher risk of cyst recurrence.

Question: What is the most common significant complication with diagnosis of an ovarian cyst antenatally?

Answer: Antenatal torsion is the most common complication and occurs most typically in large cysts. It may lead to intracystic haemorrhage and subsequent ovarian necrosis. A postnatal ultrasound scan visualising a large complex cyst is suspicious of such events. Most commonly at laparoscopy or Pfannenstiel mini-laparotomy, a large, black cyst free-floating in the pelvis is identified. It is the antenatally torted ovary that has necrosed and should be removed. It is crucial to document and identify the other solitary ovary intraoperatively and, of course, offer parental reassurance.

BIBLIOGRAPHY

1. American College of Obstetrics and Gynaecology: Guideline Number 783 (Reaffirmed 2021) Adnexal Torsion in Adolescents.
2. Aust Thomas et al. Laparoscopic Surgery in Pediatric and Adolescent Gynaecology Practice – Adnexal Torsion. Paediatric and Adolescent Gynaecology. Eds. Sarah M Creighton, Cambridge University Press 2018.
3. Manjiri S, Padmalatha SK, Shetty J. Management of complex ovarian cysts in newborns – our experience. J Neonatal Surg. 2017;6(1):3.

4. Akın MA, Akın L, Özbek S, Tireli G, Kavuncuoğlu S, Sander S, Akçakuş M, Güneş T, Öztürk MA, Kurtoğlu S. Fetal-neonatal ovarian cysts–their monitoring and management: retrospective evaluation of 20 cases and review of the literature. J Clin Res Pediatr Endocrinol. 2010;2(1):28–33.

5. Ritchie J, O'Mahony F, Garden A, on behalf of British Society for Paediatric & Adolescent Gynaecology. Guidelines for the management of ovarian cysts in children and adolescents. Accessed 07, 2020. https://britspag.org/wp-content/uploads/2019/11/Ovarian-cystmanagement-in-PAG-guideline-revised.pdf. BritSPAG Dec 2018.

6. Braungart S, Williams C, Arul SG, et al. Standardising the surgical management of benign ovarian tumors in children and adolescents: a best practice Delphi consensus statement. Pediatr Blood Cancer. 2022;69(4):e29589.

7. Pio L, Abu Zaid A, Zaghloul T, Halepota HF, Davidoff AM, Losty PD, Abdelhafeez HH. Ovarian-sparing surgery for ovarian tumors in children: a systematic review and meta-analysis. Eur J Surg Oncol. 2023. Oct;49(10):106923.

33

Acute scrotum

ALEXANDER CHO AND ZENI HAVELIWALA
Great Ormond Street Hospital for Children NHS Foundation Trust, London, UK

INTRODUCTION

Acute scrotum is a term referring to an acute change to the scrotum with or without accompanying pain. A thorough clinical history in terms of onset of symptoms and pain is key to understanding the leading pathology to guide timely investigation and management.

Scenario: A 11-year-old boy is seen at the hospital emergency department with a 9-hour history of sudden-onset right testicular pain. He describes the pain as 10/10 in terms of severity and has vomited once. Clinical examination demonstrates a 'high-riding testis' with scrotal swelling and exquisite tenderness. The patient is promptly taken to the operating theatre (**Figure 33.1**).

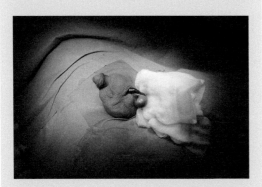

Figure 33.1 Torted testis delivered through scrotal incision.

Question: What is the diagnosis now, and how will you manage this patient?
Answer: The patient has experienced acute testicular torsion, with a twist in the spermatic cord within the tunica vaginalis (intra-vaginal). The perfusion to the testicle is severely compromised, and immediate detorsion is indicated. This is performed by the surgeon rotating the testicle away from the midline and securely placing it in warm saline-soaked swabs. Whilst the testicle makes an effort to recover and reperfuse, the contralateral side is explored and pexed (i.e. fixed to the inner scrotum) using non-absorbable sutures using a three-point fixation technique.

Question: Why do you explore the contralateral testis?
Answer: It is important to assess the contralateral healthy testis, as the 'bell-clapper deformity' is found bilaterally in 60%–80% of all cases (Osumah et al. 2018).

Question: On reassessment of the affected side, the testicle remains dusky and congested. What are your options now?
Answer: Poor perfusion post detorsion is not uncommon. A clinical decision will now need to

DOI: 10.1201/9781003182290-36

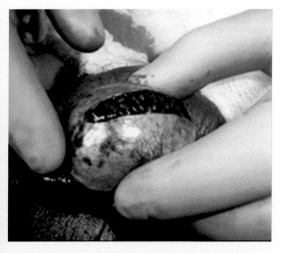

Figure 33.2 Anterior capsulotomy incision of tunica albuginea (Figueroa et al. 2012).

be made about the potential viability and survival of the testis compared with the risk of not undertaking an orchidectomy and the potential negative impact on the contralateral healthy testis. Rates of orchidectomy at the time of emergency surgery are approximately around 40% (MacDonald et al. 2018).

Impaired arterial inflow and venous outflow lead to oedema of the vasculature and supporting testicular structures, which prevents adequate venous outflow once the testicle is detorted. This represents a form of 'compartment syndrome', which can be relieved by performing a polar capsulotomy covered with a tunica albuginea flap (see **Figure 33.2**) (Figueroa et al. 2012), which is an option aimed at enhancing testicular salvage.

Question: How likely is it that the testicle will survive?
Answer: At the time of emergency presentation, this patient had pain for more than 6 hours, which decreases the likelihood of testicular salvage. More than 90% of testes survive if de-torted within 6 hours of the immediate onset of pain, which falls to less than 50% of patients with a pain history exceeding 6 hours (MacDonald et al. 2018).

Question: Does this patient need follow-up? If so when and why?
Answer: Yes, a routine follow-up after 6 months should be arranged with the surgical service, with an ultrasound scan to assess the presence and volume of the testis. Six months will allow the testicle

to recover from torsion injury and inflammation to settle so an accurate assessment of the testicle can be made. The rate of long-term testicular atrophy, defined as a testicle <50% volume of the contralateral testis, is approximately 50% in most cases (Lian et al. 2016).

At clinic follow-up, a conversation regarding future fertility and cosmesis needs to be discussed with the family if the affected side has atrophied or the testis been excised.

Question: What advice would you give regarding future fertility if the torted testicle did not survive?
Answer: In the longer term, boys with a history of testicular torsion have decreased sperm motility and reduced sperm counts (Arap et al. 2007), but there is no compelling evidence this has an impact on the final paternity rate (Gielchinsky et al. 2016).

Testicular torsion is a urological emergency which requires prompt assessment and treatment with urgent surgery. It affects 1 in 4000 males. In the pubertal age group, it usually occurs secondary to an anatomical abnormality of the insertion of the tunica vaginalis that is higher on the spermatic cord. This is referred to as a 'bell-clapper' deformity, which allows the cord to be suspended from its attachments and is prone to torsion.

Whilst the literature may suggest high levels of sensitivity and specificity with colour Doppler real-time ultrasonography, it is heavily dependent on operator experience and availability at hospital centres with the potential of false-negative reports (Baker et al. 2000). Torsion can be early, partial or intermittent in its clinical presentation, and all three possibilities may demonstrate a positive Doppler flow on imaging; therefore, surgical exploration on clinical findings is recommended. Negative surgical exploration is preferable to a missed 'late' diagnosis based on a false-negative scan. The use of ultrasound in the assessment of testicular pathology is reserved for specific cases under senior guidance in patients with atypical features or late clinical presentation (Royal College of Surgeons, 2014).

At scrotal exploration, as stated earlier, if torsion is present, the testis should be de-torted away from the midline and assessed for reperfusion by placing it in a warmed saline-soaked gauze for 30 minutes. A clearly necrotic testicle will require orchidectomy, but those with doubtful viability can be preserved with or without polar capsulotomy.

Testicular salvage is dependent on the duration of ischaemia (hours), which can be determined by an accurate history from the patient of the duration of pain. Clearly, the longer the duration of pain, the less the chance of testicular survival. Although testicular atrophy is correlated with lower sperm counts, as stated, endocrine function and paternity rates seem to be unaffected (Yang et al. 2011).

Scenario: A 1-day-old term male newborn is brought to the attention of the hospital surgical team due to a left-sided scrotal swelling and erythema. Maternal pregnancy was uncomplicated. The baby was born by normal vaginal delivery and has been otherwise feeding well.

Question: What are the differential diagnoses possible with this male newborn?

Answer: Scrotal swelling and erythema could be due to a hydrocoele, an incarcerated inguinoscrotal hernia, a testicular mass or testicular torsion. Scrotal swelling may sometimes be the initial presentation of abdominal pathology, such as necrotising enterocolitis or spontaneous intestinal perforation, as intra-abdominal contents may travel down an open patent processes vaginalis.

On examination, the baby is stable with normal vital observations. The abdomen is unremarkable and the left scrotum is red and swollen and the underlying testicle feels uniformly enlarged with a mild hydrocoele.

Question: What are your next steps in management?

Answer: Clinically this baby seems likely to have testicular torsion, but a testicular mass or inguinal scrotal pathology may also present in this manner in newborns. A testicular and groin ultrasound would be the next useful investigation.

Question: What differentiates torsion in this very young age group from torsion in the teenage male category?

Answer: Torsion in the neonatal age group is classically termed 'extra-vaginal torsion' as the tunica vaginalis does not attach and fix to the scrotum for a few weeks after birth. This scenario means the entire testicle along with its paratesticular attachments have twisted, compromising the blood supply to the testicle.

Question: A testicular ultrasound is suggestive of a diagnosis of newborn testicular torsion and excludes other pathology. How would you now manage this patient?

Answer: The distinction between prenatal torsion with a poor chance of testicular survival versus perinatal torsion, which carries a greater probability of testicular salvage, is very difficult to make. A perinatal event would be highly suggested if signs/symptoms developed over the course of the few hours since delivery and birth. Often, the only distinguishing factor in these cases is a clear history of the onset of symptoms.

The mother recalls the infant's scrotum was normal immediately after birth. This now increases the possibility for perinatal torsion and the potential risk of synchronous contralateral testicular torsion. Although the incidence of bilateral testicular torsion is low, it can present with unilateral signs (Nandi and Murphy 2011). Given the catastrophic nature of bilateral testicular loss, urgent exploration with bilateral testicular fixation is herein recommended. Salvage rates can be up to 20% of cases if the operation is performed urgently (Nandi and Murphy 2011).

Scenario: An 8-year-old boy is referred to your hospital emergency department with a 4-hour history of sudden-onset left testicular pain.

Question: What further information do you want to know, and what are your next steps?

Answer: This is a urological emergency and assessment of this patient for possible testicular torsion should be undertaken. Other differential diagnoses would include torsion of the testicular appendage(s) and epididymitis.

A further detailed history regarding the onset of pain, current pain score and relevant past medical or surgical history should be noted. A clinical examination of the abdomen and external genitalia needs to be performed noting the position of the testis, the presence or absence of a 'blue dot', absence of the cremasteric reflex or any findings suggestive of the presence of testicular masses.

A 'blue dot' sign is readily visible through the scrotal skin with a transillumination pen torch test with point tenderness in this particular region. The remainder of the testicle is normal. A clinical diagnosis of torsion of the appendage of the testis is made. Torsion of the testicular appendage is one of the most common causes for testicular pain in the prepubertal child and occurs secondary to twisting of a vestigial remnant of the Mullerian duct, usually located in the upper pole of the testis. It accounts for more than 50% of cases presenting at emergency hospital settings. The peak age of occurrence is typically 7–12 years of age. Often the pain is localised to the upper pole of the testis and is not associated with systemic symptoms.

Question: How will you manage this patient?
Answer: Torsion of the appendage testis is usually a self-limiting condition and is often usually managed conservatively with simple oral analgesia, bed rest and anti-inflammatory medication. Inflammation and pain usually resolve within a week. Surgical exploration is rarely required, but can be considered if the pain does not resolve with conservative measures. If there is any diagnostic uncertainty, the patient requires an urgent surgical exploration.

Scenario: A 2-year-old boy presents to the hospital emergency department with a 12-hour history of unilateral scrotal redness and swelling. The child has a low-grade temperature. On examination, the testis is normal to palpation and is not tender whilst the cord feels somewhat thickened and tender (**Figure 33.3**).

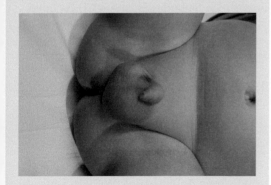

Figure 33.3 Left sided scrotal erythema and non tender swelling.

Question: How will you manage this patient?
Answer: The history and clinical examination are consistent with a possible diagnosis of epididymitis. Epididymitis is usually self-limiting at this age group and secondary to viral infection, and the treatment is mainly conservative. I would request a urine dipstick exam, though a normal urinalysis does not exclude epididymitis. A Doppler ultrasound would additionally be requested to confirm or refute the working diagnosis. Antibiotics are reserved for children with a positive urine dipstick test for leucocytes and/or nitrites or a positive culture from the testicular swab at exploratory operation. If there is any uncertainty of the diagnosis, I would proceed to urgent surgical exploration.

Epididymitis is encountered in 11%–26% of children with acute scrotal pain (Mushtaq et al. 2003, Murphy et al. 2006). There is a bimodal age distribution, with a peak incidence observed in infancy and those over 6 years of age (Cappèle et al. 2000). The aetiology includes ascending infection, viral, retrograde urine reflux into the vas and seminal vesicles, haematogenously spread bacteria and other rare urological abnormalities. Infants may have a higher incidence of urinary tract abnormalities (70%) (Merlini et al. 1998), but the overall requirement for detailed or invasive urological intervention is small. Therefore, investigation with follow-up ultrasound is reserved for those children who have recurrent attacks of epididymitis (Cappèle et al. 2000).

Scenario: A 3-year-old boy is referred to you from your accident and emergency department with a right-sided scrotal swelling associated with erythema and pain. On further questioning, the swelling was reportedly noted 4 hours ago when the mother was changing the boy's underclothes and initially only seen in the perineum region. The patient's observations are normal. On examination, the boy appears well, with no palpable groin pathology. The testes are non-tender on examination and lying normally. The right hemi-scrotum skin and ipsilateral perineal region are reddened and erythematous. The urine dipstick test is normal.

Question: What is your working differential diagnosis for this presentation?
Answer: Testicular torsion is the most important differential to consider. This presentation is not concerning as the young patient is not experiencing testicular pain or tenderness. Other differential diagnoses include epididymitis, torsion of the

appendix testis, acute hydrocoele, incarcerated hernia, trauma, testicular or paratesticular tumour, vasculitis and idiopathic scrotal oedema.

This boy's history and clinical examination point towards idiopathic scrotal oedema, which is a poorly understood condition that leads to redness, swelling and oedema of the scrotal tissues, with no effect on the testicle.

Question: How would you treat this patient?
Answer: Idiopathic scrotal oedema is a self-limiting disorder, and no specific treatment is indicated. Antihistamine agents may be given if pruritus is a troublesome symptom, and an anti-inflammatory can be used to hasten patient recovery.

BIBLIOGRAPHY

Arap MA, Vicentini FC, Cocuzza M, Hallak J, Athayde K, Lucon AM, et al. Late hormonal levels, semen parameters, and presence of antisperm antibodies in patients treated for testicular torsion. J Androl. 2007;28:528–532.

Baker LA, Sigman D, Mathews RI, Benson J, Docimo SG. An analysis of clinical outcomes using color doppler testicular ultrasound for testicular torsion. Pediatrics. 2000;105(3 pt 1): 604–607.

Cappèle O, Liard A, Barret E, Bachy B, Mitrofanoff P. Epididymitis in children: is further investigation necessary after the first episode? Eur Urol. 2000;38(5):627–630. doi: 10.1159/000020343. PMID: 11096248.

Figueroa V, Pippi-Salle JL, Braga LHP et al. Comparative analysis of detorsion alone versus detorsion and tunica albuginea decompression (fasciotomy) with tunica vaginalis flap coverage in the surgical management of prolonged testicular ischemia. J Urol 2012; 188(4 Suppl.):1417–1422.

Gielchinsky I, Suraqui E, Hidas G, Zuaiter M, Landau EH, Simon A, et al. Pregnancy rates after testicular torsion. J Urol. 2016;196:852–855.

Lian BS, Ong CC, Chiang LW, Rai R, Nah SA. Factors predicting testicular atrophy after testicular salvage following torsion. Eur J Pediatr Surg. 2016;26:17–21.

MacDonald C, Kronfli R, Carachi R, O'Toole S. A systematic review and meta-analysis revealing realistic outcomes following paediatric torsion of testes. Journal Pediatric Urology. 2018;14(6):503–509.

Merlini E, Rotundi F, Seymandi PL, Canning DA. Acute epididymitis and urinary tract anomalies in children. Scand J Urol Nephrol. 1998;32(4):273–275. doi: 10.1080/003655998750015449. PMID: 9764455.

Murphy FL, Fletcher L, Pease P. Early scrotal exploration in all cases is the investigation and intervention of choice in the acute paediatric scrotum. Pediatr Surg Int. 2006;22(5):413–416. doi: 10.1007/s00383-006-1681-0. Epub 2006 Apr 7. PMID: 16602024.

Mushtaq I, Fung M, Glasson MJ. Retrospective review of paediatric patients with acute scrotum. ANZ J Surg. 2003;73(1–2):55–58. doi: 10.1046/j.1445-2197.2003.02612.x. PMID: 12534742.

Nandi B, Murphy FL. Neonatal testicular torsion: a systematic literature review. Pediatr Surg Int. 2011;27(10):1037–1040. doi: 10.1007/s00383-011-2945-x. Epub 2011 Jul 8. PMID: 21739126.

Osumah TS, Jimbo M, Granberg CF, Gargollo PC. Frontiers in pediatric testicular torsion: an integrated review of prevailing trends and management outcomes. J Pediatr Urol. 2018;14:394–401.

The Royal College of Surgeons. Commissioning Guide on Management of Paediatric Torsion for Consultation. 2014. https://www.rcseng.ac.uk/library-and-publications/rcs-publications/docs/commissioning-guide-paediatric-torsion/

Yang C, Song B, Tan J, Liu X, Wei GH. Testicular torsion in children: a 20-year retrospective study in a single institution. Scientific World Journal. 2011;11:362–368.

34

Disorders of the breast

VICKY WONG
Hong Kong Children's Hospital, Hong Kong, China

JENNIFER MOU
CUHK Medical Centre, Hong Kong, China

Scenario: A 10-day-old full-term male newborn was referred from a regional health centre to the neonatal intensive care unit (NICU) with bilateral breast enlargement. Neonatal physical examinations were within normal limits until day 9 of life, when the infant was found to have bilateral symmetrical breast enlargement. On examination, the baby is noted to have soft tissue swelling over bilateral breast buds and a whitish discharge but no tenderness was evident (**Figure 34.1**).

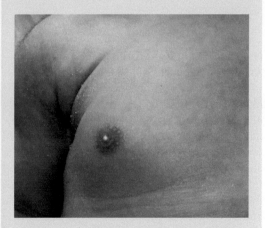

Figure 34.1 Soft tissue swelling over right breast with a white coloured discharge at the nipple. Similar physical findings were detected with the left breast.

Question: What is the most likely diagnosis? Are any further investigations needed?

Answer: Neonatal breast enlargement, or physiological breast hypertrophy, is the most likely clinical diagnosis in this baby. It is a benign condition that is commonly seen in healthy newborns and is reported to occur in approximately 70–80% of infants. The postulated mechanism is secondary to maternal oestrogen hormone levels in the fetal circulation, which in turn trigger the secretion of prolactin causing proliferation of the breast glandular tissue. The terminology or definition of neonatal breast development is also unclear, as it is without a definite cut-off measurement. A working group recommended to use the term "mastauxe" and further subdivided the groups into neonatal mastauxe (breast bud diameter ≤3 cm) and giant mastauxe (breast bud diameter >3 cm). This benign condition usually presents in the first or second week of life and later involutes within a few months of age. Sometimes the whitish secretion may be seen upon breast expression, and it is then called "witch's milk" with a composition resembling maternal milk. There is no sinister clinical significance for this benign disorder, which will resolve without

DOI: 10.1201/9781003182290-37

active treatment. Hence, management consists of simple observation and parental reassurance. As it is considered a benign physiological condition in healthy newborns, further laboratory workup or imaging would not be necessary.

> **Scenario:** A 15-year-old girl noted her right breast growing asymmetrically larger over a few months. She thought it was the normal development of her breasts initially. Later on, she was aware that it is weird to have asymmetrical breasts but she was too embarrassed to talk about it with her friends or parents. As a result, she covered her breasts discretely with a cardigan or loose-fitting jackets even in summer months. It was not until her right breast became so heavy and also stretched the skin causing so much discomfort that she told her mother about it. Her mother brought her to a family doctor physician without delay.

Question: What are the differential working diagnoses? How would you differentiate them?

Answer: The girl may either have juvenile breast hypertrophy or a phyllodes breast tumour.

Juvenile breast hypertrophy is a benign yet rapidly growing condition which can involve one or both breasts. The exact mechanism is unknown, but it is believed to be related to end-organ hypersensitivity to normal circulating levels of female gonadal hormones.

Fibroadenoma is a common, benign condition in young women and teenagers. It can present as a small (usually <3 cm), firm, mobile and rubbery mass sometimes termed 'breast mouse'. Fibroadenomas can be multiple too; however, if the breast mass is rapidly growing to a size >5 cm, it should be considered a phyllodes tumour until proven otherwise.

Breast examination should be conducted on the normal side first to allow the surgeon to understand the texture of normal breast tissue better – which varies among individuals and within the same individual during different periods of the female menstrual cycle. In this girl, a huge firm irregular mass of 8 cm was detected in her right breast involving both the lower inner and lower outer quadrants. Like most cases of phyllodes tumours, the diagnosis can be made by history and physical examination alone.

Question: What investigations will be needed? Is fine needle aspiration (FNA) or core needle biopsy (CNB) required in all cases?

Answer: Ultrasonography can be arranged for this girl to document the size, margins and other features of the tumour. FNA or CNB may be offered in the same exam setting under sonographic guidance in order to gain histological information of the lesion. If phyllodes tumour is suspected clinically, FNA or CNB may not always be useful, and the result can even be misleading because of diagnostic sampling errors. Excisional biopsy should be offered instead.

Phyllodes tumours can be benign, borderline or malignant. They can all grow very fast, breaking aggressively through the skin to cause pain and discomfort. Therefore, surgical excision is advised in all cases. Surgeons should also actively watch out for recurrence in malignant tumours with after-care patient follow-up health surveillance.

> **Scenario:** A healthy 8-year-old girl is admitted to the surgical ward with a painful right breast mass for 1 week. She was initially cared for by her family doctor with a course of oral antibiotics and then referred to the regional hospital when fever developed. On physical examination, her right breast was swollen, tender, erythematous and fluctuant. Inflammatory markers including white blood cell count, erythrocyte sedimentation rate and C-reactive protein were all raised.

Question: What is the diagnosis?

Answer: A tender and fluctuant breast mass with signs and symptoms of systemic infection is highly suggestive of a breast abscess. We can diagnose breast abscess confidently by physical examination. With breast sonography the surgeon will obtain further information about the size of the abscess, the extent of inflammatory changes and involvement of regional axillary lymph nodes. Breast abscess in the adolescent is uncommon, and predisposing factors include trauma; underlying skin conditions, e.g. atopic dermatitis; and allied medical problems, e.g. immunodeficiency, poorly controlled diabetes mellitus, and occasionally is seen in the young lactating adolescent (**Figure 34.2**).

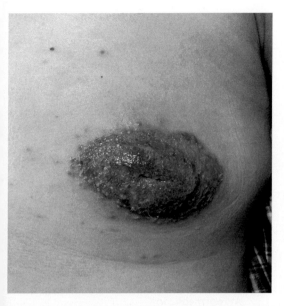

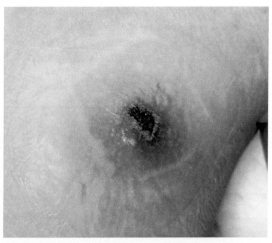

Figure 34.3 Left breast abscess with incision and drainage performed. The photo shows the wound condition 4 weeks after the operative procedure. Daily wound dressings, including vacuum-assisted wound closure therapy, were applied.

Figure 34.2 Atopic dermatitis or other skin conditions are risk factors for the development of breast abscess with an untreated skin infection.

Question: What are the next steps in management?
Answer: The optimal management of paediatric breast abscess is unclear, as published studies are few in number. As a result, current principles are mostly based on adult populations, which include abscess drainage and antibiotic therapy. *Staphylococcus aureus* is the most common organism found in mastitis or breast abscess. In general, the penicillin group or cephalosporins would be the best choice of antibiotics until microbiology sensitivity tests are available from pus culture.

Two types of abscess drainage techniques are used in clinical practice:

a. *Surgical incision and drainage*: This is the classical standard management for a breast abscess, which involves operation with general anaesthesia. Surgical techniques include incision over the pointed area, radical deloculation and drainage of the pus from the abscess cavity. The cavity is then irrigated and then loosely packed with ribbon gauze. Daily wound dressings are necessary until the cavity contracts. The disadvantages of open drainage methods include poor cosmetic outcome, a long healing time and postoperative pain with regular postoperative wound dressings and increased financial hospital costs (**Figure 34.3**).

b. *Percutaneous drainage*: A popular alternative in recent years is percutaneous drainage by needle aspiration or insertion of a small-calibre catheter under guided local anaesthesia. This procedure can be performed in an outpatient clinic setting. Repeated aspiration may be required before complete resolution in most cases, and occasionally conversion to open drainage may be necessary if the infection is not adequately controlled. The reported cure rate in the literature is around 50–90%, and higher success rates are documented with the aid of ultrasound scan to look for residual loculi. Other risk factors identified for failure are larger abscess (>5 cm), higher pus volume and longer duration of symptoms. Several small-sized randomized controlled trials have demonstrated advantages of this technique over surgical open drainage methods, including it being more cost-effective and having a better cosmetic outcome and shorter healing time, and theoretically may minimize the risk of breast bud damage in the female prepubertal breast.

Based on the principles of modern surgical practice, first-line treatment for a paediatric breast abscess is percutaneous drainage, as it is the least invasive method. Open drainage should therefore be reserved for patients with persistent or recurrent disease after multiple attempts at aspiration, those with large abscess lesions (>5 cm) or where systemic sepsis needs immediate control.

BIBLIOGRAPHY

1. Lee EJ, Chang YW, Oh JH, Hwang J, Hong SS, Kim HJ. Breast lesions in children and adolescents: Diagnosis and management. Korean J Radiol. 2018;19:978–91.
2. De Silva NK. Breast development and disorders in the adolescent female. Best Pract Res Clin Obstet Gynaecol. 2018;48: 40–50.
3. Murphy BL, Glasgow AE, Ubl DS, Habermann EB, Lemaine V. Surgical treatment of adolescent breast disorders: Institutional experience and national trends. J Pediatr Adolesc Gynecol. 2018;31: 299–303.
4. Frazier AL, Rosenberg SM. Preadolescent and adolescent risk factors for benign breast disease. J Adolesc Health. 2013;52:S36–40.
5. Gao Y, Saksena MA, Brachtel EF, terMeulen DC, Rafferty EA. How to approach breast lesions in children and adolescents. Eur J Radiol. 2015;84:1350–64.
6. Valerio E, Palatron S, Vanzo V, Vendramin S, Cutrone M. Breast disorders of the newborn. Arch Dis Child Educ Pract Ed. 2016;101:236–8.
7. Dekonenko C, Shah N, Svetanoff WJ, Osuchukwu OO, Sobrino JA, Oyetunji TA, Fraser JD. Characterization of pediatric breast abscesses and optimal treatment: A retrospective analysis. J Surg Res. 2021;257:195–202.

35

Ectopic pregnancy

CARA WILLIAMS
Alder Hey Children's Hospital, Liverpool, UK

Scenario: A 14-year-old girl is brought to the hospital emergency department by ambulance with a 24-hour history of worsening right iliac fossa pain and diarrhoea. Her urinary pregnancy test on arrival is positive. She is tachycardic and hypotensive.

Question: What is your differential diagnosis?
Answer: A diagnosis of ectopic pregnancy should be considered in any postpubertal girl presenting to the emergency department with collapse, acute abdominal/pelvic pain or gastrointestinal symptoms, particularly diarrhoea, vomiting and dizziness. An urgent urinary pregnancy test should be performed on admission, and if not possible catheterisation to obtain a specimen of urine should be performed.

An ectopic pregnancy is any pregnancy implanted outside of the endometrial cavity. In the UK, the incidence is approximately 11/1000 pregnancies. Risk factors include tubal damage from previous surgery or infection, including sexually transmitted infections, smoking and in vitro fertilisation. The majority of girls and women, though, do not have any identifiable risk factors.

Ectopic pregnancies have a potential to rupture causing rapid significant intra-abdominal haemorrhage. This can lead to cardiovascular collapse and even untimely death. There were five maternal deaths in the UK from ruptured ectopic pregnancies in 2015–2017, with all deaths occurring within

some 48 hours of presentation with their ectopic pregnancy.

Other gynaecological differential diagnoses should include ovarian cyst torsion or rupture, endometriosis, obstructed Mullerian duct anomalies, miscarriage, sexually transmitted infections and pelvic inflammatory disease. Non-gynaecological differential diagnoses include appendicitis, urinary tract infection and constipation.

Question: What is your immediate management?
Answer: If a ruptured ectopic pregnancy is suspected, initial management includes emergent IV access, IV fluids, nil by mouth and analgesia as required. Bloods should be requested for urgent full blood count (FBC), cross-match and serum beta-human chorionic gonadotropin (βHCG). A bedside Haemacue can be done to look for anaemia. Haemodynamic resuscitation should be expeditiously performed with IV fluids and blood transfusion if required. The gynaecology team should be called to review the patient urgently, but if the girl has presented to a community hospital with no resident on-call gynaecology, the attending surgeons should and must review. If the patient is haemodynamically very unstable, she should not be transferred to another hospital trust to see gynaecology, but she should be managed emergently by the surgeons where she is.

The gold-standard imaging modality for diagnosing an ectopic pregnancy is a transvaginal ultrasound. If this is not available or there is any haemodynamic instability to suggest rupture, a focussed

DOI: 10.1201/9781003182290-38

assessment with sonography in trauma (FAST) scan should be performed to look for any evidence of intra-abdominal haemorrhage from a ruptured ectopic pregnancy.

Question: What are the different types of ectopic pregnancy?

Answer: The majority of ectopic pregnancies are tubal, but they can also be cervical, ovarian, interstitial (within the interstitial portion of the fallopian tube), cornual (within a non-communicating uterine horn), abdominal and in a caesarean section uterine scar. A heterotopic pregnancy is defined as the simultaneous presence of an intrauterine pregnancy and an ectopic pregnancy, with an incidence of 1:30,000.

Most ectopic pregnancies will present during the first trimester as the pregnancy outgrows the surrounding structures, leading to pain and eventual rupture and haemorrhage. Cornual ectopic pregnancies occurring in a non-communicating uterine horn often present much later, nearer 20 weeks' gestation, as the uterine horn can accommodate more growth of the ectopic pregnancy.

Question: If a FAST scan shows intra-abdominal haemorrhage, what should the management be?

Answer: Evidence of intra-abdominal haemorrhage with a positive pregnancy test and haemodynamic instability suggests a ruptured ectopic pregnancy. The patient should be taken to the operating room theatre straight away (National Confidential Enquiry into Patient Outcome and Death [NCEPOD] category immediate) for a laparoscopy or laparotomy. Laparoscopy is preferable to laparotomy due to its many advantages including shorter operating time, less intraoperative blood loss, less risk of adhesion formation, shorter hospital stay, lower cost, quicker recovery time, lower analgesic requirements and better cosmetic appearance. However, evidence would suggest there is no difference in the outcome of subsequent successful pregnancy between laparoscopy and laparotomy. The decision regarding route of surgery will depend on the expertise of the surgeon and the haemodynamic stability of the patient.

Question: How are the different ectopic pregnancies treated surgically?

Answer: If a tubal ectopic pregnancy is diagnosed at laparoscopy/laparotomy, a unilateral salpingectomy should be performed. If there are other fertility-reducing factors in the patient's history (previous ectopic pregnancy, previous complex abdominal/pelvic surgery, previous pelvic inflammatory disease or contralateral tubal damage), a salpingotomy can be considered. However, this can be associated with persistent trophoblast and requires after-care follow-up with serum βHCG levels and may require further treatment with methotrexate or salpingectomy.

If the ectopic pregnancy is located in the interstitial portion of the tube, the cornual aspect of the uterus will need to be resected along with the tube. This can be associated with significant haemorrhage. Diluted vasopressin can be injected into the myometrium below the interstitial pregnancy to help reduce blood loss.

A cornual ectopic pregnancy, located in a non-communicating uterine horn, requires complete excision of the rudimentary uterine horn to prevent recurrence. Cornual pregnancy rupture often occurs later, in the second trimester, when the uterus is much larger, making surgery more difficult. Care must be taken to identify the ureter nearby, as Mullerian duct anomalies are often associated with urinary tract anomalies.

Ovarian ectopic pregnancies should be managed by enucleation of the gestational products from the ovary or wedge resection if there is a large ectopic mass. Haemostasis can be achieved with sutures or electrocautery. Damage to surrounding normal ovarian tissue should be minimised. Oophorectomy may occasionally be required if there is suspicious ipsilateral ovarian pathology or excessive haemorrhage.

Laparoscopic treatment is an option in abdominal pregnancies that are of an early gestation where the site of implantation does not involve a highly vascular area. Advanced abdominal ectopic pregnancies are associated with significant maternal and fetal morbidity and mortality, and therefore laparotomy is required. Incision of the placenta should be avoided. If the placenta is attached to major vessels or vital structures, it can be left in situ to await spontaneous resorption. However, this can be associated with significant morbidity (ileus, bowel obstruction, fistula formation, haemorrhage and peritonitis). Methotrexate and selective arterial embolization have been used as adjunctive treatments to surgery.

In a heterotopic pregnancy, surgical removal of the ectopic pregnancy is advised, especially if the patient is haemodynamically unstable. Care must be taken not to manipulate the uterus during the procedure.

Traditional management of a cervical pregnancy was with dilatation and curettage. This was associated with significant bleeding and a high risk of hysterectomy. This is usually reserved for the haemodynamically unstable patient where there is excessive bleeding. The later the gestation that a cervical pregnancy presents, the higher the risk of hysterectomy. Adjunctive methods to control haemorrhage include uterine artery ligation and uterine artery embolization.

Surgical management of a caesarean section scar pregnancy includes suction evacuation, hysteroscopic resection or excision of the pregnancy via open or laparoscopic surgery.

Question: If an unruptured tubal ectopic pregnancy is diagnosed and the girl is haemodynamically stable, what would the management options be?
Answer: Medical and conservative options can be used for the management of ectopic pregnancy in haemodynamically stable patients. Medical management is with a single intramuscular injection of methotrexate at a dose of 50 mg/m². Success rates for single-dose methotrexate for tubal ectopic pregnancy range from 65% to 95% with 3–27% of patients requiring a second dose.

Criteria for use of methotrexate include haemodynamic stability, minimal/no pain, βHCG <5000, no fetal heart activity seen on scan and no evidence of intrauterine pregnancy. Patients must be willing to attend for regular follow-up, which can be quite protracted. The most common side effects include nausea, bloating, stomatitis and a transient elevation in liver enzymes. Patients are advised to best avoid pregnancy for 3 months following treatment with methotrexate.

Expectant management is an option for patients who are haemodynamically stable with minimal or no pain and a low and declining βHCG level. They will require regular follow-up with serial βHCG monitoring. Success rates of expectant management range from 57% to 100% depending on case selection, with success being inversely proportional to the serum βHCG level.

Question: What else needs to be considered in this girl?
Answer: Anti-D prophylaxis should be offered to all RhD-negative girls and women who have had

surgical management of ectopic pregnancy to prevent against alloimmunisation and haemolytic disease of the fetus and newborn in a subsequent pregnancy. Evidence is lacking for the risk of allo-immunisation following medical or conservative management of ectopic pregnancies, but if there has been significant bleeding or pain in early pregnancy, anti-D prophylaxis should be offered.

A sexual health risk assessment should be performed. The patient should be offered opportunistic screening for sexually transmitted infections (STIs). Vaginal swabs or urine can be sent for *Chlamydia, Gonorrhoea* and *Trichomonas*. The female patient should also be offered HIV/syphilis/hepatitis screening, but this may need to be done at the local sexual health centre or genitourinary medicine clinic. Future contraceptive choices should be fully discussed, and the patient should be signposted to a local adolescent sexual health clinic where required.

It is important to consider the possibility of child sexual exploitation or child sexual abuse in all sexually active young people. 'Spotting the Signs' is a national proforma produced by the British Association of Sexual Health and HIV (BASHH) and Brook. If the girl is considered to be at risk, the local safeguarding lead should and must be informed.

The psychological impact of the pregnancy and pregnancy loss should not be underestimated. The patient should be made aware of how to access psychological support via patient support groups such as the Ectopic Pregnancy Trust or local bereavement counselling services.

Question: What is her risk of recurrence and effect on long-term fertility?
Answer: Most long-term follow-up studies suggest a recurrence rate of ectopic pregnancy of approximately 18.5%. Randomised controlled trials have shown no difference in fertility outcomes for women managed with surgical, medical or conservative treatment. The patient should therefore be offered an early pregnancy scan at around 6–7 weeks' gestation to locate the pregnancy in any future subsequent pregnancy.

BIBLIOGRAPHY

Knight M, Bunch K, Tuffnell D, Shakespeare J, Kotnis R, Kenyon S, Kurinczuk JJ, On behalf of MBRRACE-UK. Saving Lives, Improving Mothers' Care - Lessons learned to inform maternity care from the UK and Ireland Confidential Enquiries into Maternal Deaths and Morbidity 2015–17. Oxford: National Perinatal Epidemiology Unit, University of Oxford 2019.

Elson CJ, Salim R, Potdar N, Chetty M, Ross JA, Kirk EJ On behalf of the Royal College of Obstetricians and Gynaecologists. Diagnosis and management of ectopic pregnancy. BJOG 2016; 123: e15–e55.

Qureshi H, Massey E, Kirwan D, Davies T, Robson S, White J, Jones J, Allard S. BCSH guideline for the use of anti-D immunoglobulin for the prevention of haemolytic disease of the fetus and newborn. Transfusion Medicine. 2014; 24(1): 8–20.

Ashby J, Browne R, Dwyer E, Fifer H, Forsyth S, Hamlyn E, Rayment M, Rogstad K, Ward C, Wilkinson D. BASHH national guideline on the management of sexually transmitted infections and related conditions in children and young people. BASHH 2021.

Rogstad K, Johnston G. Spotting the Signs. A national proforma for identifying risk of child sexual exploitation in sexual health services. BASHH 2014.

36

Sexually transmitted infections

CARA WILLIAMS
Alder Hey Children's Hospital, Liverpool, UK

Scenario: A 14-year-old girl attends the hospital emergency department with a 2-day history of lower abdominal pain, pyrexia (38.5°C) and an offensive purulent vaginal discharge. She is sexually active and is currently taking the combined oral contraceptive pill.

Question: What are the important aspects of history taking in this situation?

Answer: All patients under 16 years of age should have their competency to consent to history taking, examination and treatment assessed and clearly documented at the outset. Young people presenting with symptoms suggestive of a sexually transmitted infection (STI) should have a thorough sexual and gynaecological history and holistic sexual risk assessment. This should be performed in a safe, confidential and private environment. They should be asked about specific symptoms including dysuria, postcoital bleeding, intermenstrual bleeding, abnormal discharge, abdominal pain and deep dyspareunia. Contraceptive use and compliance should be assessed to ascertain pregnancy risk. Use of recreational drugs including alcohol and chemsex are also important in the sexual risk assessment. Past medical history should include human papilloma virus (HPV) vaccination history. Any vulnerabilities should be identified, such as self-harm, mental health issues, special educational needs and domestic violence.

Information about their sexual relationship should be ascertained, including when they last had sexual intercourse, if the intercourse was consensual, age of partner, gender of partner, number of sexual partners in the last 3 months, type of sex (anal, oral or vaginal) and use of condoms.

A full risk assessment for child sexual exploitation (CSE) should be performed, using the 'Spotting the Signs' proforma. A young person may perceive their situation as consensual when in fact they are being groomed, as this is the nature of sexual exploitation. If a young person is considered to be at risk, local safeguarding policy should be followed and the case discussed with the safeguarding lead. Confidentiality must be explained properly to young people, including its parameters and the potential need to seek advice if they are believed to be at risk of significant harm.

Question: What examination and investigations should be performed in this case?

Answer: Fully informed consent should be obtained prior to examination, which should include abdominal palpation, speculum and bimanual examination. Speculum may reveal a mucopurulent cervicitis with or without contact bleeding. On bimanual examination, there may be pelvic tenderness and/or cervical motion tenderness. Vulvovaginal swabs should be taken for *Neisseria gonorrhoeae*, *Chlamydia trachomatis* and *Trichomonas vaginalis* and other causes of vaginal discharge such as *Candida* and bacterial vaginosis. If there has been any oral or anal penetration, oropharyngeal and anal swabs should also be considered. If a speculum and swabs are declined by the adolescent girl, a first-void urine for nucleic acid amplification test (NAAT) can be used, although it has a lower sensitivity compared with cervical or vaginal swabs. A pelvic ultrasound should be scheduled to look for other causes of acute abdominal pain and to assess for hydro/pyosalpinx or tubo-ovarian abscess.

Question: What are the differential diagnoses?
Answer: The differential diagnosis includes STIs such as *Chlamydia* or *Gonorrhoea*, pelvic inflammatory disease (PID), tubo-ovarian abscess, gastroenteritis, appendicitis and urinary tract infection. Other causes of acute abdominal pain such as ovarian cyst torsion or rupture and endometriosis should be considered.

PID is usually the result of infection ascending from the endocervix causing endometritis, salpingitis, parametritis, oophoritis, tubo-ovarian abscess and/or pelvic peritonitis. *N. gonorrhoeae* and *C. trachomatis* account for a quarter of all UK cases of PID. A positive test for *N. gonorrhoeae* or *C. trachomatis* supports the diagnosis of PID, but the absence of infection does not exclude PID. Elevated erythrocyte sedimentation rate (ESR) or C-reactive protein (CRP) also supports the diagnosis but is non-specific. The absence of endocervical or vaginal pus cells has a good negative predictive value (95%) for a diagnosis of PID, but their presence is non-specific (poor positive predictive value – 17%).

Her bloods show a raised white cell count and CRP. Speculum reveals a mucopurulent cervicitis, and she has cervical motion tenderness on bimanual examination. Her ultrasound shows a normal uterus, bilateral normal ovaries, normal appendix and some free fluid in the pouch of Douglas. The working diagnosis is PID, and she is admitted for analgesia and antibiotics.

Question: What are the antibiotics of choice?
Answer: The British Association of Sexual Health and HIV (BASHH) guidelines should be used in conjunction with discussion with the local specialist genitourinary medicine, infectious diseases and paediatric pharmacy teams for anyone under

the age of 16 years. Delaying treatment is likely to increase the risk of long-term sequelae such as ectopic pregnancy, infertility and pelvic pain. Because of this and the lack of definitive diagnostic criteria, a low threshold for empiric treatment of PID is recommended.

Broad-spectrum antibiotic therapy is required to cover a wide variety of aerobic and anaerobic bacteria. Intravenous therapy is recommended in severe clinical disease including pyrexia >38°C, presence of tubo-ovarian abscess or pelvic peritonitis. Intravenous therapy should be continued until 24 hours after clinical improvement and then switched to oral. Treatment for a female child over 12 years weighing more than 45 kg is as follows:

- Intravenous ceftriaxone 2 g daily
- Intravenous doxycycline 100 mg BD (oral if tolerated)

Followed by:

- Oral doxycycline 100 mg BD for 14 days
- Oral metronidazole 400 mg BD for 14 days

Or

- Intravenous clindamycin 900 mg TDS
- Intravenous gentamicin* 2 mg/kg loading dose followed by 1.5 mg/kg TDS

Followed by:

- Oral clindamycin 450 mg QDS to complete 14 days OR oral doxycycline 100 mg BD to complete 14 days
- Oral metronidazole 400 mg BD to complete 14 days
    (*Gentamicin levels need to be monitored if this regimen is used.)

If there is a tubo-ovarian abscess present and no clinical improvement after 24–48 hours of intravenous broad-spectrum antibiotics, drainage of the abscess should be considered, either with interventional radiology or laparoscopy. Positive swabs should be treated appropriately as per BASHH guidelines.

Management of specific STIs according to BASHH guidelines are as follows:

Condition/ Infection	Suggested treatment
Chlamydia	Neonate • Azithromycin 20 mg/kg/day PO od for 3 days* OR • Erythromycin 12.5 mg/kg PO qd for 14 days* (*Erythromycin and azithromycin in neonates under 2 weeks) Increases risk of hypertrophic pyloric stenosis Child weight <45 kg • Erythromycin 50 mg/kg/day PO divided into 4 doses daily for 14 days Child aged ≥2–12 years • Erythromycin 250 mg PO qd for 7 days or bd for 14 days Child >12 years • Doxycycline 100 mg PO bd for 7 days OR • Azithromycin 1 g orally as a single dose, followed by 500 mg once daily for two days OR • Erythromycin 500 mg PO bd for 14 days OR • Ofloxacin 200 mg bd or 400 mg PO od for 7 days

Condition/ Infection	Suggested treatment
Gonorrhoea	Gonococcal ophthalmia (neonates) This is an ophthalmic emergency, and ophthalmology input and hourly eye irrigation are essential to prevent visual loss from corneal ulceration and scarring. • Ceftriaxone 50 mg/kg IV or IM single dose (maximum dose 125 mg*) OR • Cefotaxime 100 mg/kg IM single dose (maximum dose 1 g) (*Ceftriaxone is contraindicated in premature neonates up to a corrected gestational age of 41 weeks. Ceftriaxone should be administered cautiously to hyperbilirubinemic infants. IV infusion to be administered over 60 minutes. Expert paediatric advice is required regarding dosage.) Non-ophthalmic gonorrhoea Child <2 years • Ceftriaxone 125 mg IM single dose Child <12 years and weight <45 kg • Ceftriaxone 125 mg IV or IM single dose Child 9–11 years weight >45 kg • Ceftriaxone 250 mg IV or IM single dose Child >12 years • Ceftriaxone 1 g IM single dose If declines IM injection • Cefixime 400 mg PO single dose plus azithromycin 2 g PO stat

Condition/ Infection	Suggested treatment
Trichomonas or Bacterial Vaginosis	Child 1–3 years • Metronidazole 50 mg PO tds for 7 days Child aged 3 years to <7 years • Metronidazole 100 mg PO bd for 7 days Child aged 7 years to <10 years • Metronidazole 100 mg PO tds for 7 days Child >10 years • Metronidazole 400 mg PO bd for 7 days OR • Metronidazole 2 g PO single dose
Mycoplasma genitalium	Evidence base for the treatment and management of mycoplasma genitalium is limited in children Child >12 years Uncomplicated infection: • Doxycycline 100 mg PO bd for 7 days followed by azithromycin 1 g orally as a single dose then 500 mg PO od for 2 days • Moxifloxacin 400 mg PO od for 10 days# Complicated urogenital infection (PID, epididymo-orchitis): • Moxifloxacin 400 mg PO od for 14 days# # MHRA/CHM advice: New restrictions and precautions for use due to very rare reports of disabling and potentially long-lasting or irreversible side effects

Condition/ Infection	Suggested treatment
Anogenital warts	Observation period for minimum of 3 months unless symptoms of pain, bleeding or irritation. First-line treatment cryotherapy +/− local topical anaesthetic Podophyllotoxin and Imiquimod are not licensed for use in children. Can be used in 2- to 18-year-olds with specialist advice off-licence. Excision/electro surgery under general anaesthesia can be considered if all other treatment modalities have failed.
Genital Herpes	Neonatal herpes High risk of vertical transmission, suspected or unwell neonate • IV acyclovir (20 mg/kg 8 hourly) for 10 days Acute HSV episode Treat if within 5 days of start of episode or while new lesions are still developing. Child 1 month–2 years • Acyclovir 100 mg PO five times a day for 5 days Child >2 years • Acyclovir 200 mg PO five times a day for 5 days Child weighing >40 kg • Acyclovir 400 mg PO tds for 5 days Child >12 years • Acyclovir 400 mg PO tds for 5 days OR • Valaciclovir 500 mg bd for 5 days Analgesia • 5% lidocaine ointment may be useful to apply especially prior to micturition

Condition/ Infection	Suggested treatment
Congenital Syphilis	Benzyl penicillin sodium 60–90 mg/kg daily IV (in divided doses given as 30 mg/kg 12 hourly) in the first 7 days of life and 8 hourly thereafter for a further 3 days for a total of 10 days
Acquired Syphilis	Child <12 years • IV benzyl penicillin sodium 200,000–300,000 IU/kg/day IV administered as 50,000 IU/kg every 4–6 hours × 10 days Child >12 years • IV benzyl penicillin sodium 50,000 IU/kg every 4–6 hours xx 10 days

Note: *Gentamicin levels need to be monitored if this regimen is used.

Question: The patient's swabs are positive for chlamydia. How common are chlamydia and other STIs in the adolescent female population?

Answer: Data from Public Health England and Health Protection Scotland found that between 2009 and 2014, 6394 under 16-year-olds were diagnosed with an STI per year. In England, 1.5% of those adolescents were under 13 years. In the under 16s, 87% of infections were in girls, and in the under 13s, 62% of infections were in girls. In the 16–19 age group there were 93,713 STIs diagnosed per year. The British Paediatric Surveillance Unit monitored STIs in under 13s from 2010–2012 and found an incidence of 0.075 per 100,000 children per year.

Chlamydia is the most common STI diagnosed in young people, with 128,000 new diagnoses in patients 15–24 years old in 2016. Anogenital warts are the second most common STI diagnosed, followed by genital herpes and gonorrhoea. The introduction of the HPV vaccine in 2008 has led to a significant reduction in anogenital warts: 62% reduction in first episode of anogenital warts in young men and 72% reduction in young women.

Question: What are the safeguarding considerations in this case?

Answer: Gillick competence must be assessed at the outset of the hospital consultation. A thorough risk assessment for CSE using the 'Spotting the Signs' proforma should be performed. Presence of bacterial/protozoal STI in 13- to 15-year-olds is a potential marker of CSE.

The age of her partner is important. In the UK, the age of consent (the legal age at which people can have sex) is 16 years. If the child is under 13 years, then it is classed as statutory rape. It is against the law for any person over the age of 16 years to engage in sexual activity with a child under the age of 16 years.

If there had not been a history of sexual activity, child sexual assault should then be considered and thoroughly investigated. In a girl under 13 years, an urgent referral to social services is required. In girls over the age of 13 years, cases should be assessed on an individual basis and discussed with the local safeguarding lead to decide on the need for referral to social services.

Question: After treatment of the acute episode of PID, what are the next steps?

Answer: The broad-spectrum antibiotics used to treat PID will cover *C. trachomatis*, so no further antimicrobials will be required. The girl should be referred to the genitourinary medicine team for full STI screening including HIV, hepatitis and syphilis. An assessment should be made as to the need for HIV postexposure prophylaxis (PEP) or hepatitis vaccination. Follow-up review 2–4 weeks after therapy may be useful to ensure adequate clinical response, compliance with oral antibiotics, screening and treatment of sexual contacts, awareness of the significance of PID and its sequelae and repeat pregnancy test, if indicated.

Test of cure (TOC) is not routinely recommended for uncomplicated genital chlamydia infection because residual, non-viable chlamydial DNA may be detected by NAAT for 3–5 weeks following treatment. TOC is recommended in pregnancy, where poor compliance is suspected and where symptoms persist.

Contact tracing will be carried out by the genitourinary medicine clinic. This is important because transmission rates can be up to 75%. The current male partner should be contacted and offered screening for gonorrhoea and chlamydia. Tracing of contacts within 6 months of symptom onset is recommended, but this may be influenced by sexual history.

Because many cases of PID are not associated with chlamydia or gonorrhoea, broad-spectrum empirical therapy should also be offered to male partners, e.g. doxycycline 100 mg twice daily for 1 week. Partners should be advised to avoid intercourse until they and the index patient have completed the treatment course.

The girl should be encouraged to partake in the National Chlamydia Screening Programme (NCSP), where young people under the age of 25 are encouraged to have opportunistic screening for chlamydia. She should be encouraged to have the HPV vaccine if she has not had it in school already.

Compliance with contraception should be assessed and information given about alternative long-acting reversible contraceptives. The importance of always using condoms to protect against STIs should also be discussed.

Question: What are her long-term reproductive implications from having PID?

Answer: PID is the primary cause of tubal factor infertility and is an important risk factor for ectopic pregnancy. The risk of these outcomes increases following repeated episodes of PID. Other long-term complications include pelvic adhesions, chronic pelvic pain and perihepatic adhesions secondary to Fitz–Hugh-Curtis syndrome.

BIBLIOGRAPHY

Ashby J, Browne R, Dwyer E, Fifer H, Forsyth S, Hamlyn E, Rayment M, Rogstad K, Ward C, Wilkinson D. BASHH National Guideline on the Management of Sexually Transmitted Infections and Related Conditions in Children and Young People. 2021.

United Kingdom National Guideline for the Management of Pelvic Inflammatory Disease. 2018. https://www.bashhguidelines.org/current-guidelines/systemic-presentation-and-complications/pid-2019/

Nwokolo NC, Dragovic B, Patel S, Tong CYW, Barker G, Radcliffe K. 2015 UK national guideline for the management of infection with Chlamydia trachomatis. International Journal of STD & AIDS 2016;27(4): 251–267.

Brook G, Church H, Evans C, Jenkinson N, McClean H, Mohammed H, Munro H, Nambia K, Saunders J, Walton L, Sullivan A. 2019 UK National Guideline for consultations requiring sexual history taking: Clinical Effectiveness Group British Association for Sexual Health and HIV. International Journal of STD & AIDS 2020;31(10): 920–938.

BASHH. Brook. Spotting the Signs of CSE Proforma. https://legacy.brook.org.uk/our-work/spotting-the-signs-cse-national-proforma

PART 4

Head and Neck

37

Thyroid

PAUL S. CULLIS, ALOK SHARMA, AND IAIN J. NIXON
Royal Hospital for Children and Young People, Edinburgh, UK

Scenario: A 13-year-old female presents to the paediatric endocrinology outpatient clinic for review of diabetes. The girl has a past medical history of type 2 diabetes mellitus, polycystic ovary syndrome and obesity. The doctor reviewing the teenage girl at clinic identifies a neck lump incidentally.

Question: What other examination findings would be helpful and provide clues to diagnosing the neck lump? What are the next best steps in management?

Answer: Palpation of cervical lymph nodes would be the most helpful additional aspect of clinical examination to include the central and lateral compartments. Locoregional spread via lymphatics to the cervical chain – 'lateral aberrant thyroid' – is typical of papillary thyroid carcinoma. Additionally, assessment of thyroid hormone status is essential. This patient is clinically euthyroid, which is confirmed on thyroid laboratory function tests. Assessment of laryngeal nerve function with flexible nasolaryngoscopy confirms normal vocal cord activity. An ultrasound scan with fine needle aspiration cytology (FNA) would also be a useful first-line investigation. The scan reveals a 2-cm lesion within the left lateral lobe of the thyroid gland (**Figure 37.1**). This is a solid, hypoechoic nodule with extensive

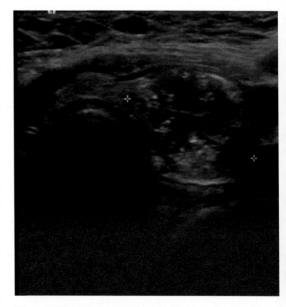

Figure 37.1 Ultrasound scan shows a 2-cm lesion within the left lateral lobe of the thyroid gland. This is a solid, hypoechoic nodule with extensive internal microcalcifications, typical of papillary cell carcinoma and is graded as U5.

internal microcalcifications, typical of papillary carcinoma, and is graded as U5. Cytology is consistent with papillary thyroid carcinoma (Thy5). MR imaging also performed in this case revealed similar findings consistent with the thyroid ultrasound scan (**Figure 37.2**).

DOI: 10.1201/9781003182290-41

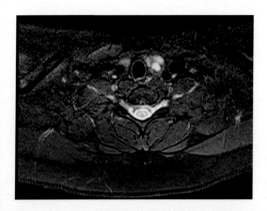

Figure 37.2 Cross-sectional MR T2 image showing multiseptated fluid-weighted cystic structure in the lower pole of the left lobe of the thyroid gland.

Question: What operation should be considered?
Answer: In a patient with a small unilateral tumour confined to the thyroid gland, operative excision is essential. For paediatric patients total thyroidectomy is best recommended. This is because of high rates of multicentric disease – typically involving both lobes of the thyroid – which results in higher reoperation rates following hemi- rather than total thyroidectomy. In this particular patient a hemithyroidectomy had been undertaken because of multiple comorbidities. Pathology revealed a 16-mm-diameter, well-circumscribed papillary thyroid carcinoma with numerous foci of micropapillary carcinoma identified additionally throughout the lobe of resected thyroid and associated small-volume lymph nodes. The tumour was staged as T1b(m)N1aM0. Subsequent later discussions at a multidisciplinary team (MDT) tumour board meeting recommended a complete thyroidectomy to remove the contralateral lobe and facilitate radioactive iodine treatment. The patient underwent complete surgery, which in this case confirmed additional microscopic foci of papillary thyroid carcinoma in the gland remnant, and has now undergone adjuvant radioactive iodine ablation therapy.

Paediatric thyroid cancers exhibit higher rates of disease multicentricity and both regional and distant metastatic disease in comparison to adult tumours. Despite these seemingly adverse prognostic factors, long-term prognosis is considered excellent (>95% survival, although ~20% recurrence risk).

Question: What are the complications of thyroid surgery, and how are these minimised?
Answer: Following thyroid lobectomy there is risk of postoperative haemorrhage with airway compromise. As a result, such patients are monitored closely for a minimum of 6 hours postoperatively. There is also a risk of injury to recurrent laryngeal nerves (<5%) which would result in a hoarse voice. Longer term, around 25% of paediatric patients having thyroid surgery may become hypothyroid, requiring L-thyroxine replacement. Bilateral total (or complete) surgery is associated with similar risks, although bilateral recurrent laryngeal nerve palsy can result in the permanent need for tracheostomy. As the parathyroid glands lie adjacent to the thyroid, patients are at risk both in the short term (20%) and long term (1–2%) of hypoparathyroidism. High-volume thyroid surgeons have notably lower risks of complications (>30 index operations/annum), and paediatric surgery with a typical low volume throughput of thyroid patients annually may therefore be associated potentially with a higher incidence of complications than in adult practice. It is emphasised strongly therefore that paediatric thyroid surgery is best only undertaken by high-volume thyroid surgeons with super-centralisation of practice where possible.

Scenario: The parents of a 12-year-old girl have reported that she has become quite anxious and her school performance has declined recently. The family attended the general practitioner who noted the teenager had weight loss and sweaty palms and palpated a smooth, firm and non-tender goitre, without cervical lymphadenopathy.

Question: What is your working diagnosis, and which blood tests may be helpful in this scenario?
Answer: The symptoms and signs are highly suggestive of hyperthyroidism with diffuse enlargement of the thyroid gland ("toxic goitre") so thyroid function tests would be helpful. A raised T_4 would be expected in this scenario, and most often, decreased thyroid-stimulating hormone (TSH) levels would be seen to suggest a primary cause, such as Graves's disease. The presence of TSH receptor antibodies would help establish the final diagnosis. In Hashimoto's thyroiditis, hypothyroidism is typically seen, and elevated antithyroid peroxidase or antithyroid microsomal antibodies will be detected. A benign colloid goitre is an alternative diagnosis, but such patients are normally euthyroid. Antibodies would not be detected. Notably this is the most common cause of diffuse thyroid enlargement in children. Inflammatory (e.g. subacute thyroiditis) and compensatory (e.g. iodine

deficiency, medications) causes are encountered less frequently than the aforementioned diagnoses. Ultrasound is a useful adjunct in making diagnosis and would be expected to show diffuse thyroid enlargement as in Graves's disease, which was this patient's underlying diagnosis.

Question: Which therapy options are available for a patient with this condition?

Answer: Thionamide derivatives, such as methimazole and propylthiouracil, are often used as first-line medical agent therapies. These inhibit thyroid hormone synthesis; some inhibit conversion of T_4 to T_3 and may have immunosuppressive activity. Side effects are usually mild, such as nausea and rash, but serious adverse drug events can occur infrequently, such as the most feared, agranulocytosis, occurring in <1% patients. If resistance to pharmacological drug therapy is apparent or severe reactions to medication were to develop, then ablative thyroid therapies are indicated. Radioiodine therapy with ^{131}I aims to induce a hypothyroid state to prevent recurrent Graves's disease, rather than achieving euthyroidism. Radioiodine is generally considered effective and safe. Vomiting and radiation-induced thyroiditis are side effects, and long-term risks of malignancy appear to be unfounded, certainly in older children and adults. In younger children ^{131}I therapy is usually avoided. Surgery is the alternative option here for treatment of Graves's disease in the very young patient. Total thyroidectomy is the operation of choice, as subtotal thyroidectomy carries significant risks of Graves's recurrence. The pitfalls of surgery have been discussed previously.

Scenario: A 12-year-old girl who is otherwise fit and well attends the paediatric surgery ambulatory clinic with a longstanding, painless, midline swelling in the neck, which the parents have noted on two occasions has become hot, red and discharged pus.

Question: What is the working differential diagnosis, and what examination findings would be helpful in narrowing this diagnostic list?

Answer: The differential diagnosis includes a thyroglossal cyst, dermoid cyst, cervical lymphadenopathy, atypical mycobacterial infection, sebaceous cyst and, less likely, carcinoma. A useful aspect of clinical examination is to request that the patient swallow, which is easily accomplished by providing a glass of water, and demonstrating that the neck mass moves on tongue protrusion. Thyroglossal cysts will typically move during these manoeuvres. A thyroglossal cyst was diagnosed at clinic. Thyroglossal cysts tend to present in childhood, with approximately 50% present <20 years of age. Complications include infection/abscess formation, and occasionally malignancy (papillary cancer) can present within a thyroglossal duct cyst. Infection is a relatively common troublesome issue and is best managed with antibiotics; incision and drainage increases the risk of recurrence after formal excision. The risk of carcinoma is considered very low (<1%), though considered more frequent amongst girls.

Question: Which imaging investigations are indicated?

Answer: An ultrasound +/− FNA cytology may be performed if there is concern of an alternate diagnosis, especially carcinoma; however, thyroglossal cyst is generally a clinical diagnosis. Ultrasound confirms the position of the neck cyst (with an orthotopic normal thyroid gland) and can facilitate FNA if indicated. FNA is generally not well tolerated in children, it may yield less information than in adult thyroid practice and there is risk of developing a chronic discharging fistula from any procedural insult with a congenital thyroid duct cyst. If significant tongue base involvement is suspected, MRI scan can also be a useful investigation. Of interest, this patient underwent MR imaging (**Figures 37.3** and **37.4**).

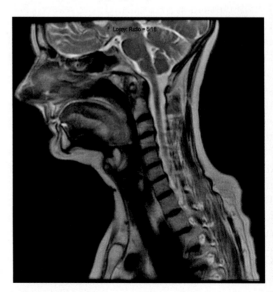

Figure 37.3 Sagittal T2 MR image showing a thyroglossal cyst.

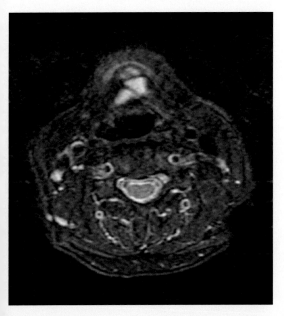

Figure 37.4 Transverse T2 MR image showing a thyroglossal cyst.

Question: What would the next best steps in management be?

Answer: A simple cystectomy or cyst enucleation will result in high rates of recurrence (>30%). Sistrunk's operation should therefore be scheduled. This involves a complete excision of the cyst and the thyroglossal duct tract from the isthmus to tongue base and central portion of the hyoid bone. This definitive procedure is preferred because of the associated low recurrence risk (3%–5%). The Sistrunk procedure has more recently been 'modified' in response to growing recognition of the aberrant ramifying nature of the thyroid duct tract, thus reducing disease recurrence rates to <1%.

Scenario: The clinical geneticist refers a 4-year-old boy to the surgical clinic after undertaking genetic testing. The boy's mother was diagnosed with multiple endocrine neoplasia type 2A (MEN2A) after presenting with thyroid cancer at aged 14 years. The child's genetic testing reveals a mutated allele of the RET proto-oncogene.

Question: What thyroid cancer may the mother have had in adolescence?

Answer: Medullary thyroid carcinoma (MTC) arises from the parafollicular C cells within the thyroid gland, which normally produces calcitonin and can be used as a vital tumour marker and accounts for about 5% of thyroid malignancies in childhood. MTC may be associated with MEN2A, MEN2B, familial MTC (FMTC) syndrome or occur sporadically. Late presentation is typical in sporadic cases, with metastases often present at diagnosis.

Question: Why has the medical geneticist referred this otherwise healthy boy to the surgeon?

Answer: Prophylactic thyroidectomy may prevent MTC from developing in asymptomatic children carrying the mutated RET proto-oncogenes. This strategy approach is especially important, as resection remains the only effective curative treatment. It is recommended that children with MEN2A and MEN2B undergo prophylactic total thyroidectomy at 5 and 1 years of age, respectively, in order to prevent development of MTC and confer normal healthy life expectancy. These practice guideline recommendations reflect the fact that MTC in association with MEN2B tends to present earlier and is more biologically aggressive. Progress to advance genetic analysis of RET mutations has allowed better risk categorization of malignant degeneration. Radical neck node dissection is not typically required in children undergoing prophylactic thyroidectomy.

BIBLIOGRAPHY

1. Francis GL, Waguespack SG, Bauer AJ, et al. *Thyroid* (2015). PMC4854274
2. Scottish Thyroid Cancer Project Board. *Consensus guidance on routine practice for differentiated thyroid cancer in Scotland* (2020). http://www.edinburghdiabetes.com/scottish-thyroid-cancer.
3. NICE. *Thyroid disease: assessment and management* (2019). https://www.nice.org.uk/guidance/ng145/chapter/recommendations.
4. British Thyroid Foundation (2021). https://www.btf-thyroid.org/guidelines-and-statements.
5. Martucci C, Crocoli A, De Pasquale MD, et al. Thyroid cancer in children: a multicenter international study highlighting clinical features and surgical outcomes of primary and secondary tumors. Front Pediatr 2022;10:914942.

6. Diesen DL, Skinner MA. In Ashcraft's Paediatric Surgery. Ch 76. Endocrine disorders and tumors 2014;1067–1085.

7. Sistrunk WE. The surgical treatment of cysts of the thyroglossal tract. Ann Surg 1920;71:121–123.

8. Seow-En I, Hong Pheng Lo A, Wen Quan Lian D, et al. Thyroid duct cyst carcinoma: diagnostic and management considerations in a 15 year old with a large submental mass. BMJ Case Rep 2015. doi 10.1136/bcr-2015-210923

38

Branchial cleft, branchial fistula and sternal cleft lesions

EMMA J. WHITEHALL AND ADAM J. DONNE
Alder Hey Children's Hospital, Liverpool, UK

Scenario: A 15-year-old boy presented to a tertiary paediatric centre with a 2-week history of a left-sided neck swelling, which was uncomfortable. He did not have any systemic symptoms or any other head and neck problems such as sore throat or voice change. He became more aware of the swelling when swallowing, but was able to eat and drink normally. He was otherwise fit and well with no prior history of any other medical problems.

On examination the patient had a visible 5 cm x 7 cm left-sided level II neck swelling, which was firm and non-fluctuant, with no overlying skin changes. There was no restriction of neck movements and no trismus.

Question: What is the likely diagnosis? What other feature should be looked for on examination?

Answer: This is most likely a branchial cyst even though it was not fluctuant in this case. Other possible differential diagnoses would include unilateral cervical lymphadenopathy. It is unlikely to be an abscess, as the swelling was not fluctuant or tender. The differential diagnoses also would include a lymphovascular lesion or a dermoid cyst. Lymphangiomas can present at any age, although they are usually apparent soon after birth.

The patient should be carefully examined for evidence of an external punctum indicating the opening of a sinus tract or fistula. Sinuses are tracts which have a blind ending and which may open either internally or externally. Fistulae by definition are a connection between two epithelial lined surfaces and so will have both internal and external openings. Branchial anomalies may be classified as either cysts, sinuses or fistulae or a combination of these, resulting from failure of the branchial cleft to fully involute during embryonic development. It is rare to find an internal opening to a branchial anomaly in the ambulatory clinic or on oral examination or at endoscopy.

Question: What type of branchial cyst is this?

Answer: This is a second branchial cleft cyst. Second branchial cleft cysts are usually located in the lateral neck anterior to the upper third of the sternocleidomastoid, which correlates to the finding of the neck swelling in the level II region of the neck in this patient. Cysts may also be found without an external sinus tract opening.[1,2] Any associated sinus is usually in the lower third of the neck just anterior to the sternocleidomastoid muscle. Abnormalities of the second branchial cleft are the most common type of branchial cleft lesion encountered in paediatric surgical practice and can be associated with the branchio-oto-renal syndrome. This particular patient did not have any diagnosis of a genetic syndrome, but investigations should best include a pure tone audiometry and renal ultrasound scan as initial screening tests.

DOI: 10.1201/9781003182290-42

Second branchial cleft cysts, sinuses and fistulae arise from remnants of the embryological second branchial arch. Second branchial cleft sinuses represent the majority of cleft sinus types. These are the most common type of branchial abnormality. Sinuses or fistulae are more commonly diagnosed in children, as they may discharge or the external punctum may be noticed.[3] Cysts are often diagnosed later in teenagers or young adults, as they are not initially evident, but the swelling increases in size with time. This was the case for this patient who presented with the cyst at the age of 15 years.

Question: What is the usual anatomical course of a second branchial cleft sinus or fistula?
Answer: As mentioned earlier, the external opening of a second branchial cleft sinus tends to appear anterior to the lower third of the sternocleidomastoid muscle. The sinus tract runs close to the glossopharyngeal (IX) and hypoglossal (XII) nerves, as well as the external and internal carotid arteries,[1] before opening internally at the tonsillar fossa. The tract may either run between the external and internal carotid arteries or deep or superficial to the carotid sheath. If a true fistula, the medial most aspect will open at the palatine tonsil.

The main differences between the four subtypes of second branchial sinuses are listed in **Table 38.1**. Note that type II is the most common subtype.

Table 38.1 Subtypes of second branchial cleft anomalies

Subtype	Relation to sternocleidomastoid muscle	Relation to carotid sheath
I	Anterior	Does not contact carotid sheath
II	Deep	May be either anterior or posterior
III	Deep, extends to the lateral wall of the pharynx	Between external and internal carotid arteries
IV	Deep, adjacent to the lateral wall of the pharynx	Deep

Question: Does this patient require any further investigations to confirm the diagnosis?
Answer: Ultrasound is a useful investigation to demonstrate the cystic nature of the lesion and can differentiate it from lymphadenopathy or abscess within a lymph node.

In order to further define the relationship of the cyst or sinus tract to other anatomical structures, cross-sectional imaging may be required. This can also be useful to assess whether a sinus tract or fistula is present, particularly if a cyst has been identified clinically or by ultrasound.[4] It may also be able to define better deeper lesions which cannot be fully appreciated by ultrasound, for example, a subtype IV cyst. MRI provides better soft tissue definition than CT scan.

This patient had both an ultrasound (**Figure 38.1**) and CT (**Figure 38.2**) at the time of his initial clinic presentation.

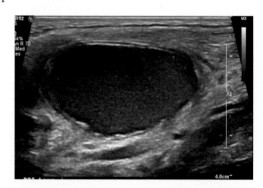

Figure 38.1 Ultrasound scan showing a second branchial cleft cyst in a 15-year-old boy.

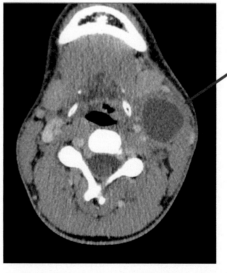

Figure 38.2 CT scan showing left-sided second branchial cleft cyst in a 15-year-old boy (*red arrow*).

Scenario: A 4-year-old girl presents with a history of malodorous discharge from the right ear. She did not have problems with hearing, and there is no pain associated with the discharge. On examination a pit is visible in the inferolateral portion of the ear canal.

Question: What is the likely working diagnosis? What else would you as the surgeon examine in the head and neck regions?

Answer: This presentation is consistent with a first branchial cleft abnormality. In the presence of discharge and a pit there is likely to be either a sinus present with an opening into the external auditory canal or a fistula connecting the internal opening in the ear canal to an external opening.

It would be important to examine the patient for any evidence of an associated cyst lesion, which may be present in close association with the nearby parotid gland. A cyst would be palpable either inferior to or just anterior to the pinna of the ear. Examination should assess for an external opening of a fistula, which may be present either just above the mandible or inferior to the mandible in the suprahyoid regions of the neck. Finally, a full head and neck examination would be indicated to assess for any associated abnormalities or dysmorphic features which may be associated with related genetic syndromes.

First branchial cleft anomalies are classified into type I (purely ectodermal) and type II (containing both ectodermal and mesodermal tissue), based on Work's classification.[4] Type I lesions are cystic without a tract. They are usually medial to the conchal bowl, and the cyst may extend to the postauricular groove. Type II lesions usually form a tract which courses from an external opening inferior to the angle of the mandible and above the hyoid bone or onto the face superior to the mandible. The tract runs through the parotid gland and passes either deep or superficial to the facial nerve. It may have a blind end inferior to the ear canal (sinus) or may open internally inside the ear canal (fistula). Approximately 10% of patients with a type II lesion have a membranous attachment between the floor of the ear canal and the tympanic membrane.[5]

Question: What are the potential differential diagnoses for first branchial cleft anomalies?

Answer: First branchial cleft sinuses or fistulae usually open internally in the external auditory canal. This can give rise to symptoms such as otorrhea (if there is discharge from the sinus) or otalgia, which may result in initial misdiagnosis and inappropriate management. Careful examination can help to distinguish first branchial cleft anomalies from otological conditions such as cholesteatoma and otitis media. A first branchial cleft may also be confused for a lesion within the parotid gland, and ultrasound imaging can be helpful here to differentiate these.

Another important differential diagnosis is preauricular sinus. Preauricular sinuses may initially appear similar on cursory examination; however, the anatomical location of the pit allows the exact diagnosis to be made. While first branchial sinuses may have an internal opening within the ear canal or an external opening which is located close to the angle of the mandible and therefore inferior to or anterior to the lower part of the pinna of the ear, preauricular sinuses open just anterior to the root of the helix. Preauricular sinuses result from incomplete fusion of the hillocks of His during development of the pinna and therefore have a different origin from first branchial cleft anomalies. Both branchial cleft anomalies and preauricular sinuses may present with infection in the sinus resulting in erythema and swelling. In this situation locating the sinus opening can be more difficult, so imaging with ultrasound and re-examination when the initial infection has been treated with antibiotics may be helpful.

Note: Atypical mycobacterial infection of a level II neck node (or a parotid node) may give a similar clinical appearance to a chronically infected type I branchial cleft cyst.

Question: How do third or fourth branchial cleft anomalies present clinically?

Answer: Third and fourth branchial anomalies usually occur in the left side of the neck. Second branchial types can be bilateral. Third branchial cleft cysts appear in a similar location to second branchial cleft anomalies, typically anterior to the sternocleidomastoid muscle. They tend to be more inferior in the neck than second variant anomalies. If there is an external sinus opening, it will also be present in the lower neck. If there is an internal opening, it will typically drain into the pyriform fossa. These lesions will usually present with neck swelling or may have symptoms of infection.

Fourth branchial cleft anomalies occur in the lateral lower third of the neck, and the majority are on the left side. The cyst is most commonly adjacent to the superior lobe of the thyroid gland. If there is an external opening, it will be located inferior to the thyroid and cricoid cartilages. As with third cleft anomalies, if there is an internal opening, it will be in the pyriform fossa. The course of the sinus or fistula tract is closely related to the course of the recurrent laryngeal nerve.[8] The most common presentation is with infection, which due to the close proximity to the thyroid gland can result in a suppurative thyroiditis. There have been some reports of fourth branchial cleft cysts causing hypoglossal nerve palsies from resultant compression.

Possible other differential diagnoses for third and fourth branchial cleft anomalies include lymphadenopathy, lymphatic or vascular malformations, dermoid cysts, thyroglossal duct cysts and primary thyroid pathology. These can usually be excluded by clinical examination and imaging.

Question: How should a patient with a branchial cleft anomaly be best managed?
Answer:

1. **Initial assessment**
   A careful history and examination should be carried out to determine how the anomaly is affecting the child and whether they have had episodes of infection. Examination will allow the surgeon to establish which type of lesion is likely to be present and if there are any current signs of infection.

   If the lesion is actively infected, the patient should be treated with antibiotics prior to definitive surgical treatment. However, if the external opening of the sinus in the lower neck is not discharging and is not causing infection, then it could be left untreated.

2. **Investigation**
   Ultrasound is often useful as an initial imaging modality as it can help to differentiate branchial cleft anomalies from other diagnoses. It is often quick to obtain, and no radiation is involved. If the diagnosis is confirmed and surgery is planned, CT or MRI (or sometimes a combination of both) will be indicated to assess how the lesion relates to other structures in the neck to help plan surgical excision safely. Many surgeons prefer to avoid CT in favour of MRI if the patient can tolerate MR examination. Incisional biopsy is contraindicated, as it will leave behind part of the lesion, which may potentially result in recurrent infections, and subsequent surgery will be more difficult due to scarring and distortion of the anatomy.

3. **Operation(s)**
   The definitive treatment for all types of branchial cleft anomaly is surgical excision. A complete excision of the cyst along with any associated sinus or fistula tract is required. The main reason for surgical excision is related to the high rate(s) of infection, which usually tend to recur if untreated. Depending on the type of anomaly, the tract can be identified either from the external or internal opening and followed carefully meticulously to resect it en-bloc.

   For second to fourth anomalies direct pharyngo-laryngoscopy at the time of excision is indicated to look for the sinus opening in the tonsillar fossa or pyriform fossa.[9] This can be carried out under the same general anaesthetic in combination with excision. Recently, for simple fistulae with no cysts, some surgeons have advocated use of internal opening monopolar cautery in efforts to seal off the opening and reduce the infection risk adequately to avoid excision completely.

   Excision of first branchial anomalies often requires superficial parotidectomy with careful preservation of the facial nerve to ensure the tract is fully excised.[6,7] Surgery for second anomalies may be combined with an ipsilateral tonsillectomy to ensure that any opening present in the tonsillar fossa has been fully removed, although this is debatable (**Table 38.2**).

Scenario: A 7-week-old baby presents to clinic with a congenital skin contracture in the midline of the neck anteriorly and an associated cystic lesion. Examination and ultrasound are suggestive of a cervical midline fusion defect.

Table 38.2 Types of branchial cleft anomalies

Type	Location of cyst	Internal opening	External opening	Management considerations
First	Anteroinferior to pinna	External auditory canal	On face superior to angle of mandible or in suprahyoid region of neck inferior to angle of mandible	May require superficial parotidectomy to completely excise sinus or fistula tract
Second	Anterior to upper third of sternocleidomastoid	Tonsillar fossa	Anterior to upper third of sternocleidomastoid	May require ipsilateral tonsillectomy to completely excise sinus or fistula tract
Third	Anterior to lower third of sternocleidomastoid	Pyriform fossa	Anterior to lower third of sternocleidomastoid	Endoscopy is useful to identify internal opening
Fourth	Lateral neck adjacent to superior lobe of thyroid	Pyriform fossa	Inferior third of neck inferior to cricoid cartilage	Endoscopy is useful to identify internal opening

Question: How will you manage this patient?

Answer: Midline fusion defects result from incomplete fusion of the branchial arches in the midline during embryological development (**Figure 38.3 a–d**). In the neck this results in a raw 'weeping area' of skin in the midline, typically in the suprasternal region. Cystic lesions can also occur here and be mistaken for arteriovenous malformations. Over time the central cleft lesion can become increasingly scarred and result in contractures. This

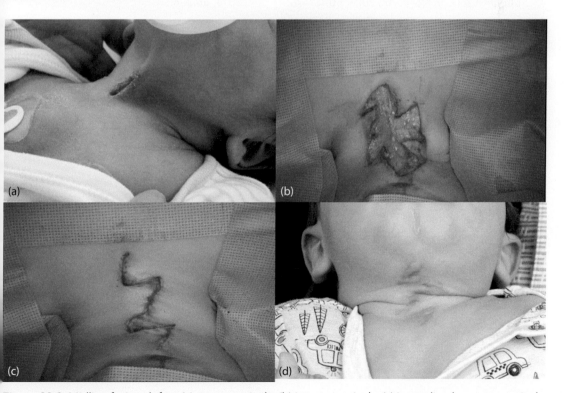

(a)   (b)   (c)   (d)

Figure 38.3 Midline fusion defect (a) preoperatively, (b) intraoperatively, (c) immediately postoperatively and (d) when healed.

will cause problems such as torticollis, restricted neck extension and tethering of the chin.

Excision requires removal of the skin lesion and associated fibrotic area, which is more extensive than the apparent size of the skin lesion. The subcutaneous tissue may extend from sternum to chin and prevent head extension. Z-plasty repair with excision is essential to prevent wound contracture.[10] This patient was therefore managed as a joint shared case between ear/nose/throat (ENT) surgeons and plastic surgery service.

BIBLIOGRAPHY

1. Ahuja AT, King AD, Metreweli C. Second branchial cleft cysts: Variability of sonographic appearances in adult cases. *Am J Neuroradiol* 2000; **21**:315–9.
2. Guldfred LA, Philipsen BB, Siim C. Branchial cleft anomalies: Accuracy of preoperative diagnosis, clinical presentation and management. *J Laryngol Otol* 2012; **126**:598–604.
3. Acierno SP, Waldhausen JHT. Congenital cervical cysts, sinuses and fistulae. *Otolaryngol Clin North Am* 2007; **40**:161–76.
4. Work WP. Newer concepts of first branchial cleft defects. *Laryngoscope* 1972; **82**:1581–93.
5. Triglia JM, Nicollas R, Ducroz V, *et al*. First branchial cleft anomalies: A study of 39 cases and a review of the literature. *Arch Otolaryngol - Head Neck Surg* 1998; **124**:291–5.
6. Chavan S, Deshmukh R, Karande P, Ingale Y. Branchial cleft cyst: A case report and review of literature. *J Oral Maxillofac Pathol* 2014; **18**:150.
7. Quintanilla-Dieck L, Virgin F, Wootten C, *et al*. Surgical approaches to first branchial cleft anomaly excision: A case series. *Case Rep Otolaryngol* 2016; **2016**:1–8.
8. Joshi MJ, Provenzano MJ, Smith RJH, *et al*. The rare third branchial cleft cyst. *Am J Neuroradiol* 2009; **30**:1804–6.
9. Nicollas R, Ducroz V, Garabédian EN, Triglia JM. Fourth branchial pouch anomalies: A study of six cases and review of the literature. *Int J Pediatr Otorhinolaryngol* 1998; **44**:5–10.
10. Helal AA, Mahmoud BA. Congenital midline cervical cleft. *J Pediatr Surg Case Reports* 2018; **36**:3–6.

39

Lymphadenopathy

AMPAIPAN BOONTHAI AND PAUL D. LOSTY
Ramathibodi Hospital, Mahidol University, Bangkok, Thailand

Scenario: A 2-year-old girl presents to your hospital with a fever and has a palpable submandibular lymph node of 1 week's duration. There is no weight loss and/or history of tuberculosis contact.

Physical examination: It shows a recorded temperature of 37°C, pulse 80/min, respiratory rate 20/min, blood pressure 100/60 mmHg. Body weight is 13.4 kg.

Head and neck examination: Multiple palpable enlarged lymph nodes are evident of varied size: 0.5–2 cm. The lymph nodes are non-tender to palpation and the overlying skin normal without erythema. Oral mouth examination shows an aphthous ulcer on the right buccal mucosa.

Question: How are lymphadenopathy sites and pathology areas correlated?

Answer: Lymph nodes filter lymph from predefined anatomical areas, and the location of the enlarged lymph node thus may give clues as to the site of underlying pathology. For example, submandibular or submental lymphadenopathy is usually resultant from pathology in the oral cavity, buccal mucosa, tongue, oropharynx and anterior neck because they filter lymph drainage from these defined areas (**Figure 39.1**).

A detailed clinical review identifying associated symptoms such as rashes, arthralgias, fever, or infectious illness contacts can greatly aid in developing a differential diagnosis. Viral lymphadenitis is often accompanied by a viral prodrome illness. The

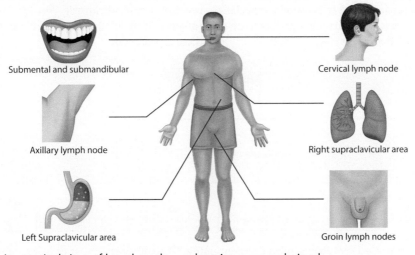

Submental and submandibular

Axillary lymph node

Left Supraclavicular area

Cervical lymph node

Right supraclavicular area

Groin lymph nodes

Figure 39.1 Anatomical sites of lymph nodes and territory areas drained.

DOI: 10.1201/9781003182290-43

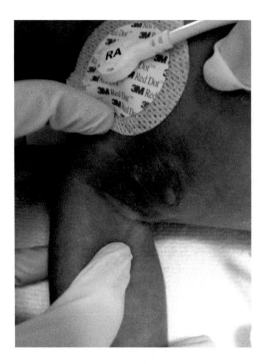

Figure 39.2 Multiple enlarged lymph nodes at the axilla. This newborn patient was later diagnosed to have congenital tuberculous lymphadenitis.

classic 'B symptoms' of fever, night sweats and unexplained weight loss should increase the surgeon's suspicion for lymphoma, whilst a clinical response to prescribed antibiotic therapies suggests a bacterial source. Confirming a patient's immunization history as well as family and social history may occasionally reveal unusual infection, autoimmune disorders or hereditary disease. In developing countries children showing signs of lymphadenopathy with firm, enlarged, painless lymph nodes especially if they are matted together, have a high incidence of *Mycobacterium tuberculosis* (**Figure 39.2**).

After obtaining a full detailed history, clinical and physical examination should be performed to delineate the characteristics and distribution of the involved lymph nodes and correlated with associated physical findings (**Figure 39.3**).

Question: What are the next appropriate steps to investigate in this patient?
Answer: Up to 90% of healthy children may have palpable lymph nodes at one time or another; thus it is important to minimize the risks of invasive procedures.

In those patients with cervical lymphadenopathy, a complete blood count and plain chest radiography are sufficient for initial investigations. Should any abnormality be detected or suspected from these early test investigations, then timely further management is key by scheduling lymph node biopsy and/or tumour marker workup (e.g. lymphoma, neuroblastoma).

Question: What are common indications for lymph node biopsy in paediatrics?
Answer: The degree of lymph node enlargement has been one of the key criteria for consideration of malignancy potential in children with lymphadenopathy. While normal lymph nodes in children can be enlarged up to 1 cm, a cut-off size of 3 cm has a sensitivity of 66% and a specificity of 80% for malignancy.

Based on the physical examination, our young patient has multiple cervical lymphadenopathy detected with submandibular lymph nodes approximately 2 cm in size. This patient may have benign cervical lymphadenopathy because of infection, inflammation, malignancy, medications or other disease processes.

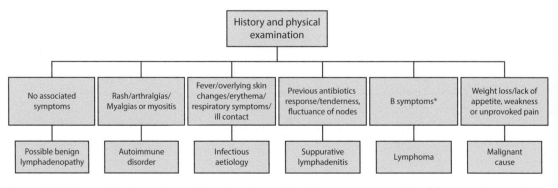

Figure 39.3 Associated symptoms in lymphadenopathy. *B symptoms consist of fever, night sweats and unexplained weight loss.

Question: Considering the patient's history and information gathered from the physical exam, do you think the child needs any specific treatment for her current condition and why?

Answer: The appropriate management in this clinical scenario is active observation only. From the patient's history the child was noted to have an unspecified viral upper respiratory tract infection before she developed cervical lymphadenopathy without any other concerning 'B symptoms' or unprovoked pain. Physical examination showed no stigmata associated with malignancy such as generalized lymphadenopathy, supraclavicular lymphadenopathy or fixed non-tender nodes.

A number of 'red flag' factors associated with malignant lymphadenopathy have been identified in which tissue biopsy is advisable (**Table 39.1**).

Table 39.1 Clinical features associated with peripheral lymphadenopathy concerning for malignancy

- Systemic symptoms (fever >1 week, fatigue, night sweats, significant weight loss >10% of body weight)
- Supraclavicular lymphadenopathy
- Generalized lymphadenopathy
- Fixed non-tender lymph nodes >1 cm with onset in the neonatal period
- Non-tender lymph nodes ≥3 cm in diameter that increase in size during treatment
- Persistent lymphadenopathy ≥4 weeks
- Firm, matted, fixed nodes
- Mediastinal mass or hilar adenopathy
- Abnormal complete blood count
- Absence of symptoms in the ear, nose and throat regions
- Persistently elevated or raising erythrocyte sedimentation rate or C-reactive protein

Source: Adapted from table 1 of Grant C, et al. Lymphadenopathy in children: a streamlined approach for the surgeon - a report from the APSA cancer committee. *Journal of Pediatric Surgery* 10/01 2020;56. Reference 2.

Question: Does excisional biopsy have better sensitivity and specificity in the diagnosis of lymphadenopathy compared to fine needle aspiration (FNA)?

Answer: FNA yields a 92%–100% specificity and 67%–100% sensitivity in determining a malignant lymphadenopathy diagnosis. However, if there are clinical concerns of malignancy, i.e. progressive growth and systemic symptoms, an excisional biopsy should be promptly arranged to confirm the diagnosis.

Scenario: An 18-month-old girl underwent excisional biopsy of a submandibular lymph node and developed an asymmetrical face when crying immediately postoperation. Physical examination is shown in **Figure 39.4**.

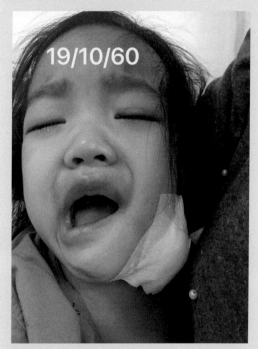

Figure 39.4 Abnormality is noted on the left side of the lower face seen immediately postoperatively.

Question: What do you think is a cause of this abnormality?

Answer: The clinical photograph shows a typical deformity 'asymmetric crying facies' resultant from iatrogenic marginal mandibular nerve (MMN) injury to the facial nerve.

The incidence of MMN branch injury depends on the surgery performed and may be seen in up to 20% patients after excision of the submandibular gland. The MMN is a terminal branch of the extracranial part of the facial nerve which has a superficial course across the body of the mandible. This nerve maintains facial symmetry during facial expression by innervating depressor muscles of the lower lip. Resultant injury will produce asymmetry of the mouth during smiling, crying, etc.

The injury may be a temporary neurapraxia which spontaneously recovers or, if permanent, require plastic surgery nerve muscle transfer reconstruction.

SUMMARY

Lymphadenopathy is a common occurrence in children of which the aetiology is usually benign, self-limiting and requires no specific active treatment. Careful history taking and physical examination will greatly aid in identifying causes and guide further investigations. Confirmatory biopsy is warranted when it is mandatory to exclude malignancy for which pathological tissue material can be obtained either by FNA or excisional biopsy.

BIBLIOGRAPHY

1. Farndon S, Behjati S, Jonas N, et al. How to use... lymph node biopsy in paediatrics. Arch Dis Child Educ Pract Ed 2017;102:244–248.
2. Grant C, Aldrink J, Lautz T, et al. Lymphadenopathy in children: A streamlined approach for the surgeon — A report from the APSA Cancer Committee. J Pediatr Surg. 2021;56(2):274–281.
3. Murphy F, Losty PD. Pediatric lymph node biopsy – an eleven year single center experience. Pediatr Blood Cancer 2016;63(S3):S1–S321.
4. Tulley P, Webb A, Chana JS, et al. Paralysis of the marginal mandibular branch of the facial nerve: treatment options. Br J Plast Surg 2000;53(5):378–385.

40

Airway disorders: Subglottic stenosis

BRONAGH LANG, RANIA MEHANNA, AND JOHN RUSSELL
Childrens Health Ireland, Crumlin, Ireland

Scenario: A full-term male with a diagnosis of trisomy 21 was admitted to our institution at 8 months of age for elective repair of an atrial septal defect, a ventricular septal defect and closure of a patent ductus arteriosus. Postoperatively he remained intubated in the paediatric intensive care unit. He was successfully extubated but 4 days later developed biphasic stridor with increased work of breathing and an oxygen requirement.

Question: What is stridor?
Answer: Stridor is derived from the Latin word stridulous, meaning a harsh, shrill sound. The presence of stridor indicates partial obstruction of the large-diameter airways. As the radius of the airway decreases by a factor of 1, the area of the airway decreases by a power of 4. Due to the smaller diameter of the paediatric airway compared to that of adults, even minor changes can lead to a marked reduction in overall airway calibre. See **Figure 40.1**.

Question: What is your differential diagnosis?
Answer: Biphasic stridor suggests a severe, fixed airway obstruction at the level of the glottis, subglottis or upper trachea. Children with trisomy 21 have midface hypoplasia, macroglossia, narrowed nasopharynx and a shortened palate. Compared to other children they also have a relatively smaller subglottis, which predisposes them to developing acquired subglottic stenosis despite being intubated with a smaller-sized endotracheal tube [1].

Given the history of intubation (although not for a prolonged period of time) and diagnosis of trisomy 21, subglottic stenosis should be considered.

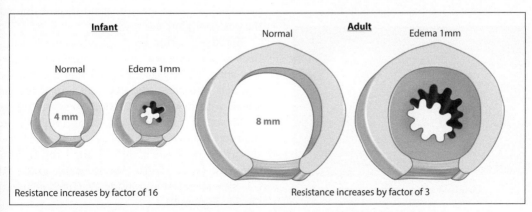

Figure 40.1 Effect of reductions in airway radius in paediatric patients versus adults.

DOI: 10.1201/9781003182290-44

Other differentials to consider in this case are post-intubation glottic granulomas, bilateral vocal cord palsy or laryngeal oedema [2].

Question: What investigations would you carry out?
Answer: Investigations of biphasic stridor will vary depending on the severity of symptoms. Given this child had a critical airway, he was taken to theatre for a microlaryngoscopy and bronchoscopy (MLB) under general anaesthesia, which is the gold-standard investigation.

If, on the other hand, the child is stable with mild stridor, investigations to consider are a plain film X-ray which may reveal a characteristic narrowed appearance at the subglottic area, known as the steeple sign. A flexible naso-endoscopy gives a good view of the supraglottis and vocal cords and allows dynamic assessment of the airway but does not visualise the subglottis or trachea.

> **Scenario:** An MLB was carried out which revealed bilateral vocal cord intubation granulomas and grade 3 subglottic stenosis. See below images.

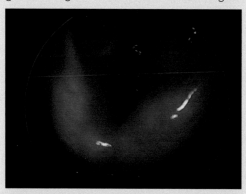

Bilateral intubation granulomas.

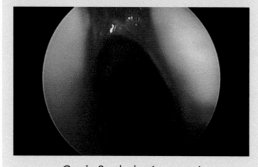

Grade 3 subglottic stenosis.

Question: What is subglottic stenosis and how is it graded?
Answer: Subglottic stenosis (SGS) can be acquired, congenital or mixed. The subglottis is the narrowest part of the paediatric laryngotracheal airway with a diameter of 4.5–5.5 mm in full-term neonates and just 3.5 mm in preterm infants.

Although the leading cause of acquired SGS is prolonged intubation, it can be a result of trauma or severe infection. The incidence of acquired SGS following neonatal intubation is reported as <1% and is usually the result of prolonged endotracheal intubation. The use of a large-diameter endotracheal tube even for a short period can lead to ischemic ulceration and scarring. Acquired SGS became an increasingly encountered entity as a direct consequence of the introduction of prolonged intubation for premature neonates with immature lungs in the 1960s. Measures taken to prevent SGS include use of an uncuffed tube placed via a nasal route, which reduces potential tube movement to a minimum. Injury to the airway is less likely with a small tube, which allows a small leak on positive pressure ventilation [3].

The increased use of microcuff endotracheal tubes with high-volume low-pressure cuffs in anaesthesia and paediatric intensive care has also reduced the incidence and prevalence of SGS [4].

During the initial assessment with MLB a careful evaluation of the stenosis is required. It is important to note the grade, the thickness and the length of the stenosis. The assessment also looks for stenosis involving the vocal cords, how near it is to the vocal cords, the presence of any other airway pathology or other areas of stenosis, for example, the posterior glottis or trachea.

The Myer Cotton grading system for SGS utilizes an endotracheal tube as a measure of airway size. The largest measured size that can be inserted into the subglottis and still maintain a leak with normal ventilation pressures (up to 25 cm water) is compared to the age-appropriate tube size for that child. The percentage of stenosis can then be calculated: Grade I (up to 50% stenosis), grade II (51–70% stenosis), grade III (71–99% stenosis) and grade IV (100% stenosis) [5]. See **Figure 40.2**.

Classification	From	To
Grade I	No obstruction	50% obstruction
Grade II	51% obstruction	70% obstruction
Grade III	71% obstruction	99% obstruction
Grade IV	No Detectable Lumen	

Figure 40.2 Cotton–Myer grading system to measure severity of subglottic stenosis.

Question: What is the first-line treatment for grade III subglottic stenosis?

Answer: The first-line treatment for an early grade III SGS is endoscopic balloon dilatation (EBD). EBD is carried out with suspension laryngoscopy under general anaesthesia with spontaneous ventilation. Direct laryngoscopy is performed using a 2.7- or a 4-mm 0° telescope, and the balloon catheter is introduced into the laryngeal lumen through the stenosis. The patient should then be preoxygenated. The balloon is then inflated to the rated burst pressure to maintain the balloon pressure for 2 minutes or until the patient's oxygen saturation level drops to 90%. The size and diameter of the balloon are selected according to the theoretical ideal diameter of the cricoid ring. The procedure can be performed two or three times during each session under general anaesthesia to achieve a satisfactory airway. See **Figure 40.3**.

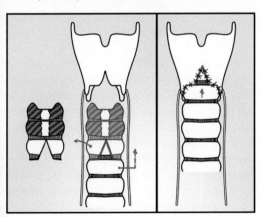

Figure 40.3 Partial cricotracheal resection.

Radial incisions with a sickle knife or carbon dioxide laser may be used in conjunction with balloon dilatation. This involves making incisions in four quadrants followed by balloon dilatation.

Topical substances such as steroids and mitomycin C (MMC) have been used to optimize endoscopic treatment. Intralesional steroid injections are known to decrease collagen synthesis and fibrosis, and though the exact mechanism of action is not completely clear, it is the most commonly used adjuvant agent currently [6]. Although controversial, MMC has been utilized in order to extend the time intervals between endoscopic treatments. MMC is a natural antibiotic produced by *Streptomyces caespitosus* and has antifibrinogenic and antineoplastic activities that have been shown to block fibroblast proliferation and thereby reduce scar formation on topical application. It has, however, fallen out of favour due to a lack of efficacy in the literature [7].

Complications of EBD are rare and include tracheitis, pneumomediastinum and tracheal laceration [8].

Scenario: The child underwent balloon dilatation with increasing size of balloons until a satisfactory airway was achieved. The posterior glottic granulomas were also removed with a cold steel technique. At the end of procedure he was nasally intubated with a size 3 microcuff endotracheal tube.

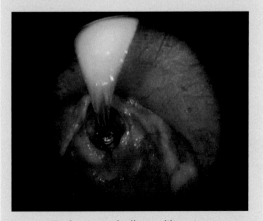

Endoscopic balloon dilatation.

Postoperatively he was successfully extubated and discharged home but presented 2 weeks later with a 2-day history of biphasic stridor. Repeat MLB revealed 88% grade III SGS. See **Figure 40.4**.

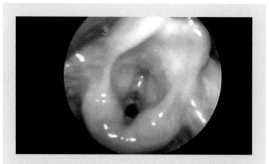

Figure 40.4 Grade III subglottic stenosis.

Question: What is the next step in management?
Answer: Given the child has failed EBD, the next step would be an endoscopic expansion procedure in the form of an anterior cricoid split (ACS).

In 1980 Cotton and Seid were the first to describe an open ACS in 12 neonates in order to avoid a tracheostomy in premature infants with SGS [9].

A cricoid split allows decompression of the oedematous submucosal glands of the subglottis and thus expansion of the airway.

When performed endoscopically, an ACS carries much less risk of accidental extubation and difficult re-intubation than with the open approach. The infant is placed in suspension laryngoscopy while spontaneously breathing under general anaesthesia. The operating surgeon places one hand externally on the neck to stabilize the cricoid and to judge the depth of the split. A microlaryngeal sickle knife or microlaryngeal scissors is used to transect the anterior cricoid mucosa and cartilage. The subglottis is then dilated with a balloon to increase the diameter [10].

The child underwent endoscopic ACS as well as balloon dilatation. He was nasally intubated with a size 3 microcuff endotracheal tube at the end of the procedure and transferred to the paediatric intensive care unit. See **Figures 40.5** and **40.6**.

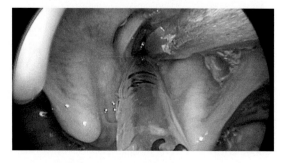

Figure 40.5 Endoscopic anterior cricoid split using microlaryngeal scissors.

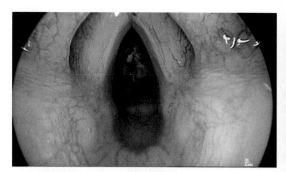

Figure 40.6 Post-endoscopic anterior cricoid split.

He was successfully extubated after 10 days. Repeat MLB 2 months later revealed a satisfactory airway and a reduction of 88% grade III to 53% grade II stenosis, which is a satisfactory result. See **Figure 40.7.**

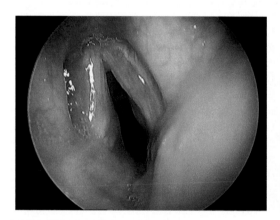

Figure 40.7 Satisfactory airway.

Scenario: An ex-premature male of 24 weeks' gestation with a history of prolonged intubation presented to our institution at corrected gestational age 38 weeks with cyanotic episodes and stridor. He also had a history of extreme low birth weight of 730 g, chronic lung disease and retinopathy of prematurity. He underwent MLB, which revealed a 70% grade III high circumferential SGS. Initially he underwent EBD. A repeat MLB 2 days later showed no improvement, and an endoscopic cricoid split was carried out. At the end of the procedure a size 3 nasal microcuff endotracheal tube was inserted. Unfortunately a repeat MLB 1 week following endoscopic ACS showed no major improvement and the patient remained intubated. See **Figures 40.8** and **40.9**.

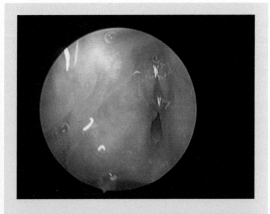

Figure 40.8 Endoscopic view post-cricoid split.

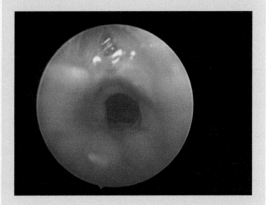

Figure 40.9 Endoscopic view post-cricoid split demonstrating high circumferential stenosis just below the vocal cords.

Question: What is your next step in management?
Answer: Tracheostomy.

This is the best option, as a laryngotracheal reconstruction is a major operation in this age group, and as he also has chronic lung disease, he would need a tracheostomy for airway protection and oxygenation anyway. It is better to wait until the baby is 2 or 3 years old to carry out airway reconstruction when they have better lung function. At this age they tolerate the surgery better, and one may also be able to correct the stenosis and remove the tracheostomy at the same time.

When compared to adult tracheostomies, paediatric tracheostomies are associated with a higher rate of complications. Early complications include accidental early decannulation, tube obstruction, positioning problems, wound breakdown and/or pneumothorax. Late complications include minor

or major bleeding from vessel erosion, granulation tissue formation, suprastomal collapse and tracheocutaneous fistula.

OPERATIVE TECHNIQUE

Under general anaesthesia with an endotracheal tube in situ, the patient is positioned with the neck extended and a shoulder roll in place. The surgical technique employed in all our patients is the horizontal skin incision marked approximately 1 cm below the cricoid cartilage.

Following skin incision, subcutaneous fat is removed to improve visualization and access and also to reduce the incidence of a false passage. The strap muscles are divided in the midline at the linea alba coli and retracted laterally. The thyroid isthmus is identified and divided, if necessary, with bipolar diathermy.

Non-absorbable stay sutures are placed above and below the intended incision site. Four quadrant absorbable maturation sutures are placed between the trachea and skin edges.

A horizontal tracheal incision is then made between the third and fourth rings. Following essential communication with the anaesthetist, the endotracheal tube is partially withdrawn and the tracheostomy tube is placed. Following confirmation of correct placement, the tube is secured with ties and the stay sutures are taped to the neck and chest and labelled.

In the immediate postoperative period, a chest X-ray is performed in the recovery room or intensive care unit (ICU) to exclude a pneumothorax. Patients are kept in the ICU postoperatively and heavily sedated until at least the first tube change, which we perform after 2–3 days at our institution. This is to promote rapid tract healing and to avoid movement which could precipitate accidental decannulation or development of a false passage. Patients are nursed with the head raised at 15° and are given a proton pump inhibitor and laxatives.

The first tube change is always carried out by the airway surgeon and an intensivist. The tube change is performed at the bedside in the paediatric intensive care unit (PICU) with the neck in extension and after a bolus of propofol (1–2 mg/kg), with enteral feeding ceased 4 hours prior. There is always a full tracheostomy set and a Frova 8.0 Fr Intubating Introducer (Cook, Inc., Bloomington,

IN) available. Once done, stay sutures are removed and patients are fit for discharge from the PICU from an airway point of view [11]. See **Figure 40.10**.

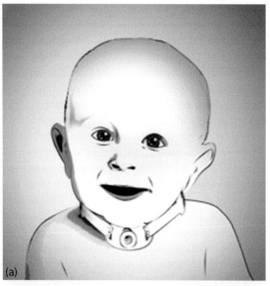

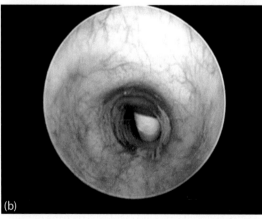

Figure 40.10 (a) External and (b) internal view of a paediatric tracheostomy.

The patient underwent tracheostomy at 4 months old with insertion of a size 3 neonatal tracheostomy tube. After several months he was discharged home with regular MLB follow-up.

Question: What reconstructive options would you consider in this case?
Answer: At this stage you would consider a laryngotracheal reconstruction (LTR) with anterior and posterior grafts at 2 or 3 years of age. LTR with costal cartilage interposition grafting was first described by Fearon and Cotton in 1972 [12].

LTR can be a single stage or double stage, and both techniques have their advantages and disadvantages. A single-stage LTR (SSLTR) allows immediate decannulation at the time of reconstruction or avoidance of tracheostomy altogether. The patient remains intubated for an extended period of time postoperatively with the tube acting as a stent. With this comes disadvantages that include care in the PICU, prolonged intubation potentiating pneumonias and the need for sedation that can induce withdrawals.

The potential for airway compromise after extubation makes the postoperative care of patients undergoing single-stage procedures very important. Contraindications for a single stage include multilevel obstruction, significant lung disease, high grade III or grade IV stenosis or in cases where reintubation is anatomically difficult [13].

A double-stage LTR (DSLTR) is where the tracheostomy tube is kept in place at the conclusion of the procedure and the patient is decannulated at a later stage [14, 15].

An LTR firstly involves exposing the laryngotracheal complex. If a double-stage procedure is planned, the incision is as noted earlier and does not communicate with the tracheostomy site. If a single-stage procedure is planned, the tracheostomy site is incorporated into the incision. A laryngofissure is then carried out, making sure to preserve the vocal cords, which is critical in order to preserve voice. At this stage, if required, a midline vertical incision is made in the posterior cricoid lamina, taking care not to incise the common wall between the airway and oesophagus.

Costal cartilage grafts are the most common graft material used today. The grafts are harvested from the fourth or fifth rib, maintaining the integrity of the deep perichondrium. A classic "boat"-shaped graft is carved to expand the airway. The grafts can be placed anteriorly and/or posteriorly depending on the extent and location of the stenosis [16]. See **Figures 40.11** and **40.12**.

In general LTR is the mainstay of surgical management in grade II and mild grade III stenosis or if the stenosis is involving or close to the vocal cords. LTR is less extensive than cricotracheal resection (CTR), as it does not require tracheal mobilization [14].

Potential complications of LTR include pneumothorax, unintentional extubation, infection or

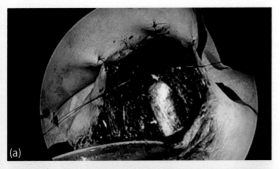

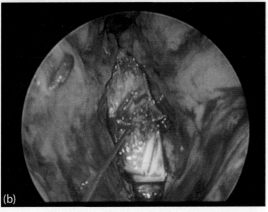

Figure 40.11 (a) Anterior costal cartilage graft and (b) posterior cartilage graft.

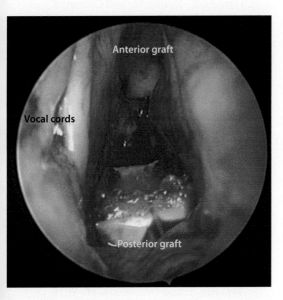

Figure 40.12 Endoscopic view of anterior and posterior grafts in situ.

failure of extubation due to oedema, restenosis or graft failure.

Scenario: At the age of 2.5 years old the patient underwent a DSLTR with anterior and posterior costal cartilage grafts. He was admitted to the PICU for 48 hours postoperatively and sedated. He recovered well postoperatively. See Figures 40.11 and 40.12.

Scenario: Unfortunately an MLB several months later demonstrated failure of the laryngotracheal reconstruction with a significant recurrence of a grade III SGS. See Figure 40.13.

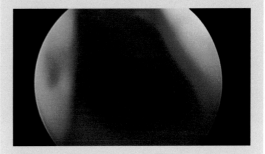

Figure 40.13 Grade 3 subglottic stenosis.

Question: What reconstructive options would you consider next?
Answer: The options include a further LTR with grafts or a partial cricotracheal resection (pCTR).

A pCTR involves segmental excision of the stenotic segment, resection of the anterior cricoid cartilage but preserving the posterior cricoid plate and completion with an end-to-end anastomosis [14]. See Figure 40.3. Monnier et al. published the first series of successful CTRs in 15 children in 1993 and followed this with an update in 1998 [17].

Similar to an LTR, a pCTR can be single stage or double stage. The choice between LTR and pCTR depends on the severity and extent of the SGS as well as the vocal cord function. It is generally accepted that a lesion very close to or involving the vocal cords is not suitable for resection and anastomosis due to the lack of tissue to suture the proximal cut end without jeopardizing the cord's function or mobility. Ideally the resection margin is a minimum of 3 mm from the vocal cords.

Complications include postoperative laryngeal oedema, restenosis, anastomotic dehiscence and recurrent laryngeal nerve injury [18].

At the age of 7 years old he underwent a single-stage pCTR. See **Figure 40.14**. Postoperatively he was nasally intubated with a size 4 microcuff endotracheal tube and kept sedated in the PICU for 2 weeks. He was successfully extubated 2 weeks postoperatively after an endoscopic assessment under general anaesthesia and was discharged home at 4 weeks post pCTR. See **Figure 40.15**. At

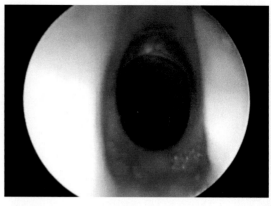

Figure 40.16 MLB at 6 months post-CTR.

his 6-month postoperative follow-up he had a normal endoscopic airway, a normal voice and normal swallowing. See **Figure 40.16**.

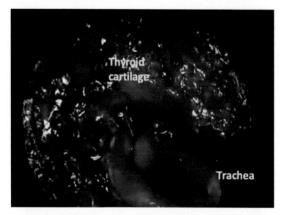

Figure 40.14 Intraoperative image during partial CTR.

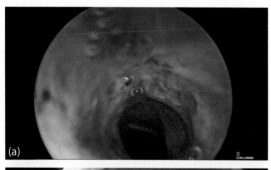

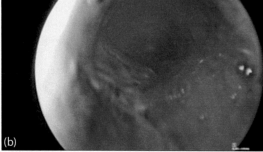

Figure 40.15 (a and b) Internal endoscopic view of the end-to-end anastomosis between the trachea and the cricoid mucosa at 2 weeks post-surgery.

BIBLIOGRAPHY

1. Mitchell, R., Call, E. and Kelly, J., 2003. Diagnosis and therapy for airway obstruction in children with down syndrome. *Archives of Otolaryngology–Head & Neck Surgery*, 129(6), p.642.
2. Pfleger, A. and Eber, E., 2016. Assessment and causes of stridor. *Paediatric Respiratory Reviews*, 18, pp.64–72.
3. Hartley, B., Rutter, M. and Cotton, R., 2000. Cricotracheal resection as a primary procedure for laryngotracheal stenosis in children. *International Journal of Pediatric Otorhinolaryngology*, 54(2–3), pp.133–136.
4. Greaney, D., Russell, J., Dawkins, I. and Healy, M., 2018. A retrospective observational study of acquired subglottic stenosis using low-pressure, high-volume cuffed endotracheal tubes. *Pediatric Anesthesia*, 28(12), pp.1136–1141.
5. Myer, C., O'Connor, D. and Cotton, R., 1994. Proposed grading system for subglottic stenosis based on endotracheal tube sizes. *Annals of Otology, Rhinology & Laryngology*, 103(4), pp.319–323.
6. Sekioka, A., Fukumoto, K., Yamoto, M., Takahashi, T., Nakaya, K., Nomura, A., Yamada, Y. and Urushihara, N., 2018. Serial intralesional triamcinolone acetonide injections for acquired subglottic stenosis in premature infants.

Pediatric Surgery International, 34(10), pp.1047–1052.

7. Ahmad Latoo, M. and Jallu, A., 2020. Subglottic stenosis in children: Preliminary experience from a tertiary care hospital. *International Journal of Otolaryngology*, 2020, pp.1–7.

8. Lang, M. and Brietzke, S., 2013. A systematic review and meta-analysis of endoscopic balloon dilation of pediatric subglottic stenosis. *Otolaryngology–Head and Neck Surgery*, 150(2), pp.174179.

9. Cotton, R. and Seid, A., 1980. Management of the extubation problem in the premature child. *Annals of Otology, Rhinology & Laryngology*, 89(6), pp.508–511.

10. Carr, S., Dritsoula, A. and Thevasagayam, R., 2018. Endoscopic cricoid split in a tertiary referral paediatric centre. *The Journal of Laryngology & Otology*, 132(8), pp.753–756.

11. Woods, R., Geyer, L., Mehanna, R. and Russell, J., 2019. Pediatric tracheostomy first tube change: When is it safe?. *International Journal of Pediatric Otorhinolaryngology*, 120, pp.78–81.

12. Fearon, B. and Cotton, R., 1972. Surgical correction of subglottic stenosis of the larynx. *Annals of Otology, Rhinology & Laryngology*, 81(4), pp.508–513.

13. Agrawal, N., Black, M. and Morrison, G., 2007. Ten-year review of laryngotracheal reconstruction for paediatric airway stenosis. *International Journal of Pediatric Otorhinolaryngology*, 71(5), pp.699–703.

14. Bajaj, Y., Cochrane, L., Jephson, C., Wyatt, M., Bailey, C., Albert, D. and Hartley, B., 2012. Laryngotracheal reconstruction and cricotracheal resection in children: Recent experience at Great Ormond Street Hospital. *International Journal of Pediatric Otorhinolaryngology*, 76(4), pp.507–511.

15. Yamamoto, K., Monnier, P., Holtz, F. and Jaquet, Y., 2014. Laryngotracheal reconstruction for pediatric glotto-subglottic stenosis. *International Journal of Pediatric Otorhinolaryngology*, 78(9), pp.1476–1479.

16. Brigger, M. and Hartnick, C., 2009. Laryngotracheal Reconstruction. *Operative Techniques in Otolaryngology Head and Neck Surgery*, 20(4), pp.229–235.

17. Monnier, P., Savary, M. and Chapuis, G., 1993. Partial cricoid resection with primary tracheal anastomosis for subglottic stenosis in infants and children. *The Laryngoscope*, 103(11), pp.1273–1283.

18. Monnier, P., 2018. Partial cricotracheal resection and extended cricotracheal resection for pediatric laryngotracheal stenosis. *Thoracic Surgery Clinics*, 28(2), pp.177–187.

PART 5

Hepatobiliary and Pancreatic Disorders

41

Biliary atresia

MARK DAVENPORT
Kings College Hospital, London, UK

Scenario: A 6-week-old infant was referred to the local paediatric unit with a history of persistent jaundice. The child was born following an uneventful pregnancy and delivery at term. She had been breastfed since and was gaining weight appropriately and was considered otherwise well. The baby was noted to be jaundiced on day 3 of life, but this faded and she was then discharged home. However, her mother and the health visitor noted the jaundice to be still evident at 6 weeks of age.

In the local unit the baby was further assessed, and later questioning suggested that her stools were inappropriately pale with dark urine. An abdominal examination did not identify any specific abnormality aside from an umbilical hernia. The examining doctor realised the importance of the clinical signs of pale stool and dark urine and initiated a series of blood tests, with the most important being a split bilirubin.

Question: Why are these clinical features important?
Answer: Persistent jaundice may be defined as jaundice occurring beyond 14 days of life, so this clearly needs further investigation, but even at this stage biliary atresia would be considered a rare cause. The history of pale, creamy or white stool is, however, strongly suggestive of a lack of bile colouring the stool. This, together with clinical evidence of a raised conjugated bilirubin, suggested that this particular bilirubin fraction is water soluble and hence can be excreted via the kidneys and hence the dark colouring of the urine. Infantile urine should be crystal-clear.

In most medical-related causes of jaundice, and physiological jaundice itself, it is the unconjugated bilirubin fraction which is elevated. A split bilirubin (total and conjugated – in older textbooks, the terms total and direct bilirubin are used) enables the paediatrician to concentrate on likely pathological causes.

Question: What are the common causes of conjugated jaundice in an infant of 6 weeks?
Answer: These can be broadly divided into medical and surgical. There is a long list of the former and a short list of the latter (**Table 41.1**).

Question: Why don't there seem to be any specific signs of liver disease in this infant?
Answer: The pathophysiology of biliary atresia can be thought of as cholestatic jaundice dating from birth with a more gradual increase in liver fibrosis as a result. This latter complication can take weeks and months to develop and is the principal cause of the liver pathophysiology such as ascites and portal hypertension. So, it would be unlikely in infants less than 6 weeks (<42 days) to have obvious hepatosplenomegaly or indeed ascites. Conversely, in infants approaching 3 months (>90 days) of life, you should now be feeling the liver and spleen, and thereafter detecting ascites.

Question: Do infants with biliary atresia present in any other way?
Answer: While jaundice is invariable (if looked for), some infants may actually present with disordered

DOI: 10.1201/9781003182290-46

Table 41.1 Medical and surgical causes of conjugated jaundice in an infant

Medical	Cause	Features	Surgical	Cause	Features
Alagille's syndrome	Genetic, biliary hypoplasia, cardiac anomalies, butterfly vertebrae	Jaundice, may present with cardiac symptoms	Choledochal malformation	Always cystic (type 1C) during neonatal period	Possible antenatal detection of a sub-hepatic cyst
Alpha-1-antitrypsin deficiency	Genetic	Jaundice	Inspissated bile syndrome/gallstones	↑Haemolysis ↑Sepsis	Usually preterm with prolonged gastrointestinal rest and use of PN
Parental nutrition–associated liver disease	Multifactorial	Usually preterm, with prolonged periods of parental nutrition. History of surgery (e.g., ileostomy)	Spontaneous perforation of bile duct	Perforation can be anterior or posterior bile duct	Fluctuating jaundice, bile ascites Pigmented hydrocele or umbilical hernia in boys
Giant-cell hepatitis	Not known	Needs liver biopsy for diagnosis	BILIARY ATRESIA		
Neonatal hepatitis	Not known	Needs liver biopsy for diagnosis			
PFIC*	Family of genetic syndromes	Progressive jaundice, itching. Usually GGT↓↓			

PFIC: Progressive familial intrahepatic cholestasis.

coagulation secondary to low vitamin K levels. This is caused because vitamin K is fat-soluble and shows impaired absorption in the absence of bile in the gut, and many countries are now abandoning routine vitamin K injections at birth. Some infants will present with abnormal bleeding, mostly minor – for example, at the umbilicus – but in others it may be serious (e.g. intracranial).

Another possible scenario is following the detection of a sub-hepatic cyst on a maternal screening antenatal ultrasound exam, which can be consistent with a variant called cystic biliary atresia (CBA). The differential diagnosis here is with a cystic choledochal malformation, which are usually larger, and patients may, in fact, not be jaundiced in the postnatal period. The more difficult discrimination is when these become obstructed and therefore jaundiced (**Figure 41.1**).

Further investigation in this infant has now included an abdominal ultrasound. This showed

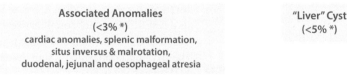

Antenatal Features

Associated Anomalies
(<3% *)
cardiac anomalies, splenic malformation,
situs inversus & malrotation,
duodenal, jejunal and oesophageal atresia

"Liver" Cyst
(<5% *)

Biliary Atresia

Conjugated Jaundice
(100%)

Acholic Stools
(95%)

Dark Urine
(90%)

Vitamin K-dependent Coagulopathy
(<3%)

Cirrhosis, ascites
(<5%)

Postnatal Features

Figure 41.1 Modes of presentation of biliary atresia.

a slightly increased liver size but with a homogenous parenchyma. The gallbladder was atrophic and did not visibly change on feeding the infant. There was no sign of dilatation of the intrahepatic bile ducts, and the portal vein and hepatic arterial flow appeared normal.

Question: Shouldn't the bile ducts increase in size in biliary atresia, as it is obstructing bile flow at the level of the extrahepatic duct?
Answer: No, this is a prime discriminator with the other surgical causes of jaundice which do feature dilated intrahepatic bile ducts. Such ducts in biliary atresia are very abnormal, being hypoplastic and disordered, and rarely exhibiting a "tree-like" pattern.

The initial laboratory blood panel shows bilirubin 150 µmol/L (conjugated 100 µmol/L); AST 150 IU/L; alkaline phosphatase 250 IU/L; and γ-glutamyl transpeptidase 500 IU/L. Viral serology is negative, and α-1-antitrypsin levels are normal. These tests confirm a biochemical "obstructive" pattern, and with the abnormal ultrasound pattern, many specialist units would continue straight to some kind of cholangiogram study (see later). Others would now do a percutaneous liver biopsy, expecting the histology to show features such as bile duct duplication, bridging fibrosis and perhaps a small cell infiltrate, again characteristic of an "obstructive" picture.

Question: Is there any role for radio-isotope studies?
Answer: These were performed far more frequently in the past certainly. The typical isotopes used are based on technetium[99m] attached to molecules designed to "track" the flow of bile (e.g. iminodiacetic acids). Absence of isotope beyond the liver is indicative of obstruction (i.e. biliary atresia), but isotope scanning has a high false-positive rate. It may be useful in a patient cohort where biliary atresia is actually unlikely – i.e. the preterm infant with a history of total parenteral nutrition (TPN) use where you are actually trying to prove it is not biliary atresia by showing isotope in the intestine.

Question: Provide more information about the spectrum of biliary atresia and its variants.
Answer: Biliary atresia is not considered a single disease, with a single uniform cause. It is probably best thought of as a final common pathway with many possible scenarios leading to it. For instance, there are variants of biliary atresia with other anomalies present, and the most representative of these, making up 10% of North American and European study series, is the biliary atresia splenic malformation syndrome (BASM). These infants have polysplenia

(though they may have no spleen at all – asplenia); vascular malformations such as a pre-duodenal portal vein and absence of the inferior vena cava; situs inversus; and, importantly, cardiac abnormalities. The genesis of all these anomalies lies within the first trimester post fertilisation, though the actual trigger is uncertain. In about 10% there is a genetic mutation (*PKD1-L-1*); in others it may arise as a result of maternal diabetes. CBA, mentioned earlier, is a distinct variant unassociated with other anomalies but having an obvious cystic component that may or may not contain bile. The third variant, though this is controversial, is biliary atresia associated with cytomegalovirus (CMV) and characterised as having CMV IgM antibodies. These infants are usually older and have more pronounced liver fibrosis.

The anatomical classification is based on a Japanese analysis of the most proximal level of biliary tract obstruction and has nothing to do with variants per se. **Figure 41.2** illustrates this. The most common by far is type 3 biliary atresia.

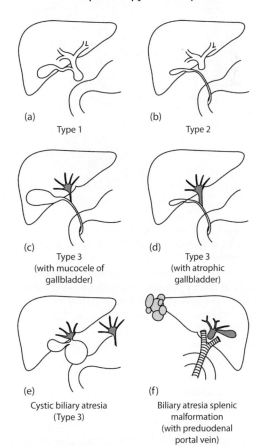

(a) Type 1
(b) Type 2
(c) Type 3 (with mucocele of gallbladder)
(d) Type 3 (with atrophic gallbladder)
(e) Cystic biliary atresia (Type 3)
(f) Biliary atresia splenic malformation (with preduodenal portal vein)

Figure 41.2 Classification of biliary atresia. (Reprinted by permission from: *Operative Pediatric Surgery* [Eds. Davenport M, Geiger J], CRC Press, 2021.)

Question: So, the baby is finally in the operating room – what next?

Answer: The first thing for the surgeon is to confirm what has, to this point, only been a suspicion. The gallbladder is the key here. Most infants have a solid, atrophic gallbladder without a lumen. This is biliary atresia, but you won't be able to do any form of cholangiogram. In others, there is clear mucus within a gallbladder lumen; again, this is biliary atresia. A cholangiogram study is possible here but will just show contrast traveling through to the duodenum. If there is bile aspirated in the gallbladder, almost certainly this is not biliary atresia. A cholangiogram might, just might, show an obstructed type 1 BA – usually a cyst – but much more likely will show a complete biliary tree with intra- and extra-hepatic parts.

The Kasai portoenterostomy (**Figure 41.3**) operation can be categorised into key phases:

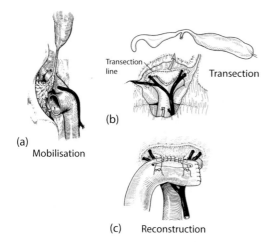

(a) Mobilisation
Transection line
Transection
(b)
(c) Reconstruction

Figure 41.3 The Kasai portoenterostomy. (a) Mobilisation of the gallbladder and extrahepatic bile ducts following division of the common hepatic duct. (b) Transection of the proximal biliary remnant from Rouviere's fossa on the right side to Rex's fossa on the left. (c) Portoenterostomy with Roux loop. (Elements reproduced by permission from Chapter 55: *Operative Pediatric Surgery* [Eds. Davenport M, Geiger J], CRC Press, 2021.)

i. *Mobilisation of the liver*: Division of the falciform and left triangular ligaments allows the liver to be dislocated from the abdominal cavity, thus providing better exposing of the porta hepatis. This does impede venous return, so careful collaboration with the anaesthetist is clearly important. Some surgeons leave the liver in situ but then usually select to sling the hepatic arteries and right and left portal veins to get decent exposure of the biliary remnants.

ii. *Dissection of the porta hepatis*: Essentially the aim is to separate vascular from biliary remnant scar tissue. Division of the common bile duct allows the proximal remnant to be freed and elevated. Most Kasai surgeons nowadays aim for an excision of all the remnant tissue in and around the interstices of the vessels, so going on to expose the Rex fossa on the left and Rouviere's fossa on the right.

iii. *Transection of the portal plate*: There is a surgical plane evident flush with the capsule of the liver that allows separation from the underlying liver. Actual 'coring out' liver tissue itself is not the aim – this simply scars up, obliterating any residual ductules.

iv. *Roux loop reconstruction*: A 40-cm Roux loop based on proximal jejunum about 5–10 cm beyond the duodenojejunal junction is raised. The actual portoenterostomy is best done in an anti-mesenteric side-to-side fashion using fine absorbable sutures – e.g. 6/0 PDS.

Question: What role (if any) does laparoscopy play in the management of biliary atresia?

Answer: Very little really. It can have a diagnostic role certainly and facilitate the cholangiogram study. There are published series where pioneers have reported its use, but in terms of actually improving the outcomes of the Kasai operation, it has absolutely no advantage, and many would say cannot it reproduce the meticulous surgery necessary for the more radical classical operation described earlier. International Pediatric Endosurgery Group (IPEG) suggested a moratorium on its use during the 2000s, but there is an increasing interest, currently particularly in large Asian centres.

Postoperatively, most hospital units use antibiotics to prevent cholangitis and high-dose steroids (which improve outcomes by 10–15%). Oral ursodeoxycholic acid may promote bile flow, but only after it is established by surgery.

Question: What are the important outcomes?

Answer: The first and most important is clearance of jaundice to normal levels of bilirubin. This can be achieved in experienced centres in approximately 50%–60% of infants. About 10%–20% really don't have any bile flow, and these should be recognisable within 2 months post-Kasai. They will need liver transplant. The other important measures of outcome are the native liver survival and true survival rates. Again, in expert centres this should be around 50% and 90%, respectively, at 5 years.

Question: What are the key factors determining success or failure of the Kasai portoenterostomy?
Answer: There are a number of these. First and foremost is actually something over which the surgeon has no control and that is the anatomy and constituents of the proximal biliary remnants. If there is no transected bile ductules or these are scant and small, then there will be a limited response. The idea behind the radical dissection proposed earlier is to maximise anatomical possibilities. Secondly, surgeon experience is considered an important determinant of outcome. It's a rare disease – something like 1 in 15–20,000 births – and only with some form of regionalisation or centralisation of care will individual surgeons build up familiarity of what is a variable disease. An 'acceptable' work volume rate has been quoted of ≥5/year. Thirdly, biliary atresia is not a static disease, and age at surgery does play a key role in outcome. Clearance of jaundice in infants ≤30 days should approach 80%, while it is, at best, about 50% or less in those ≥90 days.

The common complications are:

i. *Liver failure*: Evident with increasing jaundice, coagulopathy, ascites, failure of synthetic liver function and failure to thrive. Only treatable by liver transplantation.

ii. *Cholangitis*: Most evident within the first year post-Kasai and usually caused by gram-negative enteric organisms. Characterised by pyrexia, worsening jaundice and deranged liver biochemistry. Should be treated aggressively by intravenous antibiotics.

iii. *Portal hypertension*: Varices do take time to develop and can present as haematemesis and/or melaena from 6 to 18 months. Splenomegaly is invariable unless the baby has BASM. Varices should be treated by endoscopic sclerotherapy, and if liver function is poor then liver transplant will be required.

iv. *Malignancy*: Long-term survivors with biliary atresia inevitably have cirrhosis and so are at risk of malignant degeneration, but the risk is probably 1–2% overall.

BIBLIOGRAPHY

1. Kasai M, Suzuki S. A new operation for "non-correctable" biliary atresia – portoenterostomy. Shijitsu. 1959; 13: 733–739.
2. Davenport M, Tizzard S, Underhill J, et al. The biliary atresia splenic malformation syndrome: a twenty-eight year single centre study. J Pediatr. 2006; 149: 393–400.
3. Davenport M, Parsons C, Tizzard S, et al, Steroids in biliary atresia: single surgeon, single centre, prospective study. J Hepatol. 2013; 59: 1054–1058.
4. Davenport M, Ong E, Sharif K, et al. Biliary atresia in England and Wales: results of centralization and new benchmark. J Pediatr Surg. 2011; 46: 1689–1694.
5. Davenport M, Yamataka A. Surgery for biliary atresia: open and laparoscopic. In: Operative Pediatric Surgery 8th edition (eds Davenport M, Geiger J) pp 503–512, CRC Press, London 2020.

42

Choledochal malformation

MARK DAVENPORT
Kings College Hospital, London, UK

Scenario: A 7-year-old girl was referred to the local paediatric unit with a 3-year history of recurrent abdominal pain and two recent episodes requiring hospital admission with severe pain and vomiting. On examination, she had epigastric tenderness without guarding. No masses could be felt, and otherwise the abdomen was soft. Initial blood investigations showed a normal blood count and electrolytes but an elevated amylase level (1200, normal range: <75 IU/L). Liver biochemistry was marginally abnormal, e.g. total bilirubin 25 µmol/L, AST 75 IU/L and GGT 100 IU/L. She was treated conservatively for acute pancreatitis with intravenous fluids and settled within 3 days, with her elevated amylase and bilirubin levels returning to normal.

Further imaging using ultrasound showed a dilated biliary tree (common bile duct diameter 12 mm) and an oedematous pancreas. MRI hepatobiliary imaging (MRCP) suggested a fusiform biliary dilatation involving the extrahepatic part with a possible common channel (**Figure 42.1a**). This arrangement was later confirmed by open cholangiography (**Figure 42.1b**).

She was therefore considered to have a Type 1F choledochal malformation complicated by pancreatitis and was scheduled for elective surgery 4 weeks later.

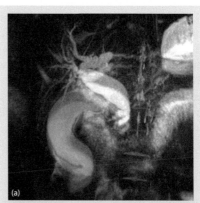
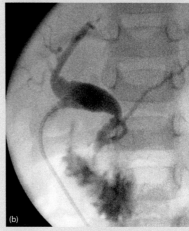

Figure 42.1 Fusiform (Type 1F) choledochal malformation presenting with pancreatitis. (a) MRCP shows biliary dilation and an obvious common channel. Note: Also, the artifact due to patient movement. (b) Confirmatory operative cholangiogram.

DOI: 10.1201/9781003182290-47

Question: Why are these clinical features important?

Answer: Pancreatitis is distinctly unusual during childhood. There is a long differential diagnosis (**Table 42.1**). However, there was no evidence of trauma, predisposing conditions suggesting gallstones, family history or abnormal drug history, so a biliary abnormality was possible. Abdominal ultrasound is a first-line investigation, and even in non-specialist centres should pick up the biliary dilatation, which is the key finding. Pancreatitis is usually fairly mild in such cases and almost invariably settles without complications (i.e. pseudocysts).

Question: How else might choledochal malformation present?

Answer: About 20% of infants these days present as an antenatally detected cyst on the maternal ultrasound scan (see later). The other common presentation is with obstructive jaundice; these may be infants and are usually Type 1C. In older children recurrent abdominal pain may lead to ultrasound and diagnosis. Some are incidental and picked up with the ubiquitous ultrasound. A small proportion seem to be related to other anomalies and specifically duodenal atresia. These are almost invariable fusiform in nature and probably congenital rather than related to previous neonatal surgery. **Figure 42.2** illustrates possible scenarios.

Antenatal Features

Sub-Hepatic Cyst
(~20%)

Choledochal Malformation

Jaundice (~30%)	Pancreatitis (~20%)	Abdominal pain (~10%)	Incidental (~10%)

Associated Anomalies e.g. Duodenal atresia (<2%)		Perforation (<5%)

Postnatal Features

Figure 42.2 Modes of presentation of choledochal malformation.

Question: What are the common types of choledochal malformation?

Answer: The first real classification (Alonso-Lej) was devised in the 1950s and based upon almost 100 cases published up to that time. This suggested three types (an extrahepatic cyst, a diverticulum of the bile duct and a localised bile duct cyst within the wall of the duodenum). This classification was further developed in the 1970s (Todani) to recognise three different types of extrahepatic dilatations (Type 1A, 1B and 1C), both extra- and intra-hepatic dilatation (Type 4A and 4B) and isolated intrahepatic dilatation (Type 5). More recently, Kings College Hospital Classification (1) simplified this further and is illustrated in **Figure 42.3**.

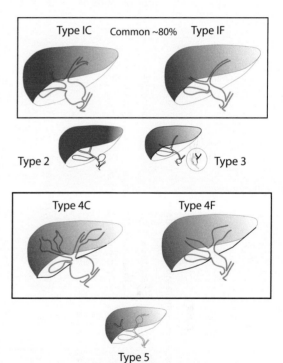

Figure 42.3 Kings College Hospital classification of choledochal malformation. (Reproduced with permission from Kronfli & Davenport. J Pediatr Surg. 2020;55[12]:2642–2646.)

Question: Is there a common cause or aetiology?

Answer: No, certainly Types 1C, 1F, 4C and 4F may be related either by varying forms of congenital bile duct stenosis and/or a common channel allowing reflux of pancreatic juice into the bile duct (2).

Table 42.1 Medical and surgical causes of pancreatitis in children

Medical	Cause	Features	Surgical	Cause	Features
Drug-related	Thiazide diuretics, anticonvulsants (e.g., valproic acid, chemotherapeutic agents, asparaginase)	Often multiple factors involved in complex patients	Trauma	Blunt abdominal trauma (e.g., bicycle handlebar) Non-accidental injury	M >> F Fracture of neck of pancreas
Hereditary pancreatitis	Genetic (e.g., SPINK1, PRSS1)	Family history, recurrent pattern	Gallstones	Haemolysis (e.g., sickle cell disease) Cholesterol stones	Usually preterm with prolonged gastrointestinal rest and use of PN
Autoimmune	Autoimmune reaction	Teenage years ↑IgG4 ↑Antinuclear antibody Associated with inflammatory bowel disease	Choledochal malformation	Fusiform > Cystic malformation Choledochocele	F > M
Viral	CMV, coxsackie virus, mumps virus, measles, EB virus Mycoplasma	Often multisystemic.	Isolated pancreatic ductal anomaly	Common channel Pancreas divisum	Diagnosed with ERCP
Cystic fibrosis	Heterozygotes **Idiopathic (up to 40%)**				

However, this is not true of the less common variants such as Types 2, 3 and 5.

Why are we using the term "choledochal malformation" and not "choledochal cyst", by the way? Because a choledochal cyst is but one specific type (Type 1C) of choledochal malformation. The word "cyst" is the Greek word for bladder and implies a certain globular, spherical shape. This does not describe the tubular, cylindrical, fusiform shape of the Type 1F choledochal malformation that is equally common and probably has a different pathophysiological profile from choledochal cysts. These are distinguishable.

Question: Where does Caroli's disease fit in here?
Answer: It doesn't really! Caroli's disease was described by a French gastroenterologist in the 1960s and has several distinct clinical features such as intrinsic hepatic fibrosis, an association with renal cysts and renal fibrosis. Furthermore, the actual biliary dilatation is confined to the intrahepatic ducts, is usually multiple, is on both sides of the liver and is relatively small and discrete. Lastly, it is definitely genetic in origin with mutations described in the *PKHD1* gene.

Question: How common are choledochal malformations?
Answer: A very difficult question to answer! There are no incidence studies – unlike biliary atresia. Not all choledochal malformations are evident at birth, and many, particularly the smaller ones, may remain completely asymptomatic for years. As a yardstick, at Kings College Hospital, UK, we would see 25–30 cases of biliary atresia annually with a known incidence of 1 in 17,000 live births. We consistently see 5–10 new cases of choledochal malformation annually, suggesting an incidence of <1 in 100,000. We do know that, like biliary atresia, there is a much greater prevalence in Asian countries (specifically Japan, Korea, China and Taiwan), although the reason is obscure.

Another possible scenario is following the detection of a sub-hepatic cyst on maternal fetal screening ultrasound. The differential here is between a variant of biliary atresia called cystic biliary atresia (CBA) and a (typically) cystic choledochal malformation. The latter are usually bigger, but there is plenty of overlap. The key to discrimination can be left until the baby is born, at which point a postnatal ultrasound should confirm the antenatal suspicion. Furthermore, it should become evident if there is functional biliary obstruction. The stools should become non-pigmented and turn white or a creamy colour, and the baby should be jaundiced with a high conjugated (split) bilirubin level.

If this is the case, then laparotomy and cholangiography should be scheduled emergently. The actual discrimination can be left to the cholangiogram to decide, and the operation tailored accordingly – a Kasai portoenterostomy or a hepaticojejunostomy.

For those detected and confirmed on ultrasound but who lose their jaundice and have normally pigmented stools, further investigations can proceed a little more slowly. This will involve an MRCP to define the anatomical features of the dilatation, and if confirmatory, a laparotomy can be scheduled electively. There is always an argument as to when this is best in the asymptomatic case. Too late, and you may be running the risk of missing ongoing yet significant liver damage. Too early, and the bile duct you are using in the anastomosis may just be too "fragile". We would favour the former approach really at some point beyond the neonatal period (>4 weeks).

Question: Is there any role for endoscopic retrograde cholangiopancreatography (ERCP) or radioisotope studies in the diagnosis?
Answer: Not really. MRCP has replaced ERCP or CT scan as the "go-to" diagnostic aid. We reserve ERCP for a small cohort of older children who present with recurrent pancreatitis yet fairly minor bile duct dilatation. These may have intrinsic pancreatic duct anomalies such as pancreas divisum, but they may also have "common channel syndrome" where there is an obvious (on ERCP) long common channel but not much bile duct dilatation. The cause of the pancreatitis in these cases (and the case described earlier) is reflux of bile into the pancreatic duct (Babbitt's observation), prompting premature activation of pancreatic enzymes and triggering pancreatitis. These children will need surgical separation of bile and pancreatic ducts.

Radioisotopes have a limited diagnostic role, though they can be used to determine functionality of the biliary system. There may be some asymptomatic children with mild fusiform dilatation, and a technetium[99m] iminodiacetic scan can show a normal bile excretion, justifying continued observation.

Question: The child finally appears in the operating room – what comes next?
Answer: The cholangiogram study (e.g. **Figure 42.1b**) is performed either directly into the dilated bile duct

or via the cystic duct. This will define the proximal intrahepatic bile duct anatomy to enable the anastomosis and also what is happening distally in the common channel. In this case (previous pancreatitis), it is imperative to clear the common channel of any debris or stones and ensure no ampullary stenosis.

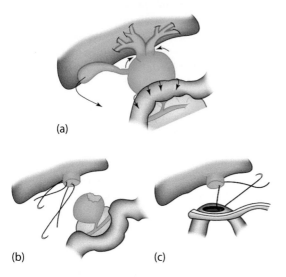

(a)

(b)   (c)

Figure 42.4 Stages of choledochal surgery. (a) Mobilisation of the dilated extrahepatic biliary tract and gallbladder. (b) Division at the level of the common hepatic duct and mobilisation of the distal bile duct within the head of pancreas. (c) Reconstruction hepaticojejunostomy using a Roux loop of jejunum. (Reproduced by permission from Choledochal malformation. In: *Surgery of the Liver, Bile Ducts and Pancreas* 3rd edition [Eds. Davenport M, Heaton ND, Superina R.] CRC Press, 2017.)

Choledochal surgery (**Figure 42.4**) can be broken into key phases (3):

i. *Excision of the dilated common bile duct and gallbladder*: Take down the gallbladder retrogradely from its bed to define the cystic duct junction, ligate the cystic artery and expose the common hepatic duct. Dissect medially and laterally along the duct/cyst. The right hepatic artery is at risk and can run in front of or behind the duct. Encircle the duct at the level of the common hepatic duct; the portal vein is at risk posteriorly. Divide and then free the duct from its bed. At the distal end, there is a dissection within the head of pancreas towards the junction with the pancreatic duct and the

common channel. You don't have to visualise this (for fear of damaging it) but leaving too great a bile duct remnant behind is similarly not a good idea. Either way, ensure the common channel is free and dilatable with a probe passed from above.

ii. *Biliary reconstruction*: Usually this involves a Roux loop. So, divide the jejunum about 10 cm from the duodenojejunal junction. Measure the length of the Roux loop, typically at about 40 cm, but certainly long enough to reach the porta hepatis via a retrocolic tunnel without tension. Restore intestinal continuity with a jejunojejunostomy (stapled or hand-sewn). The hepaticojejunostomy is performed end-to-side with the common hepatic duct near enough to the bile duct bifurcation – there is no need to go higher in most cases – to ensure a perfect anastomosis. Typically, absorbable monofilament (e.g. PDS™) is preferred. Always ensure, at minimum, that there is no debris or stones left in the intrahepatic duct system by a thorough saline lavage. A flexible choledochoscope or cystoscope can be used ideally to inspect.

Question: What role does laparoscopy/minimally invasive surgery play in the management of choledochal malformation?

Answer: The first laparoscopic excision of a choledochal cyst was reported during the 1990s in Italy. It very much has a role, if the operator is suitably experienced and accomplished in advanced endosurgical suture techniques. This is an uncommon operation in everyday practice, and the anastomosis is unforgiving if it leaks. It is better, and safer, to get this bit right rather than to store up complications for the future. Virtually all the major published series of laparoscopic choledochal operations have been reported from large Asian centres with a much higher case volume throughput than in Europe or North America (4). However, even here, replication of the open operation as described earlier is rarely achieved, and short-cuts have been developed. Fashioning a Roux loop is tricky laparoscopically, so most surgeons actually make the umbilical incision bigger and exteriorise the jejunum to do this part externally. Alternatively, some surgeons have abandoned a Roux loop as too difficult and elect to perform hepaticoduodenostomy. This is achieved by mobilising the duodenum ("Kocherising") enough so that the most cranial part can reach the transected common hepatic duct. This too has its downside, in that free reflux of duodenal content into the intrahepatic ducts can occur and bile can reflux into the stomach, aggravating chronic gastritis.

There may a role for robotic surgery, at least in children, to facilitate the proximal anastomosis with increasing precision techniques.

Postoperatively, most hospital centres use antibiotics for a period to prevent cholangitis, though that really should be rare if the restored bile flow is good.

Question: What are the important outcomes?
Answer: Restoration of normal bilirubin is a *sine qua non*. If this is not happening, then there is a complication. For the vast majority of children, they should become completely asymptomatic.

Possible complications are:

i. *Bile leaks*: This should be exceptional and <2% certainly in open surgery. They can be treated conservatively, but subsequent stenosis may follow. For those who have presented with pancreatitis, recurrent pancreatitis this is possible, and should be minimised by ensuring the pancreatic duct has free drainage. Sometimes a sphincteroplasty may be necessary at the same time as the choledochal surgery. If it occurs, then ERCP is warranted to exclude pancreatic/ampullary stenosis or a retained distal bile duct.
ii. *Persistence of intrahepatic dilatation*: This is the definition of a type 4 lesion, and certainly in children most diminish considerably over time if monitored by postoperative ultrasound. If not, they may form the nidus for stone formation which may precipitate cholangitis. This is much less likely nowadays as more care is spent clearing the ducts at the time of surgery.

iii. *Chronic liver disease*: Liver fibrosis, or even cirrhosis, is now very much less common than in former eras. If it is evident at the time of surgery, then close monitoring of liver function is mandatory, but it should hopefully be reversible.
iv. *Malignancy*: Some patients, typically middle-aged adults, will present with established malignant transformation in a pre-existing choledochal malformation. These have rarely been without a long history of symptoms though. It is possible, but highly unlikely, that malignant transformation of the biliary tract could occur in those parts left behind by surgery – the intrahepatic ducts and the remnant within the head of the pancreas. In a previous era when the surgery was simply internal drainage of a choledochal cyst to an adjacent part of the bowel, this was certainly a recognised long-term complication.

BIBLIOGRAPHY

1. Kronfli R, Davenport M. Insights into the pathophysiology and classification of type 4 choledochal malformation. J Pediatr Surg. 2020;55(12):2642–2646.
2. Turowski C, Knisely AS, Davenport M. Role of pressure and pancreatic reflux in the aetiology of choledochal malformation. Br J Surg. 2011;98:1319–1326.
3. Davenport M, Nguyen Thanh Liem. Choledochal malformation. In: Operative Pediatric Surgery 8th edition (eds Davenport M, Geiger J) pp 513–521, CRC Press, London 2020.
4. Liem NT, Pham HD, Dung le A, et al. Early and intermediate outcomes of laparoscopic surgery for choledochal cysts with 400 patients. J Laparoendosc Adv Surg Tech A. 2012;22:599–603.

43

Cholelithiasis

MARK D. STRINGER
Wellington Children's Hospital and University of Otago, Wellington, New Zealand

Gallstones (or cholelithiasis) may be found in children of any age and have even been reported in the fetus. Most studies of paediatric gallstones show a bimodal age distribution with a small peak in infancy and a steadily rising incidence from early adolescence onwards. In early childhood, boys and girls are equally affected, but a female preponderance emerges during adolescence. Western children have shown an increase in the prevalence of both gallstones and cholecystectomy during the last 50 years, which may reflect improved detection from the widespread use of diagnostic ultrasonography and an increase in the incidence of gallstones.

> **Scenario:** A previously well 13-year-old girl presents to the emergency department with a 24-hour history of progressively worsening right upper quadrant abdominal pain. She feels nauseated but has not vomited. She has a low-grade fever. On examination she is tender in the right hypochondrium, worse on deep inspiration. There is no palpable abdominal mass.

Question: What is your differential diagnosis? What initial basic investigations would you request and why?
Answer: Cholecystitis is a likely diagnosis, but other conditions to consider include acute hepatitis, acute pancreatitis, atypical appendicitis and a right-sided basal pneumonia. Initial blood tests should include a full blood count (including a blood film and reticulocyte count), biochemical liver function tests (LFTs), C-reactive protein, plasma lipase and urinalysis. An abdominal ultrasound scan should be requested urgently if the clinical picture is that of cholecystitis (acute tenderness, fever, elevated white cell count), but can be done as an out-patient if the diagnosis is more in keeping with biliary colic and the patient's pain improves with simple analgesia. A chest radiograph is necessary if there is a concern about a pneumonia, and a viral hepatitis screen sent if the LFTs suggest hepatitis.

Biliary colic is characterised by the sudden onset of severe right upper quadrant abdominal pain that may radiate to the right shoulder or back and be accompanied by vomiting. It is caused by transient gallstone obstruction of the cystic duct. If the obstruction persists for several hours, the gallbladder becomes inflamed leading to *acute cholecystitis*, which causes pain and tenderness in the right upper quadrant. Murphy's sign (right hypochondrial pain on deep inspiration) may be present together with fever and leucocytosis. The gallbladder may be palpable.

Empyema or mucocele of the gallbladder and Mirizzi syndrome (extrinsic compression and obstruction of the common hepatic duct from a gallstone impacted in the cystic duct or neck of the gallbladder) are rare in children.

This patient proceeded to have an abdominal ultrasound scan.

Question: Describe the sonographic findings in Figure 43.1.

DOI: 10.1201/9781003182290-48

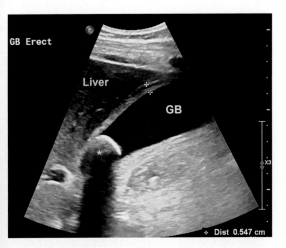

Figure 43.1 An erect study – fasting sonogram of the gallbladder (GB). *Note:* The sonogram shows a gallstone (*) impacted in the neck of the gallbladder. The gallstone casts a typical acoustic shadow. In addition, the gallbladder is distended and has an oedematous thick wall (more than 3 mm measured with the cursors). The pressure of the probe elicited tenderness (equivalent to Murphy's sign).

Question: If the echogenic focus in the gallbladder did not cast an acoustic shadow, what else could this lesion be?
Answer: A gallbladder polyp, sludge ball or blood clot, which do not typically cast an acoustic shadow. Gallbladder polyps in children are rare. They may be single or multiple (**Figure 43.2**), and numerous pathologies are possible including a cholesterol

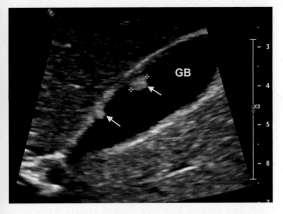

Figure 43.2 Two gallbladder polyps (arrows) in a 14-year-old boy. The largest (highlighted with the cursors) measures ~5 mm across. These echogenic lesions are contiguous with the gallbladder wall, remain fixed with changes in posture and do not cast an acoustic shadow. (GB: Gallbladder.)

polyp, adenoma, adenomatous hyperplasia, hamartoma, inflammatory polyp and heterotopic gastric or pancreatic tissue. If the polyp is symptomatic or measures 10 mm or more in size or if there are multiple smaller polyps, cholecystectomy is advisable. Asymptomatic patients with a single small polyp can simply be kept under periodic ultrasound surveillance.

Scenario: Investigations in the 13-year-old female patient showed no evidence of haemolysis, a minimally elevated aspartate aminotransferase (AST), a normal plasma lipase and a raised white cell count and C-reactive protein. Her common bile duct appeared normal on ultrasound. She was treated with an intravenous cephalosporin antibiotic and underwent a laparoscopic cholecystectomy 24 hours after admission.

Question: Describe the key operative steps in laparoscopic cholecystectomy.
Answer:

- Antibiotic prophylaxis (e.g., cefazolin), supine position, mechanical deep venous thrombosis (DVT) prophylaxis in teenagers (pharmacologic prophylaxis started postoperatively on the day of surgery if on oral contraceptive pill or other risk factors).
- Port sites: 5- or 10-mm sub-umbilical port (open Hasson technique) with three additional working ports (**Figure 43.3**). Pneumoperitoneum (8–10 mmHg). The neck of the gallbladder is retracted laterally. A laparoscopic snake liver retractor can be used to elevate the inferior surface of the liver, although some surgeons grasp the fundus of the gallbladder and push it upwards and laterally over the anterior surface of the liver. The key point is to open up the hepatocystic triangle (defined as the triangle formed by the cystic duct, the common hepatic duct and the inferior edge of the liver), which is often incorrectly referred to as Calot's triangle.
- In the 'critical view of safety' approach, the hepatocystic triangle is carefully dissected and the proximal one-third of the gallbladder is separated from the liver bed (**Figure 43.4**). Only two structures should be visible entering the gallbladder (the cystic duct and cystic artery).

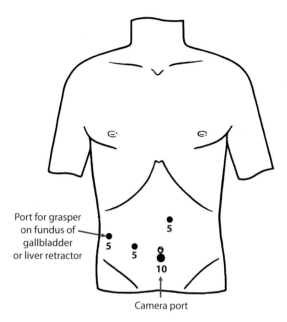

Port for grasper
on fundus of
gallbladder
or liver retractor

5

5   5

10

Camera port

Figure 43.3 Laparoscopic port positions for conventional laparoscopic cholecystectomy. A combination of 5- and 10-mm ports are used in teenagers, but smaller ports and instruments may be used in younger children. (*Note*: Single-port cholecystectomy is practised in some centres.)

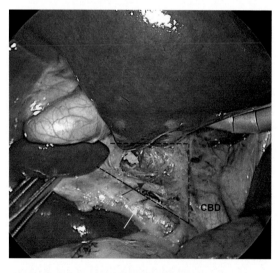

CBD

Figure 43.4 In the critical view of safety approach in laparoscopic cholecystectomy, the hepatocystic triangle (dashed lines) is carefully dissected and the proximal one-third of the gallbladder is separated from the liver bed to define the anatomy before ligating any structure. *Abbreviation*: CBD Common bile duct. (*Note*: Yellow arrow: cystic duct, red arrow: cystic artery.)

- The cystic duct must be traced laterally onto the gallbladder, but it is unnecessary (and potentially hazardous) to define its junction with the common bile duct. Before clipping the cystic duct and artery, the surgeon should verify that both structures run directly to the gallbladder and no other structures connect with the gallbladder. The cystic artery is less than 3 mm wide; if it appears larger, consider that it may be the right hepatic artery.
- The surgeon must be aware of potentially aberrant biliary and vascular anatomy such as a short cystic duct, aberrant hepatic ducts or a cystic artery crossing anterior to the common bile duct. If the biliary anatomy is unclear, intraoperative cholangiography through the cystic duct is advisable.
- The gallbladder is then dissected from its liver bed using diathermy and retrieved via the larger umbilical port. After confirming haemostasis, port sites are closed, and the gallbladder sent for histology. Routine abdominal drainage is unnecessary.

Patients with sickle cell disease undergoing cholecystectomy require careful preoperative and perioperative care to minimise the risk of perioperative complications. This includes preoperative blood transfusion to correct anaemia and reduce the proportion of haemoglobin S, together with avoidance of perioperative hypoxia, acidosis, hypovolemia and hypothermia.

Question: If the biliary anatomy is unclear or if the gallbladder is severely inflamed, what strategies should be considered to complete the operation safely?

Answer: If the anatomy is in doubt, an *intraoperative cholangiogram* should be performed to demonstrate the bile ducts. This is normally done by injecting contrast through a thin catheter inserted into the cystic duct. The operating table may need adjusting and instruments minimised to enable a clear radiolucent field of view. A normal cholangiogram shows normal extrahepatic bile duct anatomy with no filling defects and free flow of contrast through a non-dilated common bile duct to the duodenum. Bile duct injury is a rare (0.3–0.5%) but serious complication of cholecystectomy. It can arise from adverse pathology (e.g. Mirizzi syndrome, which is rare in both adults and children), variant anatomy (aberrant ductal anatomy such as a short, wide cystic duct or misinterpretation of conventional anatomy) or poor surgery technique.

Another operative strategy that is sometimes used if the gallbladder is very inflamed near the porta hepatis or the anatomy is unclear is a "fundus first" approach, beginning the dissection at the gallbladder fundus and progressively releasing the gallbladder from the liver bed towards the infundibulum.

Finally, consider the option of conversion to open cholecystectomy if the dissection is particularly difficult or hazardous.

Question: The 13-year-old girl had a single 2-cm gallstone of the type shown in Figure 43.5. What type of gallstone is this? How do the colour, size and shape of a gallstone reflect its aetiology?
Answer: These are typical cholesterol stones. Table 43.1 shows the characteristics of the varied types of gallstones found in children and common aetiologic factors. Cholesterol stones develop in static bile from cholesterol supersaturation. In children, cholesterol stones are typically seen in overweight adolescent girls, often with a family history of gallstones. Black pigment stones are typically found in haemolytic disorders, but may be associated with total parenteral nutrition (TPN) or neonatal abdominal surgery. Black pigment stones are formed from supersaturation of bile with calcium bilirubinate. Brown pigment stones are rare and associated with biliary stasis and infection; they are more often found in the bile ducts than in the gallbladder. Children can also rarely have calcium carbonate gallstones.

Biliary sludge can be a precursor to gallstone formation. It is composed of mucin, calcium bilirubinate

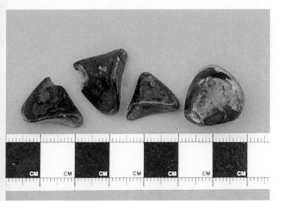

Figure 43.5 Gallbladder stones in a 13-year-old girl with symptomatic cholelithiasis.

and cholesterol crystals and appears echogenic on ultrasound (but does not cast an acoustic shadow). Gallbladder sludge is typically seen in association with TPN/fasting, sickle cell disease, treatment with ceftriaxone or octreotide and after bone marrow transplantation. Biliary sludge may resolve spontaneously or progress to gallstone formation.

Many aetiological factors are implicated in gallstone formation in children. Three dominant mechanisms are involved:

- Biliary stasis
- Excess bilirubin load
- Lithogenic bile

Some of the more common aetiological factors deserve further mention:

Haemolytic disorders

Hereditary spherocytosis, sickle cell disease and thalassemia major are associated with black pigment stones. In all three conditions, the incidence of gallstones increases with age. Haemolytic uremic syndrome, ABO or rhesus incompatibility and cardiac valve replacement may also be complicated by black pigment stones. In the newborn, an excessive bilirubin load from the breakdown of fetal haemoglobin together with an immature bilirubin excretion mechanism may promote pigment gallstone formation.

Ileal resection/disease

Ileal resection or disease (e.g., Crohn disease and/or short gut syndrome) are risk factors for black pigment gallstones. The most likely mechanism is a disturbed enterohepatic circulation of bile salts causing a relative bile salt deficiency and incomplete solubilisation of unconjugated bilirubin.

Total parenteral nutrition

The association between TPN and biliary sludge/gallstones is well established. Fasting and TPN promote biliary stasis by impairing both the enterohepatic circulation of bile acids and cholecystokinin-induced gallbladder contraction. Premature infants are particularly susceptible. Biliary sludge often clears spontaneously after enteral feeding is established, but some infants will develop gallstones.

Table 43.1 Gallstone types and characteristics in children

Type	Mixed cholesterol	Pure cholesterol	Black pigment	Brown pigment	Calcium carbonate
Appearance					
Composition	Cholesterol + Calcium salts	Cholesterol	Pigment polymer + Calcium bilirubinate	Calcium bilirubinate + Calcium salts of fatty acids	Calcium carbonate
Shape	Round or faceted	Round, smooth	Spiky or faceted	Ovoid or irregular	Ovoid or irregular
Colour	Brown pigment in rings or specks	Yellow-white	Black	Brown, soft	Grey or white
Number	Multiple	Often single	Multiple	Single or multiple	Usually, one or two only
Microbiology	Sterile	Sterile	Sterile	Infected	Sterile
Major risk factors	Female sex, obesity	Female sex, obesity	Haemolysis	Cholangitis, strictures	Neonatal intensive care

Table 43.2 Specific conditions reported to be associated with childhood gallstones

Condition	Aetiological factor(s)
Cystic Fibrosis	Abnormalities of biliary lipid and mucin composition Common bile duct stenosis
Down Syndrome	Prenatal factors may be important since calculi have been detected soon after birth
Cardiac/Liver transplantation	Multifactorial (haemolysis, cyclosporine induced changes in bile and lipid metabolism, gallbladder stasis, frusemide therapy)
Childhood cancer	Multifactorial (ileal conduit, parenteral nutrition, abdominal surgery, repeated blood transfusions and abdominal radiation therapy)
Bone marrow transplantation	Blood transfusions
Spinal surgery/Injury	Immobilisation, disturbed calcium haemostasis, blood transfusion
Hepatobiliary trauma	Haemobilia
Dystrophia myotonica	Impaired gallbladder emptying
Chronic intestinal pseudo-obstruction	Impaired gallbladder motility
Cholestatic/Cirrhotic liver disease	Alagille syndrome, Progressive Familial Intrahepatic Cholestasis, Gilbert syndrome and Wilson disease
Congenital duodenal anomalies	Fibrosis around the distal common bile duct after surgical repair

Other risk factors

Affected adolescents typically have an adult pattern of risk factors (female gender, obesity) and cholesterol gallstones. Oestrogens increase cholesterol excretion, and progesterone reduces bile acid excretion and slows gallbladder emptying. Obesity is an independent risk factor for cholelithiasis. Paradoxically, rapid weight loss also predisposes to gallstone formation. Biliary obstruction and stasis from choledochal cysts or strictures can be complicated by gallstone formation. Numerous other specific conditions have been linked to an increased incidence of gallstones in childhood (**Table 43.2**).

Question: How would you manage the following two patients with common bile duct stones?

a. **An otherwise well 6-month-old infant with mild obstructive jaundice and sonographic findings of a small gallstone and sludge in a 4-mm common bile duct?**
b. **A 14-year-old girl presenting with acute pancreatitis and multiple gallbladder stones?**

Answer: Common bile duct stones (choledocholithiasis) are relatively uncommon. They are occasionally found in infants, in children with sickle cell disease or other haemolytic disorders and in older

children with acute pancreatitis. Common bile duct calculi may be silent but can cause obstructive jaundice, cholangitis and/or acute pancreatitis.

a. An 6/12 old infant.
b. This infant has a dilated common bile duct containing biliary sludge and a small gallstone. Normal upper limits for the sonographic diameter of the common bile duct are 1 mm in neonates, 2 mm in infants, 4 mm in 1- to 10-year-olds and 6 mm in older children. The infant has mild obstructive jaundice but is otherwise well. The sensitivity and specificity of transabdominal ultrasound for gallbladder stones exceeds 98% but is only about 70–80% for common bile duct stones. Magnetic resonance cholangiography (MRC) is the investigation of choice to confirm a common bile duct stone and to rule out complex biliary disease. In this patient, an MRC confirmed the ultrasound findings and showed no evidence of underlying congenital choledochal dilatation ("choledochal cyst"). Assuming the infant has no ongoing predisposition to gallstone formation such as persistent haemolysis, he/she could initially be managed conservatively since the sludge and stone may pass spontaneously in this age group leading to normalisation of LFTs and ultrasound appearance. Oral ursodeoxycholic

acid may be helpful as a choleretic agent, and fat-soluble vitamin supplements should be given whilst there is obstructive jaundice. Indications to operate include cholangitis, deteriorating LFTs/worsening obstructive jaundice or after a few weeks of failed conservative treatment.

> **Scenario:** This 14-year-old girl patient underwent urgent investigation by MRC (**Figure 43.6**). She then proceeded to endoscopic retrograde cholangiography (ERC), sphincterotomy and extraction of the distal common bile duct stone and was readmitted 1 week later for a laparoscopic cholecystectomy.

Early ERC and sphincterotomy are recommended for common bile duct stones causing obstructive jaundice and/or cholangitis. In gallstone pancreatitis, the stone often passes spontaneously, and early laparoscopic cholecystectomy (within 2 weeks) is advisable once the pancreatitis has resolved. If there are multiple or persistent stones in the common bile duct associated with gallstone pancreatitis, ERC and stone retrieval are undertaken followed by laparoscopic cholecystectomy, as in the patient described earlier. If ERC is unavailable or unsuccessful, surgical approaches to choledocholithiasis include cholecystotomy and biliary irrigation/balloon catheters in small infants or, in older children, laparoscopic or open choledochotomy and stone removal with

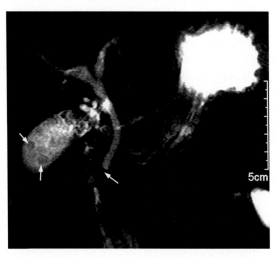

Figure 43.6 Magnetic resonance cholangiogram showing multiple gallbladder stones (short arrowheads) and a stone in the distal common bile duct (longer arrow) with some proximal bile duct dilatation.

temporary T-tube drainage. Some centres employ percutaneous radiologic retrieval techniques.

Question: A 5-year-old boy with hereditary spherocytosis is referred to you with multiple gallbladder stones. Describe your management. What factors determine whether he should have a concurrent splenectomy?

Answer: Elective laparoscopic cholecystectomy is advisable even if the gallbladder stones are asymptomatic, as they will not resolve and may cause complications. In the presence of a normal common bile duct diameter on ultrasound scan and normal LFTs, routine intraoperative cholangiography is not required. Cholecystectomy should *not* be combined with splenectomy unless the latter is indicated for haematologic reasons.

The spleen should be preserved for its immunologic function in children with hereditary spherocytosis until splenectomy is indicated for haematological reasons. The British Committee for Standards in Haematology has published helpful guidelines on the indications for splenectomy based on symptoms, haemoglobin and bilirubin concentrations and reticulocyte count. In children undergoing splenectomy for haematological reasons, cholecystectomy is advisable if gallstones are present.

Question: What is your approach to managing the child with an asymptomatic gallbladder stone?

Answer: This is a controversial area, as there are insufficient data. In infants, gallbladder stones may occasionally disappear due to a combination of dissolution and spontaneous passage. Clinical and ultrasound monitoring is sufficient provided there is no evidence of additional biliary tract disease and biochemical LFTs are normal. In older children, the optimum management of non-haemolytic gallbladder stones is uncertain. Although many children remain asymptomatic for years, the likelihood of spontaneous resolution in this age group is low, and there is a lifetime risk of complications. In the author's personal experience about 20% of patients become symptomatic within 10 years of detection. A decision to proceed to elective cholecystectomy should only be undertaken after a detailed discussion with the family regarding benefits and risks.

Children with haemolytic gallbladder stones secondary to hereditary spherocytosis are discussed in an earlier question. Opinion is divided on the management of the child with sickle cell anaemia and asymptomatic gallbladder stones.

Proponents of elective cholecystectomy argue that there is an increasing risk of complications with age, urgent surgery has a greater morbidity and it may sometimes be difficult to distinguish cholecystitis from a sickle cell abdominal crisis.

Question: Can gallstones be effectively treated without cholecystectomy?

Answer: Some parents ask about alternative therapies to treat gallstones:

1. Cholecystolithotomy with preservation of the gallbladder has been proposed as an alternative treatment of symptomatic gallbladder stones in children, but considering the safety and efficacy of cholecystectomy and the risk of recurrent gallstones after simple stone removal, this technique is not recommended.
2. Gallstone dissolution therapy is not recommended in children. Even after prolonged treatment in adults with cholesterol gallstones, rates of dissolution are low and recurrence common. Furthermore, medical therapy is ineffective for calcified and pigment stones and if the gallbladder is non-functioning.
3. Extracorporeal shock wave gallstone lithotripsy has been reported in children but requires repeated treatments under general anaesthesia, carries a risk of gallstone pancreatitis from gallstone fragments in the common bile duct and rarely yields a durable outcome. Cholecystectomy is a more efficient, reliable and permanent treatment option.

Finally, parents often ask about potential long-term ill effects from cholecystectomy. The gallbladder stores and concentrates bile but does not appear to be essential to health in humans. After cholecystectomy, the common bile duct dilates slightly to take over some bile reservoir function. Although a postcholecystectomy digestive syndrome is reported in some adults, cholecystectomy has no documented permanent serious adverse effects in children.

BIBLIOGRAPHY

Afdhal NH. Epidemiology, risk factors, and pathogenesis of gallstones. In: *Gallbladder and Biliary Tract Diseases*. Ed Afdhal NH, Marcel Dekker Inc., New York, 2000, pp. 127–146.

Alizai NK, Richards EM, Stringer MD. Is cholecystectomy really an indication for concomitant splenectomy in mild hereditary spherocytosis? *Arch Dis Child* 2010;95(8):596–599.

Bolton-Maggs PH, Langer JC, Iolascon A, et al. General haematology task force of the British Committee for Standards in Haematology. Guidelines for the diagnosis and management of hereditary spherocytosis–2011 update. *Br J Haematol* 2012;156(1):37–49.

Bruch SW, Ein SH, Rocchi C, Kim PC. The management of nonpigmented gallstones in children. *J Pediatr Surg* 2000;35:729–732.

De Caluwé D, Akl U, Corbally M. Cholecystectomy versus cholecystolithotomy for cholelithiasis in childhood: Long-term outcome. *J Pediatr Surg* 2001;36:1518–1521.

El Boghdady M, Arang H, Ewalds-Kvist M. Fundus-first laparoscopic cholecystectomy for complex gallbladders: A systematic review. *Health Sci Rev* 2022;2:100014. https://doi.org/10.1016/j.hsr.2022.100014

Kılıç ŞS, Özden Ö, Çolak ST. Comparative analysis of reliability and clinical effects of the critical view of safety approach used in laparoscopic cholecystectomy in the pediatric population. *Pediatr Surg Int* 2021;37(6):737–743.

Kumar R, Nguyen K, Shun A. Gallstones and common bile duct calculi in infancy and childhood. *Aust N Z J Surg* 2000;70:188–191.

Matos C, Avni EF, Van Gansbeke D, et al. Total parenteral nutrition (TPN) and gallbladder diseases in neonates. Sonographic assessment. *J Ultrasound Med* 1987;6:243–248.

Miltenburg DM, Schaffer R, Breslin T, Brandt ML. Changing indications for pediatric cholecystectomy. *Pediatrics* 2000;105:1250–1253.

Stringer MD. Gallbladder and biliary tree. In: Standring S. *Gray's Anatomy* 41st edn., Elsevier, London, 2015 (describes common anatomical variants)

Stringer MD, Ceylan H, Ward K, Wyatt JI. Gallbladder polyps in children–classification and management. *J Pediatr Surg* 2003; 38(11):1680–1684.

Stringer MD, Soloway RD, Taylor DR, Riyad K, Toogood G. Calcium carbonate gallstones in children. *J Pediatr Surg* 2007;42:1677–1682.

St-Vil D, Yazbeck S, Luks FI, Hancock BJ et al. Cholelithiasis in newborns and infants. *J Pediatr Surg* 1992;27:1305–1307.

44

Congenital hyperinsulinism

PABLO LAJE AND N. SCOTT ADZICK
Children's Hospital of Philadelphia, Philadelphia, Pennsylvania

Scenario: A full-term, healthy-appearing newborn who has no congenital abnormalities was transferred to the neonatal intensive care unit (NICU) due to persistent hypoglycemia that has not responded to continuous enteral feedings. The baby requires a continuous intravenous glucose infusion at a high rate through a central line. Every attempt to decrease the glucose infusion rate is quickly followed by abrupt hypoglycemia, mental status changes and a seizure. There are no abnormalities on the physical exam. Plain films and abdominal ultrasound are normal.

Question: What is the likely diagnosis of this patient? What is the pathophysiology of the disease?

Answer: The most common cause of persistent neonatal hypoglycemia is congenital hyperinsulinism (HI), an infrequent disease that has an incidence of 1 case per 50,000 live births in the general population. The key pathophysiologic feature of HI is the constant secretion of insulin independently of the plasma glucose concentration.

Question: How is HI diagnosed? Does the patient require complex laboratory tests?

Answer: Simple metabolic blood tests are required to investigate the possibility of HI. The diagnosis is confirmed when the following three criteria are present:

1. Hypoglycemia (defined as <50 mg/dL). It is important to remember that glucose in plasma needs to be measured in the absence of any drugs or clinical conditions that could lead to hypoglycemia (e.g. sepsis, trimethoprim-sulfamethoxazole).
2. Low plasma beta-hydroxybutyrate (beta-HB), acetoacetic acid (AA), and free fatty acids (FFAs), which are known as ketone bodies. The natural response of the body to hypoglycemia is the hepatic release of ketone bodies. This mechanism is naturally inhibited by insulin. Hypoglycemia with low plasma ketone bodies is a physiologic "contradiction" that can only occur if insulin is functioning in excess of its physiologic needs.
3. A positive glycemic response (≥30 mg/dL within minutes) to a 1-mg intravenous dose of glucagon. Glucagon is a natural antagonist of insulin, so a positive test proves that insulin is involved in the development of the hypoglycemia.

Question: Once the diagnosis of HI is confirmed, what is the next step in management?

Answer: The first and most important goal is to maintain euglycemia, defined as a plasma glucose concentration above 70 mg/dL, to prevent neuronal

DOI: 10.1201/9781003182290-49

hypoglycemic damage. This is generally accomplished by a continuous intravenous infusion of glucose, plus frequent or continuous enteral feedings. The glucose infusion rate (GIR) is measured in mg/kg/min. The second and critical step in the management of patients with Hi is to evaluate their response to diazoxide. Diazoxide is an agonist of the adenosine triphosphate (ATP)–dependent potassium (K-ATP) channel located on the membrane of the beta cell that inhibits the secretion of insulin and exerts a hyperglycemic effect. Patients receive diazoxide for 5 days and subsequently undergo a 12-hour fasting challenge. If they are able to maintain adequate plasma glucose levels (>70 mg/dL) with appropriate ketone body response, they are considered "diazoxide-responsive". For these patients, a long-term diazoxide regimen and a frequent feeding plan is initiated.

> **Scenario:** The patient we are managing did not respond appropriately to diazoxide and continues to require a high intravenous GIR.

Question: How are patients with severe "diazoxide resistance" HI treated?

Answer: They are managed with a pancreatectomy, the extent of which depends on the anatomical form of HI. There are two main forms of HI: focal and diffuse. The management algorithm for patients with HI is described in **Figure 44.1**.

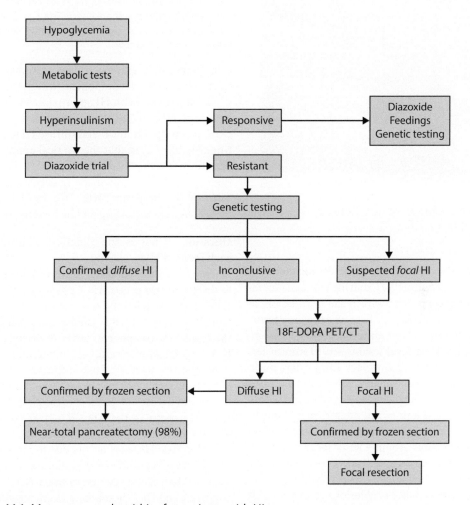

Figure 44.1 Management algorithim for patients with HI.

Question: What are the anatomical differences between focal HI and diffuse HI?

Answer: Diffuse HI affects the entire organ, although the macroscopic aspect of the pancreas is normal. On histology, however, the key finding is that 5%–10% of the beta cells have nucleomegaly. These abnormal cells are scattered evenly throughout the pancreas. The nucleomegaly can be subtle – nuclear size 3 times greater than normal is required – and expert pathology evaluation is required to confirm or exclude the diagnosis. The overall number of beta cells in diffuse HI is normal. In the following image (**Figure 44.2**) we see a beta cell with a large nucleus (black arrow) within a pancreatic islet. The black stars mark the exocrine component of the pancreas.

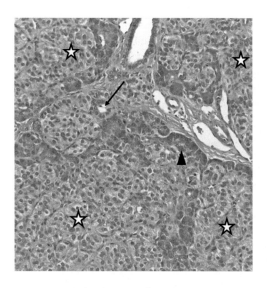

Figure 44.3 Slide showing focal lesion with beta cell hyperplasia (stars) and exocrine components within the lesion (black arrowhead) and ductal elements (black arrow).

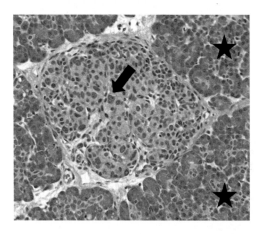

Figure 44.2 Slide showing a beta cell with a large nucleus (black arrow).

Focal HI consists of a focus of adenomatous hyperplasia of beta cells. Exocrine and canalicular cells are always present within the focal lesion, as are non-beta islet cells. The beta cells of a focal lesion are mostly normal, and nucleomegaly is occasionally present. Most focal lesions are 10 mm or less in diameter, but they can vary from a few millimeters to several centimeters. They can be located on the surface of the pancreas or embedded within the organ. Focal lesions are often firmer than the normal pancreatic tissue so they can often be identified by palpation. About 45% of focal lesions are located in the pancreatic head, 25% in the body, 15% in the tail, and about 15% involve contiguous areas of the pancreas. Focal lesions can very rarely be located within ectopic pancreatic tissue. In the following image (**Figure 44.3**) we can see the typical findings of a focal lesion: Hyperplasia of beta

cells (stars), with exocrine (black arrowhead) and ductal (black arrow) components within the lesion.

Of all patients with HI, approximately 30–40% have focal HI and 60–70% have diffuse HI. From a clinical standpoint, focal and diffuse HI are indistinguishable. Given that the surgical approach for each form is radically different, prior to the operation, all efforts must be made to determine which form of HI the patient has. This can be accomplished by genetic testing and by imaging studies.

Question: What is the genetic background of each form of HI?

Answer: The most common forms of HI occur due to defects in two genes: *ABCC8* and *KCNJ11*. These genes code, respectively, the two proteins of the K-ATP channel: SUR1 (sulfonylurea receptor-1, the regulatory component, target of diazoxide) and Kir6.2 (potassium inwardly-rectifying unit, the ion pore, sensitive to ATP). Loss-of-function mutations of the K-ATP channel keep it closed at all times, causing insulin release independent of the plasma glucose level. Mutations in the *ABCC8* and *KCNJ11* genes account for half of the cases of diffuse HI. The other half of diffuse HI cases occurs due to mutations in several other genes involved in glucose metabolism such as *GDH* (glutamate dehydrogenase), *GCK* (glucokinase), and *HK1* (hexokinase 1), among others.

Focal HI occurs through a so-called "two-hit" mechanism. The first event is the inheritance of a disease-causing mutation in the *ABCC8* or the

KCNJ11 gene on the paternal allele from a carrier father. The second event is that in a single beta cell of the pancreas, the normal maternal allele is lost. This is a post-zygotic random event called "loss of heterozygosity". To replace the lost maternal DNA, the beta cell creates a copy of the paternal DNA, which has the inherited mutation. This event is called "uniparental disomy (UPD)". With these two events, the cell is now homozygous for the mutation and has inactivated K-ATP channels. Having unregulated insulin release in a single cell is not enough to cause a clinical problem, but there is another phenomenon that occurs with the loss of the maternal *ABCC8* or *KCNJ11* allele. Next to those genes there are genes involved in the process of cell proliferation: The *H19* gene (anti-proliferation) and the insulin-like growth factor 2 gene (pro-proliferation). When the beta cell loses the maternal DNA containing the *ABCC8* and *KCNJ11* genes, it also loses the H19 and IGF2 alleles. This causes an imbalance in cellular self-regulation that leads to an adenomatous proliferation known as a focal lesion.

In general terms, patients with mutations in the K-ATP channel do not respond to diazoxide. Conversely, almost all forms of non-K-ATP HI are diazoxide-responsive. When a patient is diagnosed with HI in the absence of a family history, the parents and the patient must undergo genetic testing. In cases of diazoxide-responsive disease, the genetic testing is needed for counseling. On the other hand, in cases of diazoxide-resistant HI (K-ATP mutations), the genetic testing becomes more critical because it can help differentiate between diffuse and focal HI, determine the need for imaging studies, and help with surgical planning.

> **Scenario:** The patient we are managing underwent genetic testing, which was inconclusive. He continues to require a high GIR. It is clear that he needs a pancreatectomy.

Question: How can the two forms of HI be distinguished preoperatively with imaging studies?
Answer: The gold-standard imaging study for HI is the 18-fluoro-L-3-4-dihydroxyphenylalanine positron emission tomography study, merged with a low-dose computerized tomography (18fluoro-DOPA-PET/CT). Islet cells take up the 18F-DOPA, convert it into 18-fluoro-dopamine, and store it in vesicles that can be tracked by their gamma radiation. Lesions of focal HI are seen as bright spots

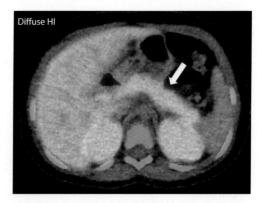

Figure 44.4 DOPA - PET CT scan showing diffuse HI.

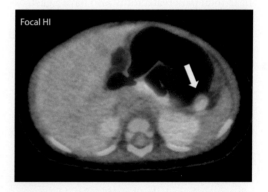

Figure 44.5 DOPA- PET CT scan showing focal HI.

of tracer over a darker background, whereas in diffuse disease, the tracer is homogeneously distributed throughout the organ. PET/CT to detect a focal lesion is about 84% accurate. When a focal lesion is identified on the 18F-PET/CT, the correlation with the actual location determined during the operation is nearly 100%. Examples of focal and diffuse HI are seen in **Figures 44.4** and **44.5**.

Question: What are the principles of the surgical management of HI?
Answer: All operations are done via a transverse supraumbilical laparotomy. The pancreas is exposed by an extended Kocher maneuver, entry into the lesser sac, and mobilization of the inferior pancreatic border. The pancreas is then inspected and carefully palpated to identify the focal lesion, if suspected. If no focal lesion is identified, 2- to 3-mm biopsies are taken with sharp scissors from the pancreatic head, body, and tail for intraoperative frozen-section analysis. Cautery should be

avoided since it distorts the frozen-section biopsy specimen.

- *Diffuse HI*: Patients with intraoperative confirmation of diffuse HI undergo a near-total (98%) pancreatectomy, which involves the resection of the entire pancreas with the exception of a small residual piece of pancreatic tissue between the common bile duct (CBD) and the duodenum. The splenic vessels must be preserved. A true near-total pancreatectomy requires a complete dissection of the intrapancreatic portion of the CBD. CBD complications (intraoperative injury or postoperative stricture) are rarely seen. Patients who undergo a near-total pancreatectomy also have a gastrostomy performed because there is a high likelihood that continuous or frequent feedings will be needed as an adjuvant to the operation.
- *Focal HI*: When the intraoperative biopsies show normal pancreatic histology, a meticulous search for the focal lesion is conducted. The preoperative 18F-DOPA PET/CT is key in orienting the search. When the genetic testing suggests focal HI but the 18F-DOPA PET/CT does not show a focal lesion, we routinely use intraoperative high-resolution ultrasound. The ultrasound can help identify a focal lesion in some cases, but it is always helpful to determine the location and course of the pancreatic duct. Focal lesions that are buried within the pancreatic tissue can be impossible to see, feel, or be detected by ultrasound. In those cases it is necessary to patiently take additional biopsies of suspicious areas for frozen-section analysis until the lesion is found. Focal lesions can have octopus-like tentacles, which make the intraoperative frozen-section confirmation of clear margins imperative. Small and superficial lesions in the body or tail are treated by simple resection using sharp scissors. Deep lesions in the body and tail are treated by distal pancreatectomy. Superficial lesions in the head of the pancreas can be treated by simple resection, but deep head lesions can be difficult to excise with clear margins without causing damage to the CBD and/or the pancreatic duct. These challenging cases are managed by a near-total pancreatic head resection, preserving the duodenal blood supply, along with a Roux-en-Y pancreaticojejunostomy to drain the pancreatic body and tail. In rare occasions a focal lesion in the pancreatic head extends into the duodenal wall, in which case a Whipple procedure may be needed.

Question: How are patients managed after the operation?
Answer: The GIR is restarted at 2 mg/kg/min and is advanced gradually to 8 mg/kg/min within the first 24–36 hours after the operation. Plasma glucose is measured hourly in the beginning and spaced out as it becomes stable. If the plasma glucose is excessively high, an insulin infusion is started. Enteral feedings are started when bowel function resumes. When patients are on full enteral feeds, a fasting test is performed. Patients who maintain euglycemia for >18 hours are considered cured. If the time to hypoglycemia is less than 18 hours, a plan of frequent feedings is developed so that patients can be safely managed at home. Patients who are unable to be weaned off the intravenous GIR rate are obviously not cured and will need further assessment to determine if additional surgery is needed.

Question: What are the outcomes of HI patients post-pancreatectomy?
Answer: Almost all patients (97% in our experience) with focal HI are cured after the operation. If this does not happen, the possibility of an incomplete resection must be considered. In the case of diffuse HI, the operation helps with patient management, since only 20% of the patients have euglycemia postoperatively without any support. Approximately 50% of patients post 98% pancreatectomy need either frequent feedings or frequent enteral glucose administration to avoid hypoglycemia. Approximately 30% of patients after near-total pancreatectomy develop insulin dependence shortly after the operation, which should not come as a surprise. Furthermore, by the age of 10 years, the vast majority of children who underwent a 98% pancreatectomy are insulin dependent. This fact underscores critically in the search for non-surgical therapies for patients with diffuse diazoxide-resistant HI.

BIBLIOGRAPHY

1. Adzick NS, De Leon DD, States LJ, et al. Surgical treatment of congenital hyperinsulinism: Results from 500 pancreatectomies in neonates and children. *J Pediatr Surg.* 2019;54(1):27–32.

2. Rosenfeld E, Ganguly A, De Leon DD. Congenital hyperinsulinism disorders: Genetic and clinical characteristics. *Am J Med Genet C Semin Med Genet.* 2019;181:682–92.

3. Lord K, Radcliffe J, Gallagher PR, et al. High risk of diabetes and neurobehavioral deficits in individuals with surgically treated hyperinsulinism. *J Clin Endocrinol Metab.* 2015;100:4133–9.

4. Thornton PS, Stanley CA, De Leon DD, et al. Recommendations from the pediatric endocrine society for evaluation and management of persistent hypoglycemia in neonates, infants, and children. *J Pediatr.* 2015;167:238–45.

5. Laje P, States LJ, Zhuang H, et al. Accuracy of PET/CT Scan in the diagnosis of the focal form of congenital hyperinsulinism. *J Pediatr Surg.* 2013;48:388–93.

6. Laje P, Stanley CA, Palladino AA, et al. Pancreatic head resection and Roux-en-Y pancreaticojejunostomy for the treatment of the focal form of congenital hyperinsulinism. *J Pediatr Surg.* 2012;47:130–5.

7. McQuarrie I. Idiopathic spontaneously occurring hypoglycemia in infants; clinical significance of problem and treatment. *AMA Am J Dis Child.* 1954;87:399–428.

8. Peranteau WH, Bathaii SM, Pawel B, et al. Multiple ectopic lesions of focal islet adenomatosis identified by positron emission tomography scan in an infant with congenital hyperinsulinism. *J Pediatr Surg.* 2007;42:188–92.

PART 6

Preparation of the Child for Surgery

45

Fluid and electrolyte balance in pediatric surgical patients

PRINCE RAJ, ABEER FARHAN, MOHAMMED AMIN AL AWADHI, AND MARTIN T. CORBALLY
King Hamad University Hospital, Kingdom of Bahrain, Bahrain

Fluid and electrolyte management of pediatric surgical patients is crucial to clinical care and requires a sound knowledge of physiology. Most protocols for pediatric fluid therapy do not always take into account the rapidly changing perioperative physiology in our vulnerable patient population.

> **Scenario:** A 4-week-old first-born male baby is brought to the hospital emergency department with a 3-day history of projectile, non-bilious vomiting after each feed. The infant is hungry in between the episodes of vomiting, irritable and lethargic.

Question: What is your working diagnosis, and what differential conditions would you also consider?

Answer: The most common surgical cause for projectile, non-bilious vomiting in a first-born male baby who was feeding well initially is infantile hypertrophic pyloric stenosis (IHPS). Other disorders to consider may be divided into medical and surgical causes of non-bilious vomiting:

Surgical:
- Gastroesophageal reflux disease (GERD).
- Pylorospasm.
- Pyloric web, diaphragm and atresia.
- Pyloro-duodenal duplication cyst.

Medical:
- Gastroenteritis.
- Raised intracranial pressure (ICP).
- Metabolic disorders: Inborn errors.

Question: The infant is examined, and vital signs are essentially stable, but there is evidence of a mild dehydration status. Abdominal examination during a test feed by the surgeon reveals a palpable mass in the epigastric region with visible gastric peristalsis observed. Blood gas lab sample shows a pH 7.46, PCO$_2$ 42, HCO$_3$ 34, BE −5, serum Na 135, K 3.1, and Cl 102. What is your interpretation of these findings?

Answer: The blood gas test shows a metabolic alkalosis associated with hypokalemia and hypochloremia. The infant's laboratory biochemical status is typical of that classically seen in IHPS, which includes:

a. Projectile, non-bilious vomiting.

b. Visible peristalsis.

c. Hypochloremic hypokalemic metabolic alkalosis.

Question: What other investigation would you undertake to help confirm your diagnosis?

Answer: The classic history of projectile, non-bilious vomiting along with the clinical finding of

DOI: 10.1201/9781003182290-51

visible peristalsis and a palpable 'lump' in the epigastric region make the diagnosis almost certain. In indeterminate cases with early presentation to hospital, the biochemical disturbance may be very mild, and consequently a small pyloric tumor may be difficult to palpate. An ultrasound scan is therefore helpful in such instances (see Chapter 12).

Question: How will you then manage an infant with IHPS?

Answer: It is important to appreciate the fact that IHPS is never a surgical emergency and IV fluid volume resuscitation and electrolyte correction are of paramount importance. Inadequate resuscitation and preparation of the patient for operation can lead to significant risks of postoperative apnea due to decreased central respiratory drive due to metabolic alkalosis (HCO_3^-).

Benson and Alpern have defined three levels of severity based on serum bicarbonate level:

Slight < 25 mEq/L.
Moderate 26–35 mEq/L.
Severe > 35 mEq/L.

The goals of early management therefore should be to correct the dehydration and electrolyte imbalance before undertaking the operation.

1. Infant should be kept nil by mouth (NPO).
2. Nasogastric tube losses should be replaced milliliter for milliliter with 0.9% NaCl (nasogastric [NG] losses depletes extra fluid and HCL loss from stomach).
3. Fluid resuscitation should be based on the degree of dehydration.
   a. Initial volume infusion rate should be 1.25–2 times the normal maintenance rate.
   b. 5% Dextrose in 0.45% normal saline solution with 20 mEq/L of KCL added per 500 mL is an optimum resuscitation regimen for fluid and electrolyte replacement. (KCL supplementation may be increased to 30 mEq per 500 mL in cases of severe hypokalemia but will require very close monitoring of serum levels.)
   c. Correction of serum bicarbonate (HCO_3) level can take several hours, up to 24 hours. The goal should be to achieve levels below 30 mEq/dL prior to operation.
   d. Urine output monitoring to assess the adequacy of resuscitation.
   e. Serial monitoring of serum electrolytes with correction of hypokalemia and hypochloremia.

Question: What is meant by the term 'paradoxical aciduria' in relation to IHPS?

Answer: Gastric outlet obstruction in IHPS leads to protracted vomiting and loss of hydrogen, chloride and potassium ions and hypochloremic hypokalemic metabolic alkalosis. Protracted vomiting also causes significant extracellular fluid losses and dehydration.

The vomiting infant tries to compensate for metabolic alkalosis by an adaptation physiology response from the respiratory and renal systems. The alkalotic state activates central chemoreceptors in the brainstem to reflexively trigger central hypoventilation with reduced respiratory drive and subsequent respiratory acidosis. The renal system makes an effort in response to expel excess bicarbonate ions, producing an alkaline urine. As sodium follows bicarbonate within the nephron unit, this results in added volume depletion to excrete a solute load. As there is established volume depletion and extracellular fluid contraction from repeated vomiting, the central nervous system (CNS) reticulo-activating system (RAS) is stimulated, and there is then heightened aldosterone secretion and subsequent sodium retention. In response, the kidneys start excreting potassium in place of sodium. Within the distal kidney convoluted tubules, potassium is exchanged with hydrogen ions through the hydrogen-potassium transport pump to reset pH balance, causing loss of potassium ions. If hypokalemia is severe, then the body has a limited capacity for excretion of potassium to maintain pH. In the cascade scenario, sodium exchange is then preferentially substituted with hydrogen ions in the distal renal tubule system, producing a paradoxical aciduria.

Question: What types of fluid management may be deployed in clinical care of the pediatric surgical patient?

Answer: This may be considered into three main categories:

1. Deficit therapy
2. Maintenance therapy
3. Replacement therapy

1. *Deficit therapy*: This is best defined as management of the fluid and electrolyte losses based on severity of dehydration. It is usually estimated from the patient's history and clinical examination. Pertinent investigations that can confirm the type of dehydration include:
   a. Serum osmolarity and serum sodium.
   b. Acid base status, pH and base deficits.
   c. Urine output.

   Weight loss in neonates and infants is a good working guide to assess the severity of deficit. Mild, moderate and severe dehydration are estimated as follows: Less than 5%, 5–10% and more than 10% of weight loss, respectively. Deficit replacement revolves around adequate restoration of CVS, CNS and renal function. Such losses should be replaced with salt solutions based on type and severity of dehydration. Potassium should be replaced only after adequate renal perfusion is established, acidosis is corrected and an infant is excreting a urine volume.

2. *Maintenance therapy*: This is designed to meet the ongoing fluid and electrolyte requirements during the perioperative period. The fluid regimen for maintenance therapy replaces insensible losses and urinary loss. Various factors affect insensible loss, including ambient temperature, gestational age, surface area exposed, type of respiration and humidity, and all these factors should be taken into account.

   Fluid requirements typically may need to be increased in babies with a fever and in hypermetabolic states such as burns or when overhead radiant heaters or phototherapy is deployed.

   The most commonly used formula to calculate maintenance fluid for children is the Holliday-Segar method:

Weight in Kilogram (kg)	Holliday Segar Method (mL/kg/day)	Holliday Segar Estimate (mL/kg/hr)
First 10 kg	100	4
Second 10 kg	50	2
Every kg thereafter	20	1

3. *Replacement therapy*: This is designed to replace ongoing abnormal fluid and electrolyte losses. It accounts here for:
   a. Third-space loss
   b. Blood loss
   c. Other losses – NG tube, ileostomy, colostomy stomas

During surgery third-space losses should be replaced with isotonic saline (0.9%). It is difficult to accurately quantify, and normally an estimate is thus made:
1–2 mL/kg/hr given for ambulatory surgery, e.g. inguinal hernia operation.
4–7 mL/kg/hr for patients having thoracotomy or ureteral reimplantation.
5–10 mL/kg/hr for major abdominal surgery, e.g. intestinal obstruction.

It is important to regularly assess clinical signs, notably heart rate, blood pressure and capillary refill time (<2 seconds) for adequacy of fluid replacement. In the postoperative period ongoing fluid losses from NG tubes and drains should all be replaced with isotonic fluids (0.9% normal saline).

Blood loss during surgery can initially be replaced with crystalloid or colloid solutions and then with blood when the hematocrit estimate has fallen to 25%.

Question: What is the definitive management for the infant with IHPS?
Answer: Once the infant has been adequately resuscitated, electrolytes are normalized and acid-base disturbance corrected (serum potassium >3 mEq/L, bicarbonate <30 mEq/L and serum chloride >90 mEq/L), operation can safely be undertaken.

Ramstedt pyloromyotomy (open or minimally invasive surgery [MIS]) involves the operating surgeon splitting the hypertrophic pylorus with blunt dissection to relieve gastric outlet obstruction.

Question: When can you start feeds postoperatively?
Answer: Feeding can be started postoperatively within approximately 4 hours of surgery in the majority of infants. Postoperative vomiting is commonly predictable, but it should not unduly delay full establishment of feeds. Many infants can be discharged from hospital within 24 hours of pyloromyotomy.

Question: What other pediatric surgical disorders may require aggressive fluid and electrolyte management in the preoperative period?
Answer:

1. Trauma victims – splenic injury, liver injury, renal injury, pancreatic injury, bowel injury.

2. Congenital abdominal wall defects – gastroschisis, cloacal exstrophy.
3. Neural tube defects – meningomyelocele.
4. Intestinal obstruction disorders – intestinal atresia, meconium ileus, Hirschsprung's disease, anorectal malformations, intussusception, malrotation with midgut volvulus.
5. Thoracic disorders – esophageal atresia, congenital chylothorax.
6. Necrotizing enterocolitis (NEC).

Question: What IV fluids should best be deployed in the immediate postoperative period?
Answer: Isotonic fluids such as 0.9% normal saline and Ringer's lactate (Hartmann's solution) should be considered in the immediate postoperative period. Intraoperative losses should have been adequately corrected, and any ongoing losses should therefore be replaced. Unrecognized hypovolemia is common, and this may also contribute to postoperative hyponatremia if there is inadequate fluid volume support with sufficient salt-containing fluids. Potassium fluids (KCL) should usually be added to IV fluid regimens after the first 24 hours. IV fluid regimens should normally also include 5% dextrose for initial glucose load replacement.

Ongoing fluid loss from the gastrointestinal tract should be replaced milliliter per milliliter according to volume and content. The electrolyte composition of the gastrointestinal fluids varies depending on the level gut involved. Chloride (Cl) ions are maximally lost from the stomach and upper jejunum, whereas biliary and pancreatic fluid losses are rich in sodium (Na). Losses from the large bowel are predominantly potassium rich (K). Therefore, the treatment of gastric fluid loss begins with normal saline (0.9%) with 20 mEq/L of KCL added per 500 mL. Biliary and intestinal tract fluid losses are replaced with Ringer's lactate/Hartmann's solution. Urine output should be monitored closely to ensure adequacy of fluid replacement.

BIBLIOGRAPHY

1. Holliday MA, Segar WE. The maintenance need of water in parenteral fluid therapy. Pediatrics. 1957: 19(5): 823–32
2. Padua AP, Macaraya JR, Dans LF, et al. Isotonic versus hypotonic saline solution for maintenance intravenous fluid therapy in children: a systematic review. Pediatr Nephrol. 2015:30(7):1163–72
3. Meyers RS. Pediatric fluid and electrolyte therapy. J Pediatr Pharmacol Ther. 2009:14(4):204–11
4. Ashcraft KW, Holcomb GW, Murphy JP, Ostlie DJ. 2010. Ashcrafts Pediatric Surgery (5th ed.). Philadelphia: Saunders Elsevier.
5. Benson CD, Alpern EB. Preoperative and postoperative care of congenital pyloric stenosis. AMA Arch Surg. 1957:75(6):877–9
6. Eaton S, De Coppi P, Pierro A. Fluid, Electrolyte and Nutritional Support of the Surgical Neonate. Rickham's Neonatal Surgery Springer Publishers 2018:191–212. Eds. PD Losty, AW Flake, RJ Rintala, JM Hutson, N Iwai.

46

Nutritional support

SIMON EATON AND DHANYA MULLASSERY
Great Ormond Street Hospital, London, UK

Children who have undergone surgery for gastrointestinal problems can have significant problems with quality and quantity of bowel for adequate absorption of nutrients. Postoperative nutritional support may therefore be necessary for short periods to await resolution of gut rehabilitative recovery. Medium- or longer-term nutritional support may be needed in other children who have inadequate bowel length, as with short gut following volvulus or NEC or for conditions affecting motility and absorption from the bowel such as gastroschisis. Understanding the methods of nutritional support and their comparative advantages and side effects is key to successful management of a paediatric surgical patient requiring calorie nutritional special requirements.

> **Scenario:** A neonate with antenatally diagnosed gastroschisis underwent staged defect closure over a period of 10 days following delivery at 38 weeks' gestation. Parenteral nutrition (PN) has been started and has reached recommended macronutrient delivery rates.

Question: What are the indications for PN? How long can infants and children tolerate a lack of enteral feeding? Was it essential for this infant to receive PN?

Answer: Indications for PN in infants and older children are prolonged postoperative ileus, mechanical obstruction/atresia, intestinal ischaemia, necrotizing enterocolitis, short bowel syndrome, gastroenterological problems such as malabsorption, intractable diarrhoea or vomiting and inflammatory bowel disease. Energy reserves are such that stable term infants can tolerate 3–4 days without enteral feeds and older children 7–10 days before starting PN, if it is anticipated that enteral nutrition may be resumed within this time period. Premature neonates have smaller energy reserves, and the time before introducing PN is thus much shorter. Some gastroschisis infants have successful primary closure with a very fast recovery of gut function and such a short duration of PN that it of necessity may be questioned. The median duration of PN, however, in gastroschisis newborns – even with protocolized feeding advancement – is around 20 days so that the vast majority of these infants will therefore require PN. However, for other surgical infants, such as those with congenital duodenal atresia, use of PN is more debatable, as the duration of PN is often typically short or can potentially be avoided completely by the use of transanastomotic tubes or tailored incremental feeding schedules. PN has risks and is financially costly, so it should not be initiated if nutritionally relevant enteral feeding can be established quickly.

Question: The baby's weight did not change during this period. Should the macronutrient content of the PN be increased?

Answer: No, unless there are other reasons for concern. In term infants the first 2 weeks of life include a period of fluid redistribution, with contraction

DOI: 10.1201/9781003182290-52

Table 46.1 Target caloric intake of enteral and parenterally fed infants and children

Age of child	Enteral feeding (kcal/k/d)	Parenteral feeding		
		Recovery phase	Stable phase ICU	Acute phase ICU
Premature	110–120	90–120		45–55
0–1 month	110			
1–3 months	100			
3 months to 1 year	80	75–85	60–55	45–50
1–4 years	80			
5–8 years	70	65–75	55–60	40–55
9–13 years	60	55–65	40–55	30–40
14–18 years	50	30–55	25–40	20–30

of the extracellular compartment and weight loss. Overfeeding of calories can lead to hyperglycaemia and fatty infiltration of the liver, and overfeeding of amino acids can potentially lead to high blood urea nitrogen.

Question: Are the caloric requirements the same for a PN-fed baby as an enterally fed baby?

Answer: Calorie requirements for PN feeding are lower than for enteral feeding (**Table 46.1**) because no calories are lost in stool and diet-induced thermogenesis is minimal.

Question: In addition to checking weight regularly, what other monitoring should be undertaken in surgical infants receiving PN?

Answer: Ideally, length and head circumference should be monitored as anthropometric measures in addition to infant weight. These should be plotted on the appropriate growth chart (UK-WHO). Electrolytes, magnesium, phosphorous and ionized calcium should be measured on a daily basis. Glucose should be monitored frequently when initiating PN, especially at times when infusion rates are increased and when PN bags are changed. Serum triglycerides should be measured after each increase in lipid infusion rate. These monitoring rates can then be decreased to less frequently (e.g. twice per week) when stable PN is established and blood urea nitrogen, creatinine and albumin measured weekly. Liver function tests (aspartate aminotransferase [AST], alkaline aminotransferase [ALT], gamma-glutamyl transferase [GGT]) and bilirubin should be monitored on a 2-weekly basis, together with alkaline phosphatase, and a full blood count.

Question: When should enteral feeding be initiated, which enteral feed should be given and how fast should it be advanced?

Answer: Many hospitals now follow a protocolized approach to feeding infants with gastroschisis, which includes initiation (which can be started with tropic feeds 24 hours after abdominal defect closure, at first signs of recovery of gut function – bowel sounds active/stool/flatus). Typically, maternal breast milk is the preferred feed, with donor breast milk or formula used if not available and advanced as tolerated. There is data to show that a standardized protocol improves outcomes, notably time to full feeds, length of hospital stay, etc., but further evidence as to which protocol is best is lacking.

Question: The infant appears to be intolerant of breast milk, and the dietician has mentioned the possibility of cow's milk protein allergy. Is this possible in an exclusively breast-fed baby, and what are the alternatives for feeding?

Answer: Bovine antigens from maternal dietary milk consumed products can be transferred from mother to baby in breast milk. If the mother wishes to continue breast-feeding, then she can try a cow's milk protein-free diet. Alternatively, extensively hydrolysed or amino acid–based formula can be used.

Question: The rate of feed advancement has been very slow due to intolerance, and liver function has started to deteriorate. Should the PN lipid infusion be discontinued?

Answer: Although PN-associated cholestasis has been linked to the lipid component of PN, lipids provide an important source of calories. As an alternative to stopping or decreasing the lipid infusion, switching the lipid from a pure soybean-based emulsion to an emulsion containing other lipid sources (e.g., olive oil, fish oil, or medium-chain triglycerides) may be effective.

Question: What are the essential constituents of PN?

Answer: The two calorie-providing components of PN are glucose (40%–60% of calories) and lipids. There is a minimum lipid requirement of 0.5 g/kg/d to meet the requirements for essential fatty acids, and the use of lipids in PN is also important, as it enables calorie needs to be met in a low fluid volume load. However, the tolerance for intravenous glucose (ability to appropriately increase insulin secretion) and lipid (ability to clear triglycerides) increases over a period of days, with tolerance for lipids increasing more slowly than that for glucose, so that stepwise increases in infusion rates are necessary with careful monitoring of glucose and triglycerides.

Question: What are the differences between central and peripheral PN?

Answer: PN required more than a few days should be best administered via centrally placed catheters in which the catheter tip is either in the vena cava or the right atrium (including peripherally inserted central catheters [i.e. PICC lines], surgically placed central catheters or centrally placed umbilical catheters). Peripheral administration, where the tip of the line is not in the vena cava or right atrium, can be used for short-term (<2 weeks) PN in stable patients whose nutritional needs can be met without using solutions >900 mOsm/l/ >12.5% dextrose.

Peripheral PN poses significant risks of complications from hyperosmolar glucose, which can cause vascular irritation or vessel damage, and thrombosis; extravasation injuries are also frequent and can be severe.

Central catheter choice depends on the catheter device already in situ and the length of time over which PN is anticipated. PICC lines have the advantage in that they can usually be placed without a general anaesthetic, but where it is anticipated that PN will be required for the medium or long term, then a tunnelled central venous catheter (CVC) should be used, placed under a general anaesthetic.

Question: What are the complications of parenteral nutrition?

Answer: *Mechanical catheter complications* include thrombosis, blockage due to calcium precipitation or lipids and incorrect placement (or displacement) of CVCs.

Metabolic complications include hyperglycaemia, hypoglycaemia, hypertriglyceridemia, electrolyte disturbances and acidosis. Monitoring on a regular scheduled basis is also important to diagnose micronutrient and vitamin deficiencies that can occur in the longer term. For children with short bowel syndrome who may be on PN (including home PN) for years, metabolic bone disease is frequent.

Fluid overload is also a potential complication of paediatric PN, especially in critically ill patients with complex

Infection/sepsis is very common in infants and children on PN (around 30% of surgical neonates will have at least one episode of clinical sepsis), and meticulous care of CVCs is important to prevent this, with use of chlorhexidine. Antibiotic prophylaxis is not recommended.

PN-associated cholestasis, which can lead to PN-associated liver disease, is also common in infants and children and seems to be related to the lipid component. This severe complication can ultimately result in liver transplantation.

Question: What are the risk factors for PN-associated cholestasis (PNAC)/liver disease?

Answer: Various clinical factors contribute to the development of PNAC, including prematurity, low birth weight, duration of PN, immature enterohepatic circulation, intestinal microflora, repeated episodes of infection, failure to implement enteral nutrition, short bowel syndrome due to resection and the number of laparotomies. Infants with gastroschisis or jejunal atresia seem to be at particular risk. This is a diagnosis of exclusion, so rather than assume that a significant elevation of bilirubin is necessarily due to PN, other diagnoses such as inborn errors of metabolism should always be considered.

Question: What are the necessary precautions to minimize the hepatic complications of PN?

Answer: The best prevention to minimize hepatic complications of PN is to try to instigate enteral feeding as early as possible. Of course, this may not be possible or may require surgical intervention to increase bowel absorptive capacity. In patients receiving PN, minimization of infection and regular review with care management by a dedicated nutrition team involving surgeons, gastroenterologists, dieticians and pharmacy has thankfully decreased the necessity for liver transplantation. In addition, modification of the lipid components of PN, by decreasing the amount of lipid administered or switching from pure soybean-based lipid emulsions to composite lipid emulsions, is recommended to minimize hepatic complications.

Question: What conditions might be indications for infants or children to receive artificial enteral feeds?
Answer: Immaturity of swallowing (e.g., prematurity), delayed gastric emptying, gastroesophageal reflux, impaired intestinal motility, Crohn's disease, neurological or metabolic comorbidity, congenital heart disease, renal disease, cystic fibrosis or sedation/intensive care are all potential reasons for receiving enteral feeds.

Question: Which feeding routes are available for enteral nutrition?
Answer: Alternative feeding routes where children are unable to feed orally include nasogastric or orogastric tubes, nasojejunal tubes, gastrostomy tubes or jejunostomy tubes. Feeding by the most physiological route possible is preferred, i.e., gastric feeding is generally preferable to jejunal feeding, as it takes advantage of salivary and gastric enzymes and stomach acid and uses the stomach as a reservoir, allowing bolus feeding. Jejunal feeding is associated with a higher frequency of diarrhoea and dumping syndrome and necessitates feeding via a pump, as boluses cannot be tolerated. Thus, transpyloric feeds are usually restricted to infants or children (1) unable to tolerate naso- or orogastric feeds; (2) at increased risk of aspiration; and (3) with anatomical contraindications to gastric feeds, such as microgastria. Nasogastric or orogastric tubes can be used for short-term feeding, but increase the risk of oral aversion, and so should be replaced by gastrostomy, gastrojejunal tube or jejunostomy feeding stoma if long-term enteral feeding is required. Where not contraindicated (e.g., aspiration risk due to an unsafe swallow) or where is no intention to attempt oral feeding (e.g. some severely neurologically impaired children), small trophic oral feeds should be considered in order to avoid oral aversion.

Question: What monitoring is recommended for children receiving long-term enteral nutrition?
Answer: As for any nutritional intervention, weight and height should be serially measured and plotted on appropriate growth centile charts. Blood chemistry (BUN, electrolytes, etc.) should be monitored, as malabsorption can result in imbalances or deficiencies. The precise monitoring regimen should be tailored to the underlying medical condition and the feeding route (e.g., monitoring for those micronutrients usually absorbed proximally in patients fed jejunally).

CONCLUSIONS

Nutrition of surgical infants and children can often be challenging and benefit from involvement of specialist paediatric dieticians, pharmacists with an in-depth understanding of parenteral nutrition, surgeons and gastroenterologists as appropriate.

BIBLIOGRAPHY

K. Joosten, N. Embleton, W. Yan, T. Senterre and ESPGHAN/ESPEN/ESPR/CSPEN working group on pediatric parenteral nutrition. *Clin Nutr* (2018). PMID: 30078715

A. Lapillonne, N. Fidler Mis, O. Goulet, C. H. P. van den Akker, J. Wu, B. Koletzko and ESPGHAN/ESPEN/ESPR/CSPEN working group on pediatric parenteral nutrition. *Clin Nutr* (2018). PMID: 30143306

D. Mesotten, K. Joosten, A. van Kempen, S. Verbruggen and ESPGHAN/ESPEN/ESPR/CSPEN working group on pediatric parenteral nutrition. *Clin Nutr* (2018). PMID: 30037708

J. B. van Goudoever, V. Carnielli, D. Darmaun, M. Sainz de Pipaon and ESPGHAN/ESPEN/ESPR/CSPEN working group on pediatric parenteral nutrition. *Clin Nutr* (2018). PMID: 30100107

Overview of enteral nutrition in infants and children S Fleet and C Duggan: https://www.uptodate.com/contents/overview-of-enteral-nutrition-in-infants-and-children. Accessed May 2022

C. Braegger, T. Decsi, J. A. Dias, C. Hartman, S. Kolacek, B. Koletzko, S. Koletzko, W. Mihatsch, L. Moreno, J. Puntis, R. Shamir, H. Szajewska, D. Turck, J. van Goudoever and ESPGHAN committee on nutrition. *J Pediatr Gastroenterol Nutr* (2010) PMID: 20453670

Aroonsaeng D, Losty PD, Thanachatchairattana P. Postoperative feeding in neonatal duodenal obstruction. BMC Pediatr (2022);22(1):467. doi:10.1186/s12887-022-03524-7

47

Special considerations for the surgical patient with allied medical disorders

KATHERINE LAU AND LISA BARNETO
Alder Hey Children's Hospital, Liverpool, UK

I – DIABETES, PERIOPERATIVE PLANNING AND COMPLICATIONS

Scenario: A 5-year-old boy has been scheduled for an incisional abdominal wall hernia repair. He has a medical history of diabetes.

Question: Is diabetes mellitus (DM) a significant comorbidity?
Answer: Yes, DM has multiple perioperative considerations, chiefly wound healing and infection, glycaemic control strategies, hypo- and hyperglycaemia, acute kidney injury (AKI), pressure ulcers, diabetic ketoacidosis (DKA) and analgesia modalities.

Question: What analgesia techniques may be considered?
Answer: Multimodal opioid-sparing analgesia is preferable, as it reduces the incidence of postoperative nausea and vomiting; for example, paracetamol, NSAIDs and regional anaesthesia

combined will reduce postoperative opioid use. However, DM increases the risk of nerve injury due to pre-existing neuropathy and infections, including epidural abscess.

Question: How may DM be managed perioperatively?
Answer: Early resumption of eating and drinking and return to normal medication has been shown to reduce length of stay in hospital and improve outcomes, whilst preventing morbidity from glycaemic variability, AKI, fluid and electrolyte imbalance. The specialist diabetes team should be involved throughout the acute hospitalised period in patients with complex treatment and needs.

DM may be managed by changes to the patient's normal medication or, if necessary, variable rate intravenous insulin infusion (VRIII), also known as sliding-scale insulin.

Question: How may DM be managed by changes to normal medication?
Answer: It has been shown that patients who are able to be safely managed by temporary changes

DOI: 10.1201/9781003182290-53

to normal medication and careful perioperative management have safer hospital admission, recovery from surgery, resumption of normal diet and medication at normal doses and safer hospital discharge.

Perioperative management of well-controlled DM may require changes to normal medication if the following criteria are met:

- Adequate long-term glycaemic control as defined by glycosylated haemoglobin measured within the last 3 months as HbA1C <69 mmol mol^{-1} or <8.5%.
- Documented normal medication with exact doses and times of administration.
- A definitive time and date for surgery to ensure that the patient will only miss one meal.
- Priority given to the diabetic patient on the operating list.
- No expected surgical reason(s) for postoperative starvation or ileus.
- Hourly capillary blood glucose (CBG) monitoring.
- Emergency treatment for hypoglycaemia and hyperglycaemia is prescribed.
- Discharge of the patient is conditional to their ability to seek medical advice (for example, 'sick day plans').
- If concerned, always involve the diabetes specialist team in the management of the patient.

Question: How may DM be managed by VRIII?
Answer: If the patient and surgical period cannot be managed with changes to medication alone or if blood glucose is >10.0 mmol/L, the initiation of VRIII is recommended. Target CBG levels have not been established in trials, but there is a consensus for a range between 6.0 and 10.0 mmol/L, which should avoid risks associated with hyperglycaemia and hypoglycaemia.

Incorrect use of VRIII can result in hypoglycaemia, rebound hyperglycaemia, excess length of hospital stay and even DKA; a safe and effective step-down to other agents should occur as soon as possible. Hospitals must have guidelines for the safe use of VRIII. Early referral of all patients to local diabetes teams for assessment of individual patients' needs ensures that VRIII is used safely and that plans are in place for glycaemic control upon cessation of VRIII.

VRIII requires:

- In-patient hospital stay.
- Hourly measurement of CBG upon starting VRIII and in the acute perioperative period.
- IV fluids containing sodium, potassium and glucose should be used if VRIII is used for >24 hours to avoid hyponatraemia and hypokalaemia (usually 5% glucose in 0.45% saline with premixed 0.15% potassium chloride).
- The patient should be given priority in the theatre operating list timing to prevent excessive starvation, which would contribute to glycaemic variability, and at an achievable time for surgery.
- Intraoperatively, hourly CBG and appropriate substrate fluids to run alongside VRIII.
- pH and lactate from blood gas sampling may be indicated.
- Daily review of insulin infusion rates to achieve CBG levels within the target range (taking into consideration interindividual variability of insulin sensitivity).
- Daily review of fluid balance, serum urea and electrolytes.
- Daily review of the continued need for VRIII.

Question: When can VRIII be stopped?
Answer: Once the diabetic patient has recovered from the acute episode and oral intake is established, background insulin (in the form of bolus or long- or intermediate-acting insulin) must be administered before stopping the VRIII. The VRIII should only be discontinued 30 minutes after subcutaneous insulin has been given, ideally at meal time. Monitoring of blood sugar should be ensured 1 hour after discontinuing VRIII and at least 4-hourly for the first 24 hours after VRIII has been discontinued. Active involvement from the diabetes team should be sought, particularly if blood sugar control has been suboptimal.

Question: What adverse events are associated with VRIII?
Answer: Well-recognised complications are hypo- and hyperglycaemia, hyponatraemia and hypokalaemia.

VRIII and the substrate solution (usually 5% glucose in 0.45% saline with premixed 0.15% potassium chloride) must be administered through a dedicated IV cannula (via which no other drugs or fluids should be administered) which includes anti-syphon one-way valves.

Hypoglycaemia (CBG falling to below 4.0 mmol/litre) would require a reduced insulin rate, administration of 5% dextrose 5 mL/kg as IV bolus and rechecking of blood glucose every 15 minutes until CBG >6 mmol/litre and then hourly.

Ketosis may result from either delayed establishment or delayed administration of subcutaneous insulin on discontinuation. The half-life of soluble insulin is approximately 5 minutes. Therefore, there will be no appreciable functioning insulin within 30 minutes of stopping a VRIII. If the patient has type 1 DM, DKA will ensue. Type 1 DM patients must never have the VRIII stopped until alternative insulin has been administered.

The diabetes specialist team should be involved if there are concerns in transferring the patient on and off VRIII.

Question: What is DKA?

Answer: DKA may mimic presentation of an 'acute surgical abdomen', and prior to performing any emergency surgery in patients with diabetes, it must be excluded as the cause of the acute abdomen.

DKA is an acute, major, life-threatening complication of DM characterised by hyperglycaemia, ketoacidosis and ketonuria. It occurs when absolute or relative insulin deficiency inhibits the ability of glucose to enter cells for utilisation as metabolic fuel, the result being that the liver rapidly breaks down fat into ketones to employ as a fuel source, resulting in overproduction of ketones. DKA occurs mainly in patients with type 1 DM, but may also be seen with type 2 DM.

Precipitating factors are intercurrent illness and reduced oral intake combined with mistaken reduction of insulin administration. The cause of the DKA must be managed, be it medical or surgical. Critical care may be required, and early involvement of diabetic specialist teams is mandatory.

BIBLIOGRAPHY

Dhatariya K, Levy N, Flanagan D et al. for the Joint British Diabetes Societies. Management of adults with diabetes undergoing surgery and elective procedures: improving standards. Revised September 2015. Available from http://www.diabetologists-abcd.org.uk/jbds/JBDS_IP_Surgery_Adults_Full.pdf (accessed 24 February 2016)

II – ANAPHYLAXIS AND MANAGEMENT

Scenario: A 5-year-old girl with spina bifida has just been transferred into the operating theatre after induction of anaesthesia for a cystoscopy. The scrub nurse notices skin flushing on the patient, and the anaesthetist records severe hypotension. A halt in the theatre procedure is called.

Question: The foremost concern is to exclude anaphylaxis. Why?

Answer: Anaphylaxis is a type I hypersensitivity reaction with an estimated incidence of 1 life-threatening reaction per 6,000 general anaesthetics. Females are affected more often than males. The anaphylactic reaction often begins 30–60 minutes after the start of the anaesthetic with an estimated mortality, once a reaction has started, of 5%. The increased mucus secretion, bronchial smooth muscle tone and vascular permeability causes airway oedema, bronchospasm and hypotension. Initial presentation may be heralded by difficulty inflating lungs, desaturation, wheeze, coughing, hypotension, flushing, skin rash, ECG changes or cardiac arrest.

Question: What is the immediate management?

Answer: Call for help, administer 100% oxygen, epinephrine and IV fluids (avoiding colloids that have a higher incidence of allergy), antihistamines (chlorpheniramine 10–20 mg by slow IV infusion), corticosteroids (100–500 mg hydrocortisone slowly IV) and bronchodilators for persistent bronchospasm.

All patients who have a serious allergic reaction should be managed or observed in a critical care area so that a biphasic response and potential end-organ damage can be recognised and treated.

Question: Should any investigations be done? If so, when and why?

Answer: Three blood test samples for mast cell tryptase concentration, which is released during degranulation, are required to assess the likelihood of an anaphylactic reaction. Its increase does not identify the causative agent, though a higher value is more likely to indicate an anaphylactic reaction. The rise in tryptase is transient; thus timing the three samples is important – immediately after the reaction has been treated and 1 hour and 5 hours after the event. Each sample should be 5–10 mL of blood in a clotted tube and sent to the laboratory, who should be informed of its arrival and the samples cooled appropriately until sent for analysis.

Later investigations to identify the causative agent should be done by referral for consultation and full testing at an allergy clinic and the likely triggers documented as alerts in the patient's medical records.

Question: What are the common triggers in the perioperative period?
Answer: Previous exposure to the drug(s) does not seem necessary, as anaphylaxis is well documented to occur by indirect sensitisation via non-drug sensitisers.

Reactions in anaesthetic practice occur most commonly with neuromuscular blocking agents (70%), latex (12.6%), colloids (4.7%) and antibiotics (2.6%). Spina bifida patients have a higher incidence of latex allergy, and latex should always be avoided.

Penicillins are most frequently implicated in type I hypersensitivity reactions. The incidence of cross-reactivity with cephalosporins is about 8%, though often incomplete and thus may be administered safely to most patients with the exception of patients with severe penicillin reactions.

Question: What is an anaphylactoid reaction?
Answer: Of note are anaphylactoid reactions which may be clinically indistinguishable. These cause a transient rise in mast cell tryptase levels, though to a lesser degree. It is a non-immunological histamine release, i.e., not mediated by sensitising IgE antibodies with previous exposure to an antigen, and is caused by direct action of a drug on mast cells. Histamine level is not usually measured in this context, as its half-life is short (3 minutes). The clinical response depends on both the drug dose and rate of delivery, but it is usually benign and confined to the skin, occurring in up to 30% of patients during anaesthesia. It is most commonly seen in reactions to contrast media. Anaesthetic drugs that release histamine directly include atracurium and morphine.

BIBLIOGRAPHY

Suspected Anaphylactic Reactions Associated with Anaesthesia. Revised Edn, 2003. The Association of Anaesthetists of Great Britain and Ireland https://www.resus.org.uk/library/additional-guidance/guidance-anaphylaxis

III – DUCHENNE MUSCULAR DYSTROPHY

Scenario: AJ is a 17-year-old boy who has Duchenne muscular dystrophy and has been seen in the scoliosis clinic for consideration of posterior spinal fixation.

Question: What is Duchenne muscular dystrophy?
Answer: Duchenne muscular dystrophy (DMD) is an X-linked neuromuscular disorder that results in abnormal formation of the dystrophin protein in muscle. Males are therefore predominantly affected, with the mean age of diagnosis around 3–5 years. Clinical presentation is progressive, severe muscular weakness affecting all muscle types with loss of gait around age 10 years, with limited to minimal ability to move limbs or grip objects by adolescence. Steroid therapy has helped limit progression by a further 2–3 years. Respiratory complications and dilated cardiomyopathy manifest in adolescence with decreased cough strength, restrictive lung disease from both muscle weakness and worsening scoliosis (see later). Global cardiac function drops between the ages of 12 and 14 yrs.

SURGICAL CRITERIA FOR SCOLIOSIS SURGERY

Children with DMD develop scoliosis when ambulation is lost, the cause of which is not fully elucidated. Progression of the scoliosis results in significant respiratory compromise, with lateral displacement of and rotation of the vertebral bodies altering the movement of the associated ribs. The muscles utilised in respiration are disadvantaged. Finally, the organs within the thoracic cage are displaced and compressed. This mechanical defect with progressive weakness of the respiratory muscles results in alveolar hypoventilation, arteriovenous shunting with type II respiratory failure and eventually cor pulmonale.

In addition to respiratory compromise, the positioning eventually makes sitting in a wheelchair uncomfortable, increasing the risk of skin breakdown and eventually children becoming bed bound. Surgery in these children therefore is intended to limit the progression of scoliosis and slow the decline in respiratory function and improve quality of life.

Question: What are the medical considerations for this patient?

Answer: DMD patients are under the care of multiple medical and surgical specialties. At the time of consideration of surgery, the child's severity of their condition will need to be assessed to determine if they will gain any benefit. Risks include long hospital admission, which may result in loss of previous level of function with poor quality of life, complications caused by the surgery requiring further operations and even death. Members of the multidisciplinary team (MDT) caring for this child will also include a respiratory physician, cardiologist and neurologist in addition to the surgical and anaesthesia teams.

Respiratory system

- Chronic pulmonary disease with a restrictive pattern is present with both respiratory and laryngeal muscle involvement.
- By adolescence, DMD patients are often on non-invasive ventilation (NIV) at night time, require regular daily physiotherapy to help clear secretions and may have a cough assist as well.
- A recent lung function test will be part of the MDT review. Patients with severe respiratory disease are unlikely to benefit from surgical treatment and are at increased risk of being ventilator dependent with a high risk of mortality.

Cardiac system

- Patients start to develop cardiomyopathy as teenagers.
- It is challenging to determine the severity of impairment due to physical limitations the disease imposes on patients. Patients may be started on an angiotensin-converting enzyme

inhibitor (ACEi) and other diuretics to try and optimise cardiac function.

- A recent echo and ECG will be part of preoperative testing required to inform decision for surgery.

Neurology

- For some children, disease progression may preclude them from scoliosis surgery.

Question: What are the anaesthesia implications for DMD children?

Answer: Individuals with DMD are at risk of many perioperative complications, both due to the primary muscle dysfunction and secondary such as cardiac/respiratory compromise.

Patients can have rhabdomyolysis with life-threatening hyperkalaemia from exposure to volatile agents and succinylcholine or from surgical stress. Of note, they are not at a higher risk of malignant hypothermia (MH), with a different etiology resulting in the previous complication. Currently it is hypothesised to be secondary to the continued attempt of atrophic muscle fibres to regenerate, and these muscles have a higher baseline intracellular calcium. On exposure to volatile anaesthesia or depolarising muscle paralysis, the intracellular calcium continues to risk promoting extravasation of intracellular potassium and creatine kinase (CK). The hypermetabolic response continues in an attempt to normalise cellular membrane stability.

DMD patients should therefore have a 'trigger-free' anaesthetic similar to MH-susceptible patients, and depolarising muscle paralysis should be avoided. Patients may present with signs and symptoms similar to an MH crisis even with a trigger-free anaesthesia. The goals of treatment would be supportive and if hyperkalaemia were present to stabilise cardiac membrane function with IV calcium and use of other therapies to shift calcium into the intracellular space.

MH is a rare autosomal dominant condition that affects the ryanodine receptor that forms part of the release to calcium from the sarcoplasmic reticulum and initiation on contraction of skeletal muscles. A triggering agent (volatile anaesthetics or succinylcholine) causes the receptor to have an uncontrolled release of calcium into the cytoplasm. Patients may be exposed to triggering agents and remain asymptomatic. Therefore, previous exposure to triggering agents does not exclude a diagnosis. The sustained rise in calcium triggers calcium adenosine triphosphate (ATP) pumps to extrude the excess intracellular calcium. The increased utilisation of ATP causes hyperthermia, hypercarbia and eventually lactic acidosis. Muscle cells eventually undergo apoptosis, causing hyperkalaemia, raised CK and myoglobinuria. Treatment includes removing the triggering agent and prioritising giving dantrolene to stop the ongoing intracellular release of calcium. Patients will require further supportive treatment including active cooling and treatment of hyperkalaemia and will require intensive care. If treatment is delayed, mortality can be as high as 70%. MH is associated with certain myopathies such as central core disease and multiminicore disease.

Question: The patient will be prone for the operation. What are the implications of this?
Answer: Prone positions have general risks that apply to all patients. DMD patients, due to their long-term steroid treatment with slow disease progression and limited mobility, are often obese, making them at risk of pressure areas. In the prone position, bolsters placed under hips and shoulders can move and impede ventilation if compression forces are exerted on the abdomen or thorax.

Access to the patient is limited, and therefore ensuring that monitoring and IV access/arterial lines/central lines are all working and can be accessed if needed is crucial. Caution is needed with regard to the face, particularly eyes and the airway, to ensure there is no compression and they can be accessed during the procedure.

Prolonged prone position may result in impaired venous drainage of the head and neck. This may cause laryngeal oedema and may result in delayed extubation in intensive care. This is a difficult consideration, as extubation postsurgery in DMD on to NIC would be ideal to minimise respiratory complications.

Turning DMD patients during operation(s) can cause haemodynamic changes that they may not be able to compensate for. When prone, the increased intrathoracic pressure may decrease preload, cause severe hypotension and in some cases cardiac arrest. Patients undergoing scoliosis repair with cardiomyopathy usually have a transoesophageal probe inserted prior to being turned prone to allow for real-time monitoring of dynamic changes occurring during surgery.

BIBLIOGRAPHY

MH Guidelines. MHANZ: https://malignanthyperthermia.org.au/malignant-hyperthermia-information/, https://malignanthyperthermia.org.au/resource-kit/

Ragoonanan V, Russell W. Anaesthesia for children with neuromuscular disease, *Continuing Education in Anaesthesia Critical Care & Pain*, Volume 10, Issue 5, October 2010, Pages 143–147, https://doi.org/10.1093/bjaceaccp/mkq028

48

Consent

PRINCE RAJ, ABEER FARHAN, AND MARTIN T. CORBALLY
King Hamad University Hospital, Kingdom of Bahrain, Bahrain

Children have the right to be informed and advised of planned interventions. If the child can be regarded as a moral agent and has the mental capacity to understand their condition and proposed treatment, then they should also be part of the consent process. This may have limited applicability in some jurisdictions, but the surgeon must still be aware of the issues in this age group.

> **Scenario:** A 15-year-old boy presents to your hospital clinic with non-specific abdominal pain. You have examined and reassured him and plan to discharge him; however, he informs you that he has lost both his unvaccinated father and uncle who died from COVID. The child wants to get the COVID vaccine; however, his mother is opposed to the vaccine and thinks that it's part of a biomedical conspiracy.

Question: How do you define consent?
Answer: It is the legal expression of the moral principle of autonomy. It underpins the propriety of treatment and provides some defence against an allegation of assault and battery and the civil wrong of bodily trespass.

Question: What is valid consent?
Answer: For consent to be valid, it must be voluntary, informed, and the person consenting must have the mental capacity to make the decision.

- *Voluntary*: The decision must be made by the person and must not be influenced by pressure from medical staff, friends, or family.
- *Informed*: All of the information about what the treatment involves, including the benefits and risks, whether there are reasonable alternative treatments, and potential negative consequences if the treatment does not go ahead.
- *Capacity*: The person must be capable of giving consent, understand the information given to them, and can use it to make an informed decision.

Question: Name the four fundamental principles of medical ethics?
Answer:

1. *Autonomy*: The ability of the person to make his or her own decisions.
2. *Beneficence*: The act is for the benefit of the patient and supports a number of moral rules to protect and defend the right of others, prevent harm, remove conditions that will cause harm, help persons with disabilities, and rescue persons in danger.
3. *Non-maleficence*: Do no harm.
4. *Justice*: Deliver fair, equitable, and appropriate treatment of all persons.

DOI: 10.1201/9781003182290-54

Question: How is mental capacity assessed?
Answer: The Mental Capacity Act 2005 governs the following:

In order to have capacity, a person must:

- Be able to understand the information related to the decision.
- Be able to retain the information for long enough to make a decision.
- Be able to weigh up or use the information to make a decision.
- Be able to communicate the decision in any way at all.

Question: Referring to the scenario listed earlier, what do you know about Gillick competence?
Answer: Before the Gillick case, the Family Law Reform Act (1969) gave young people the authority to consent to medical treatment when they reached 16 years.

It is the legal competence to give the child under 16 the right to consent to medical examination and treatment if they demonstrate sufficient maturity and intelligence to understand and appraise the nature and implications of that treatment. The aim of Gillick competence is therefore to reflect the transition of a child to adulthood. Where a child is considered Gillick competent, then the consent is as effective as that of an adult and cannot be overruled by a parent.

Question: What was the legal base behind the Gillick-competent child?
Answer: The right of a child under 16 years to consent to medical examination and treatment was decided by the UK House of Lords in *Gillick v West Norfolk and Wisbech AHA* [1986], where a mother of a girl under 16 years objected to advice that allowed doctors to give contraceptive advice and treatment to children without parental consent. Their Lordships held that a child under 16 years had the legal competence to consent to medical examination and treatment if they had sufficient maturity and intelligence to understand the nature and implications of that treatment; hence the term 'Gillick competent'.

Question: How do you assess Gillick competence?
Answer: Legal competence to make decisions is conditional on the child gradually acquiring both:

- *Maturity*: Accounting the child's experiences and ability to manage influences on their

decision making such as information, peer pressure, family pressure, fear, and misgivings.
- *Intelligence*: Accounting the child's understanding, ability to weigh risk and benefit, and consideration of longer-term factors such as effect on family life and on such things as schooling.

Decision-making competence does not simply arrive with puberty; it depends on the maturity and intelligence of the child and the seriousness of the treatment decision to be made.

Scenario: An 8-year-old boy is brought to hospital by ambulance after a fall from a playground monkey bar. He is noted to be hemodynamically unstable, with bruises around the left lower rib cage and a rigid abdomen. Focused assessment with sonography in trauma (FAST) scan confirms free fluid, and a diagnosis of a ruptured spleen is made. You determine that blood transfusion is needed to replace blood loss and advise that surgery may be necessary. You cross-match blood, but prior to the transfusion the father stops you and refuses the blood transfusion.

Question: How would you deal with this emergency scenario?
Answer: It is vital to discover the reasons behind this action by the father. In a quiet environment the parents needs to know that the child's condition is life threatening and critical and that failure to transfuse and schedule operative intervention may result in the child's death.

Question: The mother starts crying uncontrollably and the father tells you that they are Jehovah's witnesses. What is a Jehovah's Witness?
Answer: Jehovah's Witnesses are a religious faith dating back to the 1870s first founded in Pennsylvania, United States, who believe that it is against God's will to receive blood and therefore refuse blood transfusion. In 1945 blood transfusion was determined to be forbidden to Jehovah's Witnesses, as it violated God's law by their literal interpretation of the Holy Bible.

Question 3: The boy is becoming progressively unstable, and you explain that he will die without a blood transfusion. Both parents further understand the significance of this critical situation for

their child. The family ask about other alternatives to blood transfusion. What do you tell them?
Answer: Based on the Hippocratic oath, it is a medical doctor's duty of care to seek to save the child's life. The alternative options – not giving blood – may help with the child's condition temporarily; however, it will not improve the chance of overall survival, as the best treatment with significant blood loss here is a blood transfusion.

Alternatives to blood products may include:

Derivatives of primary blood components:

- Albumin
- Immunoglobulin (anti-D)
- Coagulation factors

Haemodilution:

- Intraoperative cell salvage
- Postoperative cell salvage

Crystalloids, synthetic colloids:

- Dextran
- Hydroxyethyl starch
- Gelatins (Haemacel)

Recombinant factors, e.g., FV11a
EPO, coagulation factors

Question: Based on your clinical judgment, you believe that this child is in urgent need of blood transfusion as early as possible. What can you do?
Answer: If the person with designated parental responsibility of an incompetent child is firmly opposed to the giving of blood or blood products and the clinical team believes that giving the blood or blood products is necessary to save the child's life, then the only option is to engage the hospital legal team, who will urgently petition the court to make the child a ward of the court and remove (temporarily) legal guardianship from the parents. It is essential to document all conversations with the parents and to obtain a signed statement of 'refusal of medical care' (transfusion) from the parents.

Question: The family agree on surgical intervention. Intraoperatively, the patient becomes tachycardic, and the anaesthesiologist says that the patient's haemoglobin is now only 6. What is the next course of action?

Answer: In an emergency situation the doctor can give a lifesaving transfusion after taking a further second opinion with regard to the child despite the parental refusal, as the surgeon may face criminal prosecution if a child comes to harm because treatment was deliberately withheld.

> **Scenario:** A 10-year-old boy presents to the emergency department with a 2-day history of abdominal pain and vomiting. He is febrile with tenderness and guarding in the right iliac fossa (RIF). An abdominal ultrasound scan confirms appendicitis, and you prepare the child for surgery, which includes IV antibiotics. The father will not consent to the operation.

Question: How will you act as the attending surgeon on duty?
Answer: It is important to explore the reasons behind the father's refusal of consent and to detail clearly the potential outcomes of not proceeding with appendectomy. The father may harbour concerns about surgery and/or anaesthesia, and you as the surgeon should reassure that there is adequate experienced personnel available. Involving another health care professional (second opinion) or seeking advice from a further senior colleague can offer reassurance.

Question: The father still refuses to accept surgical intervention is necessary. He thinks that his son may have gastroenteritis. He also claims that once he was treated with medications for appendicitis. What is your next step?
Answer: Acute non-perforated appendicitis can be medically treated with antibiotics. However, there is a risk of recurrence in cases of acute appendicitis. Therefore, appendectomy is considered to remain the gold standard.

Question: The father decides to leave the hospital and refuses his son's admission. He is a single father and has left his other children unattended at home. He tells you that he wants to leave. How would you act?
Answer:

1. Based on the clinical examination and investigations, the patient requires emergent admission for both medical and surgical treatment;

therefore this patient cannot be medically discharged.
2. Looking at the domestic situation, a social worker crucially needs to be involved.
3. The possible risks of leaving with his son, including the requirement for emergency operation with risks of appendiceal perforation and intra-abdominal sepsis, must be clearly explained to the father and benefits of hospital admission vs discharge highlighted.
4. The father will now have to sign a Discharge Against Medical Advice (DAMA), which is a legal document stating that he has been told about his child's illness condition, that hospital admission is advised, and that he has been informed about the risks of discharge and that he takes full responsibility for these actions.
5. 'Red flags 'must be explained and the father advised to return to the emergency department to ensure delivery of care and definitive management.

Scenario 4: A 14-year-old girl is brought to hospital by ambulance after a road traffic accident. During the primary survey, bleeding is noted from both lower limbs with evidence of bilateral lower limb deformity, and femoral fractures are diagnosed. No other injuries are noted, and following stabilization the girl is then brought to the operating room for orthopaedic surgery fixation.

Question: What is the best course of action?
Answer: Based on the principle of beneficence, saving the child's life is the immediate priority. Bleeding control, blood transfusion, and early fracture reduction is required. In an emergency situation where it is not possible to find the legal guardian(s) any lifesaving treatment can be provided without patient or parental consent, provided the treatment is considered immediately necessary to save the patient's life or to prevent a serious deterioration of their condition.

Question: The patient is hostile and disruptive, refusing surgery. What do you do?

Answer: If a young person refuses treatment which may lead to their death or severe permanent injury, the Court of Protection can overrule the patient decision.

This is the legal body that oversees operation of the Mental Capacity Act 2005. This assumes that there is time to secure this waiver. The parents of a young person who has refused treatment may consent for them, but it's usually thought best to involve the courts in this situation.

Question: Both of the child's parents are uncontactable and the patient needs urgent orthopaedic surgical fixation. How can you obtain the consent?
Answer: Only when a person designated with parental responsibility is unavailable and when there is immediate risk to 'life and limb' (necessity plus urgency equals an emergency that is both life-threatening and urgent) may a medical superintendent or clinical manager provide consent for a surgical emergency to 'preserve the child's life' or to save the child from serious and lasting physical injury or disability.

BIBLIOGRAPHY

1. Keywood K. Principles of the Mental Capacity Act 2005. In host publication. 1997.
2. Legislation.gov.uk. Family Law Reform Act 1969. 2015.
3. Airedale NHS Trust v Bland AC 1993:789
4. Gillick v West Norfolk and Wisbech Area Health Authority and Department of Health and Social Security Q.B. 581. As cited in Children's Legal Centre (1985) Landmark decision for children's rights. Childright 1984;22:11–18.
5. Smith ML. Jehovah's Witness refusal of blood products. In: Post SG, editor. Encyclopedia of bioethics. 3rd ed. Vol. 3. New York: Macmillan Reference - Thomson Gale; 2003. pp. 1341–5.
6. Thomas J. Parental refusal: legal and ethical considerations. Southern African Journal of Anaesthesia and Analgesia 2015;21(1):34–36.

49

Patient safety and WHO checklist

IAIN YARDLEY
Evelina London Children's Hospital, London, UK

Question: What is patient safety?

Answer: The World Health Organization defines patient safety as "the absence of preventable harm to a patient during the process of health care". It can be a difficult concept to grasp, as it only exists as the absence of harm; however, it is essentially the recognition that the delivery of healthcare is inherently risky, with the possibility of inadvertently injuring patients and so healthcare providers have an obligation to reduce that risk as much as possible.

The scale of harm caused by healthcare came to light in a series of landmark studies and reports published around the turn of the century, and since then patient safety has become a healthcare discipline in its own right with a significant body of research and its own nomenclature. Workers in the field of patient safety aim to identify, characterise and reduce the risks found in healthcare. A fundamental element of the philosophy of patient safety is continuous improvement and learning from past events.

Question: What is the extent of the problem?

Answer: The precise extent of the problem is difficult to define, partly due to problems identifying what harms are truly preventable; for example, is a postoperative wound infection a preventable harm or simply a consequence of treatment?

However, estimates have been made and the relevant figures are:

- One in ten patients receiving hospital care is harmed during the course of their treatment.
- The problem affects healthcare services in all countries, regardless of income level.
- Death due to adverse events occurring during healthcare is one of the top ten causes of death worldwide.

Question: Are paediatric surgical patients at increased risk of unsafe care?

Answer: Paediatric surgical patients are susceptible to the same risks as any other surgical patient such as misdiagnosis, haemorrhage and infection but do have some specific characteristics that put them at increased risk of harm, especially the smallest, most premature patients.

- They are physically smaller than adult patients, making hypothermia during surgery more likely and reducing their reserve to intraoperative insults such as haemorrhage.
- They cannot express themselves verbally as adults can, making their presentation to caregivers less specific and diagnosis more challenging.

DOI: 10.1201/9781003182290-55

- Their physiological systems may not be fully mature, making them more vulnerable to hypoglycaemia, for example.
- Paediatric surgical conditions are often rare, and so care is concentrated in a small number of centres, necessitating transfer to another hospital.

> **Scenario:** A 6-month-old boy was taken to the operating room for an inguinal herniotomy. Under general anaesthetic an incision was made in the right groin. On delivering the spermatic cord, no hernial sac was identified. The patient record was reviewed, and it was noted the hernia was recorded as being on the left side. A further incision was made on the left side and an uneventful herniotomy carried out.

Question: What has occurred here?
Answer: This is an example of wrong site surgery, where a planned procedure is carried out on the wrong body part (in this instance the wrong side) or even on the wrong patient. Wrong site surgery is a "never event". Never events are a group of adverse events that can be prevented by the application of standard safety measures, and so they should never happen; their occurrence suggests a system that is not sufficiently focussed on safety. Nevertheless, never events continue to occur, even in highly regarded healthcare institutes worldwide.

Question: Does performing the wrong site surgery mean that this was a bad surgeon?
Answer: One of the key assumptions made in patient safety is that adverse events do not happen because staff do not care or are bad at their jobs; rather, it is because it is inevitable that people will sometimes make mistakes or slips no matter how well trained or conscientious they are. In this example, no fewer than eight mental steps are necessary for the surgeon to translate their understanding and conceptualisation of the "right side" to the patient's right side and operate on the side with the hernia – a mistake in any one of these will lead to wrong site surgery. This is known as "human factors", and understanding this is critical to the success of any attempt to improve patient safety.

Reprimands and repeated education are unlikely to have any significant impact on reducing risks. What is needed are changes to the environment and procedures that care is provided in that will support staff and prevent any of the mistakes or slips they make from causing harm to the patient. This is known as a "systems approach".

Question: What could have prevented the wrong site surgery from happening?
Answer: There are a number of measures that have been proposed to prevent wrong site surgery from happening. The simplest of these is to mark the patient with an indelible skin marker near the intended site of surgery. This is standard practice for most surgeons now but is not "fool-proof", as the mark may wash off during skin preparation or be hidden under the sterile drapes.

Another measure designed to protect surgical patients is the WHO Surgical Safety Checklist.

Question: What are the elements of the checklist?
Answer: The checklist originally consisted of 19 questions in three sections, as in **Table 49.1**, but modifications and additions have been made.

Question: What additions or modifications might be helpful in a paediatric or neonatal case?
Answer: Multiple additions to the checklist are discouraged in the WHO guidance, but some modifications to fit with local or specialist practice are possible. Useful items relevant to paediatric surgery include checking the patient is securely positioned and that they are adequately warmed. A reminder to check their blood sugar level may also be appropriate, especially in neonatal cases.

Question: Other than using the checklist, what else can surgeons do to improve safety in the operating room?
Answer: Understandably, surgical training has focussed on the clinical and technical aspects of the role. Whilst technical excellence is clearly essential in ensuring good clinical outcomes and reducing complications, there are other aspects of a surgeon's makeup that are vital to ensuring their patients' safety. These have become known as "non-technical skills".

Non-technical skills for surgeons (NOTSS) are a set of cognitive and behavioural attributes that are designed to complement technical expertise and improve surgical performance. They are grouped in four domains: Situational awareness, decision making, communication and leadership. Deficiencies in these domains are commonly

Table 49.1 Content of the WHO surgical safety checklist

Sign in (before anaesthetic)	Time out (before incision)	Sign out (before the patient leaves the operating room)
Confirm patient identify, site, procedure and consent	All team members introduce themselves by name and role	Confirm: • The procedure carried out • Instrument, needle and swab counts completed • Specimens are labelled • Any equipment problems to address
Is the site marked?	Confirm the patient's identity, procedure and site of incision	What are the key concerns for recovery of the patient?
Are the anaesthetic checks complete?	Has antibiotic prophylaxis been given within 60 minutes?	
Is the pulse oximeter on the patient and functioning?	To surgeon: • Are there any critical steps to anticipate? • How long will the case take? • What is the anticipated blood loss?	
Are there any known allergies?	To anaesthetist: • Are there any patient specific concerns?	
Is there a difficult airway or aspiration risk?	To nursing team: • Has sterility of the instruments been confirmed? • Are there any equipment concerns?	
Is there a risk of >500 ml blood (>7 ml/kg in children)?	Is essential imaging displayed?	

Source: From Haynes AB, Weiser TG, Berry WR, et al. A surgical safety checklist to reduce morbidity and mortality in a global population. N Engl J Med 2009 Jan 29;360(5):491–9.

found to underlie surgical safety incidents when they are investigated. Training is available that can improve an individual's performance in each of these areas, and this is now integrated into many surgical training programmes.

Question: If a patient safety incident occurs, what can be done to prevent it from recurring?
Answer: The first step in trying to prevent an incident recurring is to understand why it happened in the first place. There are several models that can be used to investigate an incident, but the one most commonly used in healthcare and recommended by many authorities, including the UK National Health Service, is root cause analysis (RCA). Root

causes are underlying conditions that lead to errors and adverse incidents. RCA aims to identify these underlying conditions through a detailed and structured examination of the circumstances around a safety incident.

To take the example of the wrong side hernia surgery given earlier, a superficial look at the incident might simply conclude that the surgeon made a mistake, they should be reprimanded and reminded to take more care in the future. However, an RCA might discover that:

• The list order had changed and the child in question had been swapped with another boy who was scheduled to have a right inguinal hernia.

- This list order change had occurred because the incorrect fasting instructions had been sent to the patients and following the original list order would have led to a delay.
- There were no indelible marker pens available on the day case unit and so the surgeon had used a white board marker as this was available and the mark had washed off during skin preparation.
- The reason incorrect fasting instructions were issued and the stock of indelible pens had not been replenished was that the ward clerk position on the day case unit was vacant due to long-term sick leave and had not been back-filled, leaving a lack of administrative support on the unit.
- The WHO checklist had not been used for that case.
- The theatre staff on duty that day were all agency staff and did not know the hospital well and so were busy trying to find the correct kit when the "time out" section of the checklist would normally be used.

These findings cast a very different light on the error and reveal that a reprimand of the surgeon will do nothing to reduce the risk of the adverse event being repeated. Instead, more robust system changes are required, including ensuring adequate staffing levels in both clinical and non-clinical roles, to remove the underlying conditions that predisposed to the final error and patient harm. Unfortunately, these changes are inherently more difficult and expensive to implement and so often remain undone following a safety incident.

BIBLIOGRAPHY

1. Howell AM, Panesar SS, Burns EM, Donalson LJ, Darzi A. Reducing the burden of surgical harm: A systematic review of the interventions used to reduce adverse events in surgery. Ann Surg. 2014;259:630–641.
2. Youngson G. Nontechnical skills in pediatric surgery: Factors influencing operative performance. J Pediatr Surg. 2016;51:226–230.
3. Yardley I. Patient safety. In: Newborn surgery (4th edition). Ed. Puri P. CRC Press 2018.
4. Gawande A. The checklist manifesto – how to get things right. Profile Books Ltd 2011.
5. Gawande A. Complications – A surgeon's notes on an imperfect science. Picador 2002.
6. Yule S, Rowley D, Flin R, Maran N, Youngson GG, et al. Experience matters: comparing novice and expert ratings of non-technical skills using the NOTSS system. ANZ J Surg. 2009;79:154–160.
7. Corbally MT. Can we improve patient safety? Front Pediatr. 2014;2:98. doi:10.3389/fped.2014.00098
8. Yardley I, Holbrook C. Surgical safety in children. In: Pediatric surgery diagnosis and management (2nd edition). Eds. Puri P, Hoellwath ME. Springer 2023.

50

Ethical challenges of extreme preterm neonates

HIND ZAIDAN AND MARTIN T. CORBALLY

King Hamad University Hospital, Kingdom of Bahrain, Bahrain

Scenario: A 23-week-old premature male is born weighing 475 g in severe respiratory distress. He is a product of an in vitro fertilisation (IVF) pregnancy after multiple failed attempts for the last 2 years. His sibling is 10 years old, who was also a product of IVF but was born at full term. The parents want everything done for the new baby.

Question: What are the guidelines of resuscitation of a preterm infant?

Answer: The International Liaison Committee on Resuscitation (ILCR), Neonatal Resuscitation Program (NRP), Nuffield, Canadian Pediatric Society (CPS), European Resuscitation Council, Royal Collage of Obstetricians and Gynaecologists (RCOG), and British Association of Perinatal Medicine (BAPM) resuscitation algorithms all support a viability threshold above 23 weeks of age. Withholding resuscitation applies to neonates with severe congenital anomalies, anencephaly or trisomy 13 and 18. In 2010 the Dutch Paediatric Society issued guidelines for resuscitation of preterm babies above 24 + 7 weeks, whilst on the other hand in 2016 the Swedish National Guideline lowered their threshold to 22 + 7 weeks. Some guidance provides a birth weight cut-off rate – the ILCR states a 400-g policy, whereas the European Resuscitation Council advises 350 g (1–4).

Because of international variability, the age of viability is ever changeable, and a difference of 5 days can have significant consequences.

The formal decisive factors of resucitation are not strictly limited to birth weight and age alone but include first-trimester dating ultrasounds, administration of antenatal glucocorticoids, gender, multiple birth, mode of delivery and intrapartum infections, amongst other maternal, fetal and intrapartum factors.

Question: What are the chances of survival and morbidity?

Answer: The two main factors deciding cut-off points are consideration of long-term disability and realistic chance of survival. In comparing outcomes of resuscitating 'grey zone' neonates in Sweden, The Netherlands and the UK, Wilkinson et al. reported that Sweden had the lowest threshold for resuscitation. Swedish reports indicated a higher chance of survival with lower risk of severe disability at 52% when compared to UK studies, which had a low rate of survival of only 22% (5). Brumbaugh et al. reported a multicentre cohort study reviewing outcomes of 400-g extreme preterm babies including 205 neonates with a birth weight of 400 g and a gestational age between 22 and 26 weeks. Their overall survival to hospital discharge was 12% and improved to 32% with increasing gestational ages of 25 and 26 weeks. The increased survival is determined by a difference of 1 day, placing 24 + 6 (days) weeks old into a 'survivable group'. Neurodevelopmental

DOI: 10.1201/9781003182290-56

impairment was evident in 74% of the study cohort (6). When considering withholding or withdrawing treatment from an extreme preterm, Walthers compared results across three European countries to the Netherlands: The EPICure study (7) (UK and Ireland), the EPIBEL (8) (Belguim) and the EPIPAGE (9) study (France). All three studies yielded similar results when comparing survival rates for preterms born less than 26 weeks with only a 9% chance of survival in 23-week preterms. Short-term outcomes of chronic lung disease, severe retinopathy of prematurity and major neuromorbidity (where one or more were present) was found in 62% in the EPICure study and 72% in the EPIBEL study. The EPICure study showed that only 20% of children at the age of 6 years had no disability.

Question: What are the basic principles of ethics as applied to extreme prematurity?

Answer: The basic ethical principles help govern a physician's moral practice; they are as follows: Autonomy, beneficence, nonmalefecience, and justice (10, 11).

Autonomy in this subject is unique in that a preterm neonate is not autonomous over his or her body and the decision falls on the guardians. It is difficult to separate parents' wishes over the wishes of their children, and some parents may decide one way or the other for personal reasons rather than sefless reasons.

An extreme preterm will likely need long-term support in the intensive care unit and have a fluctuating hospital course. This causes serious distress for the family, who continue to live with hope that their baby will survive. But is or should, survival be the sole objecive for physicians?

The physician's goal is to do no harm (nonmalefecence) and maximise benefits (beneficience) for a healthy baby with a good quality of life (autonomy and justice).

Question: Are there conflicting moral principles in this case?

Answer: An ethical dilemma is composed of two or more conflicting moral values, where the outcome might be a 'best case scenario' but does not satisfy all obligations. The two conflicting principles are justice for the patient versus distributive justice, beneficence versus nonmalefecience.

In cases like this, serving justice for the patient often opposes distributive justice. For the patient above all, resuscitation is the first rung. Serving justice to the masses involves adequate and appropriate resource allocation to those considered most in need. From a utilitarian perspective, the likelihood of an extreme preterm infant surviving with a minor disability to becoming a functional member of society and family is relatively low. Utilitarianists question if this treatment or resuscitation is more futile than beneficial, and if outcomes are poor, then why are we going through with it? Moral obligation is the reason why.

Antenatal discussions about the baby's condition once born, therapy options and realistic prognosis help parents make a fully informed decision. Treatment options in the delivery room are guided by comparing the anticipated outcome to the condition of the baby post delivery, and large variations may warrant more or less resucitation. Physicians are morally obligated to follow the antenatal plan as discussed with the parents (9) if the baby is born in a 'grey zone'.

To maximise chances of survival for an extreme preterm, aggressive resuscitation is required. The patient's benefit lies in survival alone because of the urgency of the decision. However, in the process of aggressive resuscitation and a prolonged hospital course, they are at increased risk for complications such as retinopathy of prematurity, intraventricular hemorrhage, necrotising enterocolitis and delayed neurodevelopment. All of these potential events will affect the quality of life should the baby survive. This decision making is a lifelong commitment to potential suffering for the child and family. The intention in resuscitation is not to cause direct harm, but survival (the end goal) presumably justifies any means by which it is achieved, therefore causing indirect harm. The conflict lies in drawing the line between harm and benefit at any point during this course once resuscitative efforts have been started.

Question: What are the implications for the family?

Answer: A premature infant will likely require long-term medical after-care follow-up, may be at risk of developing other conditions as a result of their extreme prematurity, may require surgical operations and multiple hospital admissions and some will require full-time medical care at home or in a hospital setting. These possibilities are more common than not and pose a significant financial burden on the family as well as society. A growing disabled child might require a part-time nurse, tailored medical equipment such as wheelchairs or devices for posture support. Some parents may sacrifice their careers to dedicate full-time care to their disabled child; others will seek financial support from various funding agencies, but also at times mortgage their house to fund the expense. Educating other children in the family can be affected because the parents don't have funds to provide better schooling and all funds are often directed to care for the disabled child. Siblings and other members of the family are affected at an emotional level, being placed as a second priority throughout their lives, and this can harbour feelings of resentment towards their disabled sibling or even psychological consequences. In low- and middle-income countries this can prove to be catastrophic to the welfare of the entire family.

Question: What decision would you make?
Answer: Decisions like these vary greatly across nations and borders, experience and, more importantly, an individual's moral compass. Eagerly expecting parents may not understand how one day could mean life or death for a baby conceived through assisted reproduction technologies and many failed IVF trials with significant financial cost. It is the neonatologist's duty to counsel parents on morbidity and mortality rates of extreme preterm infants to help them better make a fully informed decision where resuscitation of 23- to 24-week preterm babies is then guided by parents' wishes and circumstances.

Parents' wishes may not always align with medical recommendations, but it is hugely important to take their views and reasoning into consideration when resuscitating extreme preterm babies, given they have been presented with all the facts and prognostic data. They are essentially responsible for the repercussions of this decision making for the rest of their lives – a heavy weight to bear in the delivery room. It is preferable to have these conversations at prenatal visits, but if it is not possible, then it is up to the physician's experience, clinical judgement and hospital policy (aligned with national resuscitation guidelines) to begin or withhold resuscitative efforts. For the case listed in this scenario, an appropriate management would be to assess the baby's clinical condition at birth and provide basic resuscitation. In the case that he or she deteriorates and requires advanced intensive care or aggressive resuscitation, the parents must then be consulted, since the decision will not only include advancing efforts but also seeking the permission to withhold care.

BIBLIOGRAPHY

1. Madar J, Roehr CC, Ainsworth S, Ersdal H, Morley C, Rüdiger M, et al. European Resuscitation Council Guidelines 2021: Newborn resuscitation and support of transition of infants at birth. Resuscitation. 2021;161:291–326.
2. American Academy of Pediatrics and American Heart Association. Textbook of neonatal resuscitation, 7th Ed. Weiner GM, Zaichkin J, editors 2016. 326 p.
3. Winyard A. The Nuffield Council on Bioethics Report - Critical care decisions in fetal and neonatal medicine: Ethical issues. Clinical Risk. 2007;13:70–3.
4. Management of the woman with threatened birth of an infant of extremely low gestational age. Fetus and Newborn Committee, Canadian Paediatric Society, Maternal-Fetal Medicine Committee, Society of Obstetricians and Gynaecologists of Canada. CMAJ. 1994;151(5):547–53.
5. Wilkinson D, Verhagen E, Johansson S. Thresholds for resuscitation of extremely preterm infants in the UK, Sweden, and Netherlands. Pediatrics. 2018;142(Supplement 1):S574–S84.
6. Brumbaugh JE, Hansen NI, Bell EF, Sridhar A, Carlo WA, Hintz SR, et al. Outcomes of extremely preterm infants with birth weight less than 400 g. JAMA Pediatrics. 2019;173(5):434–45.
7. Costeloe K, Hennessy E, Gibson AT, Marlow N, Wilkinson AR. The EPICure study: Outcomes to discharge from hospital for infants born at the threshold of viability. Pediatrics. 2000;106(4):659–71.

8. Vanhaesebrouck P, Allegaert K, Bottu J, Debauche C, Devlieger H, Docx M, et al. The EPIBEL study: Outcomes to discharge from hospital for extremely preterm infants in Belgium. Pediatrics. 2004;114(3): 663–75.

9. Larroque B, Bréart G, Kaminski M, Dehan M, André M, Burguet A, et al. Survival of very preterm infants: Epipage, a population based cohort study. Arch Dis Child Fetal Neonatal Ed. 2004;89(2):F139–44.

10. TL Beauchamp J Childress. Principles of biomedical ethics. New York: Oxford University Press; 2009.

11. Hazebroek FW, Tibboel D, Wijnen RMH. Ethical aspects of care in the newborn surgical patient. Semin Pediatr Surg. 2014;23(5):309–13.

51

Ethics of conjoined twins

HIND ZAIDAN AND MARTIN T. CORBALLY
King Hamad University Hospital, Kingdom of Bahrain, Bahrain

Scenario: You are called to review conjoined twins born at 36 weeks of gestation by caesarean section.

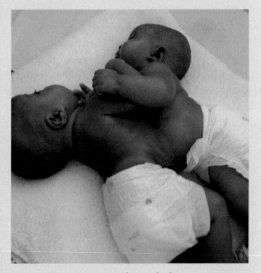

Figure 51.1 Conjoined omphalopagus twins.

Question: What is this type of fusion?

Answer: These conjoined twins are joined at the abdomen but not at the chest, pelvis or spine. They have separate respiratory, cardiovascular, spinal cords, genitalia, urinary tract systems and anal canal anatomy. The twins present with a shared portion of liver. They are classified as omphalopagus. The description of conjoined twins is best classified by the site of fusion followed by the suffix -pagus meaning 'fixed' originating from Greek. In order of prevalence, thoracopagus, including thoraco-omphalopagus, is the most common type of fusion (42% of cases reported) followed by parapagus dicephalus (11.5%), craniopagus and omphalopagus (5.5%), and the less common twinning types representing less than 3% of all cases including parapagus diprosopus, ischiopagus, pyopagus and rachipagus ('parasitic twin') (1).

Question: How will you manage these particular twins?

Answer: The initial management will include family counselling and detailed radiology investigations to better understand the twin anatomy and shared organs.

Clinical examination suggests that the hearts, lungs, spines and pelvis are separate and not considered shared. In theory, operative separation should not be challenging, and likewise there should be few ethical concerns. It is important to confirm the clinical examination with in-depth assessment of the twins' cardiovascular systems and detailed anatomical systematic imaging to confirm what organs (usually liver) are shared. Separation is not likely to cause long-term morbidity for either twin, which is an important factor in decision making, and in essence there are no ethical issues apart from the medical and surgical expertise, personnel and facilities best required to achieve safe separation.

DOI: 10.1201/9781003182290-57

Scenario: You are called to review another set of twins born at home. The parents have brought the twins to the hospital on day 3 of life.

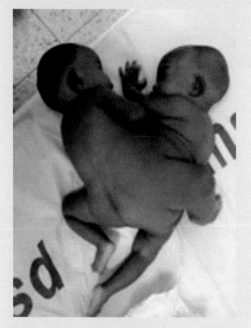

Figure 51.2 Complex Omphalo-ischiopagus twins - posterior view.

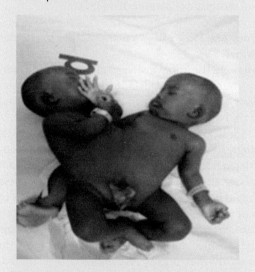

Figure 51.3 Complex Omphalo-ischiopagus twins - anterior view.

Question: What is this type of twin fusion?
Answer: These babies are classified as omphalo-ischiopagus twins. The twins are joined at the abdomen, pelvis and limbs. On closer inspection, they share three legs, one of which is conjoined (one non-functional limb and two feet), bladder exstrophy, ambiguous genitalia which appears to be a male phenotype (scrotal appearance, split phallus) and share a single anus. CT imaging confirms a shared hepatobiliary system and GI tract (small bowel and large bowel). They each have two kidneys and two separate but connected bladders (one of which is exotrophic). Workup must include CT, MRI for vascular territory mapping and contrast studies to determine bowel anatomy and 3D reconstruction.

Question: How complex is the surgery?
Answer: Separation of these twins is a major undertaking, but as discussed later poses surmountable ethical issues. The risks of separation are not only limited to the anatomical site of twin fusion but also the challenges that will be encountered intraoperatively with blood volume, anaesthetic risks, size and age of the babies. In low- to middle-income countries, access to blood products is very limited, and carefully planned scheduling of the operation is key (2). The team must include two separate anaesthetists and two surgical teams which will comprise a urologist, plastic surgeon and orthopaedic surgeon. The allocation of organs and/or limbs to the twins is largely a clinical decision based on the degree of shared anatomy. The ethical challenge is the fair distribution of organs between the separated twins to achieve the best possible functional outcomes for each. In general, this is a balance of decision making so that each twin shares an equal quality of life.

Long-term morbidity and prognosis following separation are other major ethical concerns. Healthcare systems in low- to middle-income countries are often overwhelmed, and access to effective care in a timely manner is frequently impossible. Families with twins who live in towns outside major cities are required to travel long distances to seek specialist care and sometimes even just basic medical healthcare. One or both twins will require significant aftercare such as stoma appliance supplies, long-term rehabilitation, prosthetic limbs, catheter devices and frequent aftercare follow-up and long-term management plans.

Parental wishes, anaesthetic and surgical expertise available, expected long-term quality of life and availability of resources should form the basis of reasons to separate. There should be a clear understanding of the inevitable social, educational and medical needs of such vulnerable babies and how they may be best ensured a reasonable quality of life. When all of these aspects are considered and accommodated, there is then little ethical concern.

> **Scenario:** You are asked to review conjoined ischiopagus twins who are joined at the pelvis, are tetrapus (four lower limbs), but also share a common lower vertebral column and lower spinal cord with cloacal abnormalities, hemi-vagina and hemi-uteri. One twin has dysmorphic features, a complex cardiac abnormality causing cardiac failure and other congenital abnormalities (partially absent corpus callosum, Dandy Walker malformation, severe pulmonary hypoplasia). The arterial system supplying the physiologically weaker twin is nourished mainly by the other twin's aorta.

Question: What are the ethical issues in this scenario, and how would you proceed?

Answer: It is clear that one twin is severely compromised both anatomically and functionally and that while separation is technically possible, it would likely result in the death of the weaker twin. The decisions in this case are highly complex and are somewhat similar with the UK widely publicised conjoined Manchester-Maltese babies, where separation surgery would invariably result in the immediate death of the weaker twin. The medical team (Manchester) therefore considered it ethically reasonable to offer this solution to the family, but the parents then refused and the case proceeded onwards to legal deliberation. This landmark legal case will be further discussed to highlight the pitfalls and dilemmas.

PROPOSITION 1

Ruling against separation

The parents believed that both twins should be allowed an equal chance of survival and therefore, by extension, death. If their afflictions were to cause them both to die, this was a fate they as the parents were willing to accept. For religious and other beliefs, being the twins' legal guardians, they are ultimately responsible for the medical decisions taken on behalf of their children. This right is uncontested in all consents for surgical procedures; however, in this case it was opposed. A less explored aspect to consider is the financial burden of caring for the surviving twin. Long-term rehabilitation and medical care are an expected outcome after any separation. In this case the surviving twin would face quality-of-life issues (cloacal anomaly, pelvic diastasis, and a spinal deformity) and would likely require urinary diversion, rectal washouts or a colostomy to aid bowel continence, all of which require long-term medical supplies and healthcare support. It was clear that the family may not have had easy access to long-term healthcare and lived a significant distance away from expert follow-up at a specialist hospital facility.

The outcome of death to both twins are not one easily accepted by medical professionals, and the principle of saving one life motivated the surgical position. It is still questionable where (who) this decision resides with, but ideally the parents and the medical team should be on the same side with the same goals. Although these goals may start from different perspectives, they should respect where possible the parents' views and the ultimate quality of life of the twins joined together or separated. As the medical team and parental views were not aligned, the case was unfortunately brought to court.

PROPOSITION 2

Ruling in favour of separation

The court's fundamental objective was to avoid a preventable death of one of the twins but not with the planned intent of sacrificing the other twin. Throughout the judgement it was emphasised that during their separation, no part of one twin was to be donated to the other twin and that the unhealthier twin's bodily integrity would not be compromised. It was clear that the unhealthy twin was not capable of independent existence and also not a candidate for aggressive support, such as extracorporeal membrane oxygenation (ECMO), in view of other comorbidities. Furthermore, the separation was time sensitive, with impending high-output cardiac failure (in the healthy twin). In this case, emergency separation would still result in a 60% risk of mortality to the stronger twin in comparison to a 6% mortality risk in elective twin separation. Separation here is considered the equivalent of removing life support from a terminally ill patient, which is an ethically acceptable position and legal in some countries.

However, the Court of Appeal worried that this would open a doorway forward to allow for the killing of severely disabled patients once it was determined their chance of survival was extremely low and that euthanasia (in this jurisdiction) was not lawful. It was determined that the doctrine of necessity employed in this unique twin case was to prevent the death of both twins. While the court is ultimately responsible for respecting the parents' wishes which arose from religious convictions, it was also obligated to carry out a ruling that was in the best interest of the children (3).

PRINCIPLE OF "DOUBLE EFFECT"

The principle of "double effect" deems it ethically permissible to carry out an action with a possible harmful side effect as long as the primary intention was good and the outcome is good (4). John Frame emphasises that the dying twin is alive but is in the process of (dying) an inevitable death and therefore requires care and support, not a hastened death (5). The action of purposely killing the weaker twin (in the process of separation) is considered unethical, and the effects of it are a means to an end. David H. Wenkel concluded "the action of killing one or both of the twins is not morally indifferent" (6). As moral agents, physicians are required to balance each twin's benefit and harm equally caused by the separation or lack of. The twins are separate individuals, and what is deemed beneficial for one is harmful for the other and vice versa. The principle of "double effect" falls in favour of the stronger twin but not for the weaker twin and is therefore inapplicable in this scenario. If hypothetically, the weaker twin was born independently it would not be capable of life without aggressive support, nor would it be a candidate for advanced life support because of the myriad of congenital abnormalities associated with a very poor prognosis. The twin outcome here is bleak in any situation, and a meaningful life is unsalvageable. To fulfil beneficence

to the stronger twin (who has a likelihood of survival and a potentially acceptable quality of life), the second twin is considered harmful to the sibling's prolonged survival and its existence is therefore detrimental to health (*Re A (conjoined twins) [2001] 2 WLR 480*).

A plausible solution is to wait until the imminent death of one of the twins. But as all twin separation surgery requires detailed planning, it is not at all possible to ignore the true purpose of this. Emergency separation would carry a much higher mortality risk and if not performed would result in death to both infants.

FINAL JUDGMENT

The High Court ruling considered the importance of upholding the sanctity of life for both children equally, and fulfilling that duty was choosing the lesser of two evils. The poor quality of life for both twins should they survive past 6 months, and given the circumstance of impending death to both, the decision was made therefore to save one twin, as the other would not likely survive in any given circumstance. The Court of Appeal dismissed the parents' appeal, and the twin separation took place with immediate death of the unhealthier weaker twin.

CONCLUSION

The minefield of ethical principles makes it difficult to conclude this multifaceted complex clinical case. It is an area of great uncertainty, and ethical law is constantly challenged with each new case of complex conjoined twins.

Naturally, each case is different and varied legal rulings apply in different jurisdictions, but the ultimate duty is to uphold the principles of moral conduct: To fulfil justice to the patient, respect autonomy, act with the intent of beneficence and ensure non-maleficence.

With respect to the ruling, English law and physicians, the final judgement lays a highly complex moral burden on all those involved and in particular the parents. Along with their obligations to each other, the intricacies of the family unit and their personal religious convictions cannot be assumed, predicted or understood by any court or physician. Their future has been altered by rulings in favour of a decision they were not supportive of. It is ultimately the parents' responsibility to care for the surviving twin infant with all the positive and negative outcomes and forced to accept a choice they did not make. It may be of benefit perhaps in similar future complex twin cases to listen more to the conscientious decision of the parents.

BIBLIOGRAPHY

1. Mutchinick OM, Luna-Muñoz L, Amar E, Bakker MK, Clementi M, Cocchi G, et al. Conjoined twins: A worldwide collaborative epidemiological study of the International Clearinghouse for Birth Defects Surveillance and Research. Am J Med Genet C Semin Med Genet. 2011;157C(4):274–87.

2. Barnes LS, Stanley J, Bloch EM, Pagano MB, Ipe TS, Eichbaum Q, et al. Status of hospital-based blood transfusion services in low-income and middle-income countries: A cross-sectional international survey. BMJ Open. 2022;12(2):e055017.

3. Pearn J. Bioethical issues in caring for conjoined twins and their parents. Lancet. 2001;357(9272):1968–71.

4. Beauchamp TL, Childress JF. Principles of biomedical ethics: Oxford University Press, USA; 2001.

5. Frame JM. Medical ethics: Principles, persons, and problems. 1988:10(4). Publishers Phillipsburg NJ, Presbytarian and Reformed Pub.Co.

6. Wenkel DH. Separation of conjoined twins and the principle of double effect. Christ Bioeth. 2006;12(3):291–300.

PART 7

Malignant Disorders

52

Abdominal solid tumors: Liver, renal and neuroblastic tumors

ALESSANDRO INSERRA AND ALESSANDRO CROCOLI
Bambino Gesu Hospital, University Roma Tor Vergata, Rome, Italy

In the age groups between 0 and 14 years, malignant neoplasms represent a significant cause of mortality.

The frequency of neuroblastoma is estimated at 11.3% in the 0–14 age group and 0.2% in the 15–19 age group compared to all pediatric neoplasms. For Wilms tumor these estimates are correspondingly 8.6% and 0.4%. For malignant hepatic neoplasms it is 2.3% and 1.2%, respectively.

The timely diagnosis of a tumor in pediatric patients is of enormous importance since many lesions are eminently treatable. In the event of early diagnosis, prognosis is considerably improved, and the intensity of therapy may therefore be lessened as well as the effective adequate control of metastases.

Neoplastic disease in children may have subtle findings, and the onset of symptoms most of the time (about 90% of cases) is generally linked to the effects of space by the mass which becomes evident, for example, with a volumetric increase in the size of the abdomen or with the effects of tumor compression on adjacent structures with consequent clinical symptoms.

The severity of the symptoms is closely related most of the time to the state of evolution of the disease considering that these are mostly related to disease progression.

It is important to note that almost 70–80% of pediatric cancer patients (including those with leukemia and lymphomas) will become long-term survivors. In some cases, pediatric cancer survivors may present later with second malignancies as a consequence of early treatment they have undergone in childhood, e.g., thyroid cancers.

Another challenge to consider is the role of palliative care. We must here define it as 'the best' quality of life achievable for the longest period possible or better for all the future of the child. In general, at the beginning of a patient's journey with a new cancer diagnosis, consideration should be given to organ-sparing surgery, minimally invasive surgery, and if possible, less intense chemotherapy. It is important, where possible, to try to limit or avoid radiation therapy in children and, of course, where this is required provide adequate vital organ protection from the radiotherapy field.

One of the main roles of radiological imaging in pediatric cancer care is to seek to obtain high-quality images, while minimizing trauma and distress to patients and family.

Liver tumors are uncommon in pediatrics with a frequency range between 0.5% and 2% and therefore are referred to as 'rare neoplasms'. In the United States and Europe, the expected numbers per year range from 150 to 200 new cases.

DOI: 10.1201/9781003182290-59

Scenario: A 5-year old child is referred from their family pediatrician to the hospital emergency department with an enlarged abdomen. The patient appears in fairly good general condition though they are slightly pale with some breathing difficulty noted and afebrile but has a loss of appetite.

On clinical examination the abdomen appears swollen due to the presence of a mass lesion that occupies the right hypochondrium, which is of firm to hard consistency and not mobile. Bowel sounds are normal to auscultation, and the parents state stooling behavior is normal for the child without constipation.

Question: What other tests will need to be undertaken make a diagnosis?

Answer: The presence of a space-occupying lesion in the abdomen will require investigation with laboratory blood tests and radiology imaging. Liver function tests with estimation of serum bilirubin, serum alpha fetoprotein, beta-human chorionic gonadotropin (HCG), and urinary catecholamines should be obtained. Imaging is best scheduled starting with an ultrasound exam to first clarify the origin of the mass lesion with CT and MRI scan for better information.

Blood tests later show a mild anemia with no alteration of serum transaminases and a total bilirubin within the normal limits. Serum alpha fetoprotein (AFP) is elevated, while beta HCG and catecholamines are at normal range. Ultrasound scan shows a large lesion involving the liver parenchyma without apparent involvement of the other organs. The biliary tract system is free of disease involvement.

The elevated serum AFP supports a working diagnosis of hepatoblastoma (AFP is raised in 90% of index cases).

Question: The most probable diagnosis is therefore now a hepatoblastoma. How will you proceed next?

Answer: It is now necessary to assess the extent of disease involvement with a chest CT scan with contrast to detect the presence of metastases and abdominal imaging to best define which and how many liver segments are involved.

Question: Is there a universally recognized way of assessing the extent of liver disease?

Answer: The liver is conveniently divided into eight segments according to Couinaud, which is by far the most valid reference for this definition, which sees the liver organ divided into four major sectors (2 and 3, 4a and 4b, 5 and 8, 6 and 7). Depending on the involvement of one or more liver sectors, a presurgical staging system is then performed, which will be compared later. This first staging is called the pretext stage and assesses the disease at the onset (**Figures 52.1** and **52.2**).

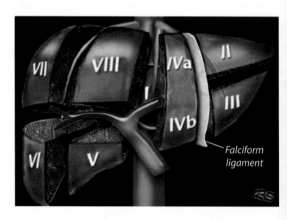

Figure 52.1 Segmental anatomy of the liver.

Question: Is all this information sufficient to indicate a therapeutic care pathway?

Answer: No. A biopsy of the liver lesion is next required for histological confirmation, which is essential to plan therapy. This can be best undertaken by an ultrasound-guided needle biopsy or by a surgical route (open biopsy) where necessary. This presurgical evaluation, called pretext, is crucially essential to assess the extent of disease at the onset (i.e., number and position of the liver segments involved), which must be compared with a posttext stage after neoadjuvant chemotherapy.

As part of this multidisciplinary evaluation, other key factors should also be noted such as invasion of the vena cava or suprahepatic veins (V), portal vein and/or its bifurcations (P), the presence of contiguous extrahepatic neoplasia (E), the presence of tumor multifocality (F), rupture of the tumor at diagnosis (R), involvement of the liver caudate lobe (C), lymph node involvement (N), and the presence or absence of distant metastases (M).

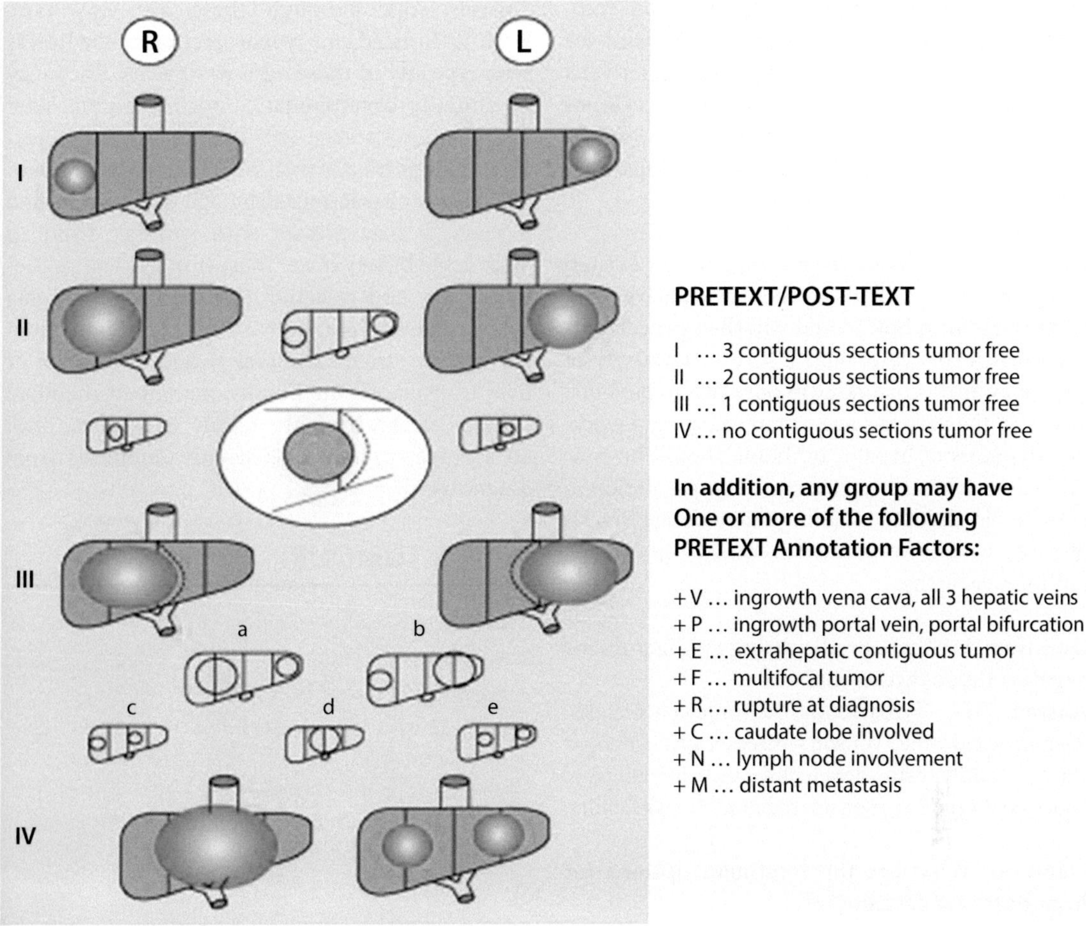

Figure 52.2 Pre-TEXT staging system based on number of segments involved at presentation.

PRETEXT/POST-TEXT

I ... 3 contiguous sections tumor free
II ... 2 contiguous sections tumor free
III ... 1 contiguous sections tumor free
IV ... no contiguous sections tumor free

In addition, any group may have One or more of the following PRETEXT Annotation Factors:

+ V ... ingrowth vena cava, all 3 hepatic veins
+ P ... ingrowth portal vein, portal bifurcation
+ E ... extrahepatic contiguous tumor
+ F ... multifocal tumor
+ R ... rupture at diagnosis
+ C ... caudate lobe involved
+ N ... lymph node involvement
+ M ... distant metastasis

Question: What are the treatment options at this point now?

Answer: It depends on the liver sectors involved and associated factors (V, P, E, F, R, C, N, M) that will guide the therapeutic approach, which now follows two possible protocols: The first SIOPEL advises neoadjuvant chemotherapy in the first instance followed by elective surgery resection, and the COG system accepts 'up-front' surgery when possible and where permitted (i.e. complete tumor resection at primary diagnosis).

A postsurgical staging (Evan's system) is possible in which the first stage includes complete resection at primary diagnosis; the second stage is the presence of microscopic residual disease; the third stage the execution of the biopsy only without resection; and finally, the fourth stage is with the presence of distant metastases.

Question: What factors will influence long-term survival?

Answer: Survival is related to the risk category stratification analysis, which takes into account pretext, AFP, and the postsurgical staging of Evans. The percentage of estimated survival outcomes are 80–85% for all hepatoblastomas, with 90%–95% achieved for those patients harboring favorable histology (i.e., fetal form or pretext 1) and 45%–80% variation for metastatic patients.

Question: Are there any other therapeutic options with chemoresistant tumors?

Answer: Yes. The first option is termed 'extreme' surgery and is reserved for those tumors in which reconstructive vascular surgery of the hepatic veins, portal vein, or hepatic artery is required – as in pretext 3 and 4. The second option is a liver transplant operation reserved for pretext 3 multifocal and pretext 4 inoperable lesions and for central hepatic tumors involving the inferior vena cava, the suprahepatic or the main portal vein, or both its branches. The presence of metastases does not contraindicate a liver transplant. Living donor (split liver) is an opportunity to be considered.

Question: If the same liver tumor lesion existed except for the AFP assay being negative in a 10-year-old boy, how would you then proceed?
Answer: In this case, with a serum negativity of AFP (may be positive value in only 50% of patients) and with the patient's age group category, a working diagnosis of hepatocarcinoma should be considered, which has a typical clinical presentation in 10-year-old children affecting the male sex in 59% of cases with an estimated frequency of 0.7 per million live births.

Question: Are there predisposing risk factors for hepatocellular carcinoma?
Answer: Yes: Tyrosinemia, chronic cholestasis, Alagille syndrome, Wilson's disease, glycogenopathies, 1-antitrypsin deficiency, and intrahepatic cholestasis type 2 are considered notable risk factors.

Question: What are the treatment options for hepatocellular carcinoma?
Answer: More than 70% of hepatocellular carcinomas are inoperable at primary diagnosis, while complete surgical resection remains the only possibility of cure. Prognosis is dependent on tumor resectability. Other possible options to consider are intra-arterial chemotherapy or a liver transplant, which is indicated in those patients with unresectable tumors and no evidence of metastatic disease.

Question: What are the outcomes of hepatocellular carcinoma?
Answer: Overall survival is poor, notably 27% survival at 2 years. Risk factors for disease recurrence include vascular invasion and the presence of a multifocal tumor. Survival after liver transplantation is approximately 86% at 1 year, 63% after 5 years, and 58% at 10 years.

Question: Are there other forms of primary malignant liver neoplasms encountered in children and adolescents?

Answer: Yes, although these are very rare. Undifferentiated embryonal sarcoma of the liver is seen typically in those aged 6–10 years. They may be initially asymptomatic; normal serum AFP and chemoresistance will require surgical resection or liver transplantation. Biliary rhabdomyosarcoma is characterized by age onset of around 5 years. It may present with jaundice from an obstructed biliary tract. These tumors require chemotherapy and resection. Hepatic angiosarcoma is a very rare tumor, with an age at onset of about 3 years. Treatment includes surgical resection or liver transplantation. Finally, malignant rhabdoid tumors of the liver are highly aggressive, with an average survival rate of only 2 months from diagnosis.

WILMS TUMOUR

Scenario: A 5-year-old child arrives to the hospital emergency room accompanied by parents who report recently noting a swollen abdomen and the passage of dark-colored urine in the last 2 days. Mild hypertension is recorded. On clinical examination a left-sided hard, firm mass is noted.

Question: How will you schedule the workup of this patient and a diagnosis?
Answer: Order basic laboratory tests, including urinalysis and abdominal ultrasound.

Lab tests appear normal. Small traces of blood are noted in the urinalysis.

Ultrasound shows a solid lesion (18 cm × 10 cm × 11 cm) in the upper pole region of the left kidney. The renal pelvis is moderately dilated. There are several enlarged lymph nodes detected along the aorta and below the celiac axis. The left adrenal gland is not readily identified.

Question: What is the leading diagnosis?
Answer: Renal neoplasm – most likely Wilms tumor given the patient age group.

Primary embryonic pediatric neoplasms of the kidney were first described by Max Wilms in 1899. The tumor originates from blastemal cells of the metanephros, which normally differentiate during development to form nephrons. Wilms tumor is considered to be the most common pediatric renal neoplasm. It can arise sporadically and has familial genetic syndromic associations, e.g. Deny Drash, hemi-hypertrophy syndrome, and Beckwith-Wiedemann syndrome.

There is a male:female ratio of 0.9. Peak incidence is 3–5 years. Seventy percent of index cases are diagnosed between 1 and 5 years. It is familial in 1% of cases, and 5% of patients present with bilateral disease – see the following figure (**Table 52.1**).

Table 52.1 Known genetic and syndromic associations

Syndrome	Locus	Implicated genes
WAGR	11p13	WT1
Denys-Drash	11p13	WT1
Beckwith-Wiedemann	11p15	IGF2, H19, p57Kp2
Simpson-Golabi-Behmel	Xq26	GPC3
Li-Fraumeni	17p13	p53
Hyperparathyroid jaw tumour	1q21–q31	HRPT2
Neurofibromatosis	17q11	NF1
Sotos	5q35	NSD1
Bloom	15q26	BLM
Perlman	?	?
Mosaic variegated aneuploidy	?	?
Trisomy 18	18	?

Question: What additional imaging is required?
Answer: Abdominal ultrasound and MRI scan. Patient evaluation must also include assessing the thorax for distant metastases. In 70% of Wilms patients, lung metastases will be present at the first presentation and are best evaluated with CT chest imaging.

Question: Are there any other evaluations that should be considered with this patient?
Answer: Yes. Echocardiography evaluation is essential before starting cancer chemotherapy. Assessment of the health of the contralateral kidney is imperative. If Wilms bilateral disease is detected, DMSA scintigraphy with renal functional assessment will help guide nephron-sparing surgery and plan staged operations.

Question: You have now defined at this point the renal origin of the neoplasm, i.e. left side, kidney tumor. The contralateral kidney has normal function and no disease involvement. No distant metastases are detected. Renal vein and inferior vena cava (IVC) shows no tumor involvement.

What will you plan next? Is ultrasound-guided needle biopsy indicated in search of diagnostic confirmation?
Answer: The treatment strategy of Wilms tumor encompasses two main themes: SIOP and COG protocols. Considering the typical age of the patient, there is no indication for renal biopsy (studies show only approximately 5% of patients or less at this typical age group will not have Wilms tumor).

Question: What are the fundamental differences between SIOP and COG protocols?
Answer: The COG protocol advocates 'upfront surgery' at primary diagnosis. The SIOP protocol advocates first chemotherapy followed by elective delayed operation.

Question: Are there substantial differences in terms of outcomes and long-term results between COG and SIOP treatment protocols?
Answer: No. Survival is equivalent: 90%–95% (COG) and 70%–80% (SIOP) in those with advanced stage disease.

Question: So, what are the main advantages and disadvantages of COG and SIOP?
Answer: Primary strengths of COG protocol:

- Up-front resection allows accurate pathology assessment of histology and extent of disease.
- Enables collection of untreated tumor tissue for biological studies.
- Avoids diagnostic errors (on SIOP 93-01 approximately 5% of renal tumor lesions were shown not to be Wilms tumor, including 1.5% of benign conditions).

Primary strengths of SIOP protocol:

- Preoperative chemotherapy reduces tumor burden volume, thereby decreasing the risk of spillage and aids 'downstaging' the tumor (introducing response to treatment as a prognostic factor for stratification).
- As a result, fewer patients receive irradiation (although slightly more may receive anthracycline therapy).

NEUROBLASTOMA

Scenario: A 2-year-old female child is referred to the hospital emergency department with a 2-week history of abdominal pain and vomiting. The parents report the child having episodes of abdominal pain with non-bilious vomiting and diarrhea. They have also noticed progressive lethargy with the child refusing to walk and play as normal, as well as limping.

Clinical exam reveals pallor with a mild tachycardia and slightly elevated blood pressure (105–80 mmHg). Laboratory blood tests show a mild anemia and high serum lactate dehydrogenase, urate, potassium, and ferritin.

An ultrasound scan and CT is ordered, which now shows a large abdominal mass spreading toward the pelvis near the common iliac arteries, reportedly encasing the IBC and both renal veins and distorting the aorta and adjacent organs.

Question: What is the likely working diagnosis in this child?
Answer: The patient has an abdominal neuroblastoma.

Neuroblastoma arises in the sympathetic nervous system and is reportedly the most common extracranial solid tumor of childhood. Approximately 600–700 new index cases are diagnosed annually in the United States. Neuroblastoma very rarely occurs in children over 10 years of age or in adults. It is estimated that approximately 2%–5% of patients will have a familial predisposition to developing neuroblastoma. Survival rates range from 40% to 90% dependent on age, site of primary tumor, disease stage, tumor biology and disease risk categorization.

Question: Are there any other neuroblastoma clinical manifestations that should be considered?
Answer: Symptoms vary with stage and tumor location:

- *Eyes*: Proptosis, ecchymosis, Horner's syndrome, heterochromia, blindness.
- *Neck*: Horner's syndrome.
- *Abdomen*: Anorexia, vomiting, diarrhea.
- *Pelvis*: Bowel, bladder dysfunction.

- *Paraspinal*: Neurological weakness, paraplegia.
- *Paraneoplastic syndromes*: WDHA syndrome with hypokalemia/chronic diarrhea, opsoclonus/myoclonus/ataxia – 'dancing eye syndrome', hypertension, headache, flushing, Harlequin sign.

Question: Are any further investigations required?
Answer: Urinary catecholamines (homovanillic acid (HVA), vanilmandelic acid (VMA)) should be assayed. Biopsy of the tumor with central venous line placement and bilateral bone marrow biopsy and trephines must be scheduled under general anesthesia. A meta-iodobenzylguanidine (MIBG) scan must be also planned to complete staging.

Question: What are the most important prognostic factors for neuroblastoma?
Answer: Prognosis is dependent on:

- Age (children older than 18 months have a worse prognosis compared to younger patients).
- Stage.
- Site of primary tumor – head and neck vs thorax vs abdomen vs pelvis.
- Pattern of metastases – MS infant vs Stage 4.
- Genetic markers – MYC N, ALK, chromosome aberration, ploidy status.

Regarding disease staging, two staging systems used for neuroblastoma.

International Neuroblastoma Staging System

INSS (1989), postsurgical staging shown in **Table 52.2**.

- **I**–Localized tumor, complete gross excision, LN negative.
- **IIA**–Localized tumor, gross residual disease, with either ipsilateral LN negative or LN sought/none found (with specific mention in operative note).
- **IIB**–Localized tumor, +/– gross residual disease, with either ipsilateral LN positive or no LN sought.
- **III**–Unresectable unilateral tumor +/– LN Localized tumor with contralateral LN (+)

Table 52.2 International Neuroblastoma Staging System (INSS, 1989) – Postsurgical staging

Stage I	Localized tumor confined to the area of origin; complete gross resection, with or without microscopic residual disease; negative lymph nodes
Stage IIA	Unilateral tumor with incomplete gross resection; negative lymph nodes
Stage IIB	Unilateral tumor with complete or incomplete gross resection; positive ipsilateral lymph nodes; negative contralateral lymph nodes
Stage III	Tumor infiltrating across midline with or without regional lymph node involvement, unilateral tumor with contralateral lymph node involvement, or midline tumor with bilateral regional lymph node involvement
Stage IV	Tumor disseminated to distant lymph nodes, bone, bone marrow, liver, or other organs (except as defined by stage IVS)
Stage IVS	Localized primary tumor as defined for stage I or II with dissemination limited to liver, skin, and/or bone marrow (under 1 year of age and <10% bone marrow involvement)

- Midline tumor (if gross resection and LN [–] or LN sought/none found, then Stage I; if gross resection and no LN sought, then Stage 3).
- **IV**–Any primary tumor, metastases to distant LN, bone, bone marrow, liver, etc.
- **IV-S**–Localized, (I, IIA, IIB) metastases to skin, liver, and/or bone marrow, <1 year of age.

International neuroblastoma risk group staging system (INRGSS)

INRGSS (**Table 52.3**) is a pre-treatment staging system designed specifically for the INRG classification system based on image-defined risk factors (IDRFs – **Table 52.4**). IDRFs are the surgical risk factors identified on radiological images (CT scans, MRI) that make complete tumor resection risky or difficult at the time of diagnosis. They are predictors of adverse surgical outcome because their presence is associated with lower complete resection rate and greater risk of surgery-related complications.

The INRG risk stratification system assigns patients into four overall risk category groups:

Very low, low, intermediate, and high risk. Risk group assignment is based on age, INRG stage (L1, L2, M, MS), and presence or absence of biological tumor characteristics including MYCN amplification, certain segmental chromosomal aberrations, and DNA ploidy. In addition, all ganglioneuroma (GN) are considered very low risk, as are ganglioneuroblastomas (GNB) with intermixed histology.

Low risk

NB patients without MYCN amplification with or without life-threatening symptoms in the following clinical situations:

- Children aged ≤18 months with localized neuroblastoma associated with IDRFs precluding upfront surgery (stage INRG L2).
- Children aged ≤12 months with disseminated neuroblastoma without bone, pleura, lung, or central nervous system (CNS) disease (stage INRG MS)

Table 52.3 International Neuroblastoma Risk Group Staging System (INRGSS)

Tumor stage	Description
L1	Localized tumor not involving vital structures, as defined by the list of IDRFs, and confined to one body compartment
L2	Local-regional tumor with presence of one or more IDRFs
M	Distant metastatic disease (except stage MS tumor)
MS	Metastatic disease in children younger than 18 months, with metastases confined to skin, liver, and/or bone marrow

Table 52.4 Image-defined risk factors (IDRFs)

Anatomic region	Description
Multiple body compartments	Ipsilateral tumor extension within two body compartments (i.e., neck and chest, chest and abdomen, or abdomen and pelvis).
Neck	Tumor encasing carotid artery, vertebral artery, and/or internal jugular vein.
	Tumor extending to skull base.
	Tumor compressing the trachea.
Cervicothoracic junction	Tumor encasing brachial plexus roots.
	Tumor encasing subclavian vessels, vertebral artery, and/or carotid artery.
	Tumor compressing the trachea.
Thorax	Tumor encasing aorta and/or major branches.
	Tumor compressing trachea and/or principal bronchi.
	Lower mediastinal tumor infiltrating costo-vertebral junction between T9 and T12 vertebral levels.
Thoracoabdominal junction	Tumor encasing aorta and/or vena cava.
Abdomen and pelvis	Tumor infiltrating porta hepatis and/or hepatoduodenal ligament.
	Tumor encasing branches of superior mesenteric artery (SMA) at the mesenteric root.
	Tumor encasing origin of celiac axis and/or origin of the superior mesenteric artery.
	Tumor invading one or both renal pedicles.
	Tumor encasing aorta and/or vena cava.
	Tumor encasing iliac vessels.
	Pelvic tumor crossing sciatic notch.
Intraspinal tumor extension	Intraspinal tumor extension whatever the location provided that more than one third of spinal canal in the axial plane is invaded, the perimedullary leptomeningeal spaces are not visible, or the spinal cord signal intensity is abnormal.
Infiltration of adjacent organs and structures	Pericardium, diaphragm, kidney, liver, duodenopancreatic block, and mesentery.
Conditions to be recorded, but not considered IDRF	Multifocal primary tumors, pleural effusion with or without malignant cells, ascites with or without malignant cells.

Intermediate risk

NB patients in the following clinical situations:

- Children aged >18 months with localized neuroblastoma without MYCN amplification, associated with IDRFs precluding upfront surgery (stage INRG L2).
- Children aged ≤12 months with disseminated neuroblastoma involving bone, pleura, lung, and/or CNS (stage INRG M), without MYCN amplification.
- Children with localized resected NB (stage INSS I) with MYCN amplification.

High risk

NB patient with disseminated disease over the age of 1 year old, or:

- INSS stage 2 and 3 disease with amplification of the MYCN proto-oncogene.
- Infants (<12 months at diagnosis) with MYCN amplified tumors.

Question: What are the surgical options for neuroblastoma?
Answer: Radical surgery should be assessed by a full consideration of extension into adjacent

structures, fixation to, or encasement of major blood vessels; risk of hemorrhage; and the patient's overall tumor burden.

Patients with unresectable tumors at primary diagnosis should have a biopsy and central venous line placement. Biopsy should be performed in order to obtain adequate tissue material for full histopathological diagnosis as well as MYCN determination, cytogenetics, and other biological studies.

The surgeon must try to obtain an adequate specimen of viable tumor tissue. Core needle biopsies may be performed under radiological image guidance or using minimally invasive surgical (MIS) procedures when indicated.

Delayed surgery for initial unresectable neuroblastoma tumors should be performed with the goal of achieving the most complete tumor resection possible, consistent with preservation of vital structures, organs, and neurologic function.

BIBLIOGRAPHY

1. Paul D. Losty, Michael La Quaglia, Sabine Sarnacki, Jörg Fuchs, Tomoaki Taguchi. Pediatric Surgical Oncology. CRC Press 2022. Eds. PD Losty, M La Quaglia, J Fuchs, S Sarnacki, T Taguchi.
2. Meyers R, Hiyama E, Czauderna P, Tiao GM. Liver tumors in pediatric patients. Surg Oncol Clin N Am. 2021;30(2):253–274.
3. Geller JI, van den Heuvel-Eibrink MM. Pediatric renal tumors – A Harmonica initiative. Pediatr Blood Cancer. 2023;70(S1–S10).
4. Neuroblastoma - Clinical And Surgical Management. 2020. Springer. Eds. S Sarnacki, L Pio.
5. La Quaglia MP, Losty PD. Pediatric surgical oncology. Semin Pediatr Surg. 2016;25(5): 249–336.
6. Losty PD. Evidence-based pediatric surgical oncology. Semin Pediatr Surg. 2016;25(5):333–335.

53

Neoplasms of the ovary and testis

SARAH BRAUNGART
Leeds Teaching Hospitals NHS Trust, Leeds, UK

PAUL D. LOSTY
Institute of Systems and Molecular Biology, University of Liverpool, Liverpool, UK
and Ramathibodi Hospital, Mahidol University, Bangkok, Thailand

Scenario: You are called to see a 4-month-old male infant in the hospital emergency department. The parents have noted that the baby's right testis appeared quite hard and clearly larger than the left side. You now undertake a full history, including the antenatal history, and conduct a clinical examination.

Question: What do you aim to determine on examination of the scrotum?
Answer: On examination the surgeon should aim to differentiate an isolated scrotal mass from other potential groin swellings such as inguinal hernia or hydrocele. Once these are excluded, it is then important to determine size and consistency of the mass, any tenderness, whether it is separate from the testis or part of the testis, if there are any skin changes such as erythema or puckering/tethering and if there is any associated inguinal lymphadenopathy.

Question: You find an isolated solid mass in the right hemiscrotum, the right testis cannot be palpated separately and there is no associated skin change or lymphadenopathy. What investigations will you arrange and why?

Answer: An ultrasound scan should be ordered and blood sampling taken for germ cell tumour markers, notably lactate dehydrogenase (LDH), alpha fetoprotein (AFP) and beta-human chorionic gonadotropin (HCG). In this very young age group the most likely diagnosis of a solid, non-tender testicular mass is a yolk sac tumour or testicular teratoma.

Yolk sac tumours are the most common prepubertal tumour, and more than 75% are encountered in the first 2 years of life. Teratomas are the second most common testicular tumour in this young age group.

Question: The ultrasound scan shows a right scrotal mass which is cystic in nature with calcification, and the tumour markers are all negative. What is the most likely diagnosis now, and how would you next proceed?
Answer: A cystic mass with calcification and negative tumour markers is most likely a teratoma. A right orchiectomy via an inguinal approach should be arranged. The specimen should be sent fresh to histopathology. Contralateral testicular fixation is a matter of debate and should be clearly discussed with the parents preoperatively.

DOI: 10.1201/9781003182290-60

Question: Histology confirms a mature testicular teratoma with no immature features. What do you tell the parents about the prognosis?
Answer: This lesion is classed as benign, and complete resection is curative.

Question: Are other surgical options available if the tumour markers are negative?
Answer: Yes – modern surgical management embraces fully the concepts of testis-sparing surgery where a lesion is notably focal and small in size (cm) and healthy adequate testicular parenchyma is evident on imaging. The lesion can be enucleated from the testis via an inguinal groin approach, frozen-section pathology reporting and the tunica capsule repaired. Note most testicular tumours in the prepubertal age group are benign.

Scenario: A 5-year-old boy is referred to your outpatient clinic with a left scrotal mass. An ultrasound scan shows a solid scrotal mass that appears separate from the testis.

Question: What is the most likely diagnosis?
Answer: The most common paratesticular neoplastic mass in this age group is paratesticular rhabdomyosarcoma.

Question: What is the treatment of paratesticular rhabdomyosarcoma?
Answer: Orchidectomy is the definitive management for a paratesticular rhabdomyosarcoma.

Question: What are the key intraoperative steps?
Answer: A radical orchiectomy should be performed via an inguinal groin incision. The cord should be carefully isolated first before any mobilisation of the scrotal tumour. The cord must be transfixed by high ligation at the internal ring, ideally with non-absorbable sutures, so that it is identifiable later in cases where the histopathological margins are considered positive or if retroperitoneal lymph node dissection is indicated.

Question: Which patients may require retroperitoneal lymph node dissection, and why is this procedure recommended?
Answer: All patients >10 years of age, or those with alveolar/fusion positive histology or with enlarged nodes on staging imaging should be considered to undergo retroperitoneal lymph node sampling. Lymph node involvement in paratesticular rhabdomyosarcoma is notably high (up to 25%), and it is a significant prognostic factor. If retroperitoneal lymph nodes are infiltrated, this will require intensification of chemotherapy as well as later need for radiotherapy.

Scenario: A 14-year old boy is referred to your outpatient clinic. He reports that he has noticed a swelling in his left testis. Upon physical examination you later note perioral freckling and gynaecomastia.

Question: What underlying condition may this boy potentially have?
Answer: Perioral mucosal freckling is one of the key diagnostic criteria for Peutz-Jeghers syndrome (PJS). A clinical diagnosis of PJS may be readily established in patients with perioral pigmentation *and* a positive family history. Patients with perioral freckling and a suspicion of PJS should always be referred to a medical clinical genetics service.

Question: Which type of testicular tumour is usually associated with PJS?
Answer: Sex cord and Sertoli Leydig cell tumours may occur in male patients with PJS. These may be active hormone-secreting and therefore may be associated with precocious puberty and male gynaecomastia.

Question: Which ovarian tumours are pathognomonic of PJS?
Answer: Sex cord stromal tumours with annular tubules (SCTATs). About one third of patients with SCTAT will have PJS.

Scenario: You are undertaking a laparoscopic appendicectomy for perforated appendicitis in a 13-year-old female. While you are undertaking pelvic lavage washout at the end of the procedure, your surgeon assistant comments on a "odd-looking" left ovary. On close inspection the left ovary is enlarged with a suspected diameter of 15 cm and appears very bulky with some obvious cystic changes. You are now concerned this may be an ovarian tumour.

Question: How will you next proceed?

Answer: This scenario highlights the incidental finding of a possible ovarian tumour and crucially needs to be managed according to strict oncological principles. Resection during the same procedure should not be undertaken because no staging investigations have yet been performed. Best practice is to complete the appendicectomy/lavage washout, allow the girl to recover from operation and then discuss the intraoperative findings with the family. Imaging, notably MRI scan, as well as blood tests for ovarian tumour markers must be arranged urgently. The case should then be discussed in the paediatric oncology multidisciplinary tumour (MDT) board meeting and further management undertaken as recommended by the MDT when all new test results are available.

Question: Which ovarian tumours are encountered in children? Are benign or malignant ovarian tumours more common in children vs. adults?

Answer: The vast majority of ovarian tumours in children are benign, with mature ovarian teratoma – a benign germ cell tumour – being the most common lesion.

Malignant ovarian tumours are typically most common around the age of 6–7 years (risk up to 30%).

Question: What is the most common malignant ovarian tumour in this age group? What tumour markers should you request in a postpubertal female patient and why? What do the individual markers specifically look for?

Answer: The most important tumour markers to request from the laboratory are germ cell tumour markers: AFP and beta-HCG. AFP is secreted by the yolk sac components of a malignant non-seminomatous germ cell tumour. The half-life is typically estimated at 5–7 days. Beta-HCG is secreted by trophoblastic cells. It is mainly raised in cases of choriocarcinoma, where there is an extraembryonic proliferation of abnormal germ cells. The half-life of beta-HCG is notably shorter at 24–36 hours. In a postpubertal female patients Ca-125 and Ca19-9 should also be assayed. These markers are important for epithelial ovarian tumours, which are very uncommon in prepubertal children but are the most common variant of ovarian malignancies in the adult population.

Question: The imaging scans shows a left-sided cystic ovarian tumour. The tumour markers are reportedly normal. What is a teratoma? How do you differentiate benign from immature lesions?

Answer: Teratomas are lesions composed of tissues derived from all three primitive germ layers (ectoderm, endoderm and mesoderm). The presence (and amount) of immature neuroectodermal tissue notably defines if a teratoma is classed as immature. Although this is fully established by histopathological analysis, imaging studies may give an indication. Mature teratomas are generally often cystic, with only small amounts of solid components. The larger the solid component, the more likely it is that the tumour is immature or malignant.

Question: What is the main purpose of an MDT board?

Answer: The main aim of an MDT board discussion is to help identify if it is likely a benign tumour. Benign tumours should be best managed by ovarian-sparing surgery wherever possible in order to preserve fertility and reduce lifetime risks of premature menopause.

Scenario: You undertake a laparoscopic procedure on an ovarian-sparing tumour. Pathology confirms a mature ovarian teratoma.

Question: What are the next scheduled follow-up arrangements and why?

Answer: Follow-up should be scheduled for all female children after resection of a benign ovarian teratoma, as there is a 5% risk of recurrent or metachronous disease. A recent consensus study recommended the first follow-up visit after 3 months with an ultrasound scan in order to check completeness of resection and as baseline imaging for further surveillance follow-up. Subsequently the patient should be reviewed regularly with ultrasound imaging every 2 years with outpatient clinic visits.

Once the patient is at pubertal age, referral to adolescent gynaecology services should be offered and arranged in order to discuss effects of ovarian surgery on fertility. This is crucially important if the patient has undergone total oophorectomy, as these females have a higher risk of premature ovarian failure.

Scenario: You are the surgical resident on call. An 8-year-old girl presents to the hospital emergency department with a 3-week history of increasing fatigue, abdominal distension and lower abdominal pelvic pain. On examination the patient is unwell and has a grossly distended abdomen. There is dullness to percussion, and you suspect abdominal ascites.

Question: What investigations will you arrange?
Answer: With these sinister clinical examination findings, malignancy must be suspected. An urgent ultrasound scan and a full set of laboratory blood tests, including tumour markers, should be arranged. Tumour markers ordered should include all germ cell tumour markers, notably LDH, AFP and beta-HCG.

Scenario: The ultrasound scan shows a mixed solid and cystic mass in the lower abdomen, which is 20 cm in diameter, and a significant amount of ascites-free fluid. LDH and AFP are markedly elevated.

Question: What is the most common malignant germ cell tumour in children?
Answer: Yolk sac tumours are the most common malignant germ cell tumour. They may occur in their pure histological forms or more commonly as a mixed malignant germ cell tumour. Presentation with rapid clinical deterioration is very typical in patients.

Histology exam of these tumours classically shows Schiller-Duvall bodies on H&E staining, which is the configuration of a central vessel surrounded by a rim of tumour cells. AFP is also generally elevated.

Question: What is the further management of this patient?
Answer: This is a malignant germ cell tumour, and therefore should be managed according to international cancer protocols (UK CCLG GCT treatment guidelines; USA North America – COG guidelines). The patient requires cross-sectional abdominal pelvic imaging and a chest X-ray at a minimum.

Management after multidisciplinary discussion at oncology tumour board will involve operation and consideration of full intraoperative staging.

Question: How will you perform the operation?
Answer: This is a large tumour (>10 cm), which is a highly likely malignant, and therefore the procedure should be best performed using an open approach in order to avoid inadvertent spillage and disease upstaging. Oophorectomy should be performed, carefully avoiding tumour rupture. At surgery, the abdominal cavity should also be fully inspected for notable suspicious lesions, and these should all be biopsied, including omentectomy. A sample of ascites fluid should be routinely sent for cytology analysis.

Question: What chemotherapy agents are used in the treatment of malignant ovarian germ cell tumours? What are the important side effects (if any)?
Answer: Chemotherapy for malignant ovarian germ cell tumours includes etoposide, carboplatin and bleomycin. Platinum-based chemotherapeutic agents are very emetogenic and ototoxic. Audiology testing should therefore be arranged prior to commencing chemotherapy. The most important side effects of bleomycin is lung toxicity with pulmonary fibrosis. Lung function tests prior to starting therapy should always be performed if the child is old enough to cooperate.

Question: Histology confirms a mixed malignant germ cell tumour stage 2. The parents ask you about the prognosis for their daughter. What are your answers?
Answer: The patient is <11 years old with a localised stage 2 tumour. Fortunately the patient has a very good prognosis, with overall survival rates estimated as high as 97%.

BIBLIOGRAPHY

1. O'Shea K, Tong A, Farrelly P, Craigie R, Cheesman E, Shukla R, Losty PD. Management and outcome of paediatric testicular tumours – A 20 experience. J Pediatr Surg. 2021;56(11):2032–6.
2. Bois JI, Vagni RL, de Badiola FI, Moldes JM, Losty PD, Lobos PA. Testis-sparing surgery for testicular tumors in children: A 20 year

single center experience and systematic review of the literature. Pediatr Surg Int. 2021;37(5):607–16.

3. Pearse I, Glick RD, Abramson SJ, Gerald WR, Shamberger RC, La Quaglia MP. Testicular-sparing surgery for benign testicular tumors. J Pediatr Surg. 1999;34(6):1000–3.

4. Howell L, Bader A, Mullassery D, Losty PD, Auth M, Kokai G. Sertoli Leydig cell ovarian tumour and gastric polyps as presenting features of Peutz-Jeghers syndrome. Pediatr Blood Cancer. 2010;55(1):206–7.

5. Hearle N, Schumacher V, Menko FH, Olschwang S, Boardman LA, Gille JJ, Keller JJ, Westerman AM, Scott RJ, Lim W, Trimbath JD, Giardiello FM, Gruber SB, Offerhaus GJ, de Rooij FW, Wilson JH, Hansmann A, Möslein G, Royer-Pokora B, Vogel T, Phillips RK, Spigelman AD, Houlston RS. Frequency and spectrum of cancers in Peutz-Jeghers syndrome. Clin Cancer Res. 2006;12(10):3209–15.

6. Latchford A, Cohen S, Auth M, Scaillon M, Viala J, Daniels R, Talbotec C, Attard T, Durno C, Hyer W. Management of Peutz-Jeghers syndrome in children and adolescents: A position paper from the ESPGHAN polyposis working group. J Pediatr Gastroenterol Nutr. 2019;68(3):442–52.

7. Rogers TN, Seitz G, Fuchs J, Martelli H, Dasgupta R, Routh JC, Hawkins DS, Koscielniak E, Bisogno G, Rodeberg DA. Surgical management of paratesticular rhabdomyosarcoma: A consensus opinion from the Children's Oncology Group, European paediatric Soft tissue sarcoma Study Group, and the Cooperative Weichteilsarkom Studiengruppe. Pediatr Blood Cancer. 2021;68(4):e28938.

8. Braungart S, Williams C, Arul SG, Bambang K, Craigie RJ, Cross KM, Dick A, Hammond P, Okoye B, Rogers T, Losty PD, Glaser A, Powis M. Standardizing the surgical management of benign ovarian tumors in children and adolescents: A best practice Delphi consensus statement. Pediatr Blood Cancer. 2022;69(4):e29589.

9. Hermans AJ, Kluivers KB, Janssen LM, Siebers AG, Wijnen MHWA, Bulten J, et al. Adnexal masses in children, adolescents and women of reproductive age in the Netherlands: A nationwide population-based cohort study. Gynecol Oncol. 2016;143(1):93–7.

10. Capito C, Galmiche-Roland L, Fresneau B, Orbach D, Sarnacki S. Tumours of the ovary. In: Pediatric Surgical Oncology. Eds. PD Losty, M La Quaglia, S Sarnacki, J Fuchs, T Taguchi. Taylor and Francis CRC Press 2022.

11. Childrens' Cancer and Leukaemia Group. Interim guidelines for the treatment of extracranial germ cell tumours in children and adolescents. 2018.

12. Frazier AL, Hale JP, Rodriguez-Galindo C et al. Revised risk classification for pediatric extracranial germ cell tumours based on 25 years of clinical trial data from the United Kingdom and United States. J Clin Onc 2015;33:195–201.

54

Head and neck malignancy

OMAR SABRA

King Hamad University Hospital, Kingdom of Bahrain, Bahrain

NECK MASS

Scenario: A 9-year-old boy presents to hospital with a right-sided parotid enlargement along with multiple bulky neck lymph nodes bilaterally. The condition was noticed a few weeks prior to hospital presentation. The patient has no associated fever or night sweats. No associated pain is reported in the head and neck area.

Question: What is your differential diagnosis?

Answer: Head and neck masses are common in the pediatric age group. Most of the time findings may relate to reactive inflammatory lymph nodes or a benign congenital neck mass such as a branchial cleft cyst or a lymphatic malformation,

Among neoplastic lesions, hemangiomas are the most common benign tumors in pediatric patients. Only a small percentage of these masses are malignant. Lymphomas, Hodgkin, and non-Hodgkin disease account for around 27% of pediatric head and neck malignancies, while neuroectodermal tumors comprise 23% of cases. The majority of epithelial tumors are thyroid in origin (around 21%), while sarcomas make up around 20% of new cases.

When located to the parotid gland, hemangiomas are still the most common benign tumors, while benign salivary epithelial tumors (mainly pleomorphic lesions) are second in prevalence.

Rhabdomyosarcomas are the most common solid malignancies within the facial region including the parotid. These tumors are common within the orbit, pharynx, and parapharyngeal spaces.

Thyroid malignancy and nasopharyngeal malignancy can involve intraparotid lymph nodes as part of the regional spread of such diseases.

Primary epithelial salivary gland tumors, mostly mucoepidermoid carcinoma, come next in incidence to primary rhabdomyosarcomas of the parotid glands.

Other rare tumors include fibrosarcomas, epithelioid sarcomas, dermatofibrosarcoma protuberans, and miscellaneous others.

Question: What are the signs to look for during examination in our patient?

Answer: A thorough clinical examination of the head and neck region is essential.

The neck examination should include locating any neck mass by its anatomical level and describing the mass in terms of size, texture, borders, and mobility. Parotid examination includes as well facial nerve function assessment.

Skin examination may show us obvious signs of infiltration by a hemangioma. Other tumors may be primary skin nodules such as dermatofibrosarcoma protuberans. Subcutaneous masses can also be present in fibrosarcomas and neuroblastoma.

Ear/nose/throat (ENT) examination should include an otological exam to rule out effusion and an ocular examination to rule out exophthalmos or oculomotor nerve paresis.

Endoscopic examination of the nasal cavity, pharynx, and larynx helps in ruling out any associated

DOI: 10.1201/9781003182290-61

occult mucosal lesion, the most common one being nasopharyngeal carcinoma.

Nasopharyngeal carcinoma presents most typically with a neck mass and, less likely, with nasal blockage and/or a conductive hearing loss secondary to Eustachian tube blockage. These presentations can frequently mimic simple adenoid hypertrophy in very young children rather than a sinister nasopharyngeal neoplasm.

Endoscopic assessment helps additionally to rule out parapharyngeal pathology such as parapharyngeal lymphatic tissue metastasis, deep lobe parotid neoplasms, or a carotid sheath mass. Such disease processes can compromise patency of the airway.

Cranial nerve examination is crucially important as well.

Oculomotor nerve function can be affected by any intraorbital tumor, frequently a lymphoma or a rhabdomyosarcoma. Parotid malignancies may invade the facial nerve when advanced. Neuroblastoma potentially affects the sympathetic chain, giving rise to Horner's syndrome, the vagus, or any other cranial nerve territories.

> **Scenario:** This patient had a normal endoscopic examination of the nose, pharynx, and larynx. Neck examination revealed a right-sided firm, hard parotid mass with irregular borders situated within the parotid tail, along with few enlarged mobile cervical lymph nodes involving level 2 and level 3 bilaterally. Facial nerve examination was normal.

Question: What are the signs that may suggest a malignant potential of such a parotid mass?
Answer: Signs of malignancy include a firm hard mass, skin infiltration, facial nerve paralysis, pain and associated pathologic palpable lymphadenopathy.

These advanced signs of malignancy are frequently absent when patients present earlier. Malignancy in the early stages for example may present with a simple small lump.

Question: How do we describe the neck lymph node compartments anatomically and what is/are the significance of such an anatomical description?
Answer: When dealing with head and neck solid malignancies, there is a surgical and a prognostic interest in localizing lymphadenopathy within certain compartments or defined levels (**Figure 54.1**).

Level I, also called the anterior neck, includes the submandibular (Ib) and submental triangles

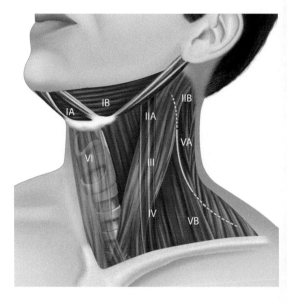

Figure 54.1 Neck lymphatic compartments, labeled from level I to VI regions. Note that the sternocleidomastoid muscle is cut to reveal the lateral chain of lymphatics. Major structures visualized include the internal jugular vein and carotid artery, spinal accessory nerve, digastric muscles, and the laryngeal framework.

(Ia). Levels II, III, and IV, also called lateral neck lymphatic regions, include the jugular chain lymphatics. The boundaries are limited by the carotid artery medially and the posterior edge of the sternocleidomastoid laterally. It extends from the skull base superiorly to the clavicle(s) inferiorly.

The hyoid bone and cricoid cartilage define the horizontal planes that divide the lateral chain into three designated levels: II, III and IV. Level II is further subdivided into IIa (anterior to spinal accessory nerve) and IIb (posterior to the spinal accessory nerve).

Level V consists of the posterior neck triangle, posterior to the sternocleidomastoid muscle.

Level VI, also called the central neck, includes lymphatic involvement from the hyoid bone to the sternum, between the two carotid arteries.

Defining lymphatic regions by their anatomical levels helps the radiologist and oncology surgeon to communicate in a more accurate way when describing and sampling lymph nodes.

Studying the lymphatic drainage pattern of the head and neck, one is able to predict the level of involvement according to the location of the primary tumor. This system thus allows radiation and surgical treatment to be targeted to high-risk levels, and thereby it is hoped to reduce the morbidity of unnecessary treatments.

Supraclavicular lymph node involvement is considered a sign of advanced lymphatic disease staging, especially in nasopharyngeal carcinomas, because of the high risk for distant metastasis in such patients.

Supraclavicular lymph nodes may reflect also distant metastasis from an intrabdominal or thoracic malignancy, i.e. look for Virchow's node and Troisier's sign.

Neck disease staging systems are well established for all head and neck mucosal and salivary tumors, except for nasopharyngeal carcinoma and thyroid cancer, which have their own pathology staging systems.

Localizing the anatomical level of lymphadenopathy is less important when dealing with certain hematological pathologies such as lymphomas, as the main therapy(ies) are directed by medical oncology not surgical resection.

Question: What are your first-line investigation plans for our patient?
Answer: Laboratory blood tests and neck ultrasound should be ordered.

Blood test investigation with a complete blood count (CBC) and differential count and infection markers will help to rule out a systemic infection. Microbial serology is useful in excluding certain infectious etiologies such as Epstein-Barr virus (EBV) virus, cytomegalovirus (CMV) virus, toxoplasmosis, and others.

Blood tests can thus help in ruling out infectious and inflammatory disorders rather than specifically confirming a malignant process.

Neck ultrasonography is frequently the only radiology study needed. It is highly reliable in detecting neck lymphadenopathy and congenital cystic masses as well as showing the degree of vascularity within solid tumors and hemangiomas. Ultrasound scan is considered a gold-standard investigative tool in the detection of thyroid pathology and lymph node disease.

CT imaging can be beneficial in better localizing a mass in relation to vital neck structures such as major blood vessels, deep fascia, and the airway, which greatly helps in planning a surgical procedure.

When the mass is located on the face, the CT scan will help detect any bone erosion.

MRI can be useful in assessing the differential diagnosis of parotid mass lesions and defining soft tissue disease involvement for the whole head and neck.

Concerning parotid malignancies, mucoepidermoid carcinomas are the most common salivary malignancy encountered in pediatric patients. Low-grade mucoepidermoid carcinomas show low T1 and high T2 intensity with localized areas of hyperintensity on T2 reflecting mucus collection, while intermediate- to high-grade tumors will show intermediate to low intensity on T2, reflecting high degrees of cellularity.

> **Scenario:** After negative blood test investigations, the patient then underwent a neck ultrasound exam which showed a hypoechoic solid irregular mass with central vascularity. Multiple reactive cervical lymph nodes were noted on both sides of the neck involving the lateral cervical chain(s).

Question: What pathological tool(s) may further aid diagnosis?
Answer: Fine needle aspiration (FNA) is usually the next step to aid pathology diagnosis.

FNA is less reliable in the young pediatric age group than in adults, as epithelial tumors are much less common in children, although with thyroid or salivary nodules, FNAC can be of significant value.

When a salivary gland is sampled by FNA, the Milan classification system is used for reporting salivary gland cytopathology. This system, published in 2018, was developed to provide a unifying reporting tool for salivary gland tumors. The system contains six main categories and resembles to a degree the Bethesda system deployed for thyroid nodules (**Table 54.1**).

Although operation is indicated in salivary neoplasms that fall under categories 3–6, planning the strategy for surgery will be different for a benign vs. a malignant tumor.

FNAC can be useful for determining suspicious lymph nodes as well as helping to stage regional metastatic disease.

> **Scenario:** Our patient's FNAC result thus showed Milan category 6, malignant. The smears showed a mixture of mucin-secreting cells, squamous cells, and intermediate cells. The specimen was labeled as a low-grade mucoepidermoid carcinoma. Ipsilateral neck lymph node FNAC was negative.

Table 54.1 Bethesda (thyroid) and Milan (salivary) cytological grading systems and consequent risks of malignancy in each grading system. Note the lower reliability of the Milan system in predicting malignancy which consequently leads to a lower threshold to operate on salivary vs thyroid mass lesions.

Grade	Bethesda system	Risk of malignancy	Milan system	Risk of malignancy
1	Non diagnostic	less than 5%	Non diagnostic	25%
2	Benign nodule	less than 5%	Non tumoral	10%
3	Atypia of unknown significance	5%–15%	Atypia of unknown significance	20%
4	Follicular neoplasm	10%–40%	Benign neoplasm	5%
			Salivary neoplams of unknown malignant potential	35%
5	Suspicious for malignancy	60%–75%	Suspicious for malignancy	60%
6	Malignant	97%–95%	Malignant	90%

Question: What imaging is now needed for tumor staging?

Answer: In view of the malignant nature of the patient's disease, further imaging is highly advisable.

MRI scan is the best modality to characterize the tumor by signal intensity and enhancement. It will help show the local extension of tumor into surrounding soft tissues and characterize the lymph nodes as well.

PET CT scan is invaluable in defining the metastatic nature of lymph nodes and distant lesions. It is less helpful in anatomically delineating the primary tumour. Low-grade tumors might show low, non-significant FDG activity, such as with low-grade mucoepidermoid, acinic cell, and adenoid cystic carcinomas. Well-differentiated thyroid malignancies have frequently non-significant FDG activity. In such low-grade tumors CT of the thorax may be a useful test to rule out distant metastasis.

Scenario: Our patient, with an MRI neck scan, was seen to have disease limited to the superficial lobe of the parotid gland. Cervical lymph nodes were described as reactive rather than having metastatic disease. CT chest was clear.

Question: What is the management plan next for our patient?

Answer: The parotid gland is separated by the facial nerve into a superficial lobe (lateral to the facial nerve) and a deep lobe (medial to the facial nerve). Most of the bulk of parotid tissue resides in the superficial lobe, which therefore makes most salivary gland tumors typically located within the superficial lobe of the gland.

Management of salivary gland tumors involves operative resection. The operation involves a superficial parotidectomy for most benign gland pathologies. Total parotidectomy (dissecting and preserving the facial nerve) is indicated in deep lobe benign parotid tumors and all malignant tumors. Our patient should undergo a total parotidectomy, attempting preservation of the facial nerve.

Rarely when the facial nerve is grossly involved by tumor, radical parotidectomy with facial nerve sacrifice is then necessary. In such a case, facial nerve reconstruction is then indicated by primary nerve anastomosis, cable grafting, or hypoglossal to facial side-to-end anastomosis, which requires the skills of a plastic reconstructive surgeon.

Deep lobe parotid tissue often contains lymph nodes that may harbor metastatic disease, which indicates that a deep lobe parotidectomy is essential in all confirmed malignant cases.

Hemangiomas within the parotid gland are treated medically in most cases like any other site hemangiomas.

Question: How is neck lymph node metastasis managed in surgically treated head and neck tumors?

Answer: Neck dissection in surgically treated head and neck malignancies is indicated in two main settings:

1. Electively, when the patient does not show lymph node metastasis, but the tumor type, grade, or its location makes the patient at high

risk of lymph node metastasis. Also termed elective neck dissection.

2. Therapeutically, when the patient already shows clinical, radiologic, or pathologic evidence of lymph node metastasis, also termed therapeutic neck dissection.

The extent or radicality of neck dissection varies according to the tumor type.

In cases termed N0 neck, only high-risk levels that are known to drain the primary tumor directly are dissected. This type of neck dissection is termed a selective neck dissection.

According to the primary disease site location, we note that the oral cavity and parts of the face anterior to the auricle drain into level 1–3 regions.

The pharynx and larynx drain into the lateral chain(s) and posterior scalp area, and the nasopharynx drains into the lateral and posterior lymphatics, while the thyroid gland drains mainly into the level 6 region.

In the case of N+ neck, a radical or modified radical neck dissection is preferred, where all neck lymph node levels are dissected. Radical neck dissection usually involves removal and sacrifice of the spinal accessory nerve (SAN), internal jugular vein (IJV), and sternocleidomastoid muscle (SCM). These non-lymphatic structures are frequently involved by tumor spread from adjacent lymph nodes.

Modified radical neck dissection consists of preserving one or more of these structures according to the extent of lymph node disease. The SAN is the most important structure to be preserved followed by the IJV then the SCM.

Cervical lymphadenectomy for salivary gland neoplasms is indicated in patients with known lymph node metastasis and in high-grade malignancies known to metastasize to lymph nodes.

Scenario: Our patient underwent a total parotidectomy with preservation of the facial nerve.

Question: What are the possible postoperative complications after salivary gland surgery and a neck dissection?

Answer: Early complications include hematoma formation, facial nerve weakness, salivary fluid collection, and wound infection.

Facial nerve recovery is almost always complete if the nerve was preserved anatomically. The marginal mandibular facial nerve branch is most commonly accidentally injured at parotid surgery.

Late patient morbidity may include Frey's syndrome (or gustatory sweating) due to aberrant innervation of the sweat glands by autonomic nerve branches, destined to the parotid gland.

Neck dissection can lead to a long list of complications other than hematoma and wound infection.

Several nerves are at risk of being injured: The SAN can be injured during dissection of level 2 or 5. The vagus nerve and its branches (recurrent laryngeal and superior laryngeal) and the sympathetic chain can also be injured during dissection of the lateral chain (level 2–4) and the central compartment (level 6).

Phrenic nerve injury can occur during a level 4 dissection.

The marginal mandibular, lingual, and hypoglossal nerves can all be injured during level 1 dissection.

Recurrent laryngeal nerves can be damaged during level 6 (central compartment) dissection.

Level 4 neck dissection on the left side may lead to thoracic duct injury with a secondary chylous leak.

Major vascular injury, intracranial hypertension (in cases of bilateral IJV sacrifice), central nervous system (CNS) stroke, and air leaks are very rare complications related to radical neck dissection.

Scenario: Pathology assessment of the patient's tumor confirmed a diagnosis of mucoepidermoid carcinoma with negative disease margins. The deep lobe of the parotid gland contained a few benign lymph nodes.

Question: Are any adjuvant treatments indicated in this patient?

Answer: Radiotherapy is indicated as adjuvant therapy in cases of intermediate- or high-grade salivary gland malignancy, adenoid cystic carcinomas, positive or close margins, presence of perineural invasion, advanced T stage, and presence of lymph node metastasis.

Radiotherapy should be used with caution in the pediatric age group, as it may lead to risks of late second new malignancy.

FACIAL MASS

Scenario: A 7-year-old boy presents to the hospital clinic with proptosis of the left eye and numbness along the left check area. He denies significant pain but has notable pressure symptoms and double vision. The patient denies having a runny nose or fever. On examination the patient has a few enlarged cervical lymph nodes involving left level 2 and 3 and the parotid area.

Question: What is the differential diagnosis?
Answer: Orbital swelling should alert the surgeon to the possibility of a complicated sinusitis, but in the absence of fever and pain, a malignant process must always be considered. Rhabdomyosarcomas are among the most common solid head and neck malignancies in the pediatric age group and by far the most common intraorbital pediatric malignancy. Intraorbital lymphomas and nerve sheath tumors are other possible differential diagnoses.

Scenario: CT scan shows an orbital vascularized mass, isodense compared to the nearby muscles, pushing on the globe anteriorly with medial orbital wall erosion into the ethmoid sinuses and inferior wall erosion into the maxillary sinus. No skull base disease erosion could be detected.

MRI shows a mass lesion that is low to intermediate intensity on T1 and hyperintense on T2, with considerable hypervascularity. No intracranial extension or dural involvement could be detected.

The patient underwent an open incisional biopsy which showed fetal muscle fiber-like cells. Immunohistochemistry for desmin, myogenin, MyoD1, and sarcomeric actin are all positive. Ultrastructural tests showed loss of heterozygosity (LOH) at 11p15.

Question: What is the pathological diagnosis?
Answer: This is a classical rhabdomyosarcoma with positive immunohistochemical staining for this tumor.

LOH at 11p15 is frequently seen in the embryonal subtype, while translocations t2-13 and t1-13 (PAX3-FOXO1 and PAX7-FOXO1 genes) are common in alveolar subtypes and represent a tendency for a more aggressive behavior.

Question: What are the clinical signs and symptoms of such a disease when located in the head and neck region? What other differential diagnosis should be considered?
Answer: Rhabdomyosarcomas are the most common type of head and neck sarcomas and the third most common solid neoplasm in the pediatric age group after Wilms tumor and neuroblastoma. It comprises approximately 50% of all pediatric sarcomas with a slight male predominance. Almost one third of head and neck rhabdomyosarcomas occur in the orbital regions.

Most children present with a localized swelling. A rapidly progressing proptosis should further prompt diagnosis. Less than half of all patients will complain of pain. Other symptoms are related to involved nearby organs such as otorrhea, rhinorrhea, nasal blockage, and cranial nerve palsy.

Cranial nerve involvement is typically common in cervical neuroblastoma, e.g. Horner's syndrome. Other sarcomas can also occur in the neck region such as fibrosarcomas, while dermatofibrosarcomas are typically skin nodules that arise in the scalp and supraclavicular area.

Question: What clinical and pathological features best define the prognosis of rhabdomyosarcoma?
Answer: Most of these tumors occur in the orbit, nose and paranasal sinuses, soft tissues, and pharynx.

These tumors are subdivided by location into parameningeal (paranasal sinuses, orbit, nasopharynx and middle ear) and non-parameningeal according to their proximity to the cranial cavity and the potential risk of CNS involvement. Parameningeal disease location holds a worse prognosis.

Orbital tumor sites have a relatively good prognosis compared to other parameningeal locations.

Metastatic disease status is a major prognostic factor. This is best investigated usually first with liver function and bony enzyme lab tests. CT chest and abdominal imaging, bone scan, and bone marrow aspirate studies will help determine metastatic disease. A PET scan is an acceptable alternative investigation for distant site disease metastatic workup.

Two major staging systems are adopted for rhabdomyosarcoma: TNM and the Clinical Grouping (CG) systems.

The CG rhabdomyosarcoma system developed by the Intergroup Rhabdomyosarcoma Study Group

(IRSG) relies mainly on the resectability of the primary tumor rather than its size. It does not include lymph node status:

i. Confined to the site of origin (completely resectable).
ii. *Local infiltration*: Gross total resection is possible, with possible microscopic residual disease.
iii. *Localized extensive tumor*: Gross residual disease is possible; usually only a biopsy is done at this stage.
iv. Metastatic rhabdomyosarcoma.

Question: What is the treatment for rhabdomyosarcomas of the head and neck region?
Answer: The treatment plan is patient individualized. Multimodality therapy is best undertaken in specialized sarcoma centers.

Resectable disease is approached surgically at first when resection morbidity is considered acceptable. Prophylactic lymph node dissection is not indicated in N0 patients. Morbidity can be reduced considerably by the availability of experienced reconstructive surgery services. Nonresectable disease is treated with systemic treatments, keeping surgery then for salvage scenarios. Radiation therapy is indicated in the alveolar disease subtypes and for patients with residual disease after initial treatment. Chemotherapeutic agents used may include vincristine, cyclophosphamide, and actinomycin D.

Question: What are the side effects of radiotherapy in the head and neck region?
Answer: Radiation therapy is highly toxic to mucosal surfaces and the salivary glands. Side effects are unavoidable most of the time if the pharynx and salivary glands are irradiated. This is manifested by dry throat, ulceration, thick crusting in the nose and pharynx, and dysphagia. Loss of taste and smell can occur with dryness of

Table 54.2 Differential listings of the most common pediatric head and neck malignancies and the main modality of treatment for each.

Type of tumors	Common location	Common histologies	Main treatment	Adjuvant treatment/ Palliative treatment
Thyroid	Thyroid	Papillary	• Hemithyroidectomy for well differentiated tumors less than 1 cm with N0 neck	Radioactive iodine for papillary and follicular
			• Total thyroidectomy for all other cases	External beam radiotherapy for other histologies
			• Prophylactic neck dissection for high stage, poorly differentiated histologies	Tyrosine kinase inhibitors for palliation
			• Therapeutic neck dissection for N+	
Salivary neoplasms	Parotid	Mucoepidermoid	• Total parotidectomy is preferred in most cases	Radiation therapy
			• Neck dissection for high grade, high stage or N+	Consider proton beam therapy as alternative
Rhabdomyosarcoma	Orbit	Embryonal subtype	• *Multimodality:* • surgery, chemotherapy, and possible radiation therapy • Sequence is defined mainly by resectability and presence of residual disease	Chemotherapy/ radiotherapy for palliation
Nasopharyngeal carcinoma	Nasopharynx	Undifferentiated carcinoma	• Radiotherapy for early disease • Chemoradiation for advanced disease, platinum based	
Neuroblastoma	Sympathetic nerves		• Surgical resection	Chemotherapy with possible radiotherapy

the nasal-oral mucosa and possibly secondary to injury of neuroepithelium.

Eye irradiation can lead to corneal opacification and optic neuropathy, while cochlear and acoustic nerve irradiation can lead to sensorineural hearing loss. Irradiation-related 'secondary new late malignancies' include salivary gland, thyroid gland malignancies, and osteosarcomas.

Table 54.2 provides a summary overview of the most common pediatric head and neck tumors and preferred treatment modalities.

BIBLIOGRAPHY

MacArthur C, Smith R. Pediatric Head and Neck Malignancies. In Cumming's Otolaryngology head and neck surgery (6th edition). Elsevier 2016: 2835–2849.

Bentz B., Hughes C, Lüdemann J, Maddalozzo J. Masses of the salivary gland region in children. Arch Otolaryngol Head Neck Surg. 2000;126(12):1435–1439.

Chadha N, Forte V. Pediatric head and neck malignancies. Curr Opin Otolaryngol Head Neck Surg. 2009;17:471–476.

Cibas ES, Ali SZ. The Bethesda system for reporting thyroid cytopathology. Am J Clin Pathol. 2009;132:658–665.

Rossi ED, Baloch Z, Pusztaszeri M, Faquin WC. The Milan System for Reporting Salivary Gland Cytopathology (MSRSGC): an ASC-IAC-sponsored system for reporting salivary gland fine-needle aspiration. J Am Soc Cytopathol. 2018;7(3):111–118.

Robbins K, Samant S, Ronen O. Neck Dissection. In Cumming's Otolaryngology head and neck surgery (6th edition). Elsevier 2016: 1702–1725.

55

Chest and mediastinal tumours

CHAN HON CHUI
Mount Elizabeth Medical Centre, Singapore

The thorax is located between the neck and the abdomen, and it includes the thoracic cavity and the chest wall. Unique to children and adolescents, tumours are usually found in the mediastinum and the chest wall. Primary lung tumours are rare. Besides malignant neoplasms, benign lesions are often encountered and should be considered.

Surgeons treating paediatric patients with chest wall and mediastinal tumours should possess a good understanding of the three-dimensional anatomy of the region and the physiology of its contained structures. The management of these patients may be especially challenging and deserves special mention.

CHEST WALL TUMOURS

Scenario: A 10-year-old boy, patient A, presented with an enlarging right lower chest swelling for 2 months. The parents had initially thought that this was a contusion sustained at a soccer game. Physical examination showed a non-tender hard mass without features of inflammation (**Figure 55.1**).

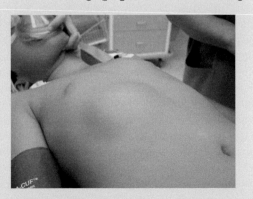

Figure 55.1 Right lower chest wall mass.

Question: What investigations would you undertake?
Answer: The possibilities of a chest wall lesion, such as a haematoma or tumour, or a chest wall deformity from an underlying pleural or peritoneal mass should be considered. Its location at the costochondral region may not be well depicted on a chest X-ray (CXR). Computed tomography (CT) of the thorax is preferred to identify the mass's origin and characteristics and the status of the underlying organs such as the lung and liver.

CT scan of the thorax (axial) showed a large mass 9 cm in diameter in the anterior right chest wall involving the sixth to eighth costochondral junctions with indentation of the right lobe of the liver (**Figure 55.2**). There was no evidence of lung or liver lesions.

Question: What are the differential diagnoses?
Answer: Tumours of the chest wall are rare in the paediatric population. Up to two-thirds of them are malignant. The most common malignant tumours are Ewing sarcoma and rhabdomyosarcoma followed by smaller numbers of osteosarcoma, fibrosarcoma, chondrosarcoma and lymphoma.

DOI: 10.1201/9781003182290-62

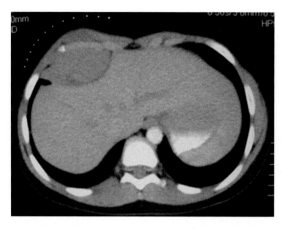

Figure 55.2 CT thorax showing right anterior chest wall mass.

Question: Besides presenting as chest wall masses, what are the other clinical presentations of chest wall tumours in children and adolescents?

Answer: Chest wall tumours also frequently present with respiratory symptoms or pain. The symptoms of respiratory compromise include tachypnoea, cough and dyspnoea on exertion that arise from pulmonary parenchymal compression by the mass and/or from a secondary pleural effusion. **Figure 55.3** shows a PET-CT scan of a 15-year-old boy, patient B, who presented only with persistent pain in the posterior left chest. It showed an invasive chest wall tumour with destruction of the left sixth, seventh and eighth ribs. Bilateral lung nodules and mediastinal lymphadenopathy consistent with metastases were also found. Bone marrow aspiration and biopsy excluded metastasis.

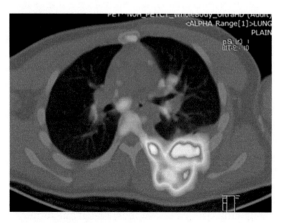

Figure 55.3 PET-CT scan showing an FDG-avid left posterior chest wall tumour with mediastinal lymphadenopathy.

Question: In both cases of chest wall tumours, what are the diagnostic methods?

Answer: Obtaining tumour tissue for diagnosis is essential. In the presence of a resectable tumour, a prior histological diagnosis of a malignant neoplasm may enable the surgeon to plan for a wide resection with negative margins. If the tumour was unresectable or metastasis was present at diagnosis, neoadjuvant chemotherapy would reduce the size of the tumour and facilitate more complete surgical resection in more patients.

The biopsy should obtain an adequate tumour sample using the least invasive technique so as to avoid treatment delay. This may be performed by image-guided coaxial core needle biopsy or an incisional biopsy. It is of paramount importance that biopsies be obtained without pleural contamination, and the incision should be placed in-line with any future resection, regardless of the technique utilized. In patient A, incisional biopsy confirmed the diagnosis of embryonal rhabdomyosarcoma. Metastatic workup, including bone marrow aspiration and biopsy, and PET-CT scan did not reveal any distant metastases. In patient B, incisional biopsy confirmed the diagnosis of Ewing sarcoma with EWS-FLI1 transcript and with the presence of metastatic lung disease and mediastinal lymph node metastases.

Question: What is the treatment advised? What are the surgical principles?

Answer: Neoadjuvant chemotherapy was administered in both patients. As expected, the tumours responded with size reduction. The lesions subsequently underwent surgical resection. The most important principle in surgical resection is the need for complete resection with negative pathologic margins, generally accepting that a 1-cm margin is required. Disruption of the tumour is to be avoided. Only the involved portion of the rib should be removed, not the entire rib. When adhesions are found between the tumour and the lung parenchyma or diaphragm, a wedge of the adherent lung or a segment of the diaphragm should be resected en bloc with the tumour so as to avoid a positive pathologic margin. In the presence of a large chest wall defect (>5 cm or involving ≥3 ribs), reconstruction with flexible prosthetic patches, such as Gore-Tex (WL Gore & Associates), Marlex mesh (C.R. Bard/Davol) and Prolene mesh (Ethicon) may be utilized (Murphy F. and Corbally

MT, 2007). In both our cases, Prolene mesh was used. After their surgeries, the patients continued to receive radiotherapy and chemotherapy.

Traditionally, both localized truncal Ewing sarcoma and rhabdomyosarcoma have been associated with decreased survival, but recent reports have shown improved survival with the use of aggressive multimodality therapy. The challenge remains to preserve form and function and achieve adequate disease-free margins.

Scenario: A 3-year-old boy presented to hospital with an enlarging painful sternal mass with overlying erythema of 3 weeks' duration. CT scan showed an osteolytic sternal mass (**Figure 55.4a** and **b**).

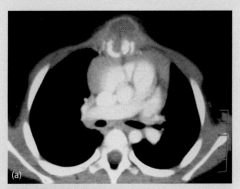

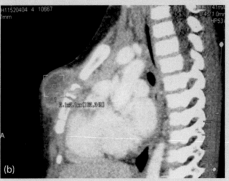

Figure 55.4 (a) Axial CT showing an osteolytic sternal tumour. (b) Sagittal CT showing a similar lesion.

Question: What is the likely diagnosis and how are you going to make the diagnosis?
Answer: Langerhans cell histiocytosis (LCH) or a destructive sternal bone neoplasm are likely diagnoses. An incisional biopsy (with curettage) will be preferred to obtain a diagnosis. Histological

examination and immunohistochemistry confirmed the diagnosis.

Question: What is LCH?
Answer: LCH is a rare disease with a prevalence of two to five cases per million in children. The aetiology remains uncertain, with recent identification of oncogenic *BRAF* or *MAP2K1* mutations in most cases of LCH suggesting that it is a clonal neoplasm and originates from the uncontrolled proliferation and accumulation of bone marrow–derived immature myeloid dendritic cells.

Question: What is the treatment strategy?
Answer: Treatment and outcome depend on the extent and severity of the disease. Unifocal involvements are usually treated locally by excision, curettage, intralesional steroid injection or radiation therapy. However, multifocal bone involvements and multisystem disease require systemic or combination therapies.

Question: Besides malignant chest wall tumours, what are the benign chest wall mass lesions that may develop in children?
Answer: Infantile haemangioma, benign osteoid osteoma, osteochondroma, fibrous dysplasia and mesenchymal hamartoma are examples of benign chest wall tumours.

Question: What are the treatment methods available for each?
Answer: Infantile haemangioma is known to spontaneously regress. Those that fail to do so may require medical therapy with propranolol or embolization and surgery. Osteoid osteoma may be self-limiting; some may require NSAIDS for pain relief or minimally invasive methods of CT-guided excision, radiofrequency or cryoablation. Osteochondroma, fibrous dysplasia and mesenchymal hamartoma may not usually require treatment unless the diagnosis is in question.

MEDIASTINAL TUMOURS

Scenario: A 15-year-old girl presents to hospital with progressively worsening shortness of breath that began 3 weeks ago. She has orthopnoea, is unable to lie flat and has required two pillows to aid sleeping. A CXR was done (**Figure 55.5**).

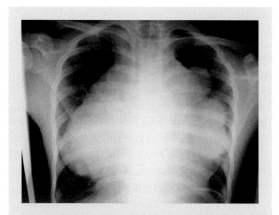

Figure 55.5 CXR showing a widened mediastinum.

Question: The mediastinum is widened, suggestive of a large mediastinal mass. What will be the next investigation?

Answer: CT scan of the thorax is required to define (1) the origin of the mass; (2) characteristics of the mass, whether solid or cystic, and the presence of unique features such as calcifications; and (3) its relationship with adjacent structures. Axial scans showed a large solid anterior mediastinal mass with areas of calcifications (**Figure 55.6**). Her serum α-fetoprotein (AFP) was grossly elevated at 21,000 μg/L. A malignant germ cell tumour (yolk sac tumour) of the mediastinum was diagnosed.

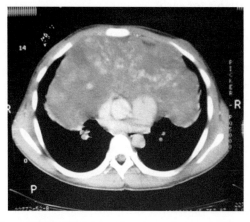

Figure 55.6 CT thorax showing a large anterior mediastinal mass.

Question: What is the clinical significance of anatomical division of the mediastinum?

Answer: The mediastinum is divided into the anterior, superior, middle and posterior compartments (**Figure 55.7**). Such anatomical division will lead

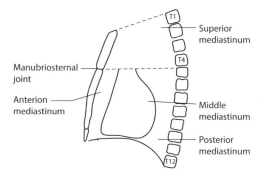

Figure 55.7 Divisions of the mediastinum.

the clinician to the appropriate differential diagnoses (**Figure 55.8**). Performing diagnostic tests based on the working differential diagnoses will reduce unnecessary procedural risks and avoid diagnostic delay (**Table 55.1**).

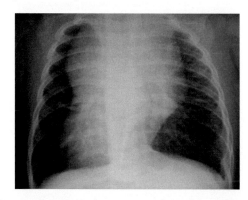

Figure 55.8 CXR showing a widened superior mediastinum.

Table 55.1 Differential diagnoses of mediastinal masses according to compartments of mediastinum

Compartment	Benign	Malignant
Anterior and Superior	• Teratoma • Lymphangioma • Haemangioma • Thymic cyst	• NHL • Hodgkin's disease • Germ cell tumour • Thymoma
Middle	• Bronchogenic cyst • Infective lymph nodes • Teratoma • Plasma cell granuloma	• NHL • Hodgkin's disease • Germ cell tumour • Sarcoma
Posterior	• Ganglioneuroma • Neurofibroma • Enterogenous cyst • Teratoma	• Neuroblastoma • Neurofibrosar-coma • Sarcoma

Abbreviation: NHL: Non-Hodgkin's lymphoma.

Question: What are the patients' clinical manifestations based on the location of the masses?

Answer: In the anterior mediastinum, they manifest with dyspnoea, orthopnoea, chest pain, cough, superior vena cava (SVC) syndrome, phrenic nerve palsy and recurrent laryngeal nerve palsy. Cardiac tamponade, pleural and pericardial effusions may also be present. In patients with lymphomas, peripheral lymphadenopathy and the typical constitutional B symptoms of fever, chills, night sweats and weight loss may be present.

Masses in the middle mediastinum present with airway obstruction and perhaps SVC syndrome. Patients with bronchogenic cysts present with cough, chest pain, dyspnoea and recurrent respiratory infections.

Posterior mediastinal masses may be asymptomatic. Large masses in close proximity to the oesophagus may present with dysphagia or odynophagia. Those that are adjacent to the airways may present with cough, haemoptysis, hoarseness of voice and wheezing. Paravertebral tumours may also present with back pain and nerve compression symptoms.

Question: What is the role of tumour markers?

Answer: Serum AFP and β-human chorionic gonadotropin (hCG) are useful tumour markers for definitive diagnosis of malignant germ cell tumours, obviating the need for tissue biopsy. In addition, such tumour markers also reflect the tumours' response to chemotherapy and are useful surveillance indicators for tumour recurrence.

Question: What is the treatment of choice for this patient?

Answer: This patient received neoadjuvant chemotherapy with good response, evident by the significant reduction in serum β-hCG and size of the mediastinal masses. Subsequently, she underwent local control with complete surgical resection by clamshell anterior thoracotomy.

Scenario: A 3-year-old boy presents with fever and was fretful for the last week worsening in the preceding 3 days. He is only willing to sleep when carried in an upright position, suggestive of orthopnoea. His face and neck were noticed to be swollen. He is unwilling to lie supine for a physical examination. There is no obvious palpable lymphadenopathy.

Question: What initial investigation will you perform?

Answer: CXR. The clinical presentation is suggestive of SVC syndrome, a group of symptoms caused by obstruction of the SVC. A CXR will be able to detect the mediastinal mass (**Figure 55.8**).

CXR should be followed by a CT scan of the thorax to confirm the presence of an anterior mediastinal mass and its characteristic (predominantly solid with minimal cystic component) (**Figure 55.9a and b**). Indeed, the SVC was obstructed together with significant compression of the trachea and bronchi.

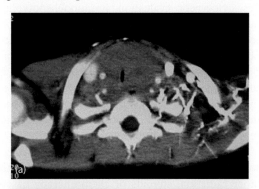

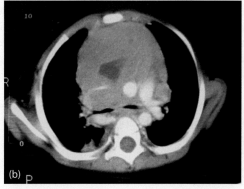

Figure 55.9 (a and b) CT (axial) scan of the thoracic inlet and the mediastinum at the level of the carina.

Question: How would you confirm the diagnosis? How would you prioritize diagnostic techniques according to risk factors?

Answer: This patient's condition warrants careful selection of diagnostic tests. Children with anterior mediastinal masses are at risk of life-threatening airway compromise during anaesthesia induction and can present a diagnostic and management challenge for paediatric surgeons. Patients with SVC syndrome, orthopnoea, tracheal cross-sectional diameter <50% and peak expiratory flow rate (PEFR) <50% (predicted) are at high risk of anaesthesia-related complications.

Evaluation using tests that do not require general anaesthesia should be performed first. Peripheral blood can be submitted for microscopy and flow cytometry, which may be diagnostic of haematological malignancies such as lymphoma. Bone marrow aspiration and biopsy performed under local anaesthesia may yield diagnostic information in lymphoma, neuroblastoma and some other malignancies. Pleural effusions may be sampled by thoracentesis using anatomic landmarks or ultrasound guidance under local anaesthesia. Cells in the effusion may be assayed by immunocytochemical studies, cytogenetic evaluation, immunophenotyping and cytology. For patients that have palpable lymph nodes, lymph node biopsy may be performed under local anaesthesia. In children with significant respiratory compromise, no pleural effusion and no lymph nodes accessible outside the chest, either a percutaneous image-guided needle tumour biopsy or an open anterior thoracotomy (Chamberlain procedure) can be performed successfully under local anaesthesia.

When the risk of obtaining a histological diagnosis outweighs that of empirical treatment with either radiation, steroids or chemotherapy based on the most likely clinical diagnosis, then the latter should be administered. This approach may prevent accurate diagnosis or immunophenotyping of the tumour due to the rapid response to treatment and should therefore be used only as a last resort.

In the previously mentioned patient, a diagnosis of acute lymphoblastic leukaemia was made based on bone marrow aspiration and biopsy. The boy received chemotherapy with good response.

Scenario: A 4-year-old girl presents with cough, fever and acute dyspnoea. CXR showed a widened superior mediastinum (**Figure 55.10**).

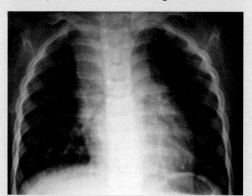

Figure 55.10 CXR showing a widened superior mediastinum.

Question: CT scan showed a large septate multicystic lesion (Figure 55.11a and b). What are the differential diagnoses?

Answer: Cystic lymphangioma is the most likely diagnosis for a multi-septate cystic lesion in the mediastinum. The density of the cystic contents resembles the signal of water or protein. Other differential diagnoses, usually solitary cysts, include bronchogenic cyst, cystic teratoma and malignant lymphoma. The majority of mediastinal cystic lymphangiomas are located in the superior and anterior compartments. CT scan remains the procedure of choice to further evaluate a mediastinal mass shown on chest radiography, with intravenous contrast delineating its vascular relationship for surgical planning.

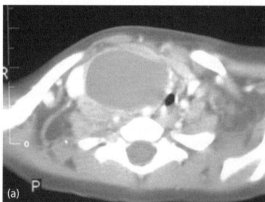

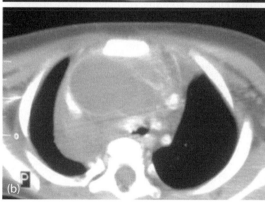

Figure 55.11 (a) CT scan (axial) at thoracic inlet; a large cystic lesion was displacing the adjacent SVC and the trachea. (b) CT scan at the superior mediastinum; a cystic lesion was encasing the SVC and branches of the aortic arch.

Question: What is the treatment of choice?

Answer: Surgical excision is the treatment of choice. Typically a progressive increase in size occurs, and in most cases, it would not be prudent to recommend observation of a cystic lymphangioma of the mediastinum. A surgical approach via a thoracotomy or median sternotomy provides excellent exposure for a meticulous dissection of all the cysts, which is essential to prevent recurrence. Since lymphangioma is benign but typically infiltrative between many adjacent vital structures, the latter should be delineated and carefully preserved.

Treatment of mediastinal lymphangioma with intralesional sclerotherapy is a limited option since reactionary increase in the size of the cysts may compromise respiration.

Scenario: A 2-year-old girl presents to her family doctor with cough and fever for 2 weeks. Physical examination showed that she was active without dyspnoea and was not debilitated. Her right chest was prominent with absence of breath sounds and dullness to percussion, suggestive of a "pleural effusion" (**Figure 55.12**).

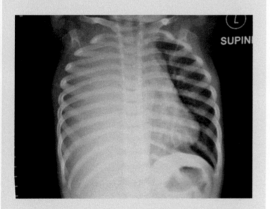

Figure 55.12 CXR with right chest opacity.

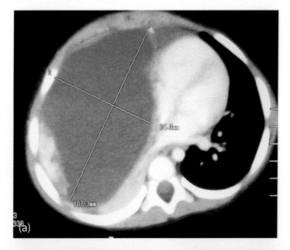

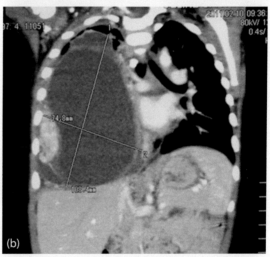

Figure 55.13 (a and b) CT scan showing a large unilocular cystic mass with displacement of the heart and compression of the lungs.

Question: CXR showed a right chest opacity; what will be the next intervention?
Answer: In view of the lack of respiratory and systemic symptoms despite the presence of a massive right "pleural effusion", CT scan of the thorax was performed that prevented an erroneous thoracentesis. CT scan showed a large cystic lesion occupying almost the entire right thorax with a small area of calcification noticed at its lateral aspect (**Figure 55.13a** and **b**). As serum AFP and β-hCG were within normal limits, a diagnosis of mature cystic teratoma was made.

Question: What is the treatment of choice?
Answer: Mature teratoma is a benign germ cell tumour. Surgical excision is the recommended treatment.

Scenario: A 3-month-old girl presented with strenuous breathing and cough. Chest auscultation revealed bilateral rhonchi. CXR showed opacity suggestive of pneumonia in the right lung. CT scan showed a cystic lesion in the posterior mediastinum (**Figure 55.14**).

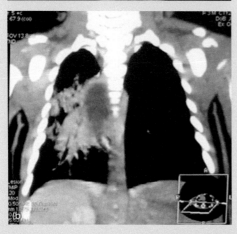

Figure 55.14 (a) CT scan showing a unilocular cyst on the right paravertebral region. (b) CT scan (coronal) showing the cystic lesion causing adjacent lung consolidation.

Question: What are the differential diagnoses?
Answer: The likelihood of a foregut duplication cyst, cystic lymphangioma or cystic teratoma should be considered.

Question: What is the next intervention?
As the cyst was causing airway compression and respiratory distress, it should be surgically excised. This was performed through a right posterolateral thoracotomy. At surgery, this was confirmed to be a foregut duplication cyst.

Question: What are foregut duplication cysts?
Answer: Foregut duplication cysts result from abnormal budding or division of the primitive foregut. Also called enterogenous cysts, they are most frequently divided into categories based on their histologic features and embryogenesis. Bronchogenic cysts occur mostly along the tracheobronchial tree and are usually found behind the carina. Most often they are unilocular and lined by ciliated columnar epithelium with focal or extensive squamous metaplasia. Oesophageal cysts are less common, and their lining may be squamous, ciliated columnar or a mixture of both. Distinction from bronchial cysts may be difficult or even impossible; the best evidence in favour of their oesophageal aetiology is when they are totally within the oesophageal wall and covered by a definite double layer of smooth muscle.

Scenario: A 2-year-old girl was found with an incidental right paravertebral tumour on CXR (**Figure 55.15a** and **b**) when she presented with 5-day-history of cough without fever. She was otherwise well. Physical examination was unremarkable. An oblique view CXR confirmed the presence of a posterior mediastinal mass.

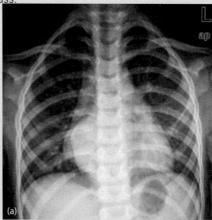

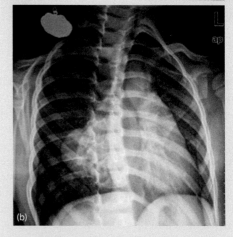

Figure 55.15 (a) CXR (PA view) shows a silhouette of a right paravertebral mass. (b) CXR (oblique view) shows a posterior mediastinal mass.

Question: How will you evaluate this finding?

Answer: CT scan of the thorax showed a solid paravertebral mass that was infiltrating the intervertebral foramina but not causing epidural compression of the spinal cord (**Figure 55.16a** and **b**). A few specks of calcification were found in the mass. The findings were consistent with a paravertebral neurogenic tumour such as neuroblastoma or ganglioneuroma.

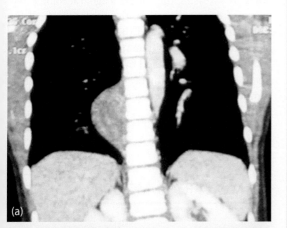

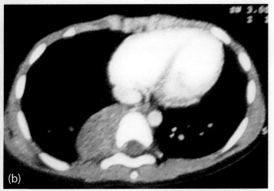

Figure 55.16 (a and b) CT scan revealing the presence of right paravertebral tumour with intervertebral infiltration.

Question: What is the therapeutic strategy in this patient?

Answer: In the presence of a surgically resectable tumour with low risk of complications, up-front tumour resection would be a reasonable option. However, in the presence of an unresectable tumour or in the presence of metastatic disease, tumour or bone marrow biopsies and neoadjuvant chemotherapy would be the preferred strategy. In the presence of a small tumour without image-defined risk factors, resection by thoracoscopy or minimally invasive surgical (MIS) technique is acceptable.

Scenario: A 3-month-old boy presents with loud noisy breathing and stridor. Other than being fretful, he is feeding well with a good body weight. A CXR was done that showed a large right cervicothoracic mass that was causing compression and displacement of his trachea.

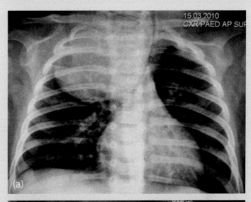

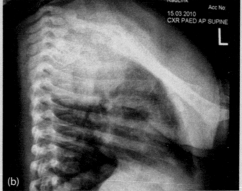

Figure 55.17 (a) CXR (PA view) showing a right thoracic inlet tumour with displacement and compression of the trachea. (b) CXR (lateral view) showing tumour occupying the superior mediastinum.

Question: What is the next investigation?

Answer: CT scan of the thorax was performed. In view of the respiratory signs it is vital that any

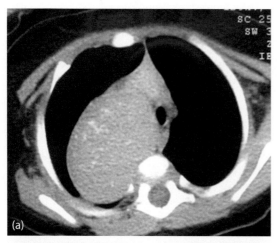

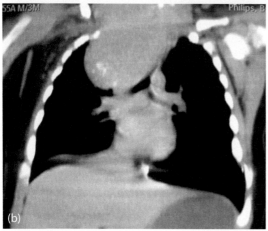

Figure 55.18 (a and b) CT scan showing calcified mass in the upper posterior mediastinum.

form of sedation should be avoided. The scan illustrates the prevertebral location of the mass that was compressing the trachea (**Figure 55.18a** and **b**). The presence of calcification suggests differential diagnoses of neuroblastoma or germ cell tumour. Normal serum AFP and β-hCG ruled out malignant germ cell tumour.

Question: What is the next course of action?
Answer: Considering the tumour's threat to the airway and the risks associated with tumour biopsy, surgical resection was chosen next, as this can be performed safely via median sternotomy. The child successfully underwent surgical resection. Histology showed a localized cervicothoracic

neuroblastoma, low-risk group. Further evaluations with bone scan, bone marrow aspiration and biopsy ruled out metastasis. Following surgery, he was monitored closely and has remained well in complete remission for 10 years.

Summary

Diagnoses of mediastinal tumours are usually made by assessing the patient's age, radiologic evidence of tumour location, the presence of calcification in the tumour and the presence of tumour markers (AFP, vanillylmandelic acid, β-hCG). Diagnosis is then verified by histologic evaluation. Resection is the mainstay treatment for benign tumours. Biopsy and chemotherapy (and/or radiation) are employed for lymphoid tumours, and resection and adjuvant therapy are used for other solid malignancies.

PULMONARY TUMOURS

Scenario: A 3-year-old girl presented with cough, wheezing and fever for the last 10 days. Bronchial breath sounds were auscultated with reduced air entry in the left chest. CXR showed opacity in the left chest (**Figure 55.19**). CT scan of the thorax found an enhancing heterogeneous mass in the left pulmonary parenchyma (**Figure 55.20**).

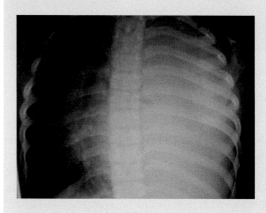

Figure 55.19 CXR showing opacity in the left chest.

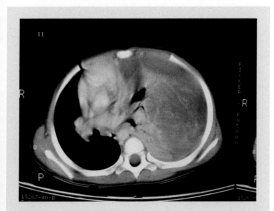

Figure 55.20 CT scan showing large mass arising from the left lung.

Question: What are the differential diagnoses? What is the management strategy approach?

Answer: The differential diagnoses here include infective pneumonia, pleuropulmonary blastoma (PPB), lymphoma and infantile fibrosarcoma, and when cystic components are present, congenital pulmonary airway malformations (CPAMs) should be considered. In this patient, PPB was the final diagnosis confirmed at left lower pulmonary lobectomy.

Diagnosis of PPB is facilitated with CT scan of the thorax, bronchoscopy and often biopsy. Biopsy can be avoided for smaller lesions, especially for type I (pure cystic) lesions in which surgical resection (pulmonary wedge resection or lobectomy) would be anticipated to achieve negative free margins. PPB can exhibit great vessel or cardiac extension, and thus an echocardiogram is indicated for advanced cases. In addition, endobronchial extension has been reported, and therefore bronchoscopy should be considered prior to surgical resection. The frequent sites of metastasis are liver, brain and spinal cord, and these sites should be evaluated.

Question: Biopsy confirmed PPB. What are the principles of management?

Answer: Primary surgical resection is a reasonable option when the lesions are small (<10 cm) and when complete, non-morbid surgical resection (pulmonary wedge resection or lobectomy) with negative margins can be anticipated. Up-front resection should also be considered when the diagnosis is not clear-cut between a PPB or a congenital pulmonary malformation. Surgical resection

alone can be curative for completely resected type I PPB with negative margins and no intraoperative tumour spillage.

For larger lesions (>10 cm), most type II or III PPB, lesions with extensive pleural involvement, or when radical, morbid resection such as pneumonectomy would be required to achieve negative margins, it is best to perform a core needle biopsy and initiate neoadjuvant chemotherapy. In this scenario, the best treatment option seems to be chemotherapy followed by complete surgical resection, adding adjuvant radiotherapy for types II and III and/or patients with disseminated disease. For metastatic or recurrent tumours, high-dose consolidation therapy with autologous stem cell rescue should be considered. The prognosis is dismally poor for most children with metastatic PPB. Overall survival is 45% at 5 years and only 8% at 10 years.

BIBLIOGRAPHY

1. Shamberger RC, Grier HE. Chest wall tumors in infants and children. Semin Pediatr Surg. 1994;3(4):267–76.
2. Shamberger RC, et al., Ewing sarcoma/ primitive neuroectodermal tumor of the chest wall: impact of initial versus delayed resection on tumor margins, survival, and use of radiation therapy. Ann Surg. 2003;238(4):563–7; discussion 567-8.
3. Saenz NC, Ghavimi F, Gerald W, Gollamudi S, LaQuaglia MP. Chest wall rhabdomyosarcoma. Cancer. 1997;80(8):1513–7.
4. Reisi N, Raeissi P, Khalilabad TH, Moafi A. Unusual sites of bone involvement in Langerhans cell histiocytosis: a systematic review of the literature. Orphanet J of Rare Dis. 2021;16:1
5. Grosfeld JL, Skinner MA, Rescorla FJ, West KW, Scherer LR 3rd. Mediastinal tumors in children: experience with 196 cases. Ann Surg Oncol. 1994;1(2):121–7.
6. Ranganath SH, Lee EY, Restrepo R, Eisenberg RL. Mediastinal masses in children. AJR. 2012; 198:197–216.
7. Rojas Y, Shi YX, Zhang W, Beierle EA, Doski JJ, Goldfarb M, Goldin AB, Gow KW, Langer M, Vasudevan SA, Nuchtern JG. Primary malignant pulmonary tumors in children: a review of the national cancer

data base. J Pediatr Surg. 2015;50(6): 1004–8.

8. Weldon CB, Shamberger RC. Pediatric pulmonary tumors: primary and metastatic. Semin Pediatr Surg. 2008;17(1):17–29.

9. Lichtenberger III JP, Biko DM, Carter BW, Pavio MA, Huppmann AR, Chung EM. Primary lung tumors in children: Radiologic-pathologic correlation from the radiologic pathology archives. RadioGraphics. 2018;38(7). https://doi.org/10.1148/rg.2018180192

10. Murphy F., Corbally MT. Chest wall reconstruction following radical resection of Ewings Sarcoma. Paediatric Surg Int. 2007, 23(4):353–6, Epub 2007 Feb 8

56

Sacrococcygeal teratoma

PAUL D. LOSTY
Institute of Systems and Molecular Biology, University of Liverpool, UK and
Ramathibodi Hospital, Mahidol University, Bangkok, Thailand

Scenario: You are called to visit the fetal medicine centre to talk with a pregnant mother and her male partner who have had a fetal MRI study undertaken at 20 weeks (**Figure 56.1**).

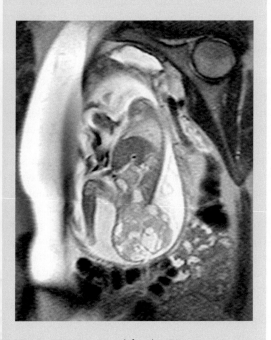

Figure 56.1 Maternal-fetal MRI scan.

Question: Upon examining the MRI study, what is your commentary?
Answer: The MRI scan shows a fetus with a large complex mass lesion arising from the pelvic extremity region. The mass from imaging extends into the pelvis from the exterior aspects of the fetus.

Question: What are the working differential diagnoses to consider?
Answer: Diagnoses include (1) sacrococcygeal teratoma (SCT), (2) a complex lymphovascular malformation, (3) chordoma and (4) other rare neoplasms.

Question: What is the most likely diagnosis?
Answer: SCT is the most likely diagnosis given the MRI image scan findings.

Question: Outline and plan your consultation with the mother and partner.
Answer: SCT is a germ cell tumour – most often benign (95% of cases) – that develops before birth and grows from the baby's coccyx or tailbone. It occurs in 1:35,000–40,000 live births and is by far the most common tumour encountered in newborns. Tumours can vary enormously in size (cm) and most often typically affect females vs males. As the fetal period continues, the tumour may show a variable pattern of biological growth and behaviour. With pregnancy progressing SCT

DOI: 10.1201/9781003182290-63

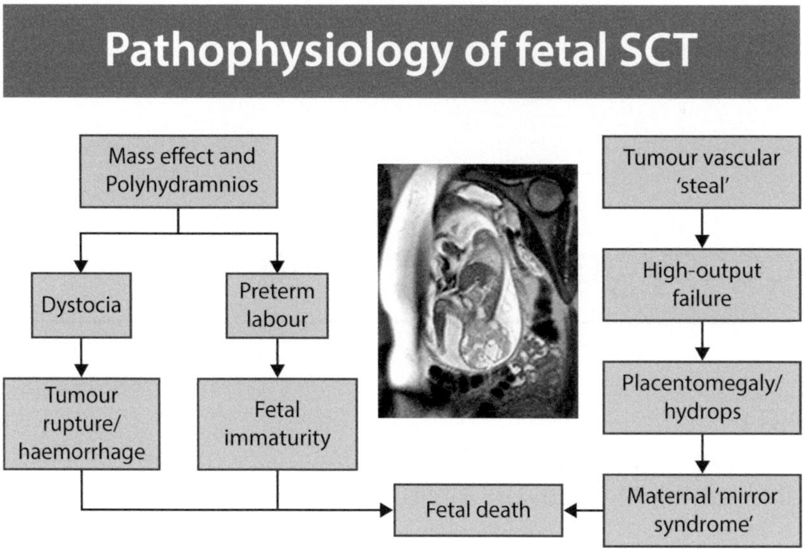

Figure 56.2 Pathophysiology of Fetal Sacrococcygeal Teratoma

lesions may thus grow to enormous and monstrous sizes, resulting in the fetus developing hydrops through 'vascular steal syndrome' in which the tumour acquires a 'parasitic circulation' leading to high-output fetal cardiac failure. Mothers can concurrently develop accelerated hypertension and a severe pre-eclampsia illness with proteinuria termed 'maternal mirror syndrome' and risk death. The fetus and mother are therefore both at 'high risk' in the antenatal period before birth delivery (**Figure 56.2**).

The pregnancy will need to be carefully monitored at the fetal medicine centre by a multidisciplinary team (MDT) with frequent surveillance imaging and maternal assessment. Elective C-section delivery near term (37 weeks) should be fully discussed with the mother and partner to avert an unplanned spontaneous labour with risks of dystocia, thus ensuring the fetus is born at a specialist centre fully equipped to provide the best care.

Reassuringly, survival is the expected norm for the fetus with SCT. Rarely SCT lesions are malignant (<5%) requiring additional multimodal chemotherapy.

Question: The mother and father want to know about the surgical plans after birth. What will you tell them?
Answer: The surgeon must discuss several major key points at the fetal medicine clinic consultation.

Details include the following: (1) Most tumours are reassuringly benign, and with complete R0 resection, including coccygectomy, recurrence is rare (<10%); (2) risks of neuropathic bladder and bowel exist with SCT neoplasms. Such risks may be linked to (a) in utero tumour growth damaging delicate neural networks innervating urinary and bowel continence mechanisms and (b) after operative surgery resultant from iatrogenic collateral injury to extirpate the SCT tumour; (3) scarring and disfigurement – with monstrous lesions resected, corrective plastic surgery in later childhood/adolescent years may be required to achieve better aesthetic outcomes, notably buttock scar revision; (4) wound breakdown/dehiscence/surgical site infection (SSI); (5) risk of impotence in males with SCT; (6) death on table during the new-born operation or in the early perioperative period secondary to gross haemorrhage, sepsis, renal and multisystem organ failure; and (7) malignancy (5%) requiring multimodal cancer therapy(ies).

Consent for the operation with the family should document and list *ALL* of these factors.

The parents are reassured by the fetal surgical counselling session and opt to continue the pregnancy. The female baby is born at 37 weeks' gestation by elective C-section, stabilised and transferred to paediatric surgery (**Figure 56.3**).

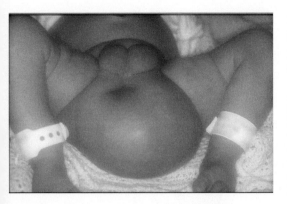

Figure 56.3 Newborn female with large SCT tumour.

Question: What are the principles of SCT operative resection step by step?

Answer: Blood laboratory tests are taken for full blood count (FBC), group X match, urea and electrolytes, along with tumour marker studies – alpha fetoprotein (AFP) and beta-human chorionic gonadotropin (HCG). Postnatal imaging investigations should include urinary tract ultrasound – pre and post voiding – to assess bladder function emptying. MRI or CT scan to reassess SCT Altman tumour stage (**Figure 56.4**) is important, as this may influence or dictate surgical strategy(ies). Informed consent is then obtained from parents by the operating surgeon detailing and re-emphasising *all* major points discussed at the fetal medicine counselling visit.

Operative surgery is undertaken after induction of general anaesthesia and full preparation, which includes securing adequate vascular access – often inserting a central venous line, arterial monitoring and ensuring urinary catheter placement. Prophylactic broad-spectrum antibiotics are routinely administered.

Depending on SCT tumour size, a midline posterior sagittal buttock crease incision may be planned, which is aesthetically superior, or in larger lesions a classical chevron approach may be adopted with the baby in a skydiver position on the table adequately protected with soft rolls under the chest and pelvis. A Pena-style nerve stimulator probe is invaluable to navigate and guide the operating surgeon to safeguard vital muscles and nerves to bladder and bowel, avoiding collateral injury. Tumour resection then proceeds carefully, avoiding rupture/spill, and coccygectomy with mass resection en bloc whilst securing a non-absorbable marking suture in the coccyx to aid its later identification with pathology lab reporting. The median and lateral sacral vessels must always first be clearly identified, suture ligated and secured before the coccyx is finally divided and resected with the SCT tumour. Beware at all times of aberrant parasitic blood vessels nourishing and feeding the tumour.

The fresh SCT specimen should be sent immediately to the pathology laboratory for later analysis. Reconstructive work then painstakingly begins aided with the nerve stimulator device on repairing pelvic floor muscles and ensuring intact sphincters. Wound closure and buttock recontouring are greatly aided by working with skilful plastic surgery services. A vacuum or suction drain is optional provided the operative field is dry (**Figures 56.5** and **56.6**)

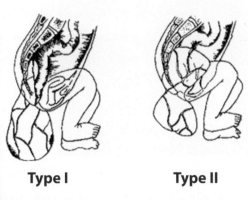
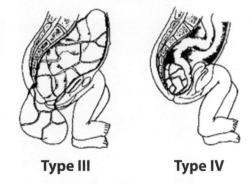

Type I   **Type II**   **Type III**   **Type IV**

Figure 56.4 Altman tumour staging system.

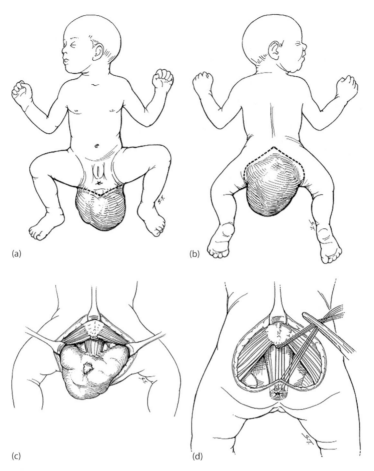

(a)

(b)

(c)

(d)

Figure 56.5 Operative SCT resection. (Adapted from PD Losty, AW Flake, RJ Rintala, JM Hutson, N Iwai. Eds. Rickham's Neonatal Surgery 2018. Springer Publishers.)

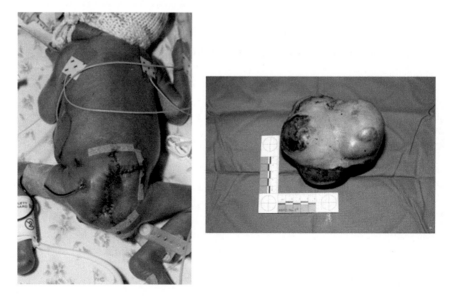

Figure 56.6 Postoperative patient. A premature birth SCT newborn. Immediate on-table wound appearance with gross specimen resected tumour.

Question: How will you plan to follow up with the patient?

Answer: The baby will require after-care health surveillance and clinic follow-up. Crucially it is important to review the final pathology lab report to confirm benign or malignant tumour status. Serial tumour marker assays, like AFP and beta-HCG, are essential ideally every 4 months in the first postoperative year. By 12 months serum AFP should normally decline to adult-range normative values. Follow-up and care plans in the second and subsequent advancing childhood years show wide surgical practice variation lacking consensus. Tumour marker assays provide reliable and early biomarker indication of tumour recurrence well ahead of imaging studies. Vigilant monitoring of urinary tract function and continence is crucial after SCT resection. Bowel function typically cannot be adequately assessed until 2–3 years in most infants and toddlers. Urinary tract infections often therefore indicate bladder malfunction with development of neuropathic bladder and co-associated vesicoureteric reflux (VUR) (**Figure 56.7**).

Ultrasound and urodynamic studies are thus a crucial aspect of surveillance health care plans with clinic follow-up. Outcome studies show 20–30% of SCT patients experience bladder and bowel problems. Urology service input is therefore vital from SCT primary diagnosis, much as is routinely practised in infants born with myelomeningocoele. Patients may require clean intermittent catheterization (CIC) therapy to aid bladder emptying to avert infection and protect urinary tract function. Bowel problems detected often much later may require laxatives, suppositories or enemas. Troublesome faecal soiling in older patients may significantly benefit from an antegrade colonic enema (ACE) appendicostomy operation. Males may be impotent if

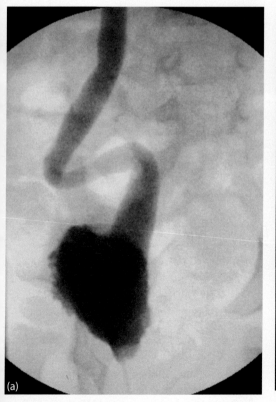
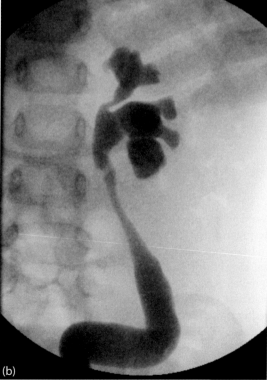

Figure 56.7 Micturating voiding cystogram study showing (a) neuropathic bladder (b) grade 3 vesico-ureteric reflux (right).

FLOW SHEET - OVERVIEW OF MANAGEMENT OF GERM CELL TUMOURS

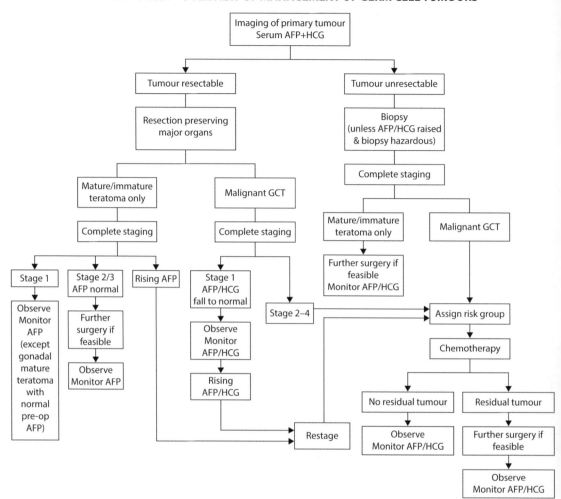

Figure 56.8 UK CCLG germ cell tumour algorithm.

sacral nerve plexus injury has occurred. Sexual dysfunction is equally reported by adult males and females. Malignant SCT new-born tumours are thankfully rare (<5%), though they require complex surgical management and multimodal platinum-based chemotherapy. SCT survivorship is thus linked with notable functional sequelae.

A UK CCLG germ cell tumour (GCT) algorithm is illustrated in **Figure 56.8**.

Late recurrences even up to 15 years later with mature benign teratomas indicate why consensus evidence-based guidelines require development and appraisal. Transitional care to adult services is clearly indicated where functional problems exist for the adolescent patients.

BIBLIOGRAPHY

1. Altman RP, Randolph JG, Lilly JR. Sacrococcygeal teratoma: American Academy of Pediatrics Surgical Section Survey – 1973. J Pediatr Surg. 1974;9:389–98.

2. Hedrick HL, Flake AW, Crombleholme TM, et al. Sacrococcygeal teratoma: Prenatal assessment, fetal intervention and outcome. J Pediatr Surg. 2004;39:430–8.

3. Gabra HO, Jesudason EC, McDowell HP, Pizer BL, Losty PD. Sacrococcygeal teratoma – A 25 year experience in a UK regional center. J Pediatr Surg. 2006;41:1513–6.

4. Rintala R, Lahdenne P, Lindahl H, et al. Anorectal function in adults operated for a benign sacrococcygeal teratoma. J Pediatr Surg. 1993:28:1165–7.

5. Braungart S, Ca James E, Powis M, Gabra H, CCLG Surgeons Collaborators, Losty PD. Sacrococcygeal teratoma: Long-term outcomes. A UK CCLG Surgeons Group Nationwide Study. Pediatr Blood Cancer. 2023;70(1)e29994. doi:10.1002/pbc.29994. Epub 2022Oct 13.

6. Salim A, Raitio A, Losty PD. Long-term functional outcomes of sacrococcygeal teratoma – A systematic review of published studies exploring 'real world 'outcomes. Eur J Surg Oncol. 2023;49(1):16–20.

57

Lymphoma

LUCA PIO

Bicêtre Hospital, Paris-Saclay University, GHU Paris Saclay Assistance Publique Hôpitaux de Paris (AP-HP), Le Kremlin Bicêtre, France

Scenario: A 9-year-old male child with no past medical history was referred from a pediatrician to the hospital emergency department with a 2-week history of fever, sweating, abdominal pain and intolerance of food. No vomiting or diarrhea was evident from the clinical history.

On examination the child was pale and noted to have right-sided abdominal pain without evidence of distension.

Question: What further study would you request to investigate this child?

Answer: A full blood count (FBC) lab test shows a lymphocytosis and a low mean corpuscular volume (MCV). Abdominal ultrasound scan reveals a right-sided mass with an ileocecal localization and without obvious peritoneal fluid collection (**Figure 57.1**).

Question: What are the next steps in management? Is there an indication for emergency operation?

Answer: No surgical procedure is urgently indicated at this stage, as the child will need further diagnostic workup.

Further history from the family reveals symptoms of a long-standing fever with sweating spells. Such findings associated with an abdominal mass should raise clinical suspicion of a lymphoproliferative disease. A full-body imaging study will now be mandatory. A total-body computed tomography (CT) scan is therefore scheduled, and further laboratory tests reveal raised lactate dehydrogenase (LDH), which is often abnormally high in 'fast growing' lymphoproliferative disorders. The FBC shows a low-level anemia, and bone marrow studies must be undertaken with aspiration and trephine biopsies. A lumbar puncture is scheduled also.

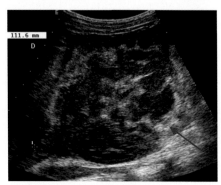

Figure 57.1 Abdominal ultrasound scan showing a solid hyperechogenic intestinal mass lesion in the context of bowel pathology (arrow).

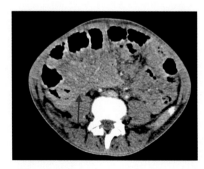

Figure 57.2 Abdominal computed tomography scan with axial views showing a right-sided solid mass lesion (arrow).

DOI: 10.1201/9781003182290-64

CT scan shows an isolated right-sided ileocecal abdominal mass (**Figure 57.2**) with no evidence of pneumoperitoneum or peritoneal fluid collections.

Question: Is there a role for surgery in a case of suspected lymphoproliferative abdominal malignancy with operative resection?

Answer: In a suspected lymphoproliferative abdominal mass with absence of surgical complications, notably intestinal perforation or obstruction, the role of surgery is strictly limited to providing an adequate tumor biopsy specimen for pathological studies.

Fine needle biopsies often do not provide adequate sampling for lymphoproliferative tumor characterization, and therefore a limited excision biopsy via laparotomy or aided by laparoscopy will be required for full molecular biology studies, immunophenotyping and cytogenetics.

Note: Surgical biopsy must avoid intestinal perforation, which would negatively impact and delay subsequent chemotherapy.

In circumstances where intraoperative findings reveal complex intestinal obstructive pathology requiring limited resection, it may be best to avoid primary intestinal anastomosis and create a temporary diverting stoma to provide a faster recovery and allow chemotherapy to be commenced as soon as possible. Medical oncology protocols may include corticosteroid treatments, which can increase the risk of intestinal anastomotic leaks. In case of ileostomy construction, attention should be directed at nutritional support for the patient replacing fluid and electrolyte losses to avoid metabolic syndrome. Stoma care management should be focused on ensuring the stoma bag appliance fits well to avoid an excoriating dermatitis.

The surgical biopsy pathology lab result now confirms Burkitt's lymphoma (BL).

Lymphomas are a group of lymphoproliferative tumors of the lymphatic reticuloendothelial system and represent the third most frequent pediatric tumor encountered in clinical practice (incidence ranging from 12% to 15%). They are classified into two distinct groups – Hodgkin's lymphoma (HL) and non-Hodgkin's lymphoma (NHL).

The World Health Organization (WHO) has further classified the different types of lymphoma, dividing HL into classic and nodular lymphocyte predominant and also dividing NHL by their cell type (B-cell and T-cell lymphomas), describing now more than 50 subtypes.

BL represents one of the most frequent NHLs; it is a B-cell neoplasm characterized by a rapid growth and divided into three distinct forms:

1. *Endemic form*: Mostly frequent encountered in equatorial Africa.
2. *Sporadic form*: Most frequent type encountered in the United States.
3. *Immunocompromised-related form*: Predominating in the immunocompromised pediatric patient, especially in transplanted children.

BL is notably the most common cause of intussusception in children over 4 years (**Figure 57.3**), which epidemiologically normally occurs below 2 years of age (so-called idiopathic intussusception).

The surgical management of intussusception BL-related disease may follow the same principles of management of lymphoproliferative solid tumors avoiding mutilating surgery (resection and anastomosis), with a predominant diagnostic role being key.

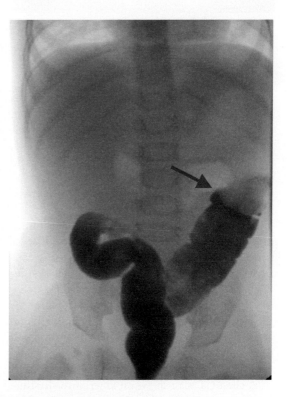

Figure 57.3 Intussusception evidenced by the contrast agent progression (arrow).

Question: A chest X-ray of a 13-year-old girl presenting with respiratory distress, weight loss and cervical lymph node enlargement showed a mediastinal enlargement (Figure 57.4). How should we manage this patient?

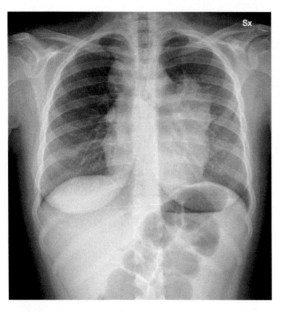

Figure 57.4 Posteroanterior chest X-ray radiograph showing a mediastinal mass lesion bulging on both sides of the mediastinum.

Answer: Evidence of lymphadenopathy requires as a first step a full clinical physical examination, checking all superficial lymph node regional territories for the following characteristics: Tenderness, size, warmth, erythema, consistency, pain and size, with the differential diagnosis including viral, bacterial and fungal infections including atypical mycobacteria.

Lymphadenopathy may also be related to immunologic diseases such as graft-versus-host disease (in patients with known transplant history), connective tissue diseases (e.g. systemic lupus erythematosus [SLE]/lupus) or Sjogren's syndrome.

A first diagnostic evaluation should be scheduled with laboratory tests such as a complete blood count (CBC), LDH titer, *Streptococcus* antigen and serologic testing (cytomegalovirus, Epstein-Barr virus, *Bartonella*, herpes, rubella, toxoplasmosis).

A chest CT scan shows an anterior mediastinal mass lesion encasing the mediastinal organs including major arterial and venous vessels (**Figure 57.5**).

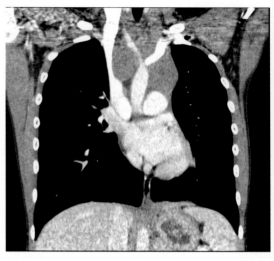

Figure 57.5 Thoracic computed tomography scan image with coronal views showing a mediastinal mass lesion encasing the aortic arch and both innominate vessel trunks.

Question: What will be the role of surgery in this case?

Answer: As for abdominal solid lymphoproliferative disease, surgery in this scenario will have a diagnostic and supportive role. In case of a mediastinal mass with tracheal airway compression >50%, even if excision biopsy is usually preferred, in order to avoid critical airway collapse during anesthesia, a fine needle biopsy under local anesthesia or pleural tap should always be considered. Orthopnea in such patients is considered a risk factor for dramatic airway collapse during induction of general anesthesia.

In cases of large pleural effusions or where there are enlarged regional superficial lymph nodes, pleural fluid tap/drainage with cytological analysis and peripheral lymph node sampling should be considered the best, first and safest approached to decrease surgical morbidity due to potential vascular injury.

A supportive role of surgery will also include securing vascular access (for chemotherapy or in the event that hemodialysis is required), including central venous line [CVL] or peripherally inserted central catheter [PICC] line insertion in the event of tumor lysis syndrome). Sometimes in high-risk situations first-line initial chemotherapy will be administered using the peripheral veins and a central venous catheter device secured at a later date.

Question: A 9-year-old male presents with a testicular mass, and laboratory tests are suspicious of a lymphoproliferative disease. What will be the surgical management?

Answer: Lymphomas may occur in a genital tract localization, notably in the ovaries or testes. The surgical management here will follow the same principles and practice as for abdominal and mediastinal sites, notably avoiding genital mutilation/castration, with tissue biopsy only needed for confirmatory diagnosis.

BIBLIOGRAPHY

1. Arber DA, Orazi A, Hasserjian R, Thiele J, Borowitz MJ, Le Beau MM, Bloomfield CD, Cazzola M, Vardiman JW. The 2016 revision to the World Health Organization classification of myeloid neoplasms and acute leukemia. Blood. 2016;127(20):2391–405.
2. Morris-Stiff G, Cheang P, Key S, Verghese A, Havard TJ. Does the surgeon still have a role to play in the diagnosis and management of lymphomas? World J Surg Oncol. 2008;6:13.
3. Bussell HR, Kroiss S, Tharakan SJ, Meuli M, Moehrlen U. Intussusception in children: lessons learned from intestinal lymphoma as a rare lead-point. Pediatr Surg Int. 2019;35(8):879–85.
4. Locke R, Comfort R, Kubba H. When does an enlarged cervical lymph node in a child need excision? A systematic review. Int J Pediatr Otorhinolaryngol. 2014;78(3):393–401.
5. Perger L, Lee E, Shamberger R. Management of children and adolescents with a critical airway due to compression by an anterior mediastinal mass. J Pediatr Surg. 2008;43(11):1990–7.
6. Ehrlich PF, Friedman DL, Schwartz CL; Children Oncology Group Hodgkin Lymphoma study section. Monitoring diagnostic accuracy and complications. A report from the Children's Oncology Group Hodgkin Lymphoma study. J Pediatr Surg. 2007;42(5):788–91.

58

Naevi

MARTIN VAN CARLEN, RONG KHAW, AND ADEL FATTAH
Alder Hey Children's Hospital, Liverpool, UK

Pigmented skin lesions are a common cause of concern in paediatric practice. This chapter will describe the management of such lesions.

Scenario: A mother attends hospital clinic with her 5-year-old daughter reporting concerns of a darkly pigmented mole on the child's face. Mum is concerned that this could be skin cancer, as recently an elderly grandmother passed away from metastatic melanoma (**Figure 58.1**).

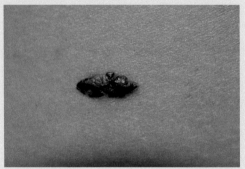

Figure 58.1 This is a histologically confirmed Spitz naevus but has features that cause suspicion: Colour variegation, diameter >6 mm and elevation.

Question: What are the concerning features suggestive of skin malignancy in children?
Answer: The top three most common skin cancers in adulthood (basal cell carcinoma, squamous cell carcinoma and melanoma) are all very rare in children, and only 1%–2% of skin lesions excised in children turn out to be frankly malignant. The ABCDE criteria for suspected skin malignancy for adults is still nonetheless applicable to the paediatric population but with several notable additions:

A is for both asymmetry and amelanotic.
   Amelanotic melanomas are more prevalent in the paediatric population.
B is for bleeding as well as border irregularity.
C is for colour variegation.
D is for diameter >6 mm.
E is for elevation and textural changes.

Question: On examination this is a 3-mm, solitary, darkly pigmented lesion with well-defined borders and uniform colour. What are Spitz naevi?
Answer: Spitz naevi are usually solitary, flesh-coloured or pink papules that occasionally have brownish pigmentation. These lesions are commonly found in the head and neck (37%), lower limbs (28%) and also the truncal region (6%). Histologically, Spitz naevi can be either spindle-cell or epithelioid-shaped and are usually symmetrical with Kamino bodies (eosinophilic globules) present. However, these features are not pathognomonic. Spitz naevi are generally benign in the paediatric population. However, there have been cases of metastasis and death with Spitz tumours, and the general term for such lesions is an atypical

DOI: 10.1201/9781003182290-65

Spitz tumour. Clinical, dermoscopic examination, and histopathological diagnosis of atypical Spitz naevi is occasionally indistinguishable from malignant melanoma; thus an urgent 2-week referral to hospital specialist clinical care services is recommended. A multidisciplinary approach is advisable here when dealing with atypical Spitz tumours in children. In general, surgical excision and careful surveillance follow-up are warranted for equivocal cases (**Figure 58.2**).

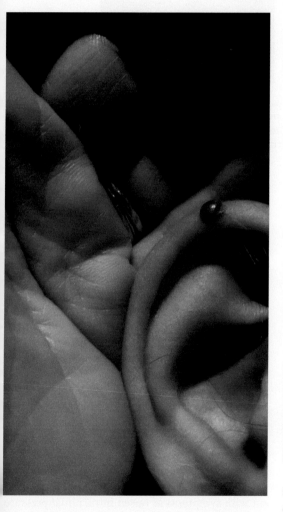

Figure 58.2 The lesion shown is a Spitz naevus with high-grade atypia and frequent mitoses. Compare the clinical features to **Figure 58.1**: There are no concerning clinical features, but in this case presentation was due to rapid growth. Consideration for dermatoscopy examination by an experienced health care practitioner and a low threshold for biopsy are prudent.

Question: How can we differentiate a benign Spitz naevi from atypical Spitz tumours?

Answer: Due to the low incidence of metastasis and mortality, there are currently no robust risk stratification systems that are able to accurately quantify the metastatic potential of atypical Spitz tumours.

Spitz et al. devised a point-based system according to patient age, presence of ulceration, tumour diameter and lesion thickness in an attempt to grade Spitz tumours into low-, intermediate- and high-risk categories.

Risk factors		Assigned score
Age	>10 years old	1
Diameter	>10 mm	1
Clark level V/ subcutaneous fat involvement		2
Presence of ulceration		2
Mitosis	<5/mm^2	0
	6–8/mm^2	2
	>8/mm^2	5

Risk classification	Total score
Low	0–2
Intermediate	3–4
High	5–11

Scenario: A full-term baby is referred shortly after birth with a large pigmented skin lesion on the trunk. On examination, there is hair growth within the lesion and several satellite lesions are also present (**Figure 58.3**).

Question: What is the diagnosis of this skin condition? What are the characteristics, and how would you classify it?

Answer: The baby has a congenital melanocytic naevi (CMN). A CMN is a black or brown mole which is present at birth or appears in the immediate weeks postnatally. CMNs constitute a benign proliferation of cutaneous melanocytes. Within the CMN group, lesions can vary in size,

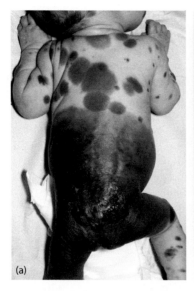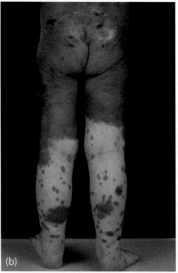

(a)　(b)

Figure 58.3 (a) Giant congenital melanocytic naevus. Note the satellite lesions, which in this context refer to the additional naevi elsewhere on the skin, not just in the locality of the primary lesion. (b) The same child approximately 3 years later. Note how the lesion may often become lighter with age. Many are reconstructive surgery conundrums, and it is often best to monitor such clinical cases rather than radically excise the whole lesion.

macroscopic appearance and histological characteristics. In addition to being cosmetically disfiguring, the larger CMNs also have an increased risk of malignant transformation into cutaneous malignant melanoma as well as being associated with non-cutaneous malignant melanoma. CMNs are usually histologically distinctly different from the more common acquired naevi, which present later in life. Histologically, CMN melanocytes can penetrate deeper into the dermis and subcutaneous tissues, as well as having the potential to involve muscle and bone.

CHARACTERISTICS AND CLASSIFICATION

CMNs generally grow in proportion to body size and are present in approximately 1% of the general population with an equal male and female distribution. One way of grouping CMNs is based on their largest diameter size (small <1.5 cm, medium 1.5–20 cm, giant >20 cm). Giant CMNs are rarer and occur in 1:20,000 newborns and have also been described as being larger than 1% total body surface area (TBSA) (i.e. surface area of palm of patient's hand) on the head and neck and 2% TBSA elsewhere on the body.

Question: What else do you look for on clinical examination?
Answer: Look at the size and number of CMNs as well as their distribution. Giant CMNs can appear in a 'swimming trunk' or glove and stocking distribution. Features that may raise concern of a malignant transformation include a new nodule or lump often presenting in the dermis or subcutaneous tissues and development of ulceration, bleeding, itching, focal growth, pain and dark pigmentation. In addition, extracutaneous malignant melanoma, referred to as 'neurocutaneous melanosis', may also occur in the mucosa of the gastrointestinal tract, in the retroperitoneum or as part of melanocyte deposits in the central nervous system. Even non-malignant neurocutaneous melanosis can be symptomatic and may present in the form of seizures. If a lesion involves the central nervous system (CNS), the patient may also present with symptoms of raised intracranial pressure such as fatigue, headaches, increased drowsiness and altered disturbed vision.

Question: The parents ask about the risk of malignant transformation What do you tell them?
Answer: Studies quote a wide percentage range of risk estimates; however, small and medium CMNs

have a relatively low lifetime risk of an estimated 1%–5% of malignant transformation. Giant CMNs have a higher risk of malignancy, approximately 5%–10%. Most of the melanomas here seem to occur in childhood, with the vast majority before the age of puberty. However, to assume that the risk disappears in adulthood is wrong, and these patients need to be carefully monitored and educated to look for the 'red flag' signs of melanoma. Most cases of patients with multiple CMNs developing melanoma have a poor prognosis, particularly those who may harbour CNS involvement.

Question: What is the immediate management?
Answer: There is usually no need for any urgent treatment at birth. The child should be referred to an appropriate multidisciplinary health care team for further management.

Question: What are the indications for treatment, and what are the options?
Answer: The treatment goals are clearly to consider cosmesis, early detection of melanoma and reduce the risk of malignant transformation of CMNs; however, there is no accepted consensus on standard treatment, and each patient must be managed individually with involvement of a multidisciplinary team (MDT) and the parents.

Factors to consider in management include:

- Malignant transformation risk
- Cosmesis
- Scarring
- Psychological effect

Superficial destructive methods such as dermabrasion, peel and laser ablation can improve the pigmentation and cosmesis while reducing the cellular burden of CMNs; however, it doesn't remove the deeper tissue layers of melanocytes, and it is not possible to submit tissue for histological analysis.

Surgical excision should be offered for any atypical CMN or suspicion of undergoing malignant transformation. In addition, facial CMNs are offered surgical excision for cosmetic reasons. Furthermore, easily excisable CMNs amenable to direct primary closure can also be treated with surgery for cosmetic reasons. If the lesion cannot be excised in one stage, then serial excision should be considered. Giant CMNs should undergo imaging to look for CNS involvement, and surgical excision of large areas may require staged surgery, e.g. tissue expansion, skin grafts or free flap tissue coverage.

Routine surgical excision has not demonstrated the risk reduction of malignant transformation; hence, it is offered on a cosmetic basis. Therefore, there is no advantage to operate on young babies, and any elective routine surgery is usually delayed until the child is at least 1 year old, when the risks of general anaesthetic are considered lower.

Occasionally, CMNs can undergo spontaneous lightening, and therefore yearly serial clinical photographs should be taken to assess for this. At times, this spontaneous lightening can be quite dramatic and improve the cosmetic appearance significantly. Furthermore, there is some evidence that traumatic disruption from surgery or thermal energy from lasers may affect CMN melanocytes adversely and trigger dysplasia and malignant transformation, and therefore this must also be clearly communicated to the parents.

Scenario: A 10-year-old boy attends the plastic surgery clinic with his mother seeking treatment, as he is concerned about the appearance of skin lesions which he has had since birth. On clinical examination, he has multiple keratotic lesions on his lower leg extending up to his thigh region that appear in whorls and seem to follow a linear pattern.

Question: What is a linear epidermal naevus?
Answer: The boy has what is termed liner epidermal naevus/keratinocytic epidermal naevi.

These are rare (0.1%–0.5%), congenital, keratotic lesions that can become verrucous as patients get older and are normally found in the extremities or truncal region. The clinical presentation has a wide spectrum ranging from solitary lesions to multiple verrucous papules that coalesce into plaques. These plaques follow the lines of Blaschko, often terminating abruptly at the midline. They affect both sexes equally. These keratotic papules can have either a unilateral or bilateral involvement and are asymptomatic. The term naevus is a misnomer, as epidermal naevi are congenital hamartomas of ectodermal origin. There have been individual case reports of malignant change into basal cell carcinoma and squamous cell carcinoma in adult patients, but the true incidence remains unknown.

Reported treatment modalities to improve cosmesis include topical treatments (steroids, 5-fluorouracil, retinoids), laser therapy and surgical excision. Although ablative laser therapy (carbon dioxide, CO_2) yields promising results, there are cases of recurrence. Current treatment options remain limited.

Question: What is epidermal naevus syndrome?
Answer: This is a broad category term that comprises epidermal naevi that have extracutaneous involvement, which could include CNS (seizures), ocular (colobomas) or skeletal abnormalities. The more common and recognized syndromes that come under this umbrella term include Schimmelpenning syndrome, Becker's naevus syndrome, phakomatosis pigmentokeratotica, naevus comedonicus syndrome, Proteus syndrome and CHILD (congenital hemidysplasia, ichthyosiform erythroderma, and limb defects) syndrome. Becker's naevus syndrome patients have muscular and skeletal abnormalities such as ipsilateral breast hypoplasia, hypoplastic upper trunk musculature, scoliosis and vertebral defects in conjunction with epidermal naevi. Of note the epidermal naevi in Becker's naevus syndrome normally does not adhere to Blashkoid lines.

Scenario: A 14-year-old girl is very keen to have a skin lesion on her scalp removed, as she has to tie up her hair all the time to attempt to conceal it. The lesion was present at birth. On examination, this is a 2 cm × 1 cm warty, pale yellow plaque which she describes as her 'bald patch' (**Figure 58.4**).

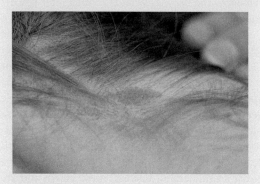

Figure 58.4 Sebaceous naevus.

Question: What is a sebaceous naevus?
Answer: Sebaceous naevi are rare, congenital, pale yellow, cerebriform plaques that commonly occur in the scalp (50%) but can also arise in the face. These lesions comprise hyperplastic sebaceous, apocrine glands, epidermis and hair follicles. They can evolve to be more verrucous and wart-like as patients get older due to hormonal changes during puberty. There is potential for malignant change into basal cell carcinoma, and the incidence is 0.8% with a lifetime risk of 5–22%. It is very rare for sebaceous naevi to undergo malignant change during childhood. However, a large-scale study involving 757 cases of sebaceous naevi in children under age 16 revealed two cases of malignant change into squamous cell carcinoma. Timing for excisional surgery remains debatable due to the low propensity for malignant change, although some authors advocate excision prior to puberty.

BIBLIOGRAPHY

1. Kinsler V, Bulstrode N. The role of surgery in the management of congenital melanocytic naevi in children: a perspective from Great Ormond Street Hospital. Journal of Plastic, Reconstructive & Aesthetic Surgery. 2009;62(5): 595–601.
2. Arneja JS, Gosain AK. Giant congenital melanocytic nevi. Plastic and Reconstructive Surgery. 2009;124(1): 1e–3e.
3. Kinsler VA, O'Hare P, Bulstrode N, Calonje JE, Chong WK, Hargrave D, Jacques T, Lomas D, Sebire NJ, Slater O. Melanoma in congenital melanocytic naevi. British Journal of Dermatology. 2017;176(5): 1131–43.

59

Vascular and lymphatic disorders

CLAIRE A. OSTERTAG-HILL, ANNA MCGUIRE, BELINDA H. DICKIE,
AND STEVEN J. FISHMAN
Boston Children's Hospital, Boston, MA

VASCULAR TUMORS WITH A FOCUS ON HEMANGIOMAS

> **Scenario:** A 2-month-old female is referred for excision of a scalp mass. On physical examination, she has a 2-cm, bright red, raised soft tissue mass on her scalp (**Figure 59.1a**) and five additional sub-centimeter red skin lesions on her trunk and extremities. What is your diagnosis?

Question: What is the expected clinical course of these lesions?
Answer: This infant has multifocal cutaneous infantile hemangiomas (IH), the most common tumor of infancy. The incidence is higher in females, premature infants, Caucasians, multiple gestations, and placental abnormalities, though the underlying etiology and pathogenesis remain unclear. Median onset is 1–2 weeks of age and most commonly occur as a focal cutaneous lesion of the head, neck, trunk, and extremities. IHs follow a predictable life cycle consisting of three phases: Proliferative (rapid neonatal growth for the first 6–7 months, typically plateauing by 10 months), involuting (fading of the shiny crimson color with softening and deflating of the mass from 1–7 years), and involuted (50% of patients have nearly normal skin at the prior lesion site, though those with larger and/or ulcerated tumors may have lax, redundant skin and scarring).

Question: What would your diagnosis be if a neonate was found to have a raised violaceous soft tissue mass at birth (Figure 59.1b)? How does the expected natural history differ from IH?
Answer: This neonate has a congenital hemangioma, characterized by being present at birth and having no postnatal growth. These lesions can be separated into rapidly involuting congenital hemangioma (RICH), partially involuting congenital hemangioma (PICH), and non-involuting congenital hemangioma (NICH). RICHs spontaneously undergo early involution, typically completed between 6 and 14 months of age. In contrast, PICHs only undergo partial involution, and NICHs do not involute and instead grow with the child.

Question: What is your differential for cutaneous vascular lesions?
Answer: Vascular anomalies are broadly divided into vascular tumors and vascular malformations, as shown in **Table 59.1**. Both can have cutaneous manifestations.

Question: What treatment is indicated, if any, for cutaneous IH, RICH, and NICH?
Answer: Most IH require only observation and reassurance. However, regular follow-up is recommended to assess for potential complications, including epithelial breakdown, ulceration, bleeding, and pain. Depending on the location of the hemangiomas, airway obstruction (cervico-facial lesion), cosmetic consequences (facial lesion), deprivation amblyopia

DOI: 10.1201/9781003182290-66

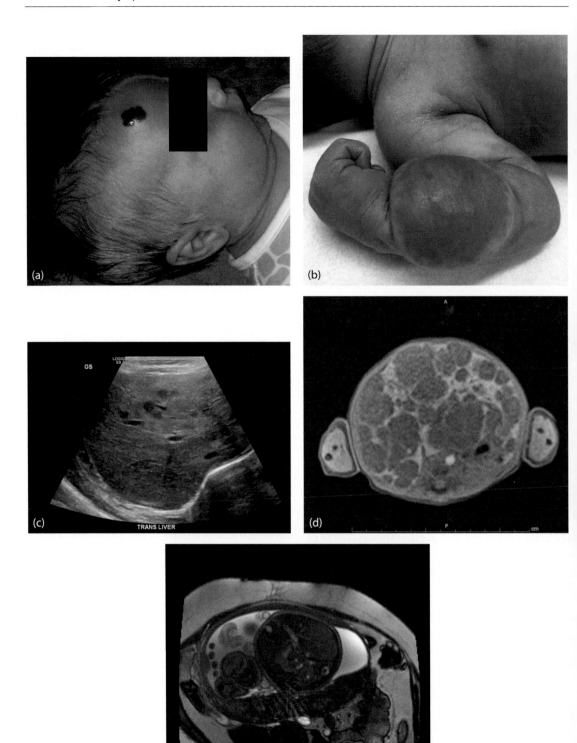

Figure 59.1 Hemangiomas can be infantile or congenital and most commonly occur on the skin and liver. (a) An infantile hemangioma in the proliferative phase. (b) A congenital hemangioma. (c) Multifocal hepatic hemangiomas. (d) Diffuse hepatic hemangiomas. (e) A large focal hemangioma seen on prenatal imaging.

Table 59.1 Abbreviated ISSVA Classification for Vascular Anomalies

Vascular anomalies				
Vascular tumors	**Vascular malformations**			
	Simple	Combined	Of major named vessels	Associated with other anomalies
Benign				
Locally aggressive or borderline	Capillary malformations Lymphatic malformations Venous malformations	CVM, CLM LVM, CLVM CAVM	Examples: ectasia, aneurysm,	Examples: Klippel-Trenaunay syndrome
Malignant	Arteriovenous malformations Arteriovenous fistula	CLAVM	stenosis	CLOVES syndrome

Source: Adapted from the 2018 ISSVA Classification of Vascular Anomalies.

(periorbital and eyelid hemangiomas), and gastrointestinal bleeding (gastrointestinal hemangiomas) may occur. IH at risk for or manifesting with these complications may warrant treatment. First-line pharmacotherapy is oral propranolol, given its high efficacy. Local therapy may include intralesional steroids and topical timolol. Indications for surgical resection of IH vary based on hemangioma stage and patient age.

In contrast, for RICH, pharmacotherapy is only indicated with high-output heart failure, vision blockage, or anatomic distortion. Early surgical resection may be indicated for necrosis, ocular obstruction, or auricular deformation, and later for aesthetic concerns. Resection of NICH for pain and/or cosmetic concerns can be considered at any time after diagnosis. Preoperative arterial embolization can be beneficial for large NICH.

Question: What congenital anomalies are associated with cutaneous hemangiomas? What additional workup should you perform with five or more cutaneous IH?
Answer: Facial hemangiomas associated with structural anomalies of the brain, cerebral vasculature, eye, aorta, and chest wall occur in the neurocutaneous disorder called PHACES syndrome. Anorectal anomalies, including PELVIS syndrome, may be associated with IH of the pelvis and perineum.

Five or more cutaneous IH are associated with an elevated risk of occult visceral hemangiomas, most commonly in the liver. Screening ultrasound is therefore indicated in these patients.

On screening ultrasound, several liver lesions are identified.

Question: Can you describe the two types of infantile hepatic hemangiomas (HHs) (Figure 59.1c and d) and which complications you should monitor for?

Answer: Multifocal infantile HHs, like their cutaneous counterpart, occur more commonly in females, are diagnosed postnatally, and stain positive for GLUT-1. They follow a natural course of involution similar to cutaneous IH, with most infants remaining asymptomatic. Infants should therefore be followed with serial abdominal ultrasounds until involution is complete. A small subset of infants develop high-output cardiac failure due to macrovascular shunting, and treatment with steroids or propranolol can often close these shunts. If HH is refractory to pharmacotherapy, embolization can be performed.

Diffuse HH are similarly associated with cutaneous IH, female gender, and GLUT-1 expression. However, these lesions have far more serious consequences, as innumerable tumors almost completely replace the normal hepatic parenchyma. Patients are at risk for abdominal compartment syndrome, respiratory distress, and multiorgan failure from the resulting massive hepatomegaly. Aggressive pharmacotherapy with propranolol, steroids, and occasionally low-dose vincristine may be required. Liver transplantation is sometimes indicated as a last resort for infants in extremis.

Diagnosis of hepatic IH warrants workup for hypothyroidism due to type 3 iodothyronine deiodinase expression in some IH.

Question: What if the focal liver mass was identified prenatally at 34 weeks of gestation on fetal ultrasound and fetal MRI shows a large solitary tumor with centripetal enhancement with central sparing (Figure 59.1e)? What is the likely diagnosis and expected postnatal course?
Answer: This fetus likely has a focal congenital HH. The hepatic counterpart of cutaneous RICH, these lesions are fully grown at birth, GLUT-1

negative, not associated with cutaneous hemangiomas, and undergo rapid spontaneous involution. These lesions typically remain asymptomatic, though intralesional thrombosis may lead to transient thrombocytopenia and anemia. A subset have macrovascular shunts from the hepatic arteries and/or portal veins to the hepatic veins and can result in high-output cardiac failure. The role of pharmacotherapy remains unclear. Embolization may be indicated for symptomatic shunts. Resection is rarely indicated.

VENOUS MALFORMATIONS AND ASSOCIATED CONDITIONS

Scenario: A 2-year-old male is referred with a bluish 'mass' on his back, which was noticed at birth and has since become larger with intermittent pain. On physical examination, he has a 3-cm soft, bluish, compressible lesion on his upper back with several small hard areas within this mass (**Figure 59.2a**).

Question: What is your diagnosis? What is the underlying pathogenesis?
Answer: This is consistent with a venous malformation (VM), the most common vascular malformation. They are present at birth but may not become apparent until later depending on the anatomic location. VMs enlarge proportionally to the patient's growth, though growth may be exaggerated during puberty. Phlebothrombosis secondary to stasis can lead to episodes of acute pain and the development of palpable phleboliths.

Glomuvenous malformations (GVMs), a variant of VM, typically occur superficially as multiple blue to deep purple nodules or plaques on the trunk or extremities.

Approximately 90% of VMs are sporadic, with half of these resulting from a somatic mutation in TIE-2 and its associated TEK gene. GVMs are frequently caused by loss-of-function mutations in glomulin, affecting vascular smooth muscle cell differentiation.

Question: What diagnosis should you consider if the child was found to have multifocal VMs diffusely spread across his body, including palms and soles (Figure 59.2b), as well as intermittent rectal bleeding?
Answer: This presentation should raise concern for blue rubber bleb nevus syndrome (BRBNS), a rare disorder of multifocal VMs primarily affecting the skin and gastrointestinal tract (**Figure 59.2c**). Chronic, sometimes occult, gastrointestinal bleeding leading to anemia is common and warrants further workup with endoscopy.

Question: What VM-related complications should you be concerned about?
Answer: Large, deep, and/or phlebolith-containing VMs can be complicated by localized intravascular coagulopathy due to stasis and stagnation of blood within the malformation. This leads to consumption of coagulation factors, causing a prolonged prothrombin time, decreased fibrinogen, and elevated D-dimers.

Additional complications may occur based on anatomic location. Cervicofacial VMs can distort facial features, synovial lining VMs can cause

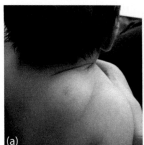
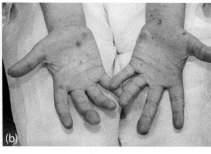
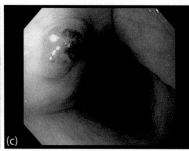

Figure 59.2 Venous malformations. (a) Venous malformation in the subcutaneous tissues of the upper back. (b) Classic cutaneous venous malformations on the palms of blue rubber bleb nevus syndrome (BRBNS). (c) Venous malformation of the colon seen in BRBNS.

hemarthrosis, gastrointestinal tract VMs can cause gastrointestinal bleeding, and rectal VMs associated with mesenteric vein ectasia portend a risk of portomesenteric venous thrombosis.

Question: When would you treat VMs? What are your treatment options?

Answer: Indications for treatment include pain, functional loss, bleeding, and appearance. Focal VMs may be successfully excised. For diffuse VMs of the extremities, compression therapy can achieve significant improvement in size and symptoms. Sclerotherapy can be an effective option for symptomatic VMs, sometimes requiring staged sessions and embolization of large draining channels. It may also be performed prior to surgical resection to allow for removal of larger lesions. Transfusion-dependent anemia secondary to gastrointestinal VMs can be treated with wedge excisions and polypectomy for multifocal VMs of BRBNS or colectomy, anorectal mucosectomy, and coloanal pull-through for diffuse colorectal VMs. Sirolimus has been demonstrated to reduce pain, bleeding, and improve quality of life (QoL) associated with VMs. The use of low-molecular-weight heparin in the setting of elevated D-dimer levels may also provide pain relief. Enoxaparin can be used preventatively to avoid disseminated intravascular coagulation in patients having surgery.

LYMPHATIC MALFORMATIONS AND ASSOCIATED CONDITIONS

Scenario: You receive a consult for a 30-year-old female at 35 weeks gestation whose fetus was found to have a complex cystic mass with septations of her right thigh (**Figure 59.3a**).

Question: What is your diagnosis and the expected postnatal course?

Answer: This is consistent with a macrocystic lymphatic malformation (LM). LMs are thin-walled vascular channels lined by lymphatic endothelial cells and can be microcystic, macrocystic, or combined. LMs represent a benign condition, though morbidity depends on the anatomic extent and location. Postnatal treatment options may include sclerotherapy, surgical debulking/resection, and pharmacotherapy with sirolimus.

Question: Postnatal imaging is consistent with an LM. The neonate undergoes debulking and intralesional sclerotherapy with doxycycline and is discharged home. What are the main complications of LM?

Answer: LMs carry a risk of intralesional bleeding from rupture of small vessels within the LM. These bleeds are typically self-limited due to

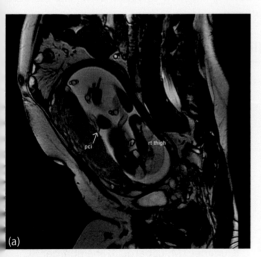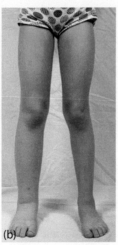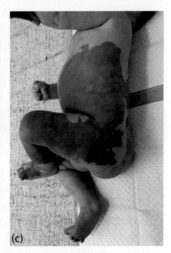

Figure 59.3 Types of lymphatic malformations. (a) Fetal MRI demonstrating a large macrocystic lymphatic malformation of the right thigh. (b) Child with congenital lymphedema of the right lower extremity (Courtesy of Dr. Arin Greene.) (c) Infant with a capillary-lymphatico-venous malformation (CLVM) of the left lower extremity and abdomen consistent with Klippel-Trenaunay syndrome.

tamponade of the causative small vessels. LMs are also at risk for infection, ranging from cellulitis to septic shock. Antibiotics should be promptly initiated.

> **Scenario:** A 3-year-old female is referred with 'swelling' of her lower extremity. On physical examination, the child has unilateral swelling of the right lower extremity, non-tender to palpation (**Figure 59.3b**). Pulse exam is normal with no skin lesions or rashes.

Question: What type of lymphatic anomaly should you consider?

Answer: The presentation is suspicious for primary congenital lymphedema. Lymphedema is marked by chronic progressive swelling due to abnormal accumulation of protein-rich fluid in the interstitial tissues secondary to abnormal development (primary) or injury to lymph nodes or lymphatic vessels (secondary).

Question: What gold-standard diagnostic test should be ordered? What treatment options can be offered?

Answer: Lymphoscintigraphy is the gold-standard study to diagnose lymphedema and quantitatively assess lymphatic function. There is no cure for lymphedema. Many patients can be managed with conservative therapy, including patient education on activities of daily living and compression therapy of the affected area. Operative intervention is considered only when conservative management fails in the following settings: The affected involved area is too heavy and prohibits participation in daily living, recurrent infection, and cosmetic concerns. Approaches may include attempts to correct the underlying lymphatic defect and excisional procedures.

Question: Again, consider a 6-month-old male being referred with 'swelling' of his lower extremity. What is your leading diagnosis if physical examination demonstrates an enlarged lower extremity with a lateral capillary malformation (CM), lymphatic vesicles, visible varicosities, and limb length discrepancy (Figure 59.3c)? Comment on the association with *PIK3CA*-related overgrowth spectrum (PROS).

Answer: The presentation is consistent with Klippel-Trenaunay syndrome (KTS), a capillary-lymphatico-venous malformation (CLVM) most commonly involving the lower extremities. The involved limb has progressive soft tissue and skeletal hypertrophy, though the severity of disease varies widely. Pelvic involvement with LM and VM may occur and can be complicated by recurrent infections, hematuria, hematochezia, and bladder outlet obstruction. Additionally, anomalous connections to the femoral or iliac veins or inferior vena cava carry a risk of pulmonary embolism. Imaging studies are important in the evaluation of these patients, including plain films to assess for limb length discrepancies, MRI to describe the type and extent of each of the vascular malformation components, and MRV to elucidate anomalous venous channels. Treatment is typically conservative and centered on symptoms. Treatment modalities include compression therapy, sirolimus (an mTOR inhibitor in the TIE2/PIK3 pathway), sclerotherapy, endovenous laser ablation or resection, and surgical debulking.

KTS harbors a mutation in the *PIK3CA* gene and is therefore included in PROS. PROS includes a number of conditions, such as CLOVES syndrome and MCAP, with shared phenotypic features of tissue overgrowth and underlying somatic mutations in *PIK3CA*. There are ongoing efforts to develop targeted therapies along the *PIK3CA* pathway.

BIBLIOGRAPHY

1. Mulliken JB, Burrows PE, Fishman SJ. Mulliken and Young's Vascular Anomalies: Hemangiomas and Malformations (second edition). Oxford University Press 2013
2. Duggan EM, Fishman SJ. Vascular Anomalies IN Holcomb III GW, Murphy JP and St. Peter SD eds. Holcomb Ashcraft's Pediatric Surgery (seventh edition). Elsevier 2020: 1147–1170
3. Kulungowski AM, Fishman SJ. Vascular Anomalies IN Coran AG, Adzick NS, Krummel TM, Laberge J, Shamberger RC and Caldamone AA eds. Pediatric Surgery (seventh edition). Elsevier 2012: 1613–1630

4. Dompmartin A, Vikkula M, Boon LM. Venous Malformation: update on ethio-pathogenesis, diagnosis & management. Phlebology. 2010; 25:224–235.
5. Maruani A, Tavernier E, Boccara O et al. Sirolimus (Rapamycin) for slow-flow malformation in children the observational-phase randomized clinical PERFORMUS trial. JAMA Dermatology. 2021; 157: 1289–1298
6. ISSVA Classification of Vascular Anomalies. 2018. www.issva.org/classification

60

Pediatric endocrine tumors

SIMONE DE CAMPOS VIEIRA ABIB
Pediatric Oncology Institute - GRAACC - Federal University of São Paulo,
São Paulo, Brazil

Pediatric endocrine tumors are tumors of the endocrine glands – hypothalamus, pineal, pituitary, thyroid, adrenal and gonads – and those that originate from neuroendocrine cells are termed neuroendocrine tumors (NETs). All are rare, and this chapter will seek to describe those which are more frequent in pediatric practice with typical scenarios outlined.

THYROID TUMORS

Thyroid cancer in children is relatively rare: 4.8–5.9 cases per 1 million people aged 0–19 years, accounting for approximately 1.5% of all cancers at this age group. They are more frequent in females.[1] The literature has shown a trend toward an increase in the incidence of thyroid cancer, particularly in children and adolescents.[2–4]

Approximately 2% of children present with palpable thyroid nodules, and most of them are benign (inflammatory lesions and follicular adenomas), but some are malignant.[5] Children and adolescents may present with nodules, palpable cervical lymph nodes and sometimes with distant metastases at diagnosis.

The papillary subtype is the most common, accounting for approximately 60% of the index cases, followed by the papillary follicular variant subtype (20%–25%), the follicular subtype (10%) and the medullary subtypes (<10%). The incidence of the papillary subtype and its follicular variant peaks between the ages of 15 and 19 years. The incidence of medullary thyroid cancer is highest in the age groups of 0–4 years and declines at older ages.[6]

Papillary carcinomas are typically multifocal, diffuse, bilateral and present with lymphadenopathies. On the other hand, follicular carcinomas, which are unifocal, metastasize to the bones and lungs and rarely to the regional lymph nodes.

The thyroid gland is susceptible to radiation; thus, thyroid cancer can present as a second late malignancy in children treated with radiotherapy or as result of environmental contamination. Thyroid cancer risks are related to the dose of radiation and are notably higher in children that were irradiated before 5 years of age and when the thyroid was near or part of the medical therapy irradiated field. For this reason, it is more frequent in Hodgkin and non-Hodgkin lymphomas than in children with leukemias and central nervous tumors.

Papillary thyroid carcinoma is the most frequent form of thyroid carcinoma diagnosed after radiation exposure. Molecular alterations, including intrachromosomal rearrangements, are frequently found, among them *RET/PTC* rearrangements being the most common.[7]

Medullary thyroid carcinoma is caused by a mutation in the *RET* proto-oncogene associated with multiple endocrine neoplasia (MEN) type 2, either MEN2A or MEN2B.[8]

Thyroid carcinomas can occur as familial cancers or be related to cancer syndromes, such as *DICER1* Carney complex, *APC*-associated polyposis, *PTEN* hamartoma tumor syndrome and Werner syndrome.

DOI: 10.1201/9781003182290-67

Thyroid cancer in children tends to present as advanced tumors and will have lymph node involvement and other metastases more frequently detected in comparison to adults and a higher recurrence rate during the first decade after diagnosis.

Workup

When a child or adolescent presents with a thyroid nodule, it is important to evaluate the lesion through ultrasound and serum thyroid-stimulating hormone (TSH) and thyroglobulin. Fine needle aspiration (FNA) and sometimes open biopsies are needed to confirm the diagnosis.

Computed tomography or magnetic resonance imaging are important for surgical planning and to evaluate the tumor relation with the aerodigestive tract. The chest should be evaluated for metastasis, especially when lymphadenopathy is detected.

Treatment

Surgery is the mainstay of treatment for thyroid cancer.[5,9] Total thyroidectomy is indicated for patients with papillary, follicular, or medullary carcinoma and should be best performed by experienced surgeons. Since medullary carcinomas are frequently associated with MEN2 syndrome, early genetic testing and counseling are indicated, and prophylactic surgery is recommended for children with the *RET* germline mutation. The rationale for total thyroidectomy is that there is an increased incidence of bilateral (30%) and multifocal (65%) disease. Additionally, it facilitates the use of radioactive iodine therapy. In patients with a small unilateral localized tumor, a near-total thyroidectomy may be considered. Evaluation of lymph nodes is of essence.

Central neck dissection (CND, also called level VI neck dissection) is recommended when there is central and/or lateral disease invasion or in case of distant metastases. Lateral neck dissection (LND) should be undertaken if there is cytological confirmation of invasion of one or more of the lateral lymph nodes. Surgical complications may include injury to one or both recurrent laryngeal nerves, which can be minimized with the use of intraoperative nerve monitoring, and hypoparathyroidism.

Postoperative treatment should then include thyroid hormone replacement. For staging purposes, the TMN system is used for pediatric thyroid cancer. Depending on staging, additional therapy with iodine I 131 (I^{131}) will be indicated. Vandetanib, cabozantinib and selpercatinib can also be used. Overall, pediatric thyroid tumors have an excellent prognosis.

ADRENAL TUMORS

Adrenal tumors in children may be linked with various conditions and may also be diagnosed prenatally or in the more advanced ages in childhood.[10–13]

By 3 years of age, the adrenal gland in children has acquired all the differentiated adrenal zone layers: Glomerulosa, reticularis and fasciculata zone. The glomerulosa zone is responsible for secreting mineralocorticoids such as aldosterone. The fasciculata zone is responsible for secreting glucocorticoids. The reticularis zone produces adrenal sex androgens, which serve as precursors for testosterone. At the center of the organ is the medulla. The chromaffin cells located here are responsible for the production of catecholamines, namely epinephrine, norepinephrine and dopamine. Tumors that originate from the cortex are frequently hormone-producing and clinically can cause combined patterns of virilization (precocious puberty, deepening voice, pubic and axillary hair, acne, genital growth) and/or Cushing syndrome (hypertension, central obesity, buffalo hump, moon face, stretch marks), hyperaldosteronism or may be asymptomatic. Since hormone-related symptoms are very important, most patients may have small adrenal masses, which are not palpable, but palpable masses can be present in patients with or without hormone-secretive adrenal tumors.

Tumors originating from the adrenal medulla are characteristically neuroblastomas/ganglioneuromas or pheochromocytomas (please refer to the section on paragangliomas and pheochromocytomas).

Differential diagnosis

The adrenal glands may also be involved in tumors originating from surrounding structures (kidney, stomach, pancreas, spleen, sympathetic chain, peritoneum and retroperitoneum) or bear metastasis from lymphomas or other rare conditions (equinococcus cysts, neurofibromas, granulomatosis, myelolipoma, xanthomatosis).[14] Thus lesions such as schwannomas, neuroblastic tumors, neurofibromas, peritoneal cysts, myofibroblastic tumors, retroperitoneal teratomas, sarcomas, lymphomas, lipomas, echinococcus cysts, granulomatosis and xanthomatosis should be considered in a wide-ranging differential diagnosis. Adrenal hemorrhages(s), congenital adrenal hyperplasia (CAH), urinary or enteric duplication cysts, adrenal heterotopia, extralobar sequestration,[15] ganglioneuroma, neuroblastoma and neonatal adrenocortical carcinomas should also be considered in the neonate and fetus.

It is therefore essential to establish the correct working diagnosis to guide effective treatment. Surgical principles for each type of tumor should be followed strictly in order to avert complications and contribute to overall better cure rate and survival.

Adrenocortical Tumors

Adrenocortical tumors (ACTs) are rare, comprising 0.2% of all pediatric malignancies.[16]

The estimated worldwide incidence is about 0.3 new cases per million individuals per year.[17] Although considered rare tumors, it is very important that surgeons are clearly aware of these rare tumors so that prompt diagnosis and effective treatments are established.

In the south and southeast regions of Brazil, ACT disease incidence rates are 15–20 times higher than those described in other countries. The ACT clustering in Brazil is due to the presence of the TP53 mutation in this native population.[18,19]

Germline TP53 mutations are present in more than 80% of ACTs in children, and they underlie signaling abnormalities that are strongly associated with ACT. ACTs are also the most frequent neoplasms identified in families afflicted with Li-Fraumeni syndrome and also are present in Beckwith-Wiedemann syndrome. De novo TP53 mutations also occur sporadically, and relatives of children with ACT may have a higher incidence of cancers.[20,21]

Workup

Most pediatric ACTs are symptomatic. Tumor biopsy is not performed to confirm diagnosis. It is crucial to avoid tumor rupture in resectable adrenal tumors. It is therefore strongly recommended that up-front biopsies not be performed.

Serum hormone levels of adrenocorticotropic hormone, cortisol, 17-hydroxyprogesterone, androstenedione, dehydroepiandrosterone sulfate (DHEA-S), testosterone, estradiol, renin and aldosterone all contribute to diagnosis and can be used to monitor and detect recurrence.[16,20,22]

Imaging studies (CT or MRI) are obtained to confirm the origin of site of the tumor, for staging and for surgical planning. Disease evaluation of surrounding structures, lymph node enlargement and vascular extension (which occurs in 20% of cases)[23] should be done. Distant metastasis should be carefully searched for in the liver, lungs and bones.

The COG ARAR0332 staging system is based on image and surgical findings (**Table 60.1**). Tumor weight, local invasion and distant metastases are the most important prognostic factors in ACT.[22,24–26]

Tumor rupture has the greatest impact on prognosis, as well as tumor weight and staging.[27]

Surgery is the only curative treatment in ACT. Patients with incomplete resection or metastatic disease have a very poor prognosis. Preoperative, intraoperative and postoperative corticosteroid supplementation is very important to avert adrenal insufficiency because of the sudden decrease in hormone production after the tumor is resected.

The aim of surgery is to achieve complete resection without rupture and lymph node evaluation. Sometimes it is necessary to resect other structures en bloc in order to achieve R0 complete resection. Although rupture can occur due to tumor friability/consistency and for anatomical reasons, i.e. the

Table 60.1 Proposed staging of adrenocortical tumors in children

Stage	Definition
I	Completely resected, small tumors (<100 g and <200 cm³) with normal postoperative hormone levels
II	Completely resected, large tumors (≥100 g or ≥200 cm³) with normal postoperative hormone levels
III	Unresectable, gross, or microscopic residual disease
	Tumor spillage
	Patients with Stage I and II tumors who fail to normalize hormone levels after surgery
	Patients with retroperitoneal lymph node involvement
IV	Presence of distant metastases

suprarenal fossa on the liver surface, just to the right of the inferior vena cava, is in close proximity with the liver capsule on the bare area of the liver and may be commonly fixed to it by loose areolar tissue. In some cases, the right adrenal gland tumor is firmly adherent to the liver by a fibrous union of the capsules[28]; the surgeon is therefore presented with a great challenge in avoiding rupture and should be extremely careful while performing gross excision of the tumor.

In general, surgical access is undertaken by open classical approaches – laparotomy or thoraco-laparotomy. Patients with ACT have inferior survival outcomes with higher disease relapse rates, especially in very large tumors. Although minimally invasive surgery (MIS) is feasible and tempting in many cases, the author strongly recommends MIS resection should always be carefully considered and performed only by experienced endoscopic surgeons at high-volume centers and with small tumors (tumors <5 cm) showing benign characteristics on imaging. Thoraco-laparotomy provides excellent access with massive tumors sited adherent to liver with better hemorrhage control.

Disease evaluation with lymph node sampling is considered a standard procedure in surgical oncology, though macroscopically enlarged lymph nodes are not frequent in ACTs. Full lymph node dissection has yet to become a formal component of radical adrenalectomy. The Children's Oncology Group (COG) ARAR 0332 prospective trial evaluated the need for retroperitoneal lymph node dissection (RPLND) in low-stage ACT. It showed it did not impact survival in stage II tumors.[24]

Vascular extension is linked to a very poor prognosis and dramatically alters the surgical strategy. In some cases, cardiac bypass may be needed to achieve R0 complete resection. It is crucially important to evaluate vascular extension preoperatively and intraoperatively at the time of operation.[23] Adrenocortical carcinoma (ACC) thrombus tends to be much more friable than those encountered in Wilms tumor.[27]

The benefits of primary tumor resection or debulking in general (including Hyperthermic Intraperitoneal Chemotherapy (HIPEC)) are yet to be clearly defined in pediatric patients with metastatic ACT. In some cases, it may be rarely indicated because of refractory/resistant hypertension and/or to relieve other symptoms of excess hormone overproduction. Although pulmonary metastectomy has also been reported as beneficial,[29] the exact indications (especially in children) have not been clearly defined. Patients harboring pulmonary metastasis have a dismal prognosis.

A multimodal therapy approach is indicated in patients deemed to have poor prognosis, including use of mitotane, cisplatin, etoposide, doxorubicin and radiotherapy, but the prognosis here remains poor with an overall 5-year survival rate of less than 50%.

It can be challenging for the pathologist to fully determine if the tumor is wholly benign (adenoma), borderline or malignant (carcinoma).[30-32]

Other prognostic factors have not been firmly established for pediatric ACT. Currently, tumor size and disease stage remain the primary prognostic features of the disease.[25,26,30,33,34]

Small tumors can behave aggressively, suggesting that more specific prognostic factors should perhaps be investigated. Obviously, the presence of metastases and/or recurrence confirms the diagnosis of carcinoma.[22,33] Adenomas have an excellent prognosis, but only about 20% of pediatric ACTs are thus classified. The Weiss histopathologic system is the most commonly used method for assessing malignancy because of its simplicity and reliability.[35,36] Distant metastases and tumor volume >200 cm^3 were associated with a poor prognosis in the EXPeRT group (European Cooperative Study Group on Pediatric Rare Tumors), and the National Cancer Data Base has also evaluated prognostic factors for pediatric ACTs.[37,38] Immunohistochemistry has not contributed to robust prognostic analysis.

In order to better define the malignant potential of ACT, a study was conducted to evaluate angiogenic and lymphangiogenic markers in ACT and controls. The first step was an effort to determine normal expression of those markers in the pediatric adrenal gland by studying adrenal glands that were resected with Wilms tumors. Following that immunohistochemistry was then evaluated in adrenal tumors. From the angiogenic perspective, combined levels of vascular endothelial growth factor, endoglin, intratumoral microvessel density (MVD) and cluster of differentiation 34 (CD34) MVD were considered better able to predict prognosis in patients with indeterminate tumor histology. Inclusion of these components in the pathologic analysis of ACT may thus refine classification in pediatric ACT.[39] Lymphatic vessel density was inversely associated with local relapse, implying that pediatric ACC may not disseminate through lymphatic vessels.[40]

Pheochromocytomas and Paragangliomas

Pheochromocytomas are catecholamine-producing tumors that originate from the adrenal medulla, whereas paragangliomas may have the same characteristics but originate from other anatomical sites. They are extremely rare tumors in children.

Paragangliomas can be classified into (1) sympathetic paragangliomas (arise from the intra-abdominal sympathetic trunk and usually produce catecholamines) and (2) parasympathetic paragangliomas (i.e. along the parasympathetic nerves of the head, neck and mediastinum and are rarely functional).[41,42]

Genetic factors and syndromes may be notably associated with paragangliomas and pheochromocytomas including Von Hippel-Lindau disease, MEN2 (pheochromocytomas are associated with mutations with the *RET* gene), neurofibromatosis type 1, familial pheochromocytoma/paraganglioma (associated with germline mutations of mitochondrial SDH genes), Carney triad syndrome, Carney-Stratakis syndrome and other susceptibility genes recently discovered including *KIF1B*, *EGLN1*, *TMEM127*, *SDHA* and *MAX*. Other subtypes depend on the presence or absence of the enzyme phenylethanolamine N-methyltransferase, responsible for conversion of norepinephrine to epinephrine.[43]

Given the higher prevalence of germline alterations in children and adolescents with pheochromocytoma and paraganglioma, genetic counseling and family kindred testing should always be considered.

Children and adolescents classically present with catecholamine overproduction symptoms, such as hypertension, headaches, sweating, palpitations, anxiety, pallor, tremor, dizziness and urinary symptoms. These can be paroxysmal or sustained and may be induced by having anesthesia or during tumor resection.[41-45] It is essential that surgeons and anesthesiologists are aware of such characteristics in order to adequately and safely prepare the patient for surgery and to monitor and deal effectively with any sudden physiologic derangements during the perioperative period.

Parasympathetic cervical paragangliomas do not secrete catecholamines and typically present as a cervical neck mass that can be asymptomatic or have compression symptoms.

Workup

Plasma-free fractionated metanephrines (metanephrine and normetanephrine), 24-hour urine collection for catecholamines (epinephrine, norepinephrine and dopamine) and fractionated metanephrines are part of the workup. Fifty percent of secreting tumors produce and contain a mixture of norepinephrine and epinephrine, while most of the rest yield norepinephrine almost exclusively, with occasional rare tumors producing mainly dopamine.

Imaging for accurate tumor localization and surgical planning includes computed tomography (CT), magnetic resonance, iodine I 123 or iodine I 131-labled metaiodobenzylguanidine scintigraphy and fluorine F 18-6-fluorodopamine positron emission tomography (PET). The latter imaging best detects metastases.[46-48]

Tumor resection is the mainstay of treatment, and patients should receive alpha and beta blockers preoperatively in order to avoid perioperative complications. For those with metastatic disease, chemotherapy with gemcitabine and docetaxel or different combinations of vincristine, cyclophosphamide, doxorubicin and dacarbazine may be used. Other therapy options include high-dose 131I-MIBG and sunitinib.[14,49-54]

It is difficult to determine malignancy in such tumors.[55,56] As some patients may develop a second tumor, postoperative surveillance is key and important with imaging, including whole-body MRI and catecholamine metabolites tests.

PEDIATRIC NEUROENDOCRINE TUMORS

NETs of the gastrointestinal tract and pancreas are extremely rare in children. The estimated incidence is 0.5 cases per million/year.[57]

NETs are sporadic in most cases, but pancreatic NETs are associated with tuberous sclerosis, MEN1, von Hippel-Lindau syndrome and neurofibromatosis type 1 (NF1).[58]

Histopathology is graded by mitotic rate, Ki-67 labeling index and presence of necrosis into well-differentiated (low grade, G1), moderately differentiated (intermediate grade, G2) and poorly differentiated (high grade, G3) tumors.[58-61]

In children, the most frequent tumor sites are notably the appendix and lung (carcinoid tumors).

Pancreatic NETs include insulinomas, gastrinomas, VIPomas and glucagonoma. The first two may be found in children, the others rarely.

Clinical presentation depends on the site, size and active hormone production. There are thus asymptomatic cases or unspecific symptoms (fatigue, weight loss, diarrhea, pain) or symptoms due to overproduction of hormones: Hypoglycemia, behavior disorders, convulsions, coma – insulinomas, Zollinger-Ellison syndrome, abdominal pain, gastroesophageal reflux – gastrinomas. A palpable abdominal mass is rare. Metastatic disease is very infrequent in children, but may present with carcinoid syndrome (flushing, diarrhea, heart failure). Appendiceal NETs are by far usually an incidental finding reported by pathologists on histology exam after appendectomy, as patients may typically present with symptoms of acute appendicitis in 63–75% of cases. Despite this, appendiceal NET is only encountered in 0.16–2.3% of all appendectomies.[62–67]

Bronchial carcinoids are typically endobronchial in location, causing a persistent cough, wheezing, shortness of breath, hemoptysis or chest pain. As such, they may be frequently overlooked and have a late diagnosis. Unlike adults, children are almost always symptomatic, with the most common presentations being pneumonia and recurrent pulmonary infections.[68]

Non-appendiceal carcinoid tumors are more likely to be larger size (cm), higher pathology grade or present with metastases.

Workup

Lab: Complete blood count, complete metabolic profile, coagulation profile. Blood LDH level, NSE, Chromogranin A and urinary 24-hours 5HIAA hydroxy indole acetic acid. For pancreatic tumors: Serum gastrin, glucagon, peptide C, VIP. Serum chromogranin A (Cg A) can help to establish the diagnosis.[69]

Image studies with CT and MRI are used to detect the primary tumor and search for metastases. In pancreatic tumors, sometimes it may not be that easy to accurately determine the tumor by imaging, as tumor nodules may be blurred. 111In-pentreotide scintigraphy, PET/CT with 11C-5-hydroxytryptophan (11C-5-HTP) and bone scintigraphy can also be used.

Surgical resection is the main aim of treatment. When R0 complete resection is not feasible or in those patients with metastatic disease, chemotherapy has limited effect.[70]

For appendiceal NET, appendectomy alone is considered curative adequate treatment for children with tumors less than 1–1.6 cm. In tumors >2 cm and when invasiveness is clinically apparent intraoperatively, then right hemicolectomy should be considered.

For pancreatic lesions, nodulectomies or pancreas resection is considered dependent on location and size of the tumor. For those with liver metastases, transarterial chemoembolization and liver transplantation may be indicated.[71–75]

For unresectable or multifocal non-appendiceal carcinoid tumors, embolization, octreotide, tyrosine kinase inhibitors and peptide receptor radionuclide therapy are valid treatment options.

BIBLIOGRAPHY

1. Golpanian S, Perez EA, Tashiro J, et al. Pediatric papillary thyroid carcinoma: outcomes and survival predictors in 2504 surgical patients. Pediatr Surg Int. 2016;32(3):201–8.
2. Vergamini LB, Frazier AL, Abrantes FL, et al. Increase in the incidence of differentiated thyroid carcinoma in children, adolescents, and young adults: a population-based study. J Pediatr. 2014;164(6):1481–5.
3. Pole JD, Zuk AM, Wasserman JD. Diagnostic and treatment patterns among children, adolescents, and young adults with thyroid cancer in Ontario: 1992–2010. Thyroid. 2017;27(8):1025–33.
4. Schmidt Jensen J, Grønhøj C, Mirian C, et al. Incidence and survival of thyroid cancer in children, adolescents, and young adults in Denmark: a nationwide study from 1980 to 2014. Thyroid. 2018;28(9):1128–33.
5. Francis GL, Waguespack SG, Bauer AJ, et al. Management guidelines for children with thyroid nodules and differentiated thyroid cancer. Thyroid. 2015;25(7):716–59.
6. Dermody S, Walls A, Harley EH. Pediatric thyroid cancer: an update from the SEER database 2007–2012. Int J Pediatr Otorhinolaryngol. 2016;89:121–6.

7. Iglesias ML, Schmidt A, Ghuzlan AA, et al. Radiation exposure and thyroid cancer: a review. Arch Endocrinol Metab. 2017;61(2):180–7.

8. Bauer AJ. Molecular genetics of thyroid cancer in children and adolescents. Endocrinol Metab Clin North Am. 2017;46(2): 389–403.

9. Spinelli C, Strambi S, Rossi L, et al. Surgical management of papillary thyroid carcinoma in childhood and adolescence: an Italian multicenter study on 250 patients. J Endocrinol Invest. 2016;39(9):1055–9.

10. Carsote M, Ghemigian A, Terzea D, Gheorghisan-Galateanu AA, Valea A. Cystic adrenal lesions: focus on pediatric population (a review). Clujul Med. 2017;90(1):5–12.

11. Słapa RZ, Jakubowski WS, Dobruch-Sobczak K, Kasperlik- Załuska AA. Standards of ultrasound imaging of the adrenal glands. J Ultrason. 2015;15(63):377–87.

12. Quinn E, McGee R, Nuccio R, Pappo AS, Nichols KE. Genetic predisposition to neonatal tumors. Curr Pediatr Rev. 2015;11(3):164–78.

13. Baudin E; Endocrine Tumor Board of Gustave Roussy. Adrenocortical carcinoma. Endocrinol Metab Clin North Am. 2015;44(2):411–34.

14. Frey S, Caillard C, Toulgoat F, et al. Non-adrenal tumors of the adrenal area: what are the pitfalls? J Visc Surg. 2020;157(3):217–30.

15. White J, Chan YF, Neuberger S, et al. Prenatal sonographic detection of intra-abdominal extralobar pulmonary sequestration: report of three cases and literature review. Prenat Diag. 1994;14(8):653–8.

16. Liou LS, Kay R. Adrenocortical carcinoma in children. Review and recent innovations. Urol Clin North Am. 2000;27:403–21.

17. Ribeiro RC, Michalkiewicz EL, Figueiredo BC, et al. Adrenocortical tumors in children. Braz J Med Biol Res. 2000;33:1225–34.

18. Ribeiro RC, Sandrini F, Figueiredo B, et al. An inherited p53 mutation that contributes in a tissue-specific manner to pediatric adrenal cortical carcinoma. Proc Natl Acad Sci U S A. 2001;98:9330–5.

19. Pinto EM, Billerbeck AEC, Villares MCBF, et al. Founder effect for the highly prevalent R337H mutation of tumor suppressor p53 in Brazilian patients with adrenocortical tumors. Arq Bras Endocrinol Metabol. 2004;48:647–50.

20. Rodriguez-Galindo C, Figueiredo BC, Zambetti GP, et al. Biology, clinical characteristics, and management of adrenocortical tumors in children. Pediatr Blood Cancer. 2005;45(3):265–73.

21. Pinto EM, Zambetti GP, Rodriguez-Galindo C. Pediatric adrenocortical tumours. Best Pract Res Clin Endocrinol Metab. 2020;34(3):101448.

22. Ribeiro RC, Pinto EM, Zambetti GP, et al. The International Pediatric Adrenocortical Tumor Registry initiative: contributions to clinical, biological, and treatment advances in pediatric adrenocortical tumors. Mol Cell Endocrinol. 2012;351:37e43.

23. Ribeiro RC, Schettini ST, Abib S de CV, et al. Cavectomy for the treatment of Wilms tumor with vascular extension. J Urol. 2006;176(1):279–83 [discussion 283–84].

24. Rodriguez-Galindo C, Pappo AS, Krailo MD, et al. Treatment of childhood adrenocortical carcinoma (ACC) with surgery plus retroperitoneal lymph node dissection (RPLND) and multiagent chemotherapy: Results of the Children's Oncology Group ARAR0332 protocol. J Clin Oncol. 2016;34(15_suppl):10515.

25. Hanna AM, Pham TH, Askegard-Giesmann JR, et al. Outcome of adrenocortical tumors in children. J Pediatr Surg. 2008;43(5):843–9.

26. Klein JD, Turner CG, Gray FL, et al. Adrenal cortical tumors in children: factors associated with poor outcome. J Pediatr Surg. 2011;46(6):1201–7.

27. Abib SCV, Weldon CB. Management of adrenal tumors in pediatric patients. Surg Oncol Clin N Am. 2021;30(2):275–90.

28. Donnellan WL. Surgical anatomy of adrenal glands. Ann Surg. 1961;154(Suppl 6):298–305.

29. Kemp CD, Ripley RT, Mathur A, et al. Pulmonary resection for metastatic adrenocortical carcinoma: the National cancer institute experience. Ann Thorac Surg 2011;92(4):1195–200.

30. Teinturier C, Pauchard MS, Brugières L, et al. Clinical and prognostic aspects of adrenocortical neoplasms in childhood. Med Pediatr Oncol. 1999;32(2):106–11.

31. Picard C, Orbach D, Dijoud F. Reply to Pathological prognostication of pediatric adrenocortical tumors: is a gold standard emerging? Pediatr Blood Cancer. 2019;66(6):e27710.

32. Weltgesundheitsorganisation, Lloyd RV, Osamura RY, et al, editors. WHO classification of tumours of endocrine organs. 4th edition. Lyon (France): International Agency for Research on Cancer; 2017.

33. Wieneke JA, Thompson LD, Heffess CS. Adrenal cortical neoplasms in the pediatric population: a clinicopathologic and immunophenotypic analysis of 83 patients. Am J Surg Pathol. 2003;27:867–81.

34. Mendonca BB, Lucon AM, Menezes CA, et al. Clinical, hormonal and pathological findings in a comparative study of adrenocortical neoplasms in childhood and adulthood. J Urol. 1995;154:2004–9.

35. Weiss LM, Medeiros LJ, Vickery AL, Jr. Pathologic features of prognostic significance in adrenocortical carcinoma. Am J Surg Pathol. 1989;13(3):202–6.

36. Aubert S, Wacrenier A, Leroy X, et al. Weiss system revisited: a clinicopathologic and immunohistochemical study of 49 adrenocortical tumors. Am J Surg Pathol. 2002;26(12):1612–9.

37. Tella SH, Kommalapati A, Yaturu S, Kebebew E. Predictors of survival in adrenocortical carcinoma: an analysis from the National Cancer Database. J Clin Endocrinol Metab. 2018;103(9):3566–73.

38. Cecchetto G, Ganarin A, Bien E, et al. Outcome and prognostic factors in high-risk childhood adrenocortical carcinomas: a report from the European Cooperative Study Group on Pediatric Rare Tumors (EXPeRT). Pediatr Blood Canc. 2016;64:e26368.

39. Dias AIB dos S, Fachin CG, Avó LRS, et al. Correlation between selected angiogenic markers and prognosis in pediatric adrenocortical tumors: angiogenic markers and prognosis in pediatric ACTs. J Pediatr Surg. 2015;50(8):1323–8.

40. Fachin CG, Bradley Santos Dias AI, Schettini ST, et al. Lymphangiogenesis in pediatric adrenocortical tumors. Pediatr Blood Cancer. 2012;59(6):1071.

41. Lenders JW, Eisenhofer G, Mannelli M, et al. Phaeochromocytoma. Lancet. 2005;366(9486):665–75.

42. Waguespack SG, Rich T, Grubbs E, et al. A current review of the etiology, diagnosis, and treatment of pediatric pheochromocytoma and paraganglioma. J Clin Endocrinol Metab. 2010;95(5):2023–37.

43. Crona J, Taïeb D, Pacak K. New perspectives on pheochromocytoma and paraganglioma: toward a molecular classification. Endocr Rev. 2017;38(6):489–515.

44. Pamporaki C, Hamplova B, Peitzsch M, et al. Characteristics of pediatric vs adult pheochromocytomas and paragangliomas. J Clin Endocrinol Metab. 2017;102(4):1122–32.

45. Pham TH, Moir C, Thompson GB, et al. Pheochromocytoma and paraganglioma in children: a review of medical and surgical management at a tertiary care center. Pediatrics. 2006;118(3):1109–17.

46. Sarathi V, Pandit R, Patil VK, et al. Performance of plasma fractionated free metanephrines by enzyme immunoassay in the diagnosis of pheochromocytoma and paraganglioma in children. Endocr Pract. 2012;18(5):694–9.

47. Timmers HJ, Chen CC, Carrasquillo JA, et al. Comparison of 18F-fluoro-L-DOPA, 18F-fluoro-deoxyglucose, and 18F-fluorodopamine PET and 123I-MIBG scintigraphy in the localization of pheochromocytoma and paraganglioma. J Clin Endocrinol Metab. 2009;94(12):4757–67.

48. Sait S, Pandit-Taskar N, Modak S. Failure of MIBG scan to detect metastases in SDHB-mutated pediatric metastatic pheochromocytoma. Pediatr Blood Cancer. 2017;64 (11).

49. Mora J, Cruz O, Parareda A, et al. Treatment of disseminated paraganglioma with gemcitabine and docetaxel. Pediatr Blood Cancer. 2009;53(4):663–5.

50. Huang H, Abraham J, Hung E, et al. Treatment of malignant pheochromocytoma/paraganglioma with

cyclophosphamide, vincristine, and dacarbazine: recommendation from a 22-year follow-up of 18 patients. Cancer. 2008;113(8):2020–8.

51. Patel SR, Winchester DJ, Benjamin RS. A 15-year experience with chemotherapy of patients with paraganglioma. Cancer. 1995;76(8):1476–80.

52. Gonias S, Goldsby R, Matthay KK, et al. Phase II study of high-dose [131I] metaiodobenzylguanidine therapy for patients with metastatic pheochromocytoma and paraganglioma. J Clin Oncol. 2009;27(25):4162–8.

53. Joshua AM, Ezzat S, Asa SL, et al. Rationale and evidence for sunitinib in the treatment of malignant paraganglioma/pheochromocytoma. J Clin Endocrinol Metab. 2009;94(1):5–9.

54. Nölting S, Ullrich M, Pietzsch J, et al. Current management of pheochromocytoma/paraganglioma: a guide for the practicing clinician in the era of precision medicine. Cancers (Basel) 2019;11(10):1505.

55. Kimura N, Takayanagi R, Takizawa N, et al. Pathological grading for predicting metastasis in phaeochromocytoma and paraganglioma. Endocr Relat Cancer. 2014;21(3):405–14.

56. Kimura N, Takekoshi K, Naruse M. Risk stratification on pheochromocytoma and paraganglioma from laboratory and clinical medicine. J Clin Med. 2018;7(9). https://doi.org/10.3390/jcm7090242.

57. C Virgone, A Ferrari, S Chiaravalli, MD De Pasquale, A Inserra, P D'Angelo, M Funmilayo Ogunleye, A Crocoli, S Vallero, S Cesaro, R Alaggio, G Bisogno, P Dall'Igna. Extra-appendicular neuroendocrine tumors: a report from the TREP project (2000–2020). Pediatr Blood Cancer. 2021;e28880. wileyonlinelibrary.com/journal/pbc, https://doi.org/10.1002/pbc.28880

58. Farooqui ZA, Chauhan A. Neuroendocrine tumors in pediatrics. Glob Pediatr Health. 2019;6:2333794X19862712.

59. Sarvida ME, O'Dorisio MS. Neuroendocrine tumors in children and young adults: rare or not so rare. Endocrinol Metab Clin North Am. 2011;40(1):65–80, vii.

60. Tang LH, Basturk O, Sue JJ, et al. A practical approach to the classification of WHO grade 3 (G3) well-differentiated neuroendocrine tumor (WD-NET) and poorly differentiated neuroendocrine carcinoma (PD-NEC) of the pancreas. Am J Surg Pathol. 2016;40(9):1192–202.

61. Rindi G, Klimstra DS, Abedi-Ardekani B, et al. A common classification framework for neuroendocrine neoplasms: an International Agency for Research on Cancer (IARC) and World Health Organization (WHO) expert consensus proposal. Mod Pathol. 2018;31(12):1770–86.

62. Virgone C, Cecchetto G, Alaggio R, et al. Appendiceal neuroendocrine tumours in childhood: Italian TREP project. J Pediatr Gastroenterol Nutr. 2014;58(3):333–8.

63. Moertel CL, Weiland LH, Telander RL. Carcinoid tumor of the appendix in the first two decades of life. J Pediatr Surg. 1990;25:1073–5.

64. Navalkele P, O'Dorisio MS, O'Dorisio TM, et al. Incidence, survival, and prevalence of neuroendocrine tumors versus neuroblastoma in children and young adults: nine standard SEER registries, 1975–2006. Pediatr Blood Cancer. 2011;56:50–7.

65. Hatzipantelis E, Panagopoulou P, Sidi-Fragandrea V, et al. Carcinoid tumors of the appendix in children: experience from a tertiary center in northern Greece. J Pediatr Gastroenterol Nutr. 2010;51(5):622–5.

66. Prommegger R, Obrist P, Ensinger C, et al. Retrospective evaluation of carcinoid tumors of the appendix in children. World J Surg. 2002;26(12):1489–92.

67. Moris D, Tsilimigras DI, Vagios S, et al. Neuroendocrine neoplasms of the appendix: a review of the literature. Anticancer Res. 2018;38(2):601–11.

68. Dishop MK, Kuruvilla S. Primary and metastatic lung tumors in the pediatric population: a review and 25-year experience at a large children's hospital. Arch Pathol Lab Med. 2008;132(7):1079–103.

69. Stawarski A, Maleika P. Neuroendocrine tumors of the gastrointestinal tract and pancreas: is it also a challenge for pediatricians?

Adv Clin Exp Med. 2020;29(2):265–70. https://doi.org/10.17219/acem/111806

70. Boston CH, Phan A, Munsell MF, et al. A comparison between appendiceal and nonappendiceal neuroendocrine tumors in children and young adults: a single-institution experience. J Pediatr Hematol Oncol. 2015;37(6):438–42.

71. Lobeck IN, Jeste N, Geller J, et al. Surgical management and surveillance of pediatric appendiceal carcinoid tumor. J Pediatr Surg. 2017;52(6):925–7.

72. Boudreaux JP, Klimstra DS, Hassan MM, et al. The NANETS consensus guideline for the diagnosis and management of neuroendocrine tumors: well-differentiated neuroendocrine tumors of the jejunum, ileum, appendix, and cecum. Pancreas. 2010;39(6):753–66.

73. de Lambert G, Lardy H, Martelli H, et al. Surgical management of neuroendocrine tumors of the appendix in children and adolescents: a retrospective French multicenter study of 114 cases. Pediatr Blood Cancer. 2016;63(4):598–603.

74. Njere I, Smith LL, Thurairasa D, Malik R, Jeffrey I, Okoye B, Sinha C. Systematic review and meta-analysis of appendiceal carcinoid tumors in children. Pediatr Blood Cancer. 2018;65(8):e27069.

75. Parikh PP, Perez EA, Neville HL, Hogan AR, Sola JE. Nationwide overview of survival and management of appendiceal tumors in children. J Pediatr Surg. 2018;53(6):1175–80.

61

Vascular access

LAURA PHILLIPS AND HANY GABRA
Great North Children's Hospital, Newcastle, UK

Scenario: A 6-year-old boy with a diagnosis of acute lymphoblastic leukaemia (ALL) is referred to the paediatric surgery services for a central vascular access device for chemotherapy.

Question: What factors need to be considered prior to insertion of a central venous access device?

Answer: Insertion of central venous access devices (CVADs) is one of the most common surgical procedures, and secure venous access is paramount for many patients' management. The various indications for CVAD insertion include chemotherapy, intravenous antibiotics/blood products, parenteral nutrition, blood sampling, haemodialysis and stem cell retrieval. It is important to know what treatment the patient will need in order to decide what type of access is required and for how long, both of which will influence the line type and number of lumens required of the device (**Figures 61.1** and **62.2**).

Various different CVADs can be used. Peripherally inserted central venous catheters (PICCs) have increasingly been popular in recent years for short- to intermediate-term access with some devices being suitable for use for up to a few months (1). In a similar way to tunnelled devices, they allow for ambulatory treatment, but tend to fail earlier and are more prone to occlusion and thrombosis (2–4), with reported complication rates of up to 40% (1). Common veins accessed in this technique, usually via ultrasound guidance, include the long saphenous, median cubital, cephalic and basilic veins. A venous cutdown can also be used to access the vein. The thin catheter is then inserted via a Seldinger technique with the tip positioned in a central venous location. They are available as both single- and double-lumen devices. PICCs labelled "power-injectable" can be deployed for high-pressure infusions such as IV contrast for CT/MRI studies.

Non-tunnelled central catheters may be used for short-term central access and are usually sited in the internal jugular, subclavian or femoral vein in critically unwell patients, either by a landmark or ultrasound-guided technique. In general, they require removal or exchange within 7–10 days.

Tunnelled CVADs may last several years and can be conveniently divided into totally implanted devices (e.g. portacath) and tunnelled external devices (Hemo-Caths, Hickman and/or Broviac). All devices require venous access either via a percutaneous Seldinger technique or via an open cut-down technique necessitating dissection and exposure of the vein with a venotomy for route of entry. Portacaths consist of a metallic or plastic reservoir with a silicone core that is placed in a subcutaneous pocket and sutured onto the chest wall, which can then be attached to a catheter tunnelled under the skin and inserted into a central venous location. The reservoir is accessed via a special Huber needle through the skin, meaning that when the device is not in use, it is completely

DOI: 10.1201/9781003182290-68

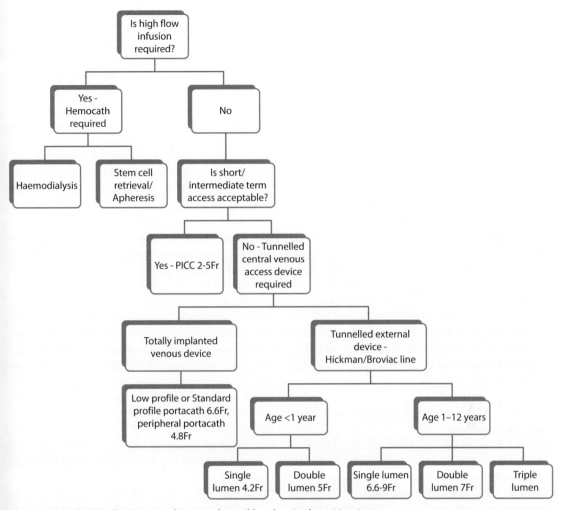

Figure 61.1 CVAD decision-making tool used by the Authors' institute.

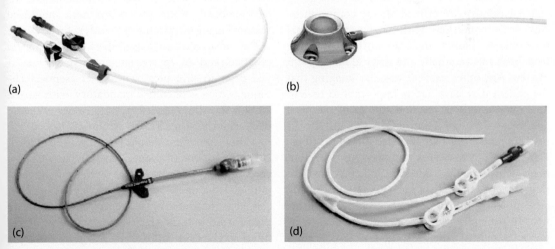

Figure 61.2 Various CVADs. (a) Hemo-Cath. (b) Portacath. (c) PICC. (d) Double-lumen Hickman/Broviac. (PICC: Peripherally inserted central catheter.)

subcutaneous and therefore allows more freedom with regard to daily activity between port use for the patient. A low-profile port can be inserted in most children and a standard-profile device in adolescents or obese patients. Peripheral ports can be conveniently sited on the non-dominant forearm and do not require a neck site puncture; they are smaller in size (4.8 Fr) and are particularly useful in older patients, for example, with mediastinal disease from Hodgkin's lymphoma.

Tunnelled external devices are manufactured from either silicone or polyurethane. They are sited in the vein and tunnelled under the skin to a distal exit site on the chest wall to minimise displacement and infection. They can have multiple lumens and sizes (Fr). A Dacron cuff on the line must be securely placed in the subcutaneous tunnel, which will then embed into the tissues to reduce risks of line displacement, but external fixation and dressings are also used for security. A Hemo-Cath is a specially designed, semi-rigid, large-bore catheter for high-flow situations with two lumens of different lengths, which can be used for treatments such as haemodialysis or apheresis.

Question: What other preoperative investigations are necessary?

Answer: Particularly in cases of lymphoma, a chest X-ray should be requested looking for mediastinal disease, as this may cause significant superior vena cava (SVC) compression. CT scan is often also required, and alternative types of access should always be considered, such as a peripherally sited port device to avoid general anaesthesia (GA) for those patients that could be challenging and hazardous with critical airway compromise. Any other conditions with known mediastinal involvement should undergo further imaging from both an anaesthetic and surgical safety point of view. Any other relevant vascular imaging that the patient may have had is important to review. This may include ultrasound studies of the head and neck, CT angiogram or MR venography. In patients who have had repeated line insertions, it is important to review the previous operation notes, which may provide vital information as to the patency of the patient's venous system and any other potential difficulties at the time of line insertion. In patients with known difficult anatomy or previous difficult line insertions, consideration

should always be given to further preoperative imaging such as an ultrasound of the neck or CT angiogram to aid operative planning and decision making. Anomalous venous anatomy, which may include left-sided SVC or double SVC, is present in up to 3% of the general population and up to 11% in those with cardiac anomalies, so it is also vitally important to note (5). Consideration should also be given to the patient's recent blood laboratory results including haemoglobin, platelet status and clotting profile, as these may need correcting before scheduling the operation and/or products available for theatre.

Question: What techniques should be used for vascular line insertion, and what equipment is required by the surgeon?

Answer: The most common approach nowadays is ultrasound-guided percutaneous puncture of either the internal jugular or the brachiocephalic vein, with reduced rates of thrombosis and vein loss compared to an anatomical landmark or classical open technique (6–8). Open insertion may still be essential in neonates and in those with failed ultrasound-guided puncture, although percutaneous insertion has been shown to be feasible and safe in newborns (8). A suitable CVAD should be chosen as discussed earlier, with the smallest appropriate gauge (Fr) chosen to reduce the risk of thrombosis and to crucially preserve the vein for future use.

Antibiotic prophylaxis is not routinely required. The patient should be positioned with the neck extended, either using a pillow or shoulder roll, and the head turned to the contralateral side for best exposure. Both sides of the neck should be scanned using ultrasound (13–6 MHz linear probe is the most commonly used device in paediatric practice) and an appropriate-sized vessel identified prior to skin prep, with strict aseptic technique, which is of course mandatory, with varied studies showing reduced infection rates with use of 2% chlorhexidine in 70% alcohol (9, 10).

Venous puncture should be ultrasound guided, either in or out of plane, generally in a supraclavicular location, dependent on the patient anatomy and the operator's skill set. Venous location should be confirmed by needle aspiration and a wire then passed into the right side of the heart or the inferior vena cava (IVC) under image fluoroscopic

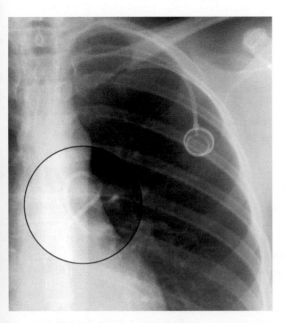

Figure 61.3 Catheter fragmented due to the "pinch off" from its acute insertion angle.

guidance for confirmation. The catheter device can then be tunnelled from the chest wall and measured prior to insertion via the Seldinger technique. Particular attention is required for left-sided CVADs, as sufficient catheter length is required to advance and pass the device along the brachiocephalic vein and prevent the line tip flipping back into the right brachiocephalic vein. The catheter tip location must always be confirmed via image intensifier, as well as the curve on the line carefully checked to ensure the angle is not too acute and to prevent the "pinch off" phenomenon (**Figure 61.3**). All lumens of the catheter must be confirmed to be flushing, working and aspirating easily. Studies have shown reduced rates of displacement with suture fixation of the device (11) and lowered chance of infection/colonisation with chlorhexidine-impregnated dressings (12, 13). Device fixation, such as use of SecurAcaths and recently skin glues and/or other securement devices, can also be considered to further reduce displacement rates (14).

Question: What is the most appropriate catheter line tip position?
Answer: Many studies have identified increased rates of venous thrombosis with proximal catheter tip misplacement, i.e. proximal (15). The ideal line tip location is the superior vena cava–right atrium (SVC-RA) junction, which can be readily identified on imaging fluoroscopy as the point at which the catheter tip crosses the right tracheobronchial angle (16). An alternative way to clearly identify the lower SVC site is its location one vertebral body distal to the main airway carina (17).

Placing the catheter tip in the RA may be associated with increased risk of perforation, cardiac tamponade and arrhythmias (16, 18); however, the distal tip of a Hemo-Cath needs to be best sited in the upper RA for adequate flow for proper use.

Central catheter tip position is also important in PICCs, as this has also been shown to reduce their complications. Upper limb PICCs should have their tip site at the SVC-RA junction and lower limb PICCs at the IVC-RA junction (19, 20).

Question: What are the potential complications of CVAD devices?
Answer: We can conveniently divide these into intraoperative, early and late postoperative complications (**Table 61.1**). CVAD complications can be extremely serious and life-threatening. No procedure should be seen by the medical teams or surgeon as "just a line insertion" and postoperative care is equally as important as the central venous line (CVL) insertion itself in maintaining the long-term function of the devices and reducing exposure to a host of potential complications. CVAD failure (mechanical and infective) prior to completion of therapy is reported in around 25% of patients (2, 21) with the lowest rates claimed with totally implanted devices such as portacaths, whereas Hemo-Caths tend to have the highest failure rates. Overall, complication rates have been recorded in up to 43% patients (21), representing a significant burden CVADs can have on the patient, as well as the economic burden on healthcare systems associated with CVAD use. Infections can occur at the line exit site as well as systemic (catheter-related bloodstream infections) and not only cause significant potential harm to the patient in terms of overwhelming sepsis but are also associated with treatment interruptions, further morbidity and significant complications for the patient. Use of systematic care bundles has been shown to reduce postoperative complications in multiple studies (22–24).

Table 61.1 CVAD complications

All CVADs		
Intraoperative	**Immediate postoperative**	**Late postoperative**
Air embolus	Infection (exit site or blood stream infection)	Infection (exit site or blood stream infection)
Arrhythmias	Mechanical failure – thrombus block or line fracture	Mechanical blockage – fibrin or thrombus, poor flow
Arterial puncture/Vessel injury	Dislodgement	Line fracture/break/"pinch off" phenomenon
Haemothorax/pneumothorax	Tip migration	Tip migration
Bleeding	Haematoma/Bleeding	Venous thrombus/Embolus/Occlusion
Cardiac tamponade	Extravasation	Line removal
Misplaced line	Tamponade/Pericardial haematoma	
Death	Haemothorax/Pneumothorax	
	Death	
Portacaths		
	Pocket haematoma/Seroma	Reservoir erosion through skin
		Line detachment from reservoir
		Reservoir damage/Blockage/Flipping

Source: Adapted from reference 25.

BIBLIOGRAPHY

1. Barrier A, Williams DJ, Connelly M, Creed CB. *Pediatr Infect Dis J* (2012) May;31(5) 519-21 doi: 10.101097/INF.06013e3182457160
2. Ullman AJ, Marsh N, Mihala G, Cooke M, Rickard CM. *Pediatrics* (2015). 26459655
3. Revel-Vilk S, Yacobovich J, Tamary H, Goldstein G, Nemet W, Weintraub M, Platiel O, Kenet G. *Cancer* (2010). 20533566
4. Chopra V, Anand S, Hickner A, Buist M, Rogers MA, Saint S, Flanders SA. *Lancet* (2013). 23697825
5. Azizova A, Onder O, Arslan S, Ardali S, Hazirolan T. *Insights Imaging* (2020). PMC7561662
6. Brass P, Hellmich M, Kolodziej L, Schick G, Smith AF. *Cochrane Database Syst Rev* (2015). PMC6517109
7. Wragg RC, Blundell S, Bader M, Sharif B, Bennett J, Jester I, Bromley P, Arul GS. *Pediatr Surg Int* (2014). 24072203.
8. Arul GS, Livingstone H, Bromley P, Bennet J. *Pediatr Surg Int* (2010). 20549506
9. Maki DG, Ringer M, Alvarado CJ. *Lancet* (1991). 1677698
10. Carson SM. *J Pediatr Nurs* (2004). 14963875
11. Barrett AM, Imeson J, Leese D, Philpott C, Shaw ND, Pizer BL, WIndebank KP. *J Pediatr Surg* (2004). 15486897
12. Lai NM, Chaiyakunapruk N, Lai NA, O'Riordan E, Pau WSC, Saint S. *Cochrane Database Syst Rev* (2016). PMC6517176
13. Ullman AJ, Cooke ML, Mitchell M, Lin F, New K, Long DA, Mihala G, Rickard CM. *Cochrane Database Syst Rev* (2015). PMC6457749
14. Macmillan T, Pennington M, Summer JA, Goddard K, Zala D, Herz N, Peacock JL, Keevil S, Chalkidou A. *Appl Health Econ Health Policy* (2018). PMC6244619
15. Geerts WH, Bergqvist D, Pineo GF, Heit JA, Samama CM, Lassen MR, Colwell CW. *Chest* (2008). 18574271
16. Vesely TM. *J Vasc Interv Radiol* (2003). 12761305
17. Albrecht K, Breitmeier D, Panning B, Troger H, Nave H. *Eur J Pediatr* (2006). 16416274

18. Askegard-Giesmann JR, Caniano DA, Kenney BD. *Semin Pediatr Surg* (2009). 19248995

19. Yamaguchi RS, Noritomi DT, Degaspare NV, Munoz GOC, Porto APM, Costa SF, Ranzani OT. *Intensive Care Med* (2017). 28584925

20. Racadio JM, Doellman DA, Johnson ND, Bean JA, Jacobs BR. *Pediatrics* (2001). 11158502

21. Ullman AJ, Gibson V, Takashima MD, Kleidon TM, Schults J, Saiyed M, Cattanach P, Paterson R, Cooke M, Rickard CM, Byrnes J, Chopra V. *Pediatr Res* (2022). 35136199

22. Chaiyakulsil C, Pharadornuwat O. *Clin Exp Pediatr* (2021). PMC7940089

23. Marsenic O, Rodean J, Richardson T, Swartz S, Claes D, Day JC, Warady B, Neu A. *Pediatr Nephrol* (2020). 31654224

24. Biasucci DG, Pittiruti M, Taddei A, Picconi E, Pizza A, Celentano D, Piastra M, Coppettuolo G, Conti G. *J Vasc Access* (2018). 29148002

25. Scott-Warren VL, Morley RB. *BJA Educ* (2015)

26. Shankar KR, Anbu AT, Losty PD. Use of the gonadal vein in children with difficult central venous access: a novel technique. J Pediatr Surg (2001);36(6):E3

27. Shankar KR, Abernethy LJ, Das KS, Roche CJ, Pizer BL, Lloyd DA, Losty PD. Magnetic resonance venography in assessing venous patency after multiple venous catheters. J Pediatr Surg (2002);37(2):175–9

https://www.smiths-medical.com/-/media/M/Smiths-medical_com/Images/Import-Images/PortACath/titaniumLoproFront_XL.png?h=391

https://www.google.com/url?sa=i&url=https%3A%2F%2Fmedcompnet.com%2Fproducts%2Flong_term%2Fhemo-cath_lt.html&psig=AOvVaw1QDzzQ71gyHZ6SI80wV40Z&ust=1649431165993000&source=images&cd=vfe&ved=0CAoQjRxqFwoTCLjKiv-ggvcCFQAAAAAdAAAAABAD

https://www.google.com/imgres?imgurl=https%3A%2F%2Favascular.com%2Fwp-content%2Fuploads%2Fhickman.jpg&imgrefurl=https%3A%2F%2Favascular.com%2Fhickman-catheter%2F&tbnid=xYBWOD1fIPGPFM&vet=12ahUKEwimu-mkoYL3AhVK-YUKHXx0AJAQMygGegUIARDgAQ.i&docid=2Wyo6gNAn1DslM&w=1500&h=750&q=hickman%20line&ved=2ahUKEwimu-mkoYL3AhVK-YUKHXx0AJAQMygGegUIARDgAQ

62

Infection and the paediatric cancer patient

OLIVER BURDALL AND TIMOTHY N. ROGERS
University Hospitals Bristol and Weston NHS Foundation Trust, Bristol, UK

INTRODUCTION

Infections frequently occur in immunosuppressed paediatric cancer patients as a consequence of cytotoxic chemotherapy that causes myelosuppression and disruption of anatomic barriers to infection including mucosal surfaces and skin. These patients are vulnerable to invasive infections caused by endogenous flora. Three vignettes illustrate specific and severe infections that the paediatric oncology surgeon is likely to encounter.

Scenario: You are asked by the oncology team to assess the perineum of a 3-year-old girl with acute lymphatic leukaemia undergoing chemotherapy. She complains of perianal

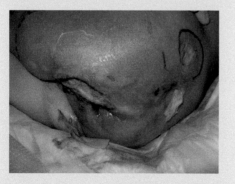

Figure 62.1 Back, buttocks and perineum of 3-year-old girl undergoing chemotherapy for leukaemia.

pain, has a temperature of 38.5 °C and her full blood count shows profound neutropenia. Examination of her perineum reveals perianal ulceration with haemorrhage and necrosis of the ulcer margins (**Figure 62.1**).

Question: What is the diagnosis?
Answer: This is characteristic of ecthyma gangrenosum (EG). There are satellite ulcerations with surrounding cellulitis. The necrosis is caused by a necrotizing bacterial vasculitis which affects the small blood vessels in the skin. The lesions start as haemorrhagic vesicles that evolve into necrotic ulcers over a course of hours to days.

Question: What is the pathogenesis of EG?
Answer: EG is separated into bacteraemic and non-bacteraemic types, where the infection occurs more commonly from haematogenous spread or less frequently by direct inoculation. Therefore, it is important to look for the source of a haematogenously spread infection (e.g. pneumonia). Gram stain of fluid from vesicles shows gram-negative, rod-shaped bacteria that can rapidly indicate the diagnosis. Blood cultures, wound cultures, urinalysis, chest X-ray (CXR) and a biopsy should be obtained.

DOI: 10.1201/9781003182290-69

Question: What is the most common causative organism?

Answer: EG is most commonly, but not exclusively, caused by *Pseudomonas aeruginosa*. Therefore, EG should alert the clinician to possible pseudomonal bacteraemia that in a neutropenic patient carries high mortality. Other causative organisms include *Staphylococcus aureus, Streptococcus* species, *Candida* and fungi. Prompt broad-spectrum antibiotics following collection of microbiology specimens is the mainstay of treatment and must include anti-pseudomonal cover, as this is a key prognostic factor for survival. Treatment must be adjusted once bacterial/fungal culture results are known.

Question: Is there any additional management you would advise?

Answer: The patient has profound neutropenia with a severe perineal infection that requires frequent surgical review. Surgical debridement is indicated if lesions show spreading necrosis. Abscess collections require drainage by aspiration or conservative incision. Granulocyte-macrophage colony-stimulating factor may be administered to aid recovery.

> **Scenario:** A 4-year-old boy presented to the emergency department after a fainting episode. Preceding this, he had a 2-month history of lethargy, tiredness and night sweats. There was no significant family history or past medical history. On physical examination he was apyrexial, was pale, had hepatosplenomegaly and has a palpable lump in the neck. An initial full blood count with differential and blood cultures were obtained, revealing a haemoglobin (Hb) of 32 g/L, platelet count 9 (×10^9/L), white cell count 32 (×10^9/L), neutrophil count 0.31 (×10^9/L) and lymphocyte count 28 (×10^9/L).

Question: What is the provisional diagnosis, and what other investigations need to be done?

Answer: He is pale and has constitutional symptoms, hepatosplenomegaly and a lump in the neck having been previously well. The concern would be that he has developed a malignancy or has an infection. Leukaemia is the most common malignancy in this age group, but lymphoma or a solid tumour would form part of the differential diagnosis. He most likely has leukaemia with haemopoietic failure demonstrated by the very low Hb, neutrophil and platelet counts associated with raised lymphoblasts/lymphocytes. Blood should be sent for flow cytometry to detect tumour cells, and a CXR requested looking for mediastinal widening and pulmonary infiltrates. A mediastinal mass, if present, should be identified before performing diagnostic bone barrow aspiration and trephines.

Question: Broad-spectrum antibiotics were started to treat possible infection. A CXR was normal. A bone barrow aspiration and trephine showed >95% blasts demonstrating infiltration by malignant cells. A lumbar puncture was normal. Fluorescent in situ hybridization (FISH) showed TEL/AML fusion (most common genetic abnormality in childhood acute lymphoblastic leukaemia), and flow cytometry of the peripheral blood confirmed a pre-cursor acute lymphoblastic leukaemia. A tunnelled central line was inserted, hyper-hydration started and chemotherapy including steroids commenced. A month into treatment he started getting abdominal pain, diarrhoea and vomiting. What is the correct initial management?

Answer: Both his leukaemia and the chemotherapy will make him immunocompromised, neutropoenic and at significant risk of infections. Abdominal pain and vomiting may signify the development of neutropenic enterocolitis (typhlitis), infective gastro-enteritis or *Clostridium difficile* enterocolitis. Initial management includes symptomatic control with analgesia and antispasmodics; appropriate fluid resuscitation and transfusion of blood products should be provided as required. Culture and virology specimens (blood/urine/stool) should be sent, followed by prompt administration of broad-spectrum antibiotics pending results to avoid fatal sepsis.

Question: What initial imaging will you request?

Answer: Abdominal radiograph (AXR) as a screening investigation is easily obtained and can show bowel dilatation, bowel wall thickening, ascites, pneumatosis and pneumoperitoneum (**Figures 62.2** and **62.3**).

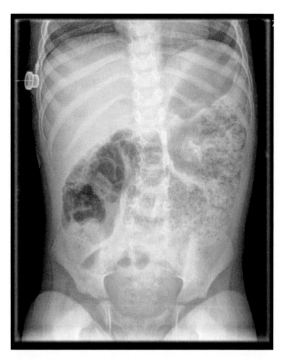

Figure 62.2 Supine abdominal radiograph showing mottled appearance of left colon, suspicious for pneumatosis. The right side of the colon also appears abnormal. There is free intraperitoneal air under the diaphragm.

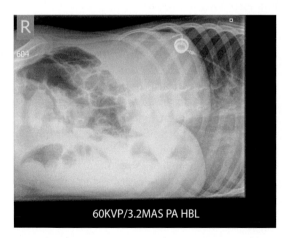

60KVP/3.2MAS PA HBL

Figure 62.3 Right-side-up lateral decubitus abdominal radiograph clearly shows free peritoneal air superior and left of the portacath.

Question: What is the pathogenesis of neutropaenic enterocolitis (NE) compared to *Clostridium difficile* colitis, and how do the radiological findings differ?

Answer: The pathogenesis of NE is multifactorial and involves mucosal injury, neutropaenia and impaired host defence to endogenous gut flora that invade the gut wall. This produces relatively non-specific findings on AXR, including thumb-printing due to bowel wall thickening and air-fluid levels from dilated aperistaltic bowel. This radiological appearance is similar to severe viral gastro-enteritis or *C. difficile* enterocolitis, which is caused by gram-positive anaerobic bacteria that produce two toxins (A and B) that have cytotoxic and enterotoxic effects on the bowel resulting in bowel dilatation, mural thickening and eventually toxic megacolon and perforation. Thus, identification of toxin in stool samples confirms the diagnosis. Pneumatosis can be a feature of both NE and *C. difficile* colitis, but may only be visible in about 10% of patients. Pneumoperitoneum is an indication for surgery. Ultrasound scan features of NE typically show bowel thickening of the caecum, right colon and terminal ileum. Pneumatosis and portal vein gas may also be seen. Abdominal computed tomography (CT scan) can be helpful in demonstrating peri - caecal oedema, fat stranding and free peritoneal fluid or air that inform when surgery is required. CT scan can be helpful in the diagnosis of appendicitis and is important because appendicectomy is the treatment for appendicitis in patients with leukaemia, as non-operative management has been associated with high mortality.

Question: How are you going to manage this patient?

Answer: Surgical intervention carries high morbidity in neutropaenic patients and should usually be avoided. However, this patient has clinical and radiological features of a perforated gut and therefore requires laparotomy. Other indications for surgery when present include uncontrollable gastro-intestinal bleeding and a deteriorating clinical course despite maximal medical therapy. Intraoperative findings of ischaemic or perforated bowel typically require right hemicolectomy with proximal diverting stoma formation. Primary anastomosis carries a high risk of anastomotic leak and should be avoided in neutropaenic cancer patients. Patients with non-perforated NE are treated conservatively with broad-spectrum antibiotics, bowel rest, total parental nutrition, correction of electrolyte imbalances and appropriate blood product transfusion. Antifungals should be considered and granulocyte-colony stimulating factor may be given. Small-volume enteral feeding is continued by some clinicians to try and provide nutrition to damaged mucosa, protect bowel flora and minimize bacterial translocation and sepsis.

At laparotomy the caecum was found to be perforated with pneumatosis and thickening of the colon. The perforation was oversewn and a dysfunctioning ileostomy was created.

Scenario: An 11-year-old girl was diagnosed with Ewing's sarcoma arising in the pelvis and has received chemotherapy and external beam radiotherapy, achieving remission (**Figure 62.4**). Six months later she develops fever and malaise and her blood count showed profound pancytopaenia.

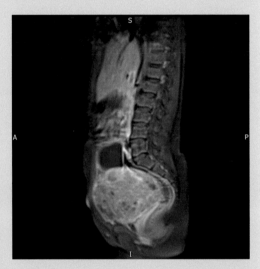

Figure 62.4 Pelvic Ewing's sarcoma filling the pelvis and displacing the bladder.

Question: What do you think has happened?
Answer: Based on the pancytopaenia and her prior history of multimodality treatment for pelvic Ewing's sarcoma, she has most likely developed a second malignancy, the most common being leukaemia (acute myeloid leukaemia). It is also possible that she has relapse of her original tumour with marrow infiltration or has an infection-related pancytopaenia (e.g. Epstein-Barr virus, cytomegalovirus, viral hepatitides).

Question: Investigations show that she has developed acute myeloid leukaemia (AML) with no evidence of recurrent Ewing's sarcoma. She receives chemotherapy and undergoes bone marrow transplantation. **On day 7 after receiving her allogenic graft you are called to the oncology ward to see her as she has developed significant haematuria over the last 24 hours and is passing clots. She has frequent and severe dysuria. What information will you want to elicit on review?**
Answer: Review should include observation of vital signs, blood results, specimens obtained for culture, treatment given and assessment of haemodynamic stability, additional oxygen requirement, haemoglobin levels, clotting profile, platelet count, venous access and pain control. Particular attention should be directed to which chemotherapy agents were used.

Question: She receives blood products to correct anaemia and thrombocytopaenia and is on broad-spectrum antibiotics with cultures (blood and urine) awaited. A patient-controlled analgesia (PCA) has been started. Chemotherapy included cyclophosphamide. What do you think is causing this presentation?
Answer: The haematuria could be caused by platelet deficiency, a urinary tract infection, haemorrhagic cystitis (HC), or radiation cystitis. Cyclophosphamide with the toxic metabolite acrolein places her at significant risk (4–36%) for HC. The BK virus (polyomavirus) subclinically infects most people and can be reactivated when the immune system is compromised and is associated with HC. Adenoviruses, JC virus and herpesviruses have also been identified in HC. Urine microscopy, culture and sensitivity (MC&S), viral culture and polymerase chain reaction (PCR) assay are used for diagnosis. Platelet transfusion corrects thrombocytopaenia. She may have radiation cystitis from her previous pelvic irradiation. Consider Mesna rescue in cyclophosphamide-induced HC.

Question: You catheterize her bladder and drain 200 mL of frank haematuria, but a bladder ultrasound shows large retained clots in her bladder. What else are you going to do for her?
Answer: In an attempt to treat bladder retention, insertion of an irrigating urethral catheter and careful bladder saline irrigations can be tried. Bladder irrigation needs very careful monitoring and should stop immediately if drainage stops (obstruction with irrigation can cause perforation). Urethral catheter irrigation may work for

small non-obstructing clots but is unlikely to effectively treat large obstructing clots. Because of the risk of bladder rupture and urinary peritonitis, there should be a low threshold to go to theatre and perform an open cystotomy, extraction of clot and insertion of a suprapubic catheter and urethral catheter. Alternatively, a gentle cystoscopy and percutaneous suprapubic catheter insertion can be attempted, but the scope view is often very poor with risk of bladder perforation.

Question: She has an open cystotomy, extraction of clots and suprapubic catheter insertion and is subsequently treated on the high-dependency unit (HDU) with continuous saline irrigation, analgesia and supportive care. Urine viral culture shows BK virus, and anti-viral treatment is given. However, she has re-accumulation of clots and multiple catheter obstructions and remains in severe discomfort 3 weeks after her cystotomy. How are you going to manage the situation now?
Answer: Re-accumulation of clots is a serious problem, and a multidisciplinary team (MDT) discussion including the parents is required to decide whether further attempts at removal of bladder clots in theatre is indicated, although it is likely they will continue to re-accumulate. Total cystectomy and ileal conduit reconstruction may be required following informed consent.

A total cystectomy and ileal conduit were performed.

BIBLIOGRAPHY

1. Long SS, Prober CG, Fisher M. Principles and Practice of Pediatric Infectious Diseases. 5th Ed, (Elsevier, 2018).
2. Steinbach WJ, Green MD, Michaels MG et al. Pediatric Transplant and Oncology Infectious Diseases. 1st Ed, (Elsevier, 2021).
3. Korte AKM, Vos JM. N Engl J Med. (2017 Dec) 7;377(23):e32. doi: 10.1056.
4. Vaiman M, Lazarovitch T, Heller L, Lotan G. Eur J Clin Microbiol Infect Dis. (2015 Apr);34(4):633–639. doi: 10.1007/s10096-014-2277-6.
5. Mullassery D, Bader A, Battersby AJ, et al. J Pediatr Surg. (2009 Feb);44(2):381–385. doi: 10.1016/j.jpedsurg.2008.10.094
6. User İR, Akbayram S, Özokutan BH. J Pediatr Hematol/Oncol. (2018 Apr);40(3):216–220.
7. Cheerva AC, Raj A, Bertolone SJ, Bertolone K, Silverman CL. J Pediatr Hematol Oncol. (2007 Sep);29(9):617–621.
8. Decker DB, Karam JA, Wilcox DT. J Pediatr Urol. (2009 Apr);5(4):254–264. doi: 10.1016/j.jpurol.2009.02.199.

PART 8

Urology

63

Prenatal urinary tract dilatation

DIANE DE CALUWÉ AND MARIE-KLAIRE FARRUGIA
Chelsea and Westminster and Imperial College Hospitals, London, UK

PRENATAL URINARY TRACT DILATATION

Prenatal diagnosis of urinary tract dilatation (UTD) occurs in 1%–2% of all pregnancies. The prenatal ultrasound identification of UTD reflects a spectrum of potential aetiologies and uropathies. In many cases, the dilatation is transient and isolated. Half of these will resolve by the end of gestation (transient) or during the first year of life (isolated) (1). Persistent and/or increasing UTD is picked up in 1:500–1:600 pregnancies. Often the aetiology is unable to be fully determined before birth and is therefore diagnosed more often in the postnatal period with additional imaging studies.

Antenatal counselling of prenatally detected urinary tract abnormalities has become an integral part of paediatric urological practice. The aim is to explain possible differential diagnoses of the fetal ultrasound findings to the parents and plan the appropriate postnatal management. Most urinary tract abnormalities are detected on the fetal anomaly scan (18–20 weeks). Progressive dilatation on follow-up (FU) scans may be associated with postnatal uropathies. The larger the size of the anteroposterior renal pelvic diameter (APRPD), the more likely it is caused by obstructive uropathy, the lower the spontaneous resolution rate and the increased possible need for surgery (2). However, this is not the case for vesico-ureteric reflux (VUR). High-grade VUR is not necessarily associated with significant UTD (**Table 63.1**).

Table 63.1 Etiology of prenatal UTD

Etiology	Incidence (%)
Transient/physiologic	50–70
Ureteropelvic junction obstruction	10–30
Vesicoureteral reflux	10–40
Ureterovesical junction obstruction/megaureter	5–15
Multicystic dysplastic kidney disease	2–5
Posterior urethral valves	1–5
Ureterocele, ectopic ureter, duplex system, urethral atresia, Prune belly syndrome, polycystic kidney diseases, l cysts	Uncommon

Source: From Nguyen et al. (3).

In 2014, a multidisciplinary consensus on the classification of prenatal and postnatal UTD was published in order to unify previous established different classification systems (3). The classification system is stratified based on gestational age and whether the UTD is detected prenatally (**Figure 63.1**) or postnatally (**Figure 63.2**).

The proposed UTD classification system is based on six categories in ultrasound findings: (1) APRPD, (2) calyceal dilation, (3) renal parenchymal thickness, (4) renal parenchymal appearance (echogenicity or presence of renal cortical cysts), (5) bladder abnormalities and (6) ureteral abnormalities.

DOI: 10.1201/9781003182290-71

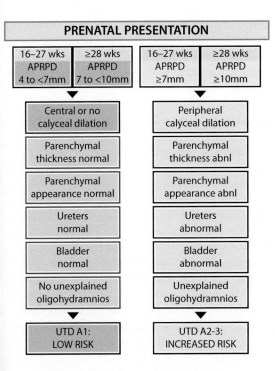

Figure 63.1 Prenatal UTD classification.
Note: *Central and peripheral calyceal dilation may be difficult to evaluate early in gestation. **Oligohydramnios is suspected to result from a GU cause.

Question: How is unilateral antenatal UTD evaluated postnatally?

Answer: Around 80% of mild antenatally detected urinary tract abnormalities will resolve, stabilise or improve on postnatal ultrasound. All babies with antenatal unilateral APRPD >10 mm should have a postnatal scan within the first month of life. A proposed investigation strategy based on the first postnatal ultrasound is the following:

- If the APRPD <10 mm without calyceal dilatation, baby can be discharged.
- If the APRPD =10–15 mm without calyceal dilatation, repeat ultrasound at 3 months and, if normal, baby can be discharged.
- If isolated APRPD >15 mm or >10 mm with dilated calyces, repeat ultrasound at 3 months and, if same or worse, organise diuretic MAG-3 renogram.
- If UTD involves a dilated ureter >4 mm, organise MCUG.

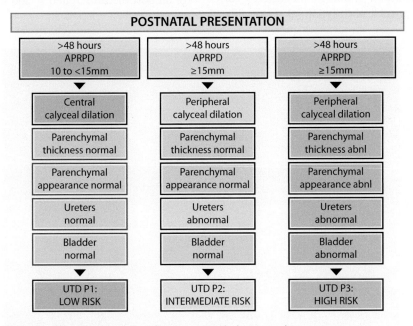

Figure 63.2 UTD classification based on first postnatal ultrasound.

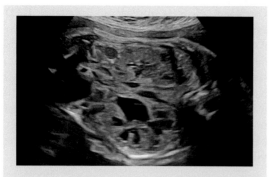

Figure 63.3 Ultrasound shows right pelvi-calyceal dilatation.

Scenario: Unilateral renal tract dilatation.
A 22-week-gestation pregnant woman has her anomaly scan with the following findings. The ultrasound in **Figure 63.3** shows right pel-vicalyceal dilatation (APRPD: 12 mm) and no dilated ureter. The contralateral kidney and the bladder are normal. An FU ultrasound at 36 weeks shows increased right pelvicalyceal dilatation (APRPD: 17 mm). The patient will be booked in clinic for antenatal counselling.

Question: What is the differential diagnosis?
Answer: The degree of dilatation is directly corre-lated with a possible obstruction (2). A non-dilated ureter suggests the obstruction to be at the level of the pelvic-ureteric junction (PUJ), whereas a dilated ureter suggests pathology at the level of the vesico-ureteric junction (VUJ), such as an obstructed or refluxing megaureter.

Question: How will you manage the baby postnatally?
Answer: The baby will be started on prophylactic antibiotics and an ultrasound will be performed between 48 hours and 4 weeks of life to reassess the degree of dilatation. Depending on the degree of dilatation, further investigations can be organised:

- *MCUG*: To confirm/rule out the presence and grade of VUR. This test can be performed at any age. The test is done under antibiotic cover.
- *MAG-3 diuretic renogram*: To assess differential function and drainage. This test is performed around 3 months of age, as the baby's glomeru-lar filtration rate (GFR) will be reduced prior to this.

The scan in **Figure 63.4** shows preserved dif-ferential function (right kidney: 47.6%, left kidney: 52.4%) and a rising, obstructive drainage curve on the left. The MAG-3 in **Figure 63.5** shows no drain-age on postmicturition and 1- and 2-hour delayed images.

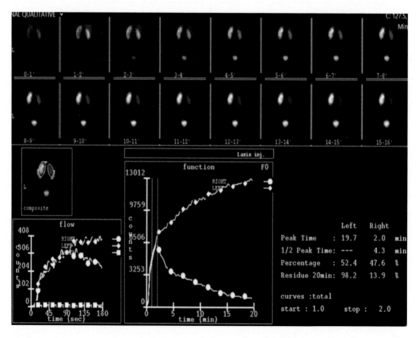

Figure 63.4 MAG-3 diuretic renogram showing obstructive (rising) on left.

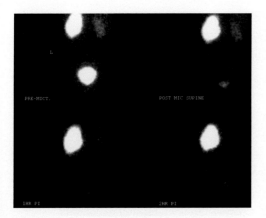

Figure 63.5 Delayed pictures from same study showing no drainage at 1 and 2 hours post injection.

Question: Will the baby require surgery in the neonatal period?

Answer: The key indication for surgery is a reduced differential function (<40%) with a rising drainage curve in the affected kidney, suggestive of PUJ obstruction. Babies with a differential function >40% may initially be safely monitored whilst maintained on prophylaxis. Increasing dilatation on serial ultrasound, break-through urinary tract infection (UTI) and an interval drop in differential function (>10%) are other indications for intervention.

Scenario: Bilateral hydroureteronephrosis in a boy. You are called to the antenatal clinic to counsel a 32-week-gestation pregnant mother with the findings shown.

Question: What is the differential diagnosis?

Answer: Figure 63.6(a) shows bilateral UTD with calyceal involvement. **Figure 63.6(b)** shows a distended thick-walled bladder and a dilated posterior urethra, also known as the "key-hole" sign. The appearance is suggestive of a lower urinary tract obstruction (LUTO) (4). Other information required would be the APRPD, renal parenchymal thickness and appearance (such as echogenicity or the presence of renal cortical cysts), presence of ureteric dilatation and the amniotic fluid index. About 20% are associated with other structural or chromosomal anomalies. The most common underlying diagnoses are posterior urethral valves (PUVs), urethral atresia or prune belly syndrome (PBS).

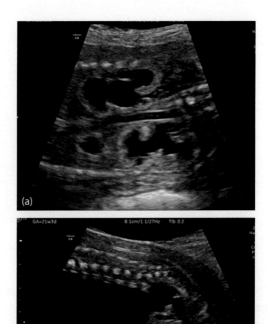

Figure 63.6(a) Ultrasound shows bilateral UTD with calyceal involvement. (b) Ultrasound shows distended thick wall bladder and dilated posterior urethra "key hole" sign.

Question: How will you manage the baby postnatally?

Answer: Following delivery, the baby will require admission to the neonatal unit for catheterisation, start of antibiotic prophylaxis, renal function assessment and renal tract ultrasound. Congenital LUTO may be associated with pulmonary hypoplasia, and hence the baby could require neonatal intensive care support. Once the creatinine stabilises, an micturating cysto-urethrogram (MCUG) should be performed.

Question: Will the baby require surgery in the neonatal period?

Answer: If the MCUG reveals a dilated posterior urethra suggestive of PUV or bladder outlet obstruction (BOO), this will require urgent surgical management. In a term baby, PUV incision may be performed using a resectoscope or hook cold knife. In smaller/premature babies, a temporary vesicostomy is an alternative option.

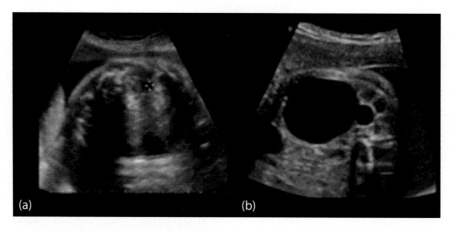

Figure 63.7 (a) Shows a multicystic dysplastic kidney. (b) Antenatal US scan shows simple renal cyst.

Question: What pulmonary changes can occur in patients with PUV?

Answer: Fetal LUTO is known to affect lung development. Although metanephric urine production begins at 12 weeks' gestation, fetal urine only makes a significant contribution to amniotic fluid after 18 weeks' gestation. Amniotic fluid is essential for bronchial branch development in the lungs; hence oligohydramnios secondary to BOO has a devastating effect on the developing lungs. Pulmonary hypoplasia associated with oligohydramnios can be caused by extrinsic compression, lack of fetal breathing movements and lack of pulmonary distension (5).

Question: What are the long-term renal and bladder implications of prenatally diagnosed PUV?

Answer: Studies exploring long-term renal outcome have revealed conflicting results. Some suggest that diagnosis before 24 weeks and prenatal diagnosis overall are associated with a higher mortality and a higher rate of chronic renal failure (CRF), while others suggest that prenatal diagnosis is beneficial to outcome. Sarhan et al. compared the outcome of 310 patients and reported development of CRF in 30% overall: 19% diagnosed prenatally vs. 40% in the postnatal group (6). Kousidis et al. suggested that prenatal diagnosis had little impact on mortality or end-stage renal disease (ESRD) in the first decade of life, as this appeared to be largely predetermined by renal dysplasia and the severity of intrauterine obstruction (7). Ylinen et al. observed no significant difference in progression to compromised renal function (35% prenatal and 26% postnatal diagnosis) in a 10-year FU study (8).

> **Scenario: Cystic changes in the kidney.** The following antenatal scans show a typical simple renal cyst (**Figure 63.7a**) and multicystic dysplastic kidney (MCDK) (**Figure 63.7b**). Contralateral kidneys were normal in each case.

Question: What is the outcome of prenatally diagnosed simple renal cysts?

Answer: Forty-two percent of simple renal cysts resolve spontaneously and are not visible on postnatal scan; 11% remain unchanged and asymptomatic. In the remainder, the postnatal scan shows unexpected findings including MCDK, renal agenesis or an adrenal lesion. Therefore, although simple renal cysts have a benign outcome, a postnatal scan is still indicated to exclude other pathology (9).

Question: What is the incidence of MCDK, and what associated anomalies would you counsel the family about?

Answer: MCDK has an incidence of 1 in 4,400 births. It is more frequently found on the left side (53%), and there is a male predominance (59%). Other urinary tract malformations are described in 31% of patients. Twenty percent have contralateral VUR, of whom 40% are high-grade. Other malformations included PUJO in 5%, ureteroceles in 1%, horseshoe kidney in 0.6% and PUV in 0.4% (10). In females, MCDK may be associated with uterine and genital malformations including obstructed hemivagina and ipsilateral renal anomaly (OHVIRA). A screening pelvic ultrasound at puberty is therefore recommended (11, 12).

Question: How will you manage the baby postnatally?

Answer: A postnatal ultrasound is performed to confirm the antenatal findings. A DMSA scan is recommended at 3 months of age to confirm that the MCDK is non-functioning or poorly functioning and that the contralateral kidney is normal. Prophylactic antibiotics and an MCUG are not indicated unless abnormal ultrasound features are present in the contralateral kidney or ureter (13). Initial management is conservative with clinical review, blood pressure monitoring and interval ultrasound. Longer-term follow-up is advisable for those with renal remnants at 10 years (13).

Question: What is the natural history?

Answer: A long-term prospective study of the outcome of MCDK over 10 years showed that on serial ultrasound, 33% had completely involuted at 2 years, 47% at 5 years and 59% at 10 years. No patients developed hypertension, significant proteinuria or malignancy (13). Indications for surgery are increase in size, change in appearance or new onset of symptoms.

Scenario: Duplex kidney with ureterocoele in the bladder. You are counselling a 36-week pregnant mother with a girl and the images in **Figures 63.8** and **63.9**. The left kidney is normal.

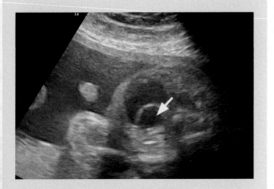

Figure 63.8 Shows a large ureterocoele (white arrow).

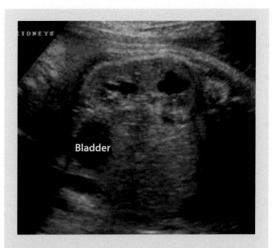

Figure 63.9 Shows a duplex right kidney with a dilated upper moiety.

Question: What is the differential diagnosis?

Answer: **Figure 63.8** shows a large ureterocoele in the bladder (white arrow). **Figure 63.9** shows a duplex right kidney with dilated upper moiety and a normal-looking lower moiety.

Duplex kidney has an incidence of 1 in 100 births, is a normal variant and can occur in one or both kidneys. If there is no dilatation of the upper and/or lower moiety, no further postnatal imaging is required.

However, in this fetus, the upper moiety and upper moiety ureter are dilated, possibly due to a ureterocoele in the bladder. A ureterocoele is a cystic dilatation of the intravesical distal ureter, usually associated with the upper moiety of a duplex system, although simplex system ureterocoeles are also possible. Sometimes there is associated VUR in the lower moiety. The ultrasound findings suggest the possibility of a non-functioning upper moiety caused by an obstructing ureterocoele.

Question: How will you manage the baby postnatally?

Answer: The baby will be started on antibiotic prophylaxis, and an ultrasound within the first month is done to reassess the degree of dilatation if the other kidney is normal. If both kidneys are dilated, there is a possibility of LUTO secondary to the ureterocele; hence the postnatal ultrasound should be done within 48 hours.

The following imaging is recommended:

- *MCUG*: To confirm/exclude BOO and/or the presence of VUR into the lower moiety.
- *DMSA*: Will show differential function of both kidneys and split function of upper and lower moiety of the duplex kidney.
- *MAG 3* (*optional*): To assess if the upper moiety is draining adequately.

Question: Will the baby require surgery in the neonatal period?

Answer: Indications for surgery are obstruction, increasing dilatation on serial ultrasound and UTIs. Cystoscopy and incision of the ureterocoele with cold knife or electrocautery is carried out to decompress the upper moiety and may be the only surgical treatment required (14–16). Asymptomatic ureteroceles may be monitored whilst maintaining prophylaxis.

If the baby re-presents with recurrent UTIs and DMSA has shown a non-functioning upper moiety, a heminephrectomy is indicated. If the DMSA shows adequate function in the upper moiety, excision of the ureterocoele and reimplantation of the upper moiety ureter or a uretero-ureterostomy are possible options.

If VUR in the lower moiety is present and the cause of recurrent UTIs, endoscopic treatment is required.

BIBLIOGRAPHY

1. Oliveira EA, Oliveira MCL, Mak RH. Evaluation and management of hydronephrosis in the neonate. Curr Opin Pediatr 2016;28:195–201.
2. Kaspar CDW, Lo M, Bunchman TE, Xiao N. The antenatal urinary tract dilatation classification system accurately predicts severity of kidney and urinary tract abnormalities. J Pediatr Urol 2017;13:485.e1–485.e7.
3. Nguyen HT, Benson CB, Bromley B, Campbell JB, Chow J, Coleman B, et al. Multidisciplinary consensus on the classification of prenatal and postnatal urinary tract dilation (UTD classification system). J Pediatr Urol 2014;10:982–98.
4. Malin G, Tonks AM, Morris RK, Gardosi J, Kilby MD. Congenital lower urinary tract obstruction: A population-based epidemiological study. BJOG An Int J Obstet Gynaecol 2012;119:1455–64.
5. Peters CA, Reid LM, Docimo S, Luetic T, Carr M, Retik AB, et al. The role of the kidney in lung growth and maturation in the setting of obstructive uropathy and oligohydramnios. J Urol 1991;146:597–600.
6. Sarhan OM, Helmy TE, Alotay AA, Alghanbar MS, Nakshabandi ZM, Hafez AT. Did antenatal diagnosis protect against chronic kidney disease in patients with posterior urethral valves? A multicenter study. Urology 2013;82:1405–9.
7. Kousidis G, Thomas DFM, Morgan H, Haider N, Subramaniam R, Feather S. The long-term outcome of prenatally detected posterior urethral valves: A 10 to 23-year follow-up study. BJU Int 2008;102:1020–4.
8. Ylinen E, Ala-Houhala M, Wikström S. Prognostic factors of posterior urethral valves and the role of antenatal detection. Pediatr Nephrol 2004;19:874–9.
9. Ng J, Loukogeorgakis S, Sanna E, Derwig I, Yu C, Paramasivam G, et al. Postnatal outcome of prenatally-detected "simple" renal cysts: Are they really simple? Early Hum Dev 2021;157:1–4.
10. Schreuder M, Westland R, van Wijk J. Unilateral multicystic dysplastic kidney: A metanalysis of observational studies on the incidence, associated urinary tract malformations and the contralateral kidney. Nephrol Dial Transpl 2009;24:1810–8.
11. Psooy K. Multicystic dysplastic kidney (MCDK) in the neonate: The role of the urologist. Can Urol Assoc J 2010;10:18–24.
12. Farrugia M-K, Hiorns MP, Mushtaq I. Multicystic dysplastic kidney and cystic accessory uterine cavity: A new prenatally diagnosed association. Pediatr Surg Int 2011;27(8):891–3.
13. Aslam M, Watson a R. Unilateral multicystic dysplastic kidney: Long term outcomes. Arch Dis Child 2006;91:820–3.
14. Chertin B, De Caluwé D, Puri P. Is primary endoscopic puncture of ureterocele a long-term effective procedure? J Pediatr Surg 2003;38(1):116–9.
15. Andrioli V, Guerra L, Keays M, Keefe DT, Tang K, Sullivan KJ, Garland K, Rafikov M, Leonard MP. Active surveillance for antenatally detected ureteroceles: Predictors of success. J Pediatr Urol 2018;14(3):243.
16. Aikins K, Taghavi K, Grinlinton M, Reed P, Price N, Upadhyay V. Cystoscopic transurethral incision in simplex and duplex ureteroceles – Is it the definitive procedure? J Pediatr Urol 2019;15(5):560.

64

Pelvi-ureteric junction obstruction

DIANE DE CALUWÉ
Chelsea and Westminster and Imperial College Hospitals, London, UK

MOHAMMED SHALABY
Bristol Royal Hospital for Children, Bristol, UK

PELVI-URETERIC JUNCTION OBSTRUCTION

Most urinary tract abnormalities are detected on the fetal anomaly scan (18–20 weeks). Progressive dilatation on follow-up (FU) ultrasound may be associated with postnatal uropathies. Pelvi-ureteric junction (PUJ) obstruction is the most common cause of urinary tract dilatation (UTD), occurring in 1:1,500 newborns. It is more common in boys and affects the left kidney more but can be bilateral. Other renal anomalies such as multicystic dysplastic kidney (MCDK), renal agenesis, duplex and horseshoe kidney can be associated with PUJ obstruction.

> **Scenario:** A term baby girl had an antenatal diagnosis of unilateral right-sided UTD. She had her first postnatal ultrasound on day 7 of life.

Question: What additional information do you want to know?
Answer: The ultrasound is showing significant dilatation of the right renal pelvis (**Figure 64.1**). You should try to determine from the rest of the ultrasound images the following information if possible:

1. The anteroposterior renal pelvic diameter (APRPD) measured at the renal hilum.
2. Presence or absence of calyceal dilatation.
3. Is there normal parenchyma or thinning of the cortex? Loss of corticomedullary differentiation is a sign of a poorly functioning kidney.
4. Is the contralateral kidney normal?
5. Is there ureteric dilatation on either side?
6. Is the bladder full or empty and does it appear normal?

The right kidney had an APRPD of 45 mm with calyceal dilatation and thinning of the cortex. There was no evidence of distal ureteric dilatation, and the contralateral kidney and bladder were normal.

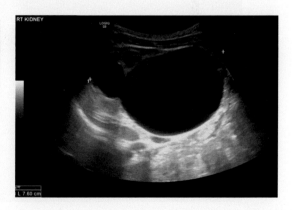

Figure 64.1 The ultrasound showing significant dilatation of the right renal pelvis.

DOI: 10.1201/9781003182290-72

Question: How will you manage the patient?

Answer: The baby will be started on antibiotic prophylaxis and an FU ultrasound at 3 months is performed to reassess the degree of dilatation. If the dilatation persists or has increased, a nuclear medicine (NM) study is performed to assess drainage and differential function of the kidneys.

Question: Which NM study would you ask for? What information are you looking for? What is the difference between MAG-3 and DMSA?

Answer: The most commonly used NM investigation to diagnose upper tract obstruction is 99m Tc MAG-3 (mercaptoacetyltriglycine) diuretic renogram. This has largely replaced 99mTc DTPA (diethylene triamine pentaacetic acid) because of its superior images, faster clearance rate and lower background activity (1).

MAG-3 diuretic renogram is performed around 3 months of age, as the baby's glomerular filtration rate (GFR) will be reduced prior to this. It is a dynamic study that gives valuable information about drainage of the kidneys (renogram curves) and differential renal function.

DMSA is a static study that provides a more precise value of differential function and will show areas of renal scarring if present. The use of DMSA here is reserved for poorly functioning obstructed kidneys where the choice of procedure lies between pyeloplasty or nephrectomy.

The MAG-3 renogram shows an obstructive drainage curve of the right kidney and a reduced differential function of 31% (**Figure 64.2**).

Question: What are the indications for pyeloplasty?

Answer: Indications for pyeloplasty and timing of surgery are not standardised. Commonly used indications are increase of APRPD on serial renal ultrasound, initial differential renal function <40%, progressive deterioration of renal function (>10%) on FU MAG-3 and bilateral PUJ (1, 2).

Babies with a differential function >40% may be safely monitored with serial renal ultrasound at 3- to 6-month intervals whilst maintained on urinary prophylaxis (3).

If the initial differential function <10% and the baby is symptomatic, nephrectomy is indicated.

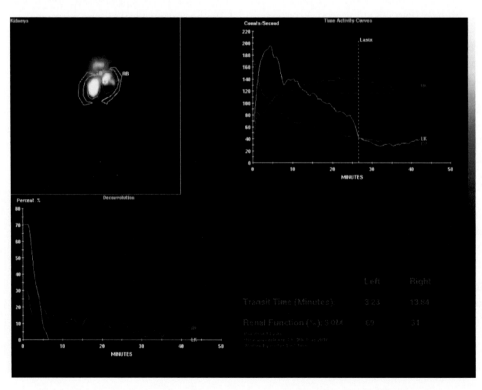

Figure 64.2 MAG-3 renogram showing an obstructive drainage curve of the right kidney.

Question: How would you perform an open pyeloplasty in infancy? What are the possible complications?

Answer: The most commonly used classical open surgical technique is the Anderson-Hynes dismembered pyeloplasty. This consists of excision of the narrowed segment, spatulation and anastomosis in the most dependant portion of the renal pelvis (4). Different approaches can be used including the anterior extraperitoneal approach, posterior lumbotomy approach and subcostal approach. The steps of open pyeloplasty include sweeping the peritoneum medially to stay in the extraperitoneal plane. Gerota's fascia is then opened. The ureter is slung, and stay sutures are placed in the ureter and caudal and cranial extents of the renal pelvis to maintain orientation followed by excision of the PUJ and spatulation of the ureter. The first three anastomotic sutures are placed at the apex, then anteriorly and posteriorly to open the ureter. First the posterior then the anterior wall of the anastomosis are completed with a running 6/0 suture, and any remaining defect is closed pelvis to pelvis.

A stent, when used, can be placed once the posterior wall is complete. Some surgeons prefer to use an external stent that can be blocked at 48 hours and removed after 7 days. Others prefer an internal double-J stent that will need to be cystoscopically removed after 6–8 weeks.

Possible complications include anastomotic leak, injury to surrounding structures, ongoing obstruction at the PUJ requiring a redo operation and stent-related complications such as bleeding, infection or stent migration.

Question: How will you FU the patient?

Answer: Postoperative FU usually includes ultrasound and MAG-3 diuretic renogram. Some paediatric urologists do not feel it is necessary to submit the child to a MAG-3 study if the ultrasound at 6–12 months clearly demonstrates resolution of the dilatation, indicating that obstruction has been successfully relieved. Others will routinely organise a MAG-3 to reassess drainage and differential function of the operated kidney in comparison to the preoperative renogram.

Assessing the postoperative ultrasound findings in a grossly dilated system can be difficult, as considerable dilatation can persist for a long time, despite a technically successful pyeloplasty.

Bilateral PUJ obstruction

The reported incidence of bilateral involvement is around 10% (5). Fewer published management study protocols exist. Patients with antenatally diagnosed bilateral UTD are of more clinical concern because of the risk of deterioration of overall renal function and require careful postnatal monitoring of renal function and urine output.

Micturating cystourethrogram (MCUG) is performed to rule out the presence of vesico-ureteral reflux (VUR) and posterior urethral valves (PUV).

If MAG-3 diuretic renogram confirms bilateral PUJ obstruction, a lower threshold for pyeloplasty is indicated, and staged pyeloplasties with initial pyeloplasty of the worst affected side has been recommended as a safe surgical modality (6).

PUJ obstruction in a duplex kidney

The reported incidence of PUJ obstruction in duplex kidneys is 2%. It tends to affect the lower pole of the duplex kidney and is more common in boys and in those with complete duplications (7).

Diagnosis can be challenging. The overlap in drainage of upper and lower moiety on MAG-3 diuretic renogram makes it sometimes difficult to confirm the diagnosis. Magnetic resonance urogram (MRU) can be helpful as shown in **Figure 64.3**.

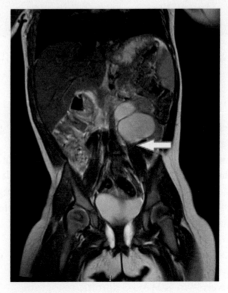

Figure 64.3 Arrow pointing to the level of the lower moiety PUJ obstruction.

Scenario: A 12-year-old boy is referred with a long-standing history of vague, intermittent left flank pain and a more recent episode of frank haematuria. He was born term, and antenatal scans did not show any abnormalities. He never had a urinary tract infection. A renal ultrasound was performed (**Figure 64.4**). The right kidney and bladder were normal.

Late presentation of PUJ obstruction is often caused by extrinsic obstruction secondary to an aberrant crossing vessel, kinks or fibrous bands. Whether the symptoms are solely related to the extrinsic obstruction remains a point of discussion (8).

Children can present with intermittent abdominal or flank pain, recurrent urinary tract infections (UTIs), abdominal mass, renal stones or haematuria.

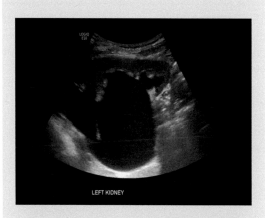

Figure 64.4 Renal ultrasound showing PUJ obstruction.

Question: Describe the findings on the ultrasound.
Answer: The ultrasound shows marked dilatation of the renal pelvis and calyces of the left kidney, with thinning of the renal cortex suggesting a possible obstruction. There was no distal ureteric dilatation.

Question: What further imaging would you organise?
Answer: 99m TcMAG-3 diuretic renogram.

The MAG-3 diuretic renogram in **Figure 64.5** shows preserved differential function (right kidney: 47.6%, left kidney: 52.4%). The uptake, transit and drainage on the right are unremarkable, whilst on the left, the drainage curve is obstructive and there is no further drainage on the delayed 1- and 2-hour images.

Question: What additional imaging can you organise to identify the possible aetiology?
Answer: Magnetic resonance urogram (MRU).

The dynamic MRU in **Figure 64.6** has the advantage of being able to demonstrate a vascular and urinary tract anatomy. It can identify one or more crossing vessels coming from the aorta or the renal artery to the lower pole of the kidney overlying the ureter causing intermittent obstruction, whilst it also will show the exact anatomy of the urinary tract (9). Here, the MRU identified one crossing vessel (yellow arrow) to the lower pole of the kidney confirming a left PUJ obstruction.

Question: How will you manage the patient?
Answer: Depending on the availability of equipment in different centres, minimally invasive surgery (MIS) and robotic pyeloplasty are now well-established procedures with similar high success rates reported in the older age patient group and have now outweighed open pyeloplasty.

The advantages are notably reduced postoperative recovery time, reduced postoperative analgesia requirements and shorter hospitalisation stay (10, 11).

Some surgeons perform laparoscopic transposition of the lower pole crossing vessels (vascular hitch), where the crossing vessel is lifted off the underlying ureter and 'hitched' within a wrap of the anterior pelvic wall. Preoperative selection of patients is critical since there are no definite preoperative or perioperative imaging techniques available to exclude an intrinsic cause (12).

Balloon dilatation and endo-pyelotomy have been described as alternative, less invasive procedures to MIS laparoscopic/robotic pyeloplasty, although reported success rates are lower and long-term FU is lacking (13).

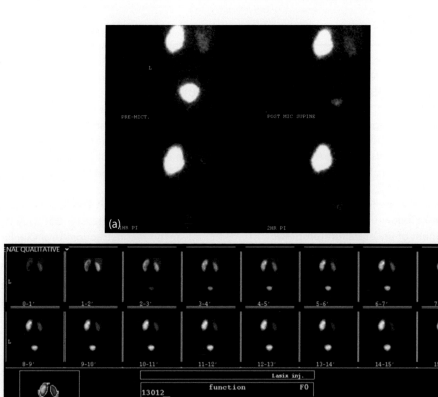

Figure 64.5 MAG-3 diuretic renogram.

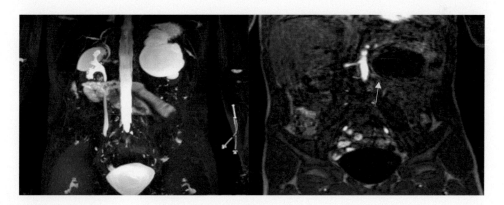

Figure 64.6 The dynamic magnetic resonance urogram.

BIBLIOGRAPHY

1. Thomas DFM (2008). Upper tract obstruction. In: Thomas DFM, Duffy PG, Rickwood AMK (eds). Essentials of Paediatric Urology (2nd ed). CRC Press.

2. Snodgrass WT, Gargollo PC (2013). Ureteropelvic junction obstruction. In: Snodgrass W (eds). Pediatric Urology. Springer, New York, NY.

3. Arena S, Chimenz R, Antonelli E, Peri FM, Romeo P, Impellizzeri P, Romeo C. A long-term follow-up in conservative management of unilateral ureteropelvic junction obstruction with poor drainage and good renal function. Eur J Pediatr. 2018;177(12):1761–1765.

4. Anderson JC, Hynes W. Retrocaval ureter: A case diagnosed pre-operatively and treated successfully by a plastic operation. BJU International (republished). 1949;21(3):209–14.

5. Duong HP, Piepsz A, Collier F, et al. Predicting the clinical outcome of antenatally detected unilateral pelviureteric junction stenosis. Urology. 2013;82:691.

6. Kim J, Hong S, Park CH, Park H, Kim KS. Management of severe bilateral ureteropelvic junction obstruction in neonates with prenatally diagnosed bilateral hydronephrosis. Korean J Urol. 2010;51(9):653–6.

7. Gonzalez F, Canning DA, Hyun G, Casale P. Lower pole pelvi-ureteric junction obstruction in duplicated collecting systems. Br J Urol Int. 2016;97(1):161–5.

8. Cancian M, Pareek G, Caldamone A, Aguiar L, Wang H, Amin A. Histopathology of ureteropelvic junction obstruction with and without crossing vessels. Urology. 2017;107:209–13.

9. Parikh KR, Hammer MR, Kraft KH, Ivancic V, Smith EA, Dillman JR. Pediatric ureteropelvic junction obstruction: Can magnetic resonance urography identify crossing vessels? Pediatr Radiol. 2015;45(12): 1788–95.

10. Tasian GE, Casale P. The robotic-assisted laparoscopic pyeloplasty: Gateway to advanced reconstruction. Urol Clin North Am. 2015;42(1):89–97.

11. Tam YH, Pang KKY, Wong YS, Chan KW, Lee KH. From laparoscopic pyeloplasty to robot-assisted laparoscopic pyeloplasty in primary and reoperative repairs for uteropelvic junction obstruction in children. J Laparoendosc Adv Surg Tech A. 2018;28(8):1012–8.

12. Esposito C, Bleve C, Chiarenza SF. Laparoscopic transposition of lower pole crossing vessels (vascular hitch) in children with pelviureteric junction obstruction. 2016 Oct;5(4):256–61.

13. Xu N, Chen S-H, Xue X-Y, Zheng Q-S, Wei Y, Jiang T, et al. Comparison of retrograde balloon dilatation and laparoscopic pyeloplasty for treatment of ureteropelvic junction obstruction: Results of a 2-year follow-up. PLoS ONE. 2016;11(3):e0152463PR. Bowlin. Pediatric Ureteropelvic junction Obstruction. June 2020

65

Posterior urethral valves

DIANE DE CALUWÉ AND NISHA RAHMAN
Department of Paediatric Surgery and Urology, Chelsea and Westminster
and Imperial College Hospitals, London, UK

POSTERIOR URETHRAL VALVES

Posterior urethral valves (PUV) are the most common cause of lower urinary tract obstruction (LUTO) in male newborns. It is widely debated whether the kidney malformations are secondary to impairment of fetal urine flow and/or manifestations of a primary defect affecting the development of the entire urinary tract (1). Oligohydramnios interferes with lung development and can consequently lead to pulmonary hypoplasia (2).

In total, 35%–55% of boys with PUV are diagnosed antenatally; the others often present in infancy or later in life (3). Postnatally, diagnosis is confirmed by micturating cystourethrogram (MCUG). Initial surgical treatment consists of cystoscopy and incision of the obstructing valves. The bladder in boys with PUV evolves from infancy into adolescence from a low-compliance hypercontractile bladder to a hypo-contractile, large-capacity bladder with poor emptying (valve bladder) as seen on video-urodynamic studies (VUDS).

Boys with PUV require long-term follow-up scheduled by a multidisciplinary team to manage bladder dysfunction and renal insufficiency, as one in three patients will progress to end-stage renal disease (ESRD). Most current studies seem to now suggest that there is little difference in progression to compromised renal function, ESRD or mortality between antenatal and postnatal diagnosed PUV, although results remain conflicting (4).

> **Scenario: Early presentation of PUV.** A 1-week-old male infant is admitted to the accident and emergency (A&E) department with a high fever and vomiting. Mid stream urine (MSU) shows >100 WBC/cm and *Escherichia coli* >10.5th CFU/mL. The baby's blood lab results show hyponatremia, hyperkalaemia, raised urea and creatinine and metabolic acidosis. The mum's antenatal scan at 20 weeks was normal. The baby is treated for urosepsis and started on corrective IV fluids and antibiotics. A urinary tract ultrasound is organised.

DOI: 10.1201/9781003182290-73

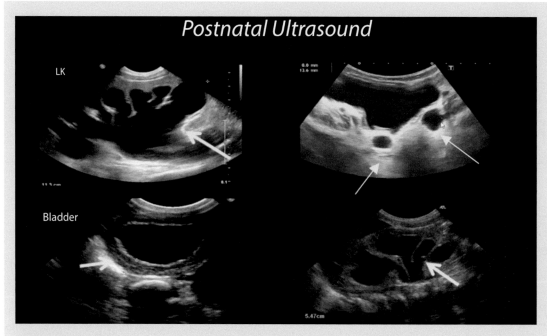

Postnatal Ultrasound

LK

Bladder

The ultrasound shows evidence of bilateral pelvicalyceal dilatation with bilateral distal dilated ureters. The bladder is notably thick walled. The baby did not pass urine during the scan. These findings in a male infant suggest bladder outlet obstruction (BOO).

Question: What would you look for when examining the urinary tract ultrasound if you suspected PUV?
Answer:

1. *Bilateral pelvicalyceal dilatation:* Are the calyces dilated? What is the measurement of the anteroposterior renal pelvic diameter (APRPD)?
2. *Renal parenchyma:* Is there normal corticomedullary differentiation? Does the parenchyma look echogenic? Are there any cortical cysts?
3. *Ureteric dilatation:* Is there evidence of distal ureteric dilatation?
4. *Thick-walled trabeculated bladder:* Normal bladder wall thickness in a male baby is 3 mm for a full and 5 mm for an empty bladder.
5. *Dilated bladder that does not empty:* Does the baby void urine? Assess prevoid and postvoid residual volumes if possible.

Question: How will you confirm the diagnosis?
Answer: Please see the following subsections.

Micturating cystourethrogram (MCUG)

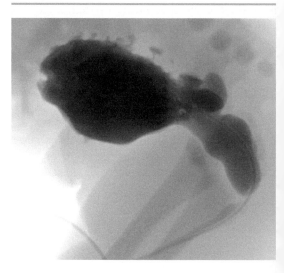

MCU: Lateral view image during voiding for the image

MCUG study has risks of introducing a urinary tract infection (UTI). The test is therefore performed under antibiotic cover (therapeutic dose for 3 days).

The MCUG image shows an irregular bladder wall with multiple diverticulae. There is no associated vesico-ureteric reflux (VUR) visualised. The posterior urethra is very dilated, and there is an abrupt transition zone into a normal-sized urethra.

Question: What would you look for in examining the MCUG study if you suspected PUV?

Answer:

1. Trabeculated bladder wall and/or presence of multiple diverticulae.

2. Presence of VUR, unilateral or bilateral, grade 1 (distal ureter) to grade 5 (intrarenal reflux VUR with clubbing of the calyces and tortuous dilated ureters).
3. Dilated posterior urethra (lateral views during urinary voiding phase with and without catheter) with acute transition zone into a normal-sized urethra.
4. Reflux of contrast into the ejaculatory ducts secondary to elevated bladder and urethral pressures.
5. Incomplete bladder emptying.

Question: What further imaging would you organise?

Answer: Please see the following subsection.

TC-dimercaptosuccinic acid (DMSA) scan

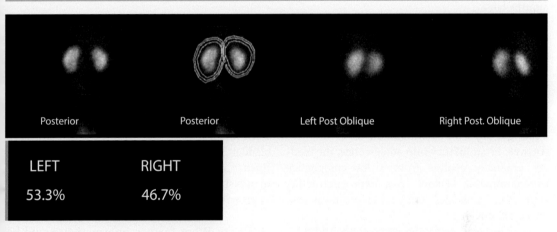

| Posterior | Posterior | Left Post Oblique | Right Post. Oblique |

LEFT	RIGHT
53.3%	46.7%

DMSA nuclear imaging is performed around 3 months of age when the kidneys are considered more mature, and hence less background field activity is present. DMSA measures differential renal function and can show the presence of renal scarring.

Question: How will you manage the baby postnatally?

Answer:

1. Baby is catheterised with a 6–8 Fr catheter to decompress the kidneys and bladder.
2. Start antibiotic prophylaxis.

3. Start IV fluids and correct any electrolyte abnormalities/acid-base balance.
4. Organise MCUG to confirm diagnosis once bloods are normalised.
5. Organise surgery once diagnosis is finally confirmed, electrolyte/acid-base imbalances corrected and creatinine stabilised.

Question: What is the timing of blood tests?

Answer: Serum chemistry in a newborn in the first 24 hours reflects maternal blood biochemistry. The newborn kidney is immature and is thus unable to concentrate urine, and newborn babies are hence prone to dehydration. Serum creatinine and blood urea nitrogen (BUN) should be tested on day 2 and repeated to identify the baby's native or "real renal function". Serum creatinine levels and glomerular filtration rate (GFR) improve with renal maturation unless significant renal dysplasia has occurred.

Question: What is the surgical management of a male newborn with confirmed PUV?
Answer: Cystoscopy is performed and the valves are incised under direct vision at 5, 7 and 12 o'clock positions with a hook cold knife or electrocautery device under antibiotic cover. A urinary catheter is left in situ for 48–72 hours. It is highly advisable to perform circumcision at the same time, especially if there is associated VUR.

In small and/or premature babies, a temporary diverting vesicostomy can be formed.

Cystoscopy and incision of the valves and closure of the vesicostomy are performed a few months later.

Most paediatric urologists will perform check surveillance cystoscopy exam after 3 months to reassess and incise any residual valves if required. VUDS can be performed to assess bladder function at around the same time.

Question: How would you manage the bladder in a younger boy with documented PUV?
Answer: From infancy into adolescence, the bladder gradually evolves from a low-compliance hypercontractile bladder to a hypo-contractile, large-capacity bladder with poor emptying as seen on VUDS imaging.

Appropriately managing overactivity and poor compliance delays the progression to renal failure (5). Anticholinergics such as oxybutynin will help with overactivity and high pressures. Botox (botulinum toxin A) injection into the bladder wall can also decrease bladder pressures, but the effect is not permanent and injections will need to be repeated. If medication fails, bladder augmentation to provide a low-pressure, high-volume compliant storage system with a Mitrofanoff stoma channel for drainage may be required.

Scenario: Late presentation of PUV. A 9-year-old male presents with a 6-month history of dribbling, difficulty in initiating urinary voiding and a prolonged urine flow. He has experienced frank haematuria on three occasions. On examination he has a palpable bladder. Renal tract ultrasound demonstrates non-dilated upper tracts and a bladder that does not empty to completion. Non-invasive urodynamics (NIUDS) show a bladder capacity of 800 mL (expected bladder capacity: 300 mL) with large post-void residuals of 200 mL and a plateau-shaped flow curve with maximum flow rate 5 mL/sec.

Question: How would you interpret these findings and how would you manage him?
Answer: This is a young male patient with features of BOO. He later underwent cystoscopy and was found to have PUV, and the valve leaflets were incised.

Boys presenting late with PUV usually have bladder storage and emptying symptoms, incontinence or recurrent UTIs. They may also have manifestations of chronic renal failure (CRF) such as growth retardation or polyuria.

Question: What further information would be helpful in planning further management?
Answer: VUDS imaging will define the nature of the lower urinary tract dysfunction in order to direct subsequent management.

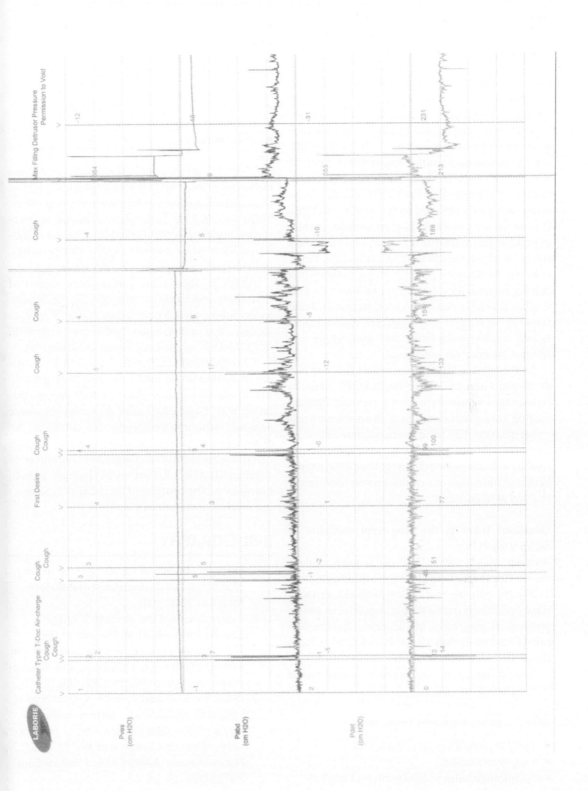

VUDS study shows a large, hypo-contractile bladder. The voiding phase was associated with poor detrusor contractions with marked abdominal straining and poor emptying ability.

Question: How would you manage the bladder in an older boy with PUV?
Answer: The bladder in boys with PUV pathologically may evolve from infancy to adolescence with the phenomenon known as the "valve bladder". Experimental studies suggest that urethral obstruction in the fetal period causes irreversible changes in the smooth muscle cells with the deposition of type III collagen in the bladder wall (6). During the early years the bladder is small, overactive and hypercontractile with high pressures. This subsequently evolves to a hypo-contractile, large-capacity bladder with poor emptying abilities in a decompensated state (myogenic failure) (7). This is often accompanied by a deterioration in renal function, so regular renal function measurement testing (creatinine, e-GFR) and monitoring any changes are crucially essential.

By the time of "late presentation" this boy had developed a decompensated bladder. This needs to be managed aggressively with a frequent double-voiding care programme and clean intermittent catheterisation (CIC) and overnight free drainage. Some boys do not tolerate CIC well, and alternatives include temporary drainage via a vesicostomy button or formation of a catheterisable Mitrofanoff channel as required.

Question: What is the long-term outcome of males with PUV?
Answer: Males with PUV will require vigilant monitoring throughout childhood into adulthood, as 20–30% patients will evolve to ESRD. Primary renal dysplasia is irreversible irrespective of timely postnatal management, but accurate characterisation of bladder dysfunction and treatment reduces the progression of renal failure.

Several criteria are used to predict unfavourable long-term outcome (8):

Prenatal poor prognostic indicators:

- Early in utero diagnosis <24 weeks.
- Oligohydramnios.
- B2 microglobulin in fetal urine >13 mg/L.

Postnatal poor prognostic indicators:

- Early clinical presentation <1 month.
- Bilateral VUR.
- Nadir creatinine (lowest serum creatinine in first year following diagnosis) >1.0 mg/dL (88.4 μmol/L) at 1 year.
- GFR <80 mL/min/1.73 m^2 at 1 year.
- Incontinence at 5 years.
- Proteinuria.

"Pop-off" mechanisms afford some protection of the upper tracts and bladder by providing release of pressure forces caused by the obstructing valves. These can include perinephric urinoma, urinary ascites, bladder diverticulae and the presence of unilateral VUR into a non-functioning kidney (valves, unilateral reflux dysplasia – VURD syndrome).

Although short-term studies have suggested that these mechanisms may offer some benefit, longer follow-up has now shown that only approximately 30% of boys aged 8–10 years of age with VURD will have a normal serum creatinine (9).

Chronic renal insufficiency can lead to a variety of metabolic abnormalities and poor growth. Treatment strategies include dietary supplementation with bicarbonate salts to correct metabolic acidosis, sodium to compensate for salt-losing nephropathy and phosphate binders such as calcium carbonate and activated vitamin D to prevent bone demineralisation. Recombinant human growth hormone can be considered for patients experiencing severe growth retardation (10).

BIBLIOGRAPHY

1. Farrugia MK, Woolf AS. Congenital urinary bladder outlet obstruction. Fetal Matern Med Rev 2010;21:55.
2. Peters CA, Reid LM, Docimo S, Luetic T, Carr M, Retik AB, et al. The role of the kidney in lung growth and maturation in the setting of obstructive uropathy and oligohydramnios. J Urol 1991;146:597–600.
3. Brownlee E, Wragg R, Robb A, Chandran H, Knight M, McCarthy L. Current epidemiology and antenatal presentation of posterior urethral valves: Outcome of BAPS CASS National Audit. BAPS CASS. J Pediatr Surg 2019;54(2):318–21.

4. Vasconcelos MA, Simões E Silva AC, Dias CS, Gomes IR, Carvalho RA, Figueiredo SV, Dumont TR, Oliveira MCL, Pinheiro SV, Mak RH, Oliveira EA. Posterior urethral valves: Comparison of clinical outcomes between postnatal and antenatal cohorts. J Ped Urol 2019;15(167):e1–167.e8.

5. Deshpande AV. Current strategies to predict and manage sequelae of posterior urethral valves in children. Pediatr Nephrol 2018;33(10):1651–61.

6. Peters CA. Congenital bladder obstruction. Prob Urol 1984;8:333.

7. Farrugia MK, Godley ML, Woolf AS, Peebles DM, Cuckow PM, Fry CH. Experimental short-term partial fetal bladder outflow obstruction: II. Compliance and contractility associated with urinary flow impairment. J Pediatr Urol 2006;2:254–60.

8. Cuckow PM. Posterior Urethral Valves. In Stringer MD, Oldham KT, Mouriquand PDE (eds). Paediatric Surgery and Urology: Long Term Outcomes Cambridge University Press, 2006:540–54.

9. Cuckow PM, Dinneen MD, Risdon RA, Ransley PG, Duffy PG. Long-term renal function in the posterior urethral valves, unilateral reflux and renal dysplasia syndrome. J Urol 1997;158(3 Pt 2): 1004–7.

10. Akchurin OM, Kogon AJ, Kumar J, Sethna CB, Hammad HT, Christos PJ, Mahan JD, Greenbaum LA, Woroniecki R. Approach to growth hormone therapy in children with chronic kidney disease varies across North America: The Midwest Paediatric Nephrology Consortium report. BMC Nephrology 2017;18:181.

66

Enuresis

FAISAL M. ALMUTAIRI AND ANJU GOYAL
Royal Manchester Children's Hospital, Manchester, UK

Scenario: A 7-year-old girl is referred to the urology clinic for bed wetting. On examination, her abdomen was soft and the bladder was not palpable.

Question: What would you like to know in her clinical history? What else do you need to focus on during the clinical examination?

Answer: Bedwetting, or nocturnal enuresis (NE), is defined as involuntary wetting during sleep. Obtaining a detailed clinical history is key, as it helps to differentiate between monosymptomatic nocturnal enuresis (MNE) and NE secondary to overactive bladder (OAB) and helps to rule out organic or anatomical causes for wetting.

The following should be asked when assessing an enuretic child:

1. Frequency of wet nights and frequency per single night.
2. Volume of wetting, whether small amounts or full soaking bed wetting. Large volume of urine in the first few hours of nighttime is typical of MNE, while variable volumes of urine, often more than once a night, is more typically associated with OAB.
3. Timing of bedwetting, whether early in the night or later, and if the child wakes up after wetting or sleeps through it.
4. Has the bedwetting been there since toilet training age (primary) or occurred after a dry period – minimum of 6 months (secondary)? One needs to carefully look for triggering factors if secondary NE.
5. Fluid intake/diet—Fluid type, frequency, total volume and pattern of intake. Diet is important, especially salt and protein intake.
6. Daytime voiding symptoms/habits—These include daytime wetting or lower urinary tract symptoms (LUTS) such as urgency and frequency.
7. History of urinary tract infections (UTIs).
8. Bowel habits.
9. Sleep disturbances—Sleep disordered breathing (SDB), including obstructive sleep apnea (OSA).
10. Social/behavioral problems.

It is uncommon to have an abnormal physical examination in monosymptomatic enuretic children. A general examination is performed including an abdominal examination, especially looking for palpable kidneys/bladder or palpable bowel for any evidence of constipation. A back examination must always be undertaken to assess for signs of spina bifida occulta such as a hyperpigmented spot, hair tufts, skin sinus or hemangioma lesions.

Genitalia examination in girls is not necessary unless there is a history of voiding difficulties such as poor stream, hesitancy or straining.

In boys, it is important to examine the penis for foreskin health (phimosis, scarring) or any meatal issues, as rarely a child with a scarred foreskin due to balanitis xerotica obliterans (BXO) may present with bed wetting.

DOI: 10.1201/9781003182290-74

Question: This girl has been bedwetting almost every night but is dry during the day with no UTI. She reports normal frequency and no urgency. Her abdominal examination is normal. What is the diagnosis of this child? How would you investigate it?

Answer: This child has NE with no history of daytime symptoms, and this would be classified as MNE, or simply enuresis as per the International Children's Continence Society (ICCS) terminology. Using the term "monosymptomatic" helps to differentiate it from non-MNE, where there is an OAB (bladder reservoir dysfunction), which may cause daytime urinary symptoms. Daytime/diurnal enuresis is not a valid terminology and should not be used.

There are clear hereditary factors in NE. NE is considered normal under the age of 5 years. It has been a common practice to consider such children for treatment only when they reach 7 years of age, but younger children should not be excluded from offering treatment. NE has a prevalence of 5%–10% at 7 years of age with a yearly spontaneous resolution rate of 15%. Children who have bed wetting every night have a low rate of spontaneous resolution, and 7 out of 100 children who are wetting the bed at the age of 7 years will take this condition onwards into adulthood. NE is more common among boys than girls. NE is notably more common in children with developmental, attention or learning difficulties.

NE can be attributed to three main factors: High arousal threshold, bladder dysfunction and nocturnal polyuria (NP). There is usually an overlap of factors in any one child and one, two or all three factors may be present. Recently, attention has been given to the chronobiology of micturition in which there is existence of a circadian rhythm in kidney, brain and bladder. This causes decreased arousal in the brain, a decreased urine production rate in the kidneys and increased functional bladder capacity during sleep. Absence of arousal is thought to be a major contributor to NE, as many parents report that their child sleeps through bed wetting. Children with NE are known to have disturbed sleep with raised arousal threshold, though the exact mechanisms are unclear.

NP is defined as nocturnal urine production (sum of amount of urine in nappies/sheets and first morning void) of at least 130% of estimated bladder volume capacity:

Estimated bladder capacity (EBC)
= (Age in years × 30) + 30 mL

OAB is usually associated with daytime urinary symptoms such as frequency, urgency and daytime wetting.

After obtaining a detailed clinical history and establishing the diagnosis, a bladder diary (BD) should be obtained. The BD is a very important tool in enuresis workup and includes a frequency/volume chart for 2 days and 7-day record of nighttime urine production. BD helps to assess for OAB and NP.

Other investigations should include:

- *Urine analysis*: Important in refractory NE to rule out any other pathology such as diabetes mellitus, diabetes insipidus or UTI.
- Blood tests are usually not required.
- Imaging studies are usually not needed in MNE workup, but ultrasonography of the urinary tract is helpful to rule out any pathology in therapy-resistant cases.

In therapy-resistant cases, further investigations may be performed to assess bladder dysfunction including uroflowmetry studies and urodynamic studies.

Question: The BD shows nocturnal polyuria (Figure 66.1), and urinalysis is normal. How will you manage enuresis?

Answer: The management of enuresis begins with a full explanation to the child and parents that NE is not behavioral and is not the child's fault. Motivation of the child together with active family support has a crucial major role in successful management of enuresis.

Urotherapy: Physiological fluid intake in the daytime with regular voiding habits are keys to successful management. It is common to find children who are not drinking enough fluids in the morning but taking most of their fluid intake in the second half of the day. Advice on good and regularly spaced fluid intake and regular voiding is the first line of management. Any constipation, if present, must be identified and managed. In children with daytime symptoms, management of these symptoms should be started first before addressing NE. OSA can contribute to NE and should be treated if present.

After urotherapy, the next options include either an enuresis alarm or desmopressin. The enuresis alarm is an effective tool in the management of NE with high success rates (50%–70%) in MNE. It is a device that has two components: Alarm and sensor for wet clothes/bedsheets. The device delivers a strong arousal stimulus, vibrational or acoustic,

Time	Day 1				Day 2			
	In	Out	Wet	Urgency	In	Out	Wet	Urgency
Time of waking up		07:24			Time of waking up		07:24	
07.00			860m				750ml	
08.00						200ml		No
09.00	250ml	220ml		No				
10.00								
11.00	200ml				150ml			
12.00	200ml	250ml		No	250ml			
13.00		250ml		No		300ml		Yes
14.00					250ml			
15.00		200ml		No	400ml			
16.00								
17.00	250ml					170ml		
18.00	250ml							
19.00		320ml		Yes	150ml			
20.00		170ml		No		200ml		No
21.00								
22.00								
23.00								
Midnight to waking up								
Time of going to bed		21:00			Time of going to bed		21:00	

	Day 1	Day 2	Day 3	Day 4	Day 5	Day 6	Day 7
Poo – Yes/No	No	Yes	No	Yes	Yes	Yes	No
If bed wetting, please complete below							
	Day 1	Day 2	Day 3	Day 4	Day 5	Day 6	Day 7
Pull – up/bed wet (weight) = a	500ml	585ml	550ml	710ml	500ml	600ml	720ml
First morning wee = b	160ml	200ml	220ml	200ml	220ml	180ml	180ml
Total night urine production = a+b	660ml	785ml	770ml	910ml	720ml	780ml	900ml

Figure 66.1 Bladder diary (BD).

after activation of its sensor component which is attached to child's clothes/bedsheets. It is crucial that both the child and their family are motivated. It is important to counsel parents that the purpose of the alarm is to train the child to recognize the need to empty the bladder and develop a conditioning behavioral reflex. Therefore, it is important that the child is woken up by parents when the alarm goes off, as children themselves usually sleep through the alarm. This therapy program should be undertaken for at least 6 weeks before deciding on final efficacy.

Initial response to the alarm may consist of smaller wet patches, waking to the alarm, the alarm going off later, fewer alarm times per night or fewer wet nights. Full dryness may come much later. Alarms may be discontinued after 14 consecutive dry nights. Enuresis alarm therapy has low relapse rates, and it is especially effective when there is no evidence of NP or small bladder capacity. An alarm may be inappropriate if the bedwetting is infrequent (fewer than one to two wet nights per week).

Question: The girl does not respond to the enuresis alarm and continues to wet every night after 2 months of daily usage. What are your next steps in management?

Answer: As the BD completed earlier confirmed NP, desmopressin therapy should be considered as the next option. Desmopressin is a selective vasopressin receptor type 2 agonist and has the antidiuretic effects of vasopressin without its pressor activity. There are two formulations: Oral tablets (200/400 mcg) and sublingual melts (120/240 mcg). Nasal spray is no longer recommended. Better results are seen with desmopressin melts, and this is explained partly by improved patient compliance with melts and better therapeutic absorption. Medication is best taken 60 minutes before bedtime with restriction of fluid intake from 1 hour before taking the drug agent to avoid fluid retention and water intoxication. It can be started with a low dose (60 mcg), and the dosage then can be escalated to 240 mcg depending on response. Alternatively, start with a high dose of 240 mcg and then reduce accordingly when a good response is seen. Desmopressin is generally safe with only a minor side effect profile. Around 30% of children with enuresis are full responders to desmopressin, and 40% have a partial response. If there is no response with high-dose therapy for 2 weeks, then it may be stopped.

Question: How would you proceed if there is no response to desmopressin?

Answer: If NE has not responded to urotherapy, alarms and desmopressin, it is good practice then to evaluate afresh with a new BD, urinalysis and an ultrasound of the urinary tract. It is important to remember that NP may mask daytime symptoms of OAB due to much reduced daytime urine production. See the completed BD in **Figure 66.2**, which shows

Time	Day 1 Date: In	Out	Wet	Urgency	Day 2 Date: In	Out	Wet	Urgency
Time of waking up		08:00				08:50		
07.00								
08.00			533ml				659ml	
09.00	200ml	30ml				75ml		
10.00								
11.00		125ml			200ml	100ml		
12.00	200ml	125ml						
13.00					200ml	25ml		
14.00		100ml						
15.00						140ml		
16.00						100ml		
17.00	200ml	125ml						
18.00	500ml				200ml	100ml		
19.00		75ml			200ml	50ml		
20.00		100ml			200ml			
21.00						100ml		
22.00		100ml			200ml			
23.00								
Midnight to waking up								
Time of going to bed		22:30				22:00		

Figure 66.2 Bladder diary.

maximal voided volume (MVV) of only 125 mL in a 9-year-old child with an EBC of 300 mL, even though the girl denied any symptom of daytime urgency/wetting/frequency. Also note NP.

Reduced urine production in the daytime may impede the development of an adequate bladder capacity. In addition, some children may have isolated nocturnal bladder dysfunction with resultant reduced nocturnal bladder capacity but normal daytime bladder function. There is usually an overlap of factors in any one child.

A combination of desmopressin and an anticholinergic agent (ACh) may be tried. Ach will improve NE due to its effects on nocturnal bladder dysfunction, and beneficial effects are enhanced with the antidiuretic effect of desmopressin. ACh effect is better if there are associated daytime symptoms. However, not all NP cases are responsive to desmopressin.

Question: If a child has NP and it has not responded to the previous treatments, what are your further options for management?
Answer: Solute load affects the volume of urine production and may cause NP and subsequent resistance to desmopressin alone. Advice on diet including reduction in protein and salt intake is important. Indomethacin is a prostaglandin synthesis inhibitor and has an antidiuretic effect that reduces water and solute (sodium, urea and others) diuresis. When indomethacin 50 mg/day is combined with desmopressin, it has been shown to cause significant reduction in nocturnal urine production.

Diuretics, such as furosemide, have been also found to be beneficial in children with NP when combined with desmopressin. Morning administration of furosemide at 0.5 mg/kg will enhance diuresis and sodium excretion, and this will lead to decreased nighttime diuresis, and this effect will be potentiated by the antidiuretic effects of desmopressin.

Question: How would you approach enuresis refractory to this medical management?
Answer: Children with therapy resistance should be evaluated with a urodynamic study to evaluate their bladder function. If OAB is confirmed, then further measures such as adrenoreceptor agonists (mirabegron) can be added to ACh. In severe cases, intradetrusor injection of botulinum toxin A is an option.

Other strategies that can be offered include:

1. Going back to the first- or second-line therapy (alarm and desmopressin, respectively), as the pathological mechanism may change over time.
2. Alarms can be tried with any other medical therapy.
3. *Tricyclic antidepressants* (*TCAs*): Although the exact mechanism of action of TCAs such as imipramine in treating enuresis is unknown, it is thought to be due to a combination of noradrenergic, serotoninergic and anticholinergic action on the bladder and its effects on urine production and arousal mechanisms. Imipramine is not indicated in children younger than 6 years. Recommended starting dosage is 25 mg at bedtime, and the dose can be increased to 50 mg if required. TCAs have rare but significant side effects, including cardiotoxicity and hepatotoxicity, in addition to minor anticholinergic side effects such as dry mouth, constipation and postural hypotension. It is recommended to have a pretreatment ECG to detect any abnormalities if there are any suspicions of a cardiac history in the child or family. It can be combined with desmopressin if the effect is incomplete after 4 weeks of therapy initiation. Among therapy-resistant enuretic children, 30–50% may be expected to benefit from imipramine, and this proportion increases if desmopressin is added. Gradual withdrawal of the imipramine dosage is necessary when discontinuation of therapy is intended. However, there can be a high relapse rate, and there is a tendency for tolerance, i.e. efficacy may wane with time. Other TCAs that have been shown to have antienuretic effects include atomoxetine and reboxetine. TCAs should not be offered in combination with anticholinergic agents.

BIBLIOGRAPHY

1. Nevéus T, Fonseca E, Franco I, Kawauchi A, Kovacevic L, Nieuwhof-Leppink A, Raes A, Tekgül S, Yang SS, Rittig S. Management and treatment of nocturnal enuresis-an updated standardization document from the International Children's Continence Society. J Pediatr Urol. 2020;16(1):10–19.

2. National Institute for Health and Care Excellence (NICE) (2010) Bedwetting in under 19s, CG111.

3. Dossche L, Walle JV, Van Herzeele C. The pathophysiology of monosymptomatic nocturnal enuresis with special emphasis on the circadian rhythm of renal physiology. Eur J Pediatr. 2016;175(6):747–54.

4. Caldwell PH, Nankivell G, Sureshkumar P. Simple behavioural interventions for nocturnal enuresis in children. Cochrane Database Syst Rev. 2013; 7:CD003637.

5. Deshpande AV, Caldwell PH, Sureshkumar P. Drugs for nocturnal enuresis in children (other than desmopressin and tricyclics). Cochrane Database Syst Rev. 2012;12:CD002238.

6. Kamperis K, Hagstroem S, Faerch M, Mahler B, Rittig S, Djurhuus JC. Combination treatment of nocturnal enuresis with desmopressin and indomethacin. Pediatr Nephrol. 2017;32(4):627–33.

67

Neuropathic bladder

FAISAL M. ALMUTAIRI AND ANJU GOYAL
Royal Manchester Children's Hospital, Manchester, UK

Scenario: A full-term male newborn was noted to have a lump in the lumbosacral area and has not passed urine for the last 18 hours. On examination the bladder is palpable. External genitalia are normal, and the back examination showed a lump (**Figure 67.1**). The newborn has bilateral club feet with limited mobility of the lower limbs. Head circumference is recorded on the 50th centile. You are now called to see the newborn for urological assessment.

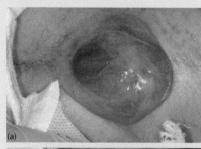

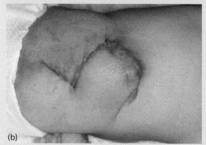

Figure 67.1 Myelomeningocoele – preoperative and postoperative repair (flaps were used to cover the defect).

Question: What is the diagnosis? How would you manage this baby?

Answer: The baby has a lumbosacral myelomeningocoele (MMC). MMC is a major neural tube defect (NTD), which also includes variant pathologies such as lipomyelomeningocoele, meningocoele and spina bifida occulta. Many of the affected children have the associated Arnold-Chiari malformation and develop hydrocephalus. Most newborns with NTD will have neuropathic bladder physiology. Other causes of neuropathic bladder include congenital sacral agenesis and less commonly may be seen in patients with anorectal malformation, spinal tumours and transverse myelitis.

NTD can be readily diagnosed on maternal fetal imaging as early as the first trimester, and suggestive signs include the 'lemon sign' (scalloping of frontal cranial bones due to backward shift of the hindbrain from herniation) and 'banana sign' (anterior concavity of cerebellar hemispheres due to partial cerebellar herniation). The NTD can be visualised and evaluated in subsequent antenatal scans taken during pregnancy.

Patients with spina bifida occulta may present with clinical findings of a lump, dermal sinus, atypical skin dimple (defined as a dimple that is larger than 5 mm and >2.5 cm away from the anus), hairy skin patch, port wine stain or a small tail.

Urological management: A palpable bladder suggests that the baby is in urinary retention and will need an indwelling catheter to effectively drain the bladder. A dedicated nursing team should be involved to give practical information and advice

DOI: 10.1201/9781003182290-75

to the parents regarding clean intermittent catheterisation (CIC), helping train them with the aim to start CIC early after MMC closure. CIC training can be delayed by a few days while the back wound heals. The baby should be commenced on antibiotic prophylaxis, usually with trimethoprim at a dosage of 2 mg/kg every night. A baseline ultrasound scan of the urinary tract should be done in the first few days. Ultrasound scans in the neonatal period invariably show normal kidneys, as associated congenital renal tract abnormalities are rare in NTD. The only abnormality that may be seen on initial early scanning is the distended bladder in newborns with urinary retention.

Question: Can NTD be prevented?

Answer: Yes – NTD has a multifactorial pathogenesis. Folic acid has a crucial and pivotal role in methylation metabolism which is involved in the aetio-pathogenesis of NTD. Studies have demonstrated that maternal folic acid supplementation reduces the risks of occurrence of NTD in offspring. The Medical Research Council (MRC-UK) published the results of a large randomised clinical trial which showed that 72% of NTDs were prevented with folic acid supplementation (4 mg/day) in 'high-risk' women that had previous pregnancies associated with spina bifida. NICE guidelines now recommended 400 mcg/day of folic acid for all women of reproductive age who are planning for pregnancy and to start taking the supplements before becoming pregnant and throughout the first 12 weeks of a confirmed pregnancy. If folic acid supplement is started 'too late' after the pregnancy is confirmed, the critical stage of neural development has already been missed.

National food fortification programmes have been established in many countries to enhance the delivery of adequate folic acid. The UK is the latest country to launch this health care programme in 2021. Multiple studies have evaluated the result of food fortification and shown significant reduction in NTD incidence rates.

Question: Is there a role for antenatal intervention?

Answer: Prenatal MMC closure with fetal surgery has been shown to reduce the need for ventriculo-peritoneal (VP) shunting in addition to claiming improvements of lower extremity neuromuscular function as reported by the Management of Myelomeningocele Study (MOMS) published in the *New England Journal of Medicine* in 2011. Later subsequent reporting of urological outcomes noted that those fetuses who had prenatal closure were more likely to have better voluntary urinary voiding compared to newborns who had postnatal repair (24% vs 4%). Children may, however, still require CIC to manage urinary continence. It therefore remains somewhat controversial at the time of writing this chapter whether fetal surgery will ultimately allow improved long-term urological outcomes

Questions: What information would you give to parents of a newborn with spina bifida?

Answer: Given the deleterious effects of NTD on the spine, brain, urinary tract, bowel and limbs, the affected child will require multidisciplinary team (MDT) care lifelong into adulthood to achieve the best outcomes. The MDT should ideally include health care professionals from urology, colorectal service, neurosurgery, orthopaedics, orthotics, physiotherapy and psychology. At specialist centres NTD monthly clinics can provide excellent services including holistic and quality after-care plans.

Urological care:

- *Neurogenic bladder and bowel*: Bladder and bowel dysfunction are a sequela of NTD. Only 12% of newborns have normal bladder function at birth, and this may further change on later follow-up. It is not fully possible to predict the extent and nature of bladder involvement based on the level of the NTD lesion. Bladder function can be variably affected, and this requires assessment by urodynamic study (UDS), and management can then be directed towards the unique pathology in that affected child. Management plans can be conservative, pharmacological and/or surgical. CIC is likely to be an integral part of whatever management is required and hence is started in all MMC newborns. Despite active management, more than 50% of affected children may have associated urinary and faecal incontinence, with approximately 25% having renal damage at adolescence.
- *Long-term goals*: Management here aims to preserve renal function from the damaging effects of a high-pressure bladder, prevent

recurrent urinary tract infections (UTIs) and seek to achieve socially acceptable continence.

- Institution of prophylactic CIC early in infancy is a proven strategy that helps to reduce upper urinary tract deterioration, prevent UTIs and achieve better continence.
- *Prophylactic antibiotics*: Are best initiated at birth, and further decision on continued usage should be based on bladder findings from a UDS. Generally, prophylactic antibiotics are not required while a patient is on a CIC programme if they have a good compliant bladder and there is no associated vesicoureteral reflux (VUR).
- *Latex allergy*: NTD patients are at 'high risk' of latex sensitisation, and hence it is best recommended to avoid using latex-containing products.

Question: After institution of a CIC programme, how will you manage the child?

Answer: A minimum of two catheterisations per day should be performed initially while awaiting a UDS exam. More frequent CIC is needed if the baby is unable to void urine without a catheter. In this infant with urinary retention, we advise 3-hourly CIC during the daytime with an indwelling overnight catheter. Overnight continuous bladder drainage can also be added to care plans if daytime CIC does not improve urinary tract dilatation or UTIs. In male babies with a tight foreskin, steroid ointment can be applied, and occasionally circumcision may be required in those with scarred tight foreskin. CIC is usually well tolerated in MMC patients, as most will lack urethral sensation.

UDS should be scheduled early, allowing some 6 weeks following back defect closure for any element of neurogenic shock to resolve. In newborns with antenatal MMC repair, UDS can be scheduled early after delivery and ideally should be done before first hospital discharge.

A video-urodynamic study should be undertaken, but if this facility is not available, then a VCUG may be combined with UDS. UDS will assess bladder capacity, compliance, detrusor overactivity and detrusor-sphincter dyssynergia (DSD). Imaging crucially helps to evaluate the appearance of the bladder, particularly noting if there is any evidence of trabeculations/diverticulae, VUR and bladder neck status.

- *Bladder capacity*: Expected bladder capacity (EBC) can be measured using the formula:

$$(Age \ (in \ years) +1) \times 30 \ mL$$

- *Compliance (mL/cm of water)*: Defined as change in bladder volume divided by change in bladder pressure. There is no consensus on compliance figures for children; hence, end detrusor filling pressure may be a better indicator of bladder compliance. Ideally filling pressures should be below 20 cm of water, and end detrusor pressures reaching above 40 cm of water strongly suggest an 'unsafe bladder'.
- *Detrusor-sphincter dysynergia (DSD)*: This is suggested by increased sphincter activity during bladder contractions or failure of the sphincter to relax at the maximum bladder capacity. Up to 53% of patients will have DSD.
- *Detrusor leak point pressure (DLPP)*: DLPP is the intravesical pressure at which urethral leakage occurs. A DLPP of more than 40 cm of water is associated with high risk of upper urinary tract deterioration.

On UDS, detrusor and sphincter activity may be identified as either overactive or underactive, resulting in different pathophysiology scenarios which may be categorised as 'safe' (incontinent) or 'high risk':

1. *Overactive sphincter and overactive detrusor*: 'High risk' (requires anticholinergics and regular CIC).
2. *Overactive sphincter and underactive detrusor*: 'High risk' (usually presents with urinary retention and only requires regular CIC).
3. *Underactive sphincter and overactive detrusor*: Incontinent (requires CIC once per day to keep the child used to the CIC intervention, as regular CIC is likely to be needed at the time of a later continence operation procedure; also requires anticholinergics).
4. *Underactive sphincter and underactive detrusor*: Incontinent (may have incomplete emptying causing UTIs; therefore, CIC is required at least two to three times per day).
5. *Normal*: Stable bladder without leakage (requires active surveillance).

In 'high-risk' bladders, there is a danger of renal tract damage from high detrusor pressure, incomplete emptying and recurrent UTI. Early urodynamic assessment studies in those fetuses who had antenatal closure showed that 52% had a 'high risk' bladder, 25% had incontinence and 4% had hypocontractile bladders, while normal bladders were present in only 18.5% of cases.

A baseline DMSA scan should be scheduled in the first 3–6 months of life, and a repeat ultrasound scan should be arranged at 3 months of age.

Question: Baseline ultrasound is normal, and UDS (Figure 67.2) at age of 8 weeks showed detrusor overactivity (DO) at 10 mL filling and leakage at 25 mL with a detrusor pressure of 76 cm of water. What would you do now at this stage (Figure 67.2)?
Answer: This is a 'high-risk' bladder, as there is a high detrusor filling pressure and DLPP of 76 cm of water. Anticholinergic medication should be started with oxybutynin at 0.1–0.4 mg/kg/day in three divided doses. CIC frequency should be increased accordingly to 3-hourly in the daytime with an overnight indwelling catheter.

The patient requires vigilant surveillance follow-up, and a repeat ultrasound scan and UDS should be performed 3 months later to assess patient response to oxybutynin and any upper urinary tract changes. If bladder pressures do not improve with anticholinergics, then intravesical injection of botulinum toxin A (BtA) should be considered. Vesicostomy may be warranted if there is no improvement in

pressures with BtA or the family finds it difficult to adhere to a CIC programme schedule or the patient has upper tract changes or recurrent UTI.

- Oral anticholinergic agents are the recommended first-line medical therapy for high-pressure neuropathic bladders. Anticholinergic agents block muscarinic receptors, and therefore inhibit involuntary bladder contractions. These agents help to increase bladder capacity and reduce DO. Oxybutynin is the most commonly used agent (also available in transdermal and intravesical forms). Adverse effects mainly include facial flushing and constipation. Tolterodine, trospium and solifenacin are other anticholinergic medications with a more selective action than oxybutynin and thus have a better side effect profile, though they are not licensed for use in children. Oxybutynin is approved for use in children above 5 years of age only.
- Mirabegron is a β3 adrenergic receptor agonist and was approved for children above 3 years of age for neurogenic detrusor overactivity in 2021. Mirabegron acts as a detrusor muscle relaxant and improves compliance in addition to improving cystometric capacity. The adverse effects profile is good with minimal reported side effects. It can be used in combination with anticholinergics.
- BtA (Botox or Xeomin or Dysport) is a neurotoxin produced by *Clostridium botulinum*

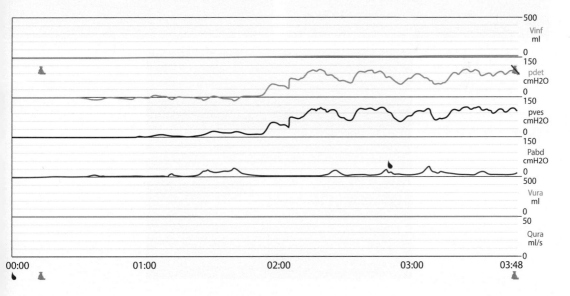

Figure 67.2 Urodynamic study at age of 8 weeks.

bacteria and acts by inhibiting presynaptic release of acetylcholine, which results in bladder muscle paralysis. The dose varies with the ona or abo isomer and for different preparations. The recommended dose for Botox is 5–10 IU/kg with a maximum dose of 300 IU and is delivered over 20–40 injection sites. Its effect usually lasts for approximately 6 months. Botox helps to reduce detrusor pressure, increase bladder capacity and improve compliance. Though there is not enough data available, it is anticipated in the long term, that repeated BtA injections, if commenced early enough, may help to avoid the need for bladder augmentation operations being required in older NTD patients

Question: What are the other considerations in the management of this child?

Answer: Bowel management should be proactive to avoid constipation and includes the use of stool softeners/stimulant laxatives along with emptying aids such as rectal suppositories or enema wash-outs. A combination of low-dose Movicol (if the patient has hard stools) with a suppository may be the first line of management. This may be escalated to enemas and trans-anal irrigation systems (e.g. Peristeen, Qfora). Management should be tailored to the child's ability and unique social conditions.

Question: Follow-up surveillance ultrasound shows a new left-sided hydroureteronephrosis (Figure 67.3) despite a CIC programme and anticholinergics. BtA was injected, but bladder pressures did not improve; hence, a vesicostomy was performed. What should be done next?

Answer: Vesicostomy is the safest option to protect the kidneys, and it is relatively easy to manage in infants and small children, as the urine drains freely into nappies. Antibiotic prophylaxis and anticholinergics can be discontinued. When the

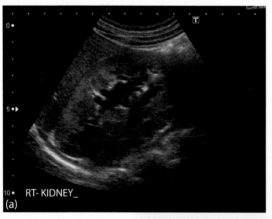
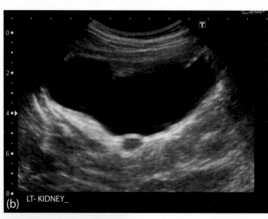
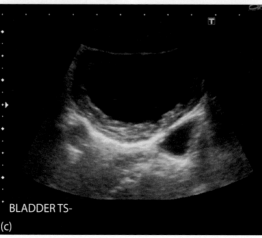

Figure 67.3 Ultrasound urinary tract surveillance study at follow-up.

child grows older, further options for social continence can be better explored as discussed later.

A follow-up DMSA scan study should be performed to detect any renal scarring, and renal function tests should be checked to evaluate for any deterioration in biochemical renal function. Cystatin C is considered a better indicator of kidney function, as children with spina bifida usually have a low muscle mass.

Question: What are the surgical options if the medical bladder management has failed?
Answer: Surgical management depends on the status of the bladder and bladder neck.

a. **Bladder management:**
   - *Diversion:*
   Vesicostomy is suitable for specific conditions in infants and young children as listed later (usually with a 'high-risk' bladder):
     - Those who have failed medical management.
     - Medical management compliance issues.
     - Failure to institute CIC programme.
   Vesicostomy is employed as a temporary option in infants and young children as stated earlier. It is not suitable for older children, as it does not allow easy application of a stoma bag. In these situations, an ileovesicostomy (a loop of small bowel is interposed between the bladder and the abdominal wall and then is fashioned into a stoma) may be a better option, as a stoma bag can be more securely applied. However, it is a valid option for social continence only if the bladder neck is competent. If the bladder neck is open, an ileal conduit diversion is a better option. An ileal conduit can be a good long-term option for those patients who are not suitable for bladder augmentation, such as those with the inability to adhere to a schedule of regular bladder emptying/CIC.
   - *Bladder augmentation:*
   Enterocystoplasty: A bowel segment can be used to augment a small bladder with high pressure/poor compliance to achieve a low-pressure reservoir and eventually protect the upper urinary tract. The stomach, jejunum, ileum and colon have all been used in bladder augmentation operations, though ileum is the most commonly used segment. Haematuria-dysuria syndrome is a unique complication when a gastric segment is deployed, and hence its use is not so common. The bladder is opened widely before securing placement of the adjunct segment, which is then detubularised to disrupt its intrinsic contractions. The operation can be accompanied by construction of a catheterisable channel conduit, typically using the appendix (Mitrofanoff) or an ileal segment (Monti-Mitrofanoff) if urethral CIC is not feasible. Most low-grade VUR will resolve with bladder augmentation alone.

Short-term complications of bladder augmentation include bleeding, intestinal adhesive obstruction, bowel anastomotic leakage or a urinary leak. Long-term complications are usually metabolic, secondary to use of the bowel segment and include metabolic acid-base disturbance, vitamin B_{12} deficiency, abnormalities in bone metabolism, renal impairment and growth retardation. Other long-term morbidity includes bladder perforation, recurrent UTIs, stone formation and risks of cancer. Stone formation is related to the excessive mucus production, especially when an ileal segment is used, and these risks can be reduced by introducing regular cycles of bladder irrigation. The estimated risks of bladder cancer in patients who have augmented bladders is between 1.2% and 3.8%. It is therefore recommended to schedule annual endoscopic surveillance at 10 years after an enterocystoplasty operation, though the utility of these examinations in the early detection of malignancy is debatable.

Bladder auto-augmentation/others: Complications of using a bowel segment for bladder augmentation have resulted in the search for alternatives such as:
   - *Detrusor myotomy (bladder auto-augmentation):* This increases bladder capacity, improves bladder compliance and decreases end filling detrusor pressures but is only useful when bladder capacity is at least 70% of the EBC. Postoperative continuous distention of the bladder for the next 7–10 days after operation is crucial and may be difficult to achieve when a simultaneous Mitrofanoff is required. It needs meticulous careful patient selection. However,

bladder auto-augmentation does not preclude the possibility of enterocystoplasty or other surgical procedures later.

– *Ureterocystoplasty*: If there is a single non-functioning kidney with a dilated ureter, then this ureter segment can be used in children with borderline capacity (at least 70% of EBC) and compliance. However, it is important to remember that ureters best suited here for this are those which are typically congenital, i.e. dysplastic and dilated. Those which undergo dilatation from high bladder pressures are unlikely to provide the required compliance and capacity.

b. **Bladder neck management:**
Urethral pressure profile (UPP) assessment during a UDS gives vital information on the status of the bladder neck. It is not a very commonly evaluated parameter on UDS exam. Supporting/corroborative evidence for sphincteric incompetence (SI) can be readily obtained by history, evidence of an open bladder neck on video UDS and by simple manoeuvres such as asking the patient to be in an erect standing position if possible and raising intra-abdominal pressure by coughing, etc. There is no evidence-based medical therapy treatment for SI. Bladder neck resistance needs to be increased surgically to provide continence, and options include insertion of an artificial urinary sphincter (AUS), fascial slings, artificial slings, injection of bulking agents or bladder neck reconstruction. None of the techniques listed have uniformly good results. Different urology centres will have their own preferred bladder neck procedure, with purported good results which cannot be replicated by others!

a. Bladder neck reconstruction with a Young Dees operation or its variations are not recommended for neurogenic bladder due to high failure rate.

b. Injection of bulking agents is used more often as an accessory option in children with residual incontinence after another continence procedure and generally does not have encouraging results.

c. Autologous fascial slings have been advocated by some urologists, but their good results have not been replicated at other centres!

d. Artificial slings (AdVance) have also been used, but experience has mainly been in adults.

e. AUS has good continence outcomes when it is successfully implanted; however, there is a 30–40% revision rate due to device erosion (of pump/cuff), infection and mechanical failure.

f. Bladder neck division/closure along with creation of a catheterisable channel is best reserved for a failed bladder neck reconstruction.

Question: What are the surgical options if a medical bowel management programme has failed?
Answer: If trans-anal irrigation is not working or not acceptable to the patient then creation of an antegrade continence enema (ACE) channel is an effective option to better manage constipation and faecal incontinence. An ACE channel can be created in various ways including by appendicostomy, cecostomy or percutaneous cecostomy.

When patients are wheelchair bound, trans-anal irrigation systems which have worked perfectly well in childhood may no longer be acceptable during adolescence and later years. To provide patients with independence and a better dignity of self-care, the ACE operation is a better option.

A permanent colostomy may be used as an option of last resort.

Question: What steps would you consider if there is worsening of neurological and urological symptoms?
Answer: MRI spine scan should be considered in cases of worsening urological, neurological or orthopaedic symptoms to rule out tethered cord syndrome (TCS). Early diagnosis and timely management of TCS are vital and necessary to avoid irreversible damage.

Question: What are the pubertal and postpubertal urological considerations for individuals born with spina bifida?
Answer: During puberty, many changes occur in patients born with spina bifida with a desire to achieve independence in self-care, particularly self-catheterisation, and bowel management. Ensuring compliance and a good routine/protocol adherence during this transitional period for

patients is essential to avoid serious complications such as bladder perforation, as mentioned earlier in those with enterocystoplasty, which may occur when CIC is not done regularly. Active supporting patient organisations such as SHINE (Spina bifida Hydrocephalus Information Networking Equality) can be very helpful in providing support.

Postpubertal sexual function and fertility concerns are now becoming important, as most NTD patients now survive well into adulthood following major advancements in health care management.

Men with spina bifida may have sexual dysfunction, especially affecting ejaculatory function. Erectile dysfunction is common, and phosphodiesterase 5 (PDE5) inhibitors are effective treatment for these men. The degree of sexual dysfunction has been correlated to many factors, notably including the level of neurological lesion (the lower-level neurological lesion is associated with more intact sexual function), impaired sacral reflexes or presence of hydrocephalus. Apart from ejaculatory dysfunction, multiple genetic and pathological factors also contribute to infertility. Assisted reproductive techniques (ARTs) such as intrauterine insemination (IUI), in vitro fertilisation (IVF) or intracytoplasmic sperm injection (ICSI) have all been used but require sperm retrieval by either rectal probe electro-ejaculation or surgery.

Sexual dysfunction in women with spina bifida is understudied; however, sexual arousal and orgasm appear to be affected. Generally, fertility is not affected.

Fear of urinary or faecal incontinence during sexual intercourse will affect having a healthy sex life and can lead to avoidance of sex in both men and women.

In women with spina bifida, contraception needs individualised professional counselling. Barrier contraception may not be appropriate with the increased risk of latex allergy sensitisation, while hormonal contraception is associated with increased risk of thrombosis. Risks of women becoming pregnant with a new baby with spina bifida is increased; therefore, folic acid supplementation must be actively encouraged when pregnancy is being planned (4 mg/day).

Pregnant women with spina bifida will clearly need to be monitored in high-risk pregnancy clinics with experienced obstetricians. Elective maternal C-section is recommended especially in those women who have an abnormal pelvis or have had previous bladder neck surgery. The presence and location of a Mitrofanoff and ACE channel stoma need to be considered when planning the C-section.

BIBLIOGRAPHY

1. Prevention of neural tube defects: results of the Medical Research Council Vitamin Study. MRC Vitamin Study Research Group. Lancet. 1991;338(8760):131–137.
2. Adzick NS, Thom EA, Spong CY, et al. A randomized trial of prenatal versus postnatal repair of myelomeningocele. N Engl J Med. 2011;364(11):993–1004.
3. Brock JW 3rd, Thomas JC, Baskin LS, Zderic SA, Thom EA, Burrows PK, Lee H, Houtrow AJ, MacPherson C, Adzick NS; Eunice Kennedy Shriver NICHD MOMS Trial Group. Effect of prenatal repair of myelomeningocele on urological outcomes at school age. J Urol. 2019;202(4):812–818.
4. National Institute for Health and Care Excellence (NICE) Guidance, (2008), Maternal and Child Nutrition. PH11.
5. Park JS, Lee YS, Lee CN, Kim SH, Kim SW, Han SW. Efficacy and safety of mirabegron a β3-adrenoceptor agonist for treating neurogenic bladder in pediatric patients with spina bifida: a retrospective pilot study. World J Urol. 2019;37(8):1665–1670.
6. Macedo A Jr, Ottoni SL, Garrone G, Liguori R, Cavalheiro S, Moron A, Leal Da Cruz M. In utero myelomeningocoele repair and urological outcomes: the first 100 cases of a prospective analysis. Is there an improvement in bladder function? BJU Int. 2019;123(4):676–681.
7. Shankar KR, Losty PD, et al. Functional results following the antegrade continence enema procedure. Br J Surg. 1998;85(7):980–982.
8. Soergel TM, Cain MP, Misseri R, Gardner TA, Koch MO, Rink RC. Transitional cell carcinoma of the bladder following augmentation cystoplasty for the neuropathic bladder. J Urol. 2004;172(4 Pt 2):1649–1651; discussion 1651-2.
9. Stein R, Bogaert G, Dogan HS, Hoen L, Kocvara R, Nijman RJM, Quadackers JSLT, Rawashdeh YF, Silay MS, Tekgul S, Radmayr C. EAU/ESPU guidelines on the management of neurogenic bladder in children

and adolescent part I diagnostics and conservative treatment. Neurourol Urodyn. 2020;39(1):45–57.

10. Stein R, Bogaert G, Dogan HS, Hoen L, Kocvara R, Nijman RJM, Quaedackers J, Rawashdeh YF, Silay MS, Tekgul S, Radmayr C. EAU/ESPU guidelines on the management of neurogenic bladder in children and adolescent part II operative management. Neurourol Urodyn. 2020;39(2):498–506.

11. Streur CS, Corona L, Smith JE, Lin M, Wiener JS, Wittmann DA. Sexual function of men and women with spina bifida: a scoping literature review. Sex Med Rev. 2021;9(2):244–266.

68

Hypospadias

AHMED T. HADIDI
Head of Hypospadias Center and Paediatric Surgery Department, San Offenbach Teaching Hospital, Goethe University, Germany

INTRODUCTION

The term hypospadias was first introduced by Galen (129–199 AD) in his book *Methodus Medendi* to describe the condition hypospadias where the urethral opening is on the undersurface of the penis (hypo means below, spadias means rent or opening).

GENERAL CONSIDERATIONS

- Hypospadias is the most frequent urogenital anomaly, occurring in 3 per 1,000 live births or 1 in 125 live males; it was usually defined as a condition characterized by the urethral opening being on the undersurface of the penis or glans.
- Recently, it is defined as a wide spectrum that may include the urethral opening on the undersurface, incomplete prepuce, chordee (penile curvature), rotation, bifid scrotum, penoscrotal transposition, and occasionally undescended testis.
- Circumcision must be avoided, and early counseling of the parents should be provided.
- May be associated with ventral penile curvature or "chordee".
- There is a familial tendency in 5%–10%.
- Standard textbooks suggest that the human urethra develops through fusion of the lateral edges of the urethral plate, like closing a zipper, and hypospadias is due to a failure of fusion.
- Recent publications suggest that the human penile urethra develops due to distal migration of the ventral mesenchyme including the urethral opening (the "Migration Hypothesis") and hypospadias is due to defective distal migration (the "Disorganization Hypothesis").
- Hypospadias in general may be divided into two main categories: Penile forms (grade I, II, and III) and perineal hypospadias (grade IV).
- Penile hypospadias (90%) have usually a good-sized penis and glans and mild chordee (less than 30 degrees) that can usually be corrected by degloving and/or dorsal plication.
- Perineal hypospadias (10%) is a syndrome associated with small-sized penis and glans, severe chordee, bifid scrotum, narrow hypoplastic urethral plate, short ano-scrotal distance (ASD), penoscrotal transposition, and occasionally undescended testis. In this form, the urethral plate needs to be divided and the underlying hypoplastic tissue excised to avoid shortening of the penis. This is the most challenging form and should be referred to specialized hypospadias centers.
- If hypospadias is associated with undescended testis, the diagnosis of disorders of sexual development (DSD) should be considered.
- The penis grows less than 1 cm in the first 4 years of life: The phallus that is small at 6 months will still be small at 3 years.
- Sexual identity is determined by 3 years of age. In older children the psychological burden relating to this must not be underestimated (in some patients, this amounts to the sensation of being

DOI: 10.1201/9781003182290-76

"different" from one's peers; in other patients, it means repeated operations on genitalia).

- Recent studies evaluating emotional, psychosexual, cognitive, and surgical risks identified that there is an optimal window for surgery at 3–18 months of age.

CLASSIFICATION

- Consistent classification is necessary in order to standardize the terminology of hypospadias and to enable improved treatment and comparison of results across centers and surgeons.
- There have been several classifications in use and are included in **Figure 68.1(b)**.
- Confusion stems from the fact that the deformity is usually described according to the site of meatus (M). The degree of chordee (C) is not usually evaluated and may go unnoticed except by urologists with experience in hypospadias.

- The Hypospadias International Society (HIS) has agreed in 2018 to adopt the Hypospadias International Classification (MCGU) based on location of the meatus (M), chordee (C), glans configuration and size (G), and the quality of the urethral plate (U). This international classification may help to compare similar forms of hypospadias in different centers and to make a rough prognosis about the success and complication rates (**Figure 68.2**).
- According to the position of the meatus, four grades are defined (**Figure 68.1a**).
- A proposed classification sheet which includes further findings including related anomalies is shown in **Figure 68.3**.
- It is suggested that the form proposed in **Figure 68.3** is always filled out at the first evaluation and, if necessary, after follow-up examinations.

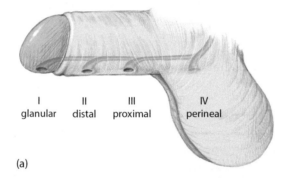

	I	II	III		IV
	glanular	distal	proximal		perineal

(a)

Kaufmann 1886	Schaefer 1950	Avellan 1975		Duckett 1996	Hadidi 2004	Hadidi 2018
Grade I	Glanular	Glanular		Glanular	Glanular	Glanular
				Sub-coronal		
				Distal penile	Distal	Penile
Grade II	Penile	Penile		Mid shaft		
Grade III				Proximal penile		Proximal
		Penoperineal		Penoscrotal		
	Perineal	Perineal		Midscrotal	Proximal	
		Perineal w/o Bulb				
Grade IV				Perineal		Perineal

(b)

Figure 68.1 (a) Classification of primary hypospadias into four grades: Glandular (grade I), distal (grade II), proximal (grade III), and perineal (grade IV). Complicated, cicatricial hypospadias with inadequate skin and scarred tissue (inappropriately called crippled hypospadias) is classified as grade V hypospadias. (b) Current classification of hypospadias. (©Ahmed T. Hadidi 2021. All rights reserved.)

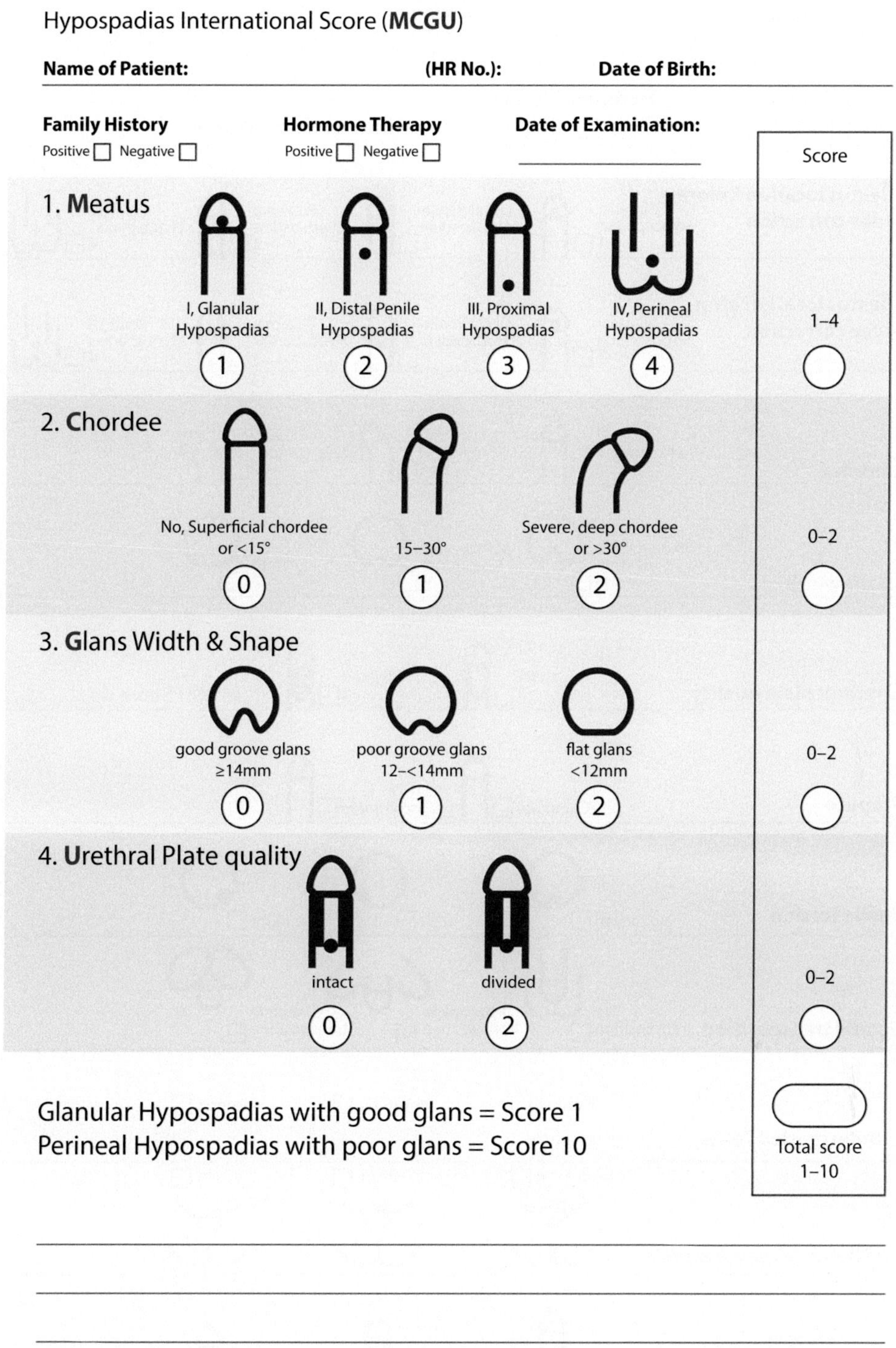

Hypospadias International Score (**MCGU**)

Name of Patient: (HR No.):   Date of Birth:

Family History   **Hormone Therapy**   **Date of Examination:**

Positive ☐ Negative ☐   Positive ☐ Negative ☐ | Score

Figure 68.2 The MCGU score that gives an idea of the difficulty of the hypospadias and the possibility of complications. The higher the score, the more difficult the hypospadias and the higher the incidence of complications. (©Ahmed T. Hadidi 2021. All rights reserved.)

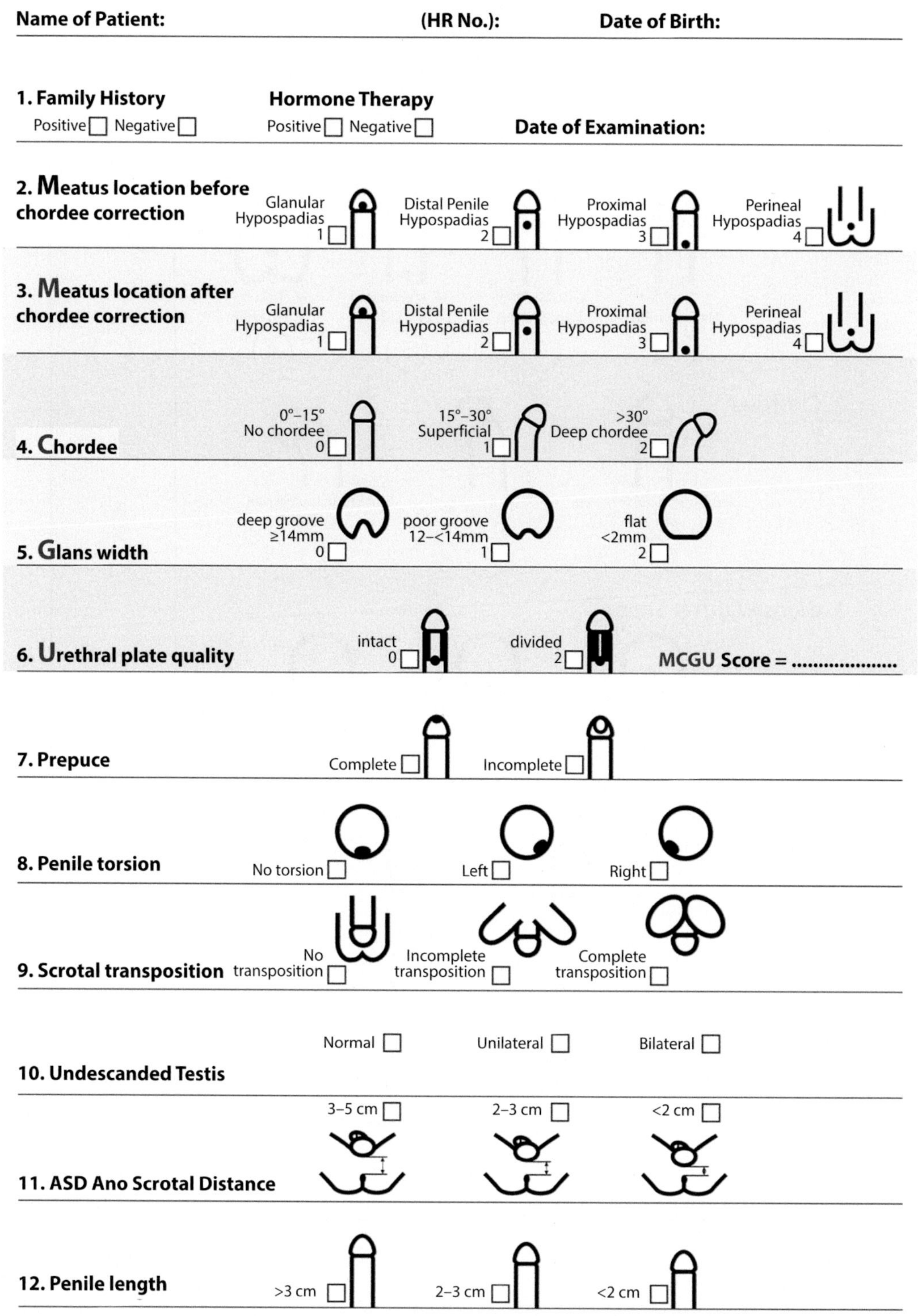

Name of Patient: **(HR No.):**   **Date of Birth:**

1. Family History   **Hormone Therapy**
   Positive ☐ Negative ☐   Positive ☐ Negative ☐   **Date of Examination:**

2. Meatus location before chordee correction

Glanular Hypospadias 1 ☐	Distal Penile Hypospadias 2 ☐	Proximal Hypospadias 3 ☐	Perineal Hypospadias 4 ☐

3. Meatus location after chordee correction

Glanular Hypospadias 1 ☐	Distal Penile Hypospadias 2 ☐	Proximal Hypospadias 3 ☐	Perineal Hypospadias 4 ☐

4. Chordee

0°–15° No chordee 0 ☐	15°–30° Superficial 1 ☐	>30° Deep chordee 2 ☐

5. Glans width

deep groove ≥14mm 0 ☐	poor groove 12–<14mm 1 ☐	flat <2mm 2 ☐

6. Urethral plate quality

intact 0 ☐	divided 2 ☐	**MCGU Score = ...**

7. Prepuce   Complete ☐   Incomplete ☐

8. Penile torsion   No torsion ☐   Left ☐   Right ☐

9. Scrotal transposition   No transposition ☐   Incomplete transposition ☐   Complete transposition ☐

10. Undescanded Testis   Normal ☐   Unilateral ☐   Bilateral ☐

11. ASD Ano Scrotal Distance   3–5 cm ☐   2–3 cm ☐   <2 cm ☐

12. Penile length   >3 cm ☐   2–3 cm ☐   <2 cm ☐

Figure 68.3 The Hypospadias Initial Score (HIS) that provides the data needed about the hypospadias patient and the possible associated malformations. It combines the MCGU in addition to information about the prepuce, rotation, testis, scrotum, and ano-scrotal distance (ASD). (©Ahmed T. Hadidi 2021. All rights reserved.)

SIGNS

- Hypospadias is usually asymptomatic.
- Signs are usually caused by a narrow meatus and downward direction of the urine stream (voiding troubles).

PREOPERATIVE WORKUP

- Clinical examination, with evaluation of:
  - The meatus size and location
  - Glans width (GW), glans dorsal length (GDL), glans ventral length (GVL)
  - ASD
  - Width of urethral plate
  - Presence of chordee
  - Prepuce
  - Penile torsion
  - Scrotal transposition and width
- Classify the form of hypospadias according to **Figure 68.3(a)**.
- Ultrasonography of kidneys and bladder (to rule out the presence of associated congenital anomalies and to evaluate the residual volume after voiding).
- Flowmetry (voiding troubles).
- If hypospadias is associated with undescended testis, chromosomal analysis is mandatory.

TECHNICAL RECOMMENDATIONS

- Gentle tissue handling is essential to get good results.
- Fine surgical instruments are essential in hypospadias repair.
- Optical magnification is advisable.
- Operation may be performed using a tourniquet, which should be released every 40 minutes or preferably without a tourniquet to reduce postoperative bleeding and edema.
- Only bipolar diathermy should be used for hemostasis.
- The repair should be performed around a large catheter (at least 10 Fr).
- The duration of the transurethral catheter should be restricted and silastic catheters should be used whenever possible to avoid tissue irritation. A suprapubic catheter may be needed if urinary diversion is desired for more than 10 days.
- For hypospadias surgery only very fine sutures must be used for the urethroplasty (6-0 or 7-0).
- Every operation should start with calibration and dilatation of the meatus.
- An artificial erection test is performed to identify and, if appropriate, correct chordee, preferably without a tourniquet.
- More than 300 techniques and modifications have been described for hypospadias correction. There are techniques that are designed for each grade of hypospadias.
- The following recommendations (**Table 68.1**) must be regarded only as a suggestion.

SURGICAL PROCEDURES

Meatotomy

- The meatus is dilated with a bougie à boule (e.g. bulb-tipped bougie).
- A longitudinal incision on the meatus of adequate length is performed, putting into consideration that the meatus will contract again with healing.
- The urethral epithelium is sutured to the glans.

Table 68.1 Techniques of hypospadias repair after chordee correction

Glanular (grade I)	Distal (grade II)	Proxima (grade III)	Perineal (grade IV)
DYG	SLAM	LABO	CEDU
Double Y glanuloplasty	Slit-like adjusted Mathieu	Lateral-based Onlay	Chordee excision and distal urethroplasty
Meatal advancement	Thiersch	Onlay island flap	BILAB
MAGPI	TIP		Bilateral-based flap
Meatal advancement glanuloplasty incorporated	Tubularized incised plate, with or without graft (GTIP)		Two-stage graft repair

Chordee correction

- Chordee may be classified into mild, moderate, and severe.
  - **Mild** superficial chordee is usually mild (<15 degrees) and is corrected in general by ventral skin degloving.
  - Many surgeons prefer to perform dorsal plication in **moderate chordee** (between 15 and 30 degrees).
  - In **severe**, deep chordee (>30 degrees), the urethral plate must be divided and the hypoplastic ventral fascia including the longitudinal fibers of the tunica albuginea, Tunica Albuginea Externa Excision (TALE), need to be excised. Others may use multiple corporotomies.
- The residual curvature is evaluated with the artificial erection test (**Figure 68.4**). To induce an artificial erection, inject 0.9% saline solution into the corpora cavernosa using a 21-G butterfly needle (Gittes's maneuver). It is less recommended now to use a tourniquet. Another approach is to use the natural erection test, where the surgeon exerts pressure at the penopubic angle with one finger and pushes the blood into the penis from the perineum.
- If chordee more than 30 degrees persists in spite of the previous procedure, a deep transverse incision in the tunica albuginea at the maximum level of curvature and a dermal graft, small intestinal submucosa (SIS), or tunica vaginalis flap from the testis are commonly used.

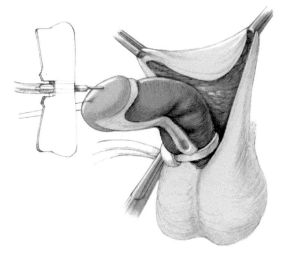

Figure 68.4 The artificial erection test.

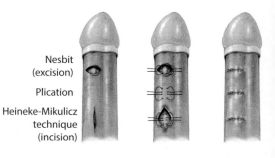

Figure 68.5 Schematic presentation of different approaches of dorsal plication. (©Ahmed T. Hadidi 2021. All rights reserved.)

Dorsal plication

- Different methods for dorsal plication were proposed as shown in **Figure 68.5**:
  - Nesbit first described plication without incision but the recurrence rate was high.
  - Nesbit then performed the plication with an excision without suture.
  - Lateral tunica albuginea plication (TAP).
  - Midline TAP.
  - Heineke Mikulicz incision.

DOUBLE Y GLANULOPLASTY (DYG)

- This technique is only suitable for patients with glanular hypospadias and a mobile urethra that can be pulled to the tip of the glans. If these conditions are not strictly observed, there may be retraction of the meatus.
- An inverted Y incision is outlined on the glans. The center of the inverted Y is located at the tip of the meatus, and the tip of the longitudinal limb is at the tip of the glans. The two oblique limbs embrace the meatus.
- The three limbs are incised and deepened creating two glandular flaps laterally and the meatus and urethra downward in the middle.
- The meatus and urethra are mobilized, pulled upward, and fixed to the tip of the glans.
- The second Y is incised as shown in the figure to allow adequate mobilization of the urethra around a catheter size Fr 12 whenever possible.
- The glandular wings are sutured around the meatus in its new position.
- The operative steps are illustrated in **Figure 68.6**.

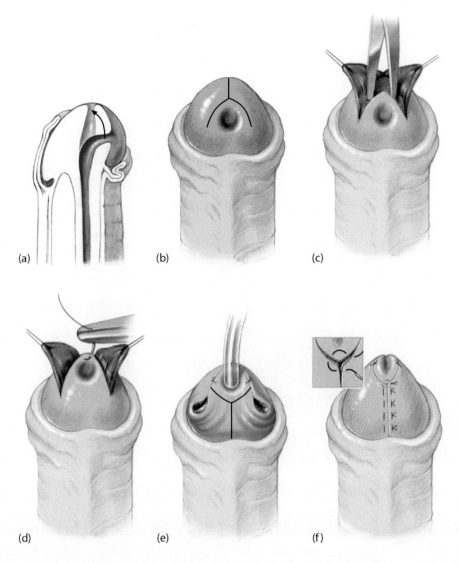

Figure 68.6 (a) Glandular hypospadias with mobile meatus. (b) Inverted Y incision. (c) The three flaps are elevated. (d) The apex of the meatus is sutured to the tip of the glans. (e) A catheter Fr 12 is introduced inside the urethra and a Y incision is made that surrounds the meatus and extends down to the coronal sulcus. (f) The glandular wings are mobilized deep enough to wrap around the urethra and are approximated in the midline. The 6 o'clock stitch is a three-point stitch that brings the urethra and the two medial edges of the glandular wings together and is magnified in the inset. (©Ahmed T. Hadidi 2021. All rights reserved.)

MEATAL ADVANCEMENT

- A circular incision in the meatus is performed and held with a stay suture.
- The urethra is dissected longitudinally along the shaft, if necessary as far as the penoscrotal junction.
- Careful coagulation with bipolar electro-cautery reduces bleeding and postoperative edema.
- The two glanular wings are sutured over the urethra from the top distally.
- The operative steps are illustrated in **Figure 68.7**.

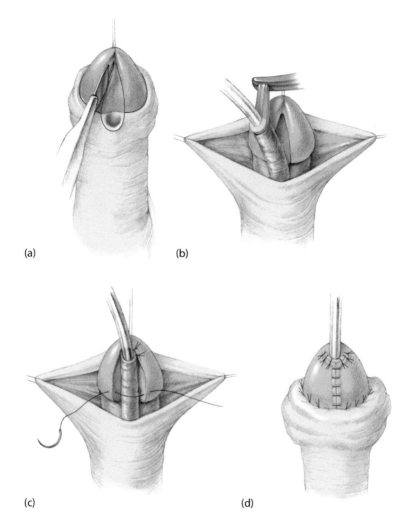

(a)

(b)

(c)

(d)

Figure 68.7 (a–d) Meatal advancement of the urethra. (©Ahmed T. Hadidi 2021. All rights reserved.)

MEATAL ADVANCEMENT AND GLANULOPLASTY INCORPORATED (MAGPI)

- A circular incision in the prepuce is performed at the level of the coronal sulcus.
- A longitudinal incision at the inner aspect of the meatus is performed as far as the tip of the glans.
- This longitudinal incision is sutured transversally with single stitches.
- The anterior aspect of the newly created meatus is secured with a stay suture and pulled up to the tip of the glans.
- A sharp incision is performed in both glanular wings in an inverted V-shape.

- The glanular wings are sutured in the apical to distal direction to enclose the urethra within the glans.
- The outer layer of the prepuce is sutured to the coronal sulcus.
- Preputial reconstruction, though possible, is not recommended at this stage.
- The operative steps are illustrated in **Figure 68.8**.

SLIT-LIKE ADJUSTED MATHIEU REPAIR (SLAM)

- This is the most popular technique for distal hypospadias repair (**Figure 68.9**).
- The SLAM modification avoids the drawback of the original Mathieu repair, which results

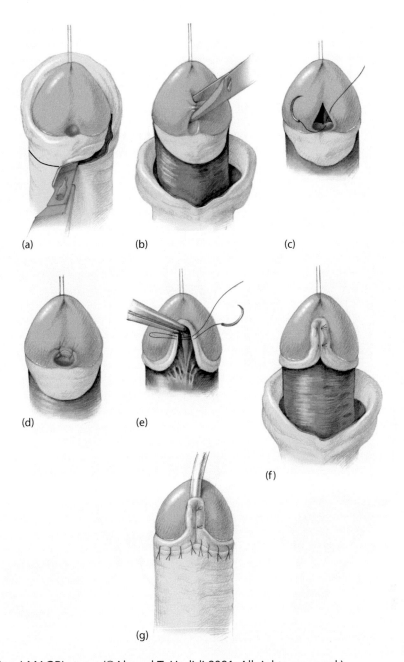

Figure 68.8 (a–g) MAGPI steps. (©Ahmed T. Hadidi 2021. All rights reserved.)

in a circular meatus that is not at the tip of the glans.

- A U-shaped incision is outlined, which differs from the classic Mathieu incision in that the distal ends of the U incision are converging and the widest point of the flap is at the meatal location.
- The flap is elevated with the underlying fascia. This is important, as this is the main blood supply to the flap.

- The new urethra is reconstructed around a catheter size Fr 12 whenever possible using three layers of sutures. Please notice that the urethra is not reconstructed to the very tip of the glans (leaving 3 mm from the incision).
- A "V" is excised from the tip of the new urethra to achieve a slit-like meatus.
- If the flap is thin or the fascia is underdeveloped, fashion a protective intermediate layer, using preputial fascia.

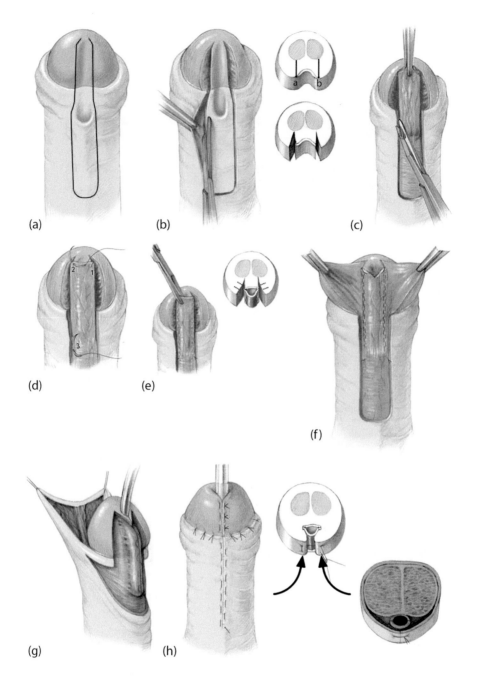

(a)

(b)

(c)

(d)

(e)

(f)

(g)

(h)

Figure 68.9 (a–h) The slit-like adjusted Mathieu (SLAM). (©Ahmed T. Hadidi 2021. All rights reserved.)

- Both granular wings are sutured together around a neo-urethra using interrupted mattress sutures.
- The technique can be successfully used when the meatus lies in the middle of the penis (so-called mid-penile hypospadias) by adopting the so-called "lateral SLAM", thus avoiding hair-bearing scrotal skin.

TUBULARIZED INCISED PLATE URETHROPLASTY (TIP URETHROPLASTY)

- The operative steps are illustrated in **Figure 68.10**.
- A circumscribing skin incision 1–2 mm proximal to the meatus is performed.

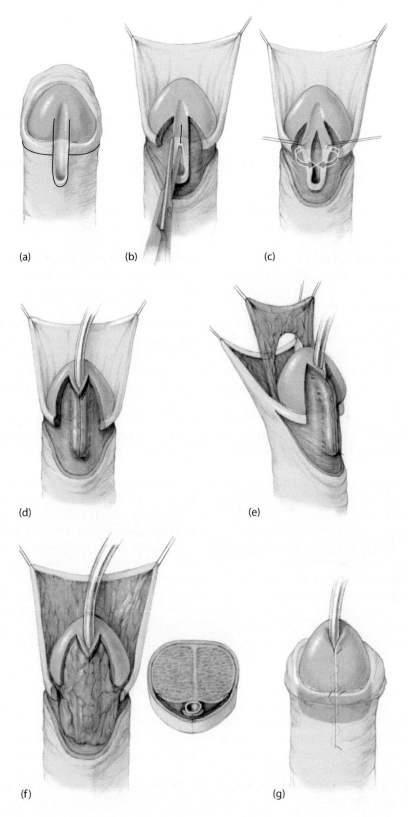

(a)

(b)

(c)

(d)

(e)

(f)

(g)

Figure 68.10 (a–g) Tubularized incised plate urethroplasty (TIP urethroplasty). (©Ahmed T. Hadidi 2021. All rights reserved.)

- The penis skin is degloved to the penoscrotal junction.
- The urethral plate is separated from the glans wings by parallel incisions.
- The glans wings are mobilized, avoiding damage to the margins of the urethral plate.
- A relaxing incision is performed using scissors in the midline from within the meatus to the tip of the glans.
- The depth of this relaxing incision depends on the plate width and depth.
- The urethra is tubularized on the inserted catheter, placing the first stitch at the mid glans, preferably with 7-0 polyglactin.
- The tubularization is completed with a two-layer running sub-epithelial closure.
- A dartos pedicle is developed from the dorsal shaft skin; it is then button-holed and transposed to the ventrum to cover the repair additionally.
- The skin edges of the tubularized glans are sutured together with the meatus.
- This method has become popular because of its simplicity; however, it may be associated with meatal stenosis, functional urethral obstruction (FUO), and fistula.
- Some surgeons prefer to cover the epithelial defect resulting from the urethral plate incision with a preputial graft in an attempt to reduce the incidence of urethral strictures (referred to as dorsal inlay draft or DIG) in an attempt to reduce stenosis and persistent fistula following the TIP repair.

LATERAL-BASED ONLAY FLAP (LABO)

- The lateral-based Onlay flap is suitable for proximal hypospadias without deep chordee that necessitates division and excision of the urethral plate.
- It has the same principle of SLAM, but it uses the lateral penile skin instead to avoid the hair-bearing skin or the scrotum.
- A U-shaped incision is outlined. The two lateral incisions go very deep into the glans and converge distally. The left lateral incision stops at the coronal sulcus and continues distally in the prepuce at the muco-cutaneous junction and constitutes the medial border of the LABO flap. The flap is designed to have a wide base as shown in **Figure 68.11(b)**.

- The right incision is deepened starting near the coronal sulcus, and the tip of the medial border is sutured to the urethral plate 2 mm proximal to the edge (A).
- The medial border of the LABO flap is sutured to the left edge of the urethral plate.
- The LABO flap is turned over catheter size Fr 12, and the second apical suture is fixed 2 mm from the tip.
- Urethroplasty is completed using continuous subcuticular 6/0 Vicryl suture on a cutting needle.
- A second and preferably third protective layer is employed from the penile fascia or dartos fascia from the scrotum.
- The glanular wings are approximated over catheter size Fr 12 and the penile skin is closed.
- The operative steps are illustrated in **Figure 68.11**.

Transverse preputial island flap (Duckett operation)

- A neourethra is created utilizing the inner preputial layer and anastomosed distally with the native urethra and apically with the glans.
- A circular incision is made of the meatus and of the inner preputial layer along the coronal sulcus.
- The urethra is dissected and a chordectomy is performed.
- The length of the urethral defect is estimated while the penis is erect.
- The prepuce is fixed with four holding sutures, so that its inner layer lies flat.
- Once the length of the neourethra is determined, the inner layer is incised accordingly.
- The inner layer is separate from the outer one, taking particular care not to injure its blood supply.
- The dissection is conducted of the vascular pedicle in such a way that rotation of the neourethra, in the craniocaudal direction, is possible without tension.
- The neourethra is created by rolling up the inner preputial layer on a catheter as a tube and closing it with a running suture.
- On the anterior aspect of the penis a channel from the coronal sulcus beyond the frenulum is performed as far as the tip of the glans, through which a passage is formed.

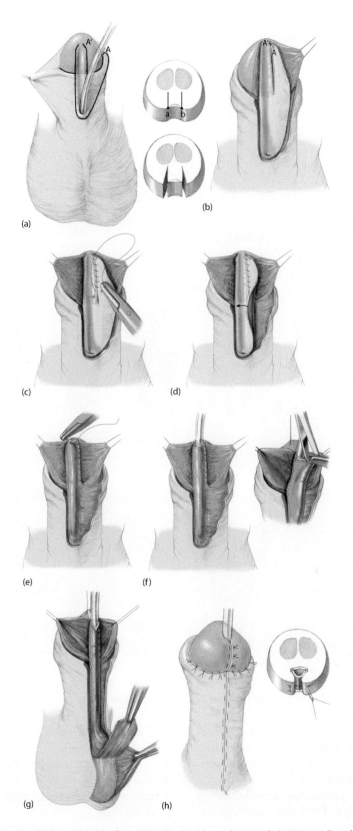

Figure 68.11 (a–h) Lateral-based Onlay flap (LABO). (©Ahmed T. Hadidi 2021. All rights reserved.)

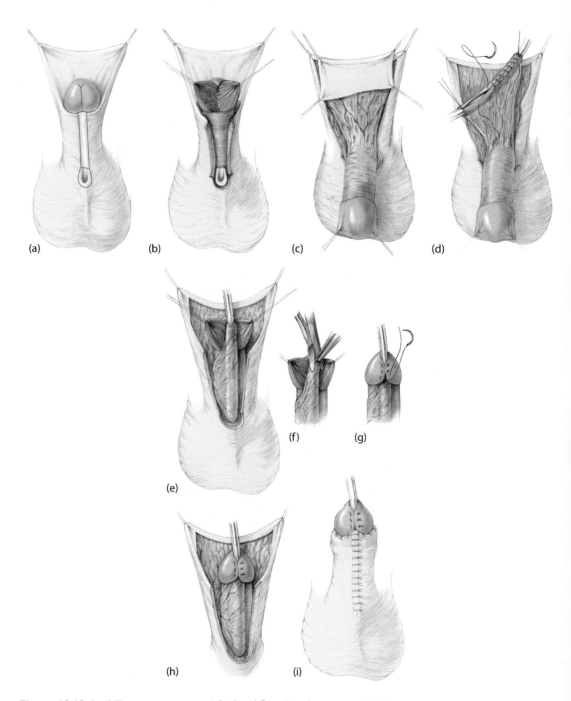

Figure 68.12 (a–i) Transverse preputial island flap (Duckett operation).

- An oblique anastomosis between the neourethra and the native urethra is performed in such a way that the suture line on the neourethra lies on the penis shaft.
- The neourethra is pulled through the channel previously developed up to the glans tip and fixed to the glans.

- The skin of the penis is closed on the shaft with a running suture.
- The outer layer is sutured to the inner one.
- It is recommended to avoid reconstruction and removal of the prepuce until a successful result is obtained.
- The operative steps are illustrated in **Figure 68.12**.

Onlay island flap

- Instead of creating a complete neourethra from the inner preputial layer only, it is possible to complete the urethral plate with the inner preputial layer.
- Semicircular skin incision along the urethral plate around the meatus.
- A pedicle flap from the inner preputial layer is dissected in the same way as for the Duckett's operation (see earlier).
- The glans is split in line with the urethral plate.
- The flap on the ventral aspect of the penis shaft is transposed and both flap borders are sutured with the free borders of the urethral plate.

- Skin closure and glanular wings closure.
- The operative steps are illustrated in **Figure 68.13**.

Bilateral-based flap (BILAB) for perineal hypospadias

- BILAB is designed to reconstruct a new urethra from the penile and preputial skin when the urethral plate has to be divided and excised in order to correct deep severe chordee (more than 30 degrees).
- A transverse subcoronal incision is performed and all the hypoplastic tissues are removed, including the longitudinal layer of the tunica

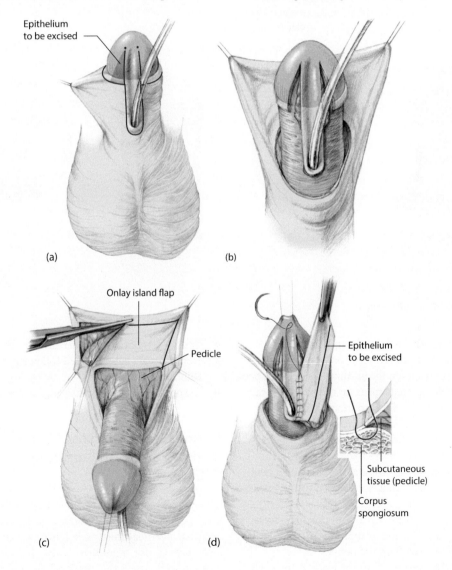

(a)

(b)

Epithelium to be excised

Onlay island flap

Pedicle

Epithelium to be excised

Subcutaneous tissue (pedicle)

Corpus spongiosum

(c)

(d)

Figure 68.13 (a–h) Onlay island flap. (*Continued*)

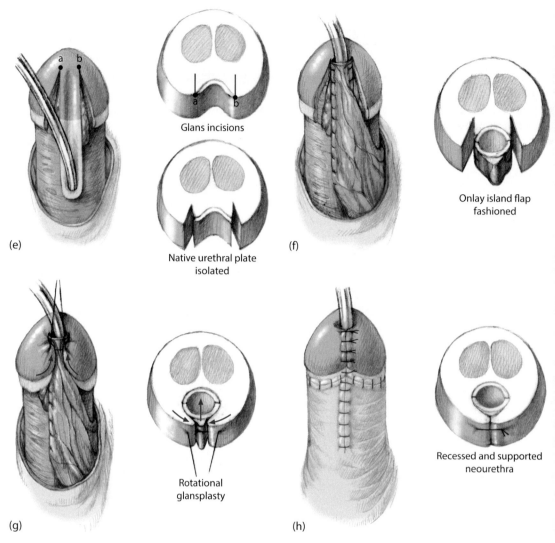

(e)

Glans incisions

Native urethral plate isolated

(f)

Onlay island flap fashioned

(g)

Rotational glansplasty

(h)

Recessed and supported neourethra

Figure 68.13 (Continued)

albuginea. The proximal edge is usually retracted back to the scrotum.

- The glans is split in the midline like an open book to provide adequate space for the new urethra.
- A transverse lateral skin incision in the prepuce is performed at the junction between the outer skin and inner mucosa on both sides.
- Both medial edges are fixed together in the midline at the tip of the glans creating a new "urethral plate" that is well fixed to the tunica albuginea in the midline (inset).
- A 4/0 Ethilon suture through the glans fixes the penis to the abdominal wall for 2–3 weeks to help to straighten the penis.
- A catheter is inserted in the bladder for a week.

- After 3–6 months, tabularization of the new urethral plate is performed following the Thiersch principle.
- The operative steps are illustrated in **Figure 68.14.**

Perineal hypospadias: Chordee excision and distal urethroplasty (CEDU)

The concept of the CEDU operation and steps are the same. The only difference that in CEDU, the original perineal meatus is left intact as a "perineal fistula" for 3 months until the wound has healed well; then the perineal fistula is closed

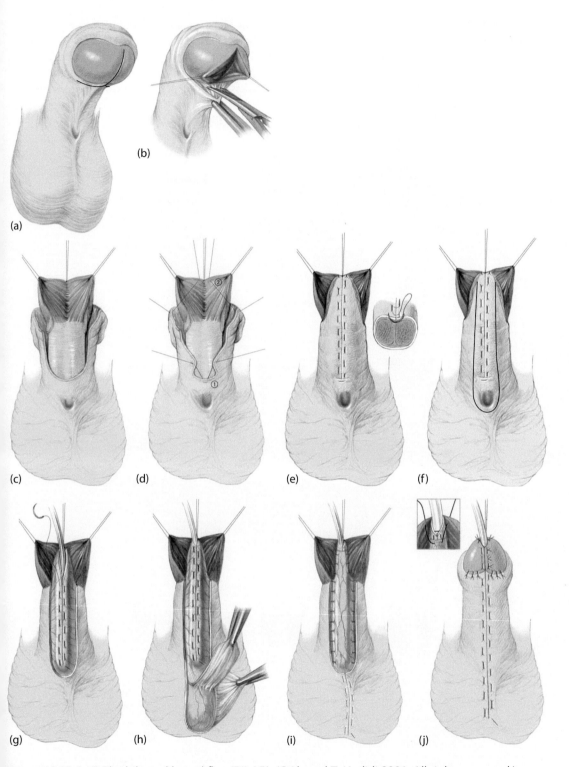

Figure 68.14 (a–j) The bilateral based flap (BILAB). (©Ahmed T. Hadidi 2021. All rights reserved.)

and final adjustment of the shape of the penis is performed.

- A transverse subcoronal incision is performed and all the hypoplastic tissues are excised, including the longitudinal layer of tunica albuginea (**Figure 68.15a,b**).

- The glans is split in the midline like an open book (**Figure 68.15c**).
- The proximal skin edge usually retracts to the proximal penis, and a transverse lateral skin incision in the preputial skin separates the outer skin from the inner mucosal layer in both sides (**Figure 68.15d**).

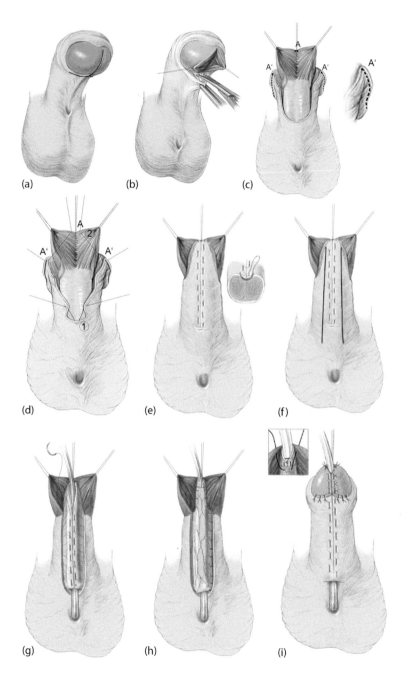

Figure 68.15 (a–i) The chordee excision and distal urethroplasty (CEDU) technique. The perineal fistula is closed 3–6 months later. (©Ahmed T. Hadidi 2021. All rights reserved.)

- Both medial edges are fixed together in the midline to the tip of the penis creating a new "urethral plate" that is well fixed to the tunica albuginea in the midline as well as laterally (**Figure 68.15e**).
- A catheter size Fr 12 is inserted into the bladder. Two longitudinal incisions are made that stop 1 cm before the meatus (**Figure 68.15f**).
- Distal urethroplasty is performed using Vicryl 6/0 around a catheter size Fr 12 (**Figure 68.15g, h**).
- Two protective layers are mobilized from both sides.
- The remaining skin is tailored to cover the glans and penis. The catheter is replaced with a silastic catheter size 10 Fr at the end of the procedure. The glans is fixed to the abdominal wall to stretch the penis and provide stability for 2–3 weeks after surgery (**Figure 68.15i**).
- The operative steps are illustrated in **Figure 68.15**.

Neourethra from buccal mucosa/ non-hairy skin

- In complicated hypospadias where there is no adequate healthy local skin, the surgeon may need to import healthy epithelium (buccal mucosa, lingual mucosa, or non-hairy skin from behind the ear or inner arm) to form a wide urethral plate as a first stage.
- A neourethra is reconstructed in the second stage.
- Bladder mucosa and one-stage repair using buccal mucosa are becoming less popular in complicated proximal hypospadias due to the high incidence of contraction.

COMPLICATIONS

- Meatal stenosis.
- Fistula formation (5–30%).
- Anastomotic urethral stenosis.
- Diverticulum formation.
- Persistent/recurrent chordee (penile curvature).
- Smegma inclusion cysts.
- Functional urethral obstruction.
- Infection.

SURGICAL PROCEDURES FOR COMPLICATIONS

Meatal stenosis/urethral stricture

- Meatal stenosis and urethral stricture have become the most common complication after hypospadias repair after the increasing popularity of the TIP technique.
- Modifications to reduce the incidence of stenosis include urethral reconstruction to the mid-glans and the insertion of a graft, referred to as "Snodgraft".

Fistula

- Fistula used to be the most frequent postoperative complication. However, meatal stenosis and urethral strictures have become the most common complications following the TIP procedure.
- Several factors may be responsible:
  - Distal stenosis.
  - Technique applied.
  - Skin damage.
  - Bleeding.
  - Edema.
  - Tension on the sutures.
  - Overlapping of suture lines.
- There are three important steps to the correction of urethral fistula:
  - Exclusion and correction of distal stenosis.
  - Wide excision of the fistula tract.
  - The use of a vascular protective intermediate layer between the urethra and skin closure.

Functional urethral obstruction (Figure 68.16)

- This is the condition where the child complains of dysuria, pain with micturition, or has recurrent fistula after simple closure.
- When the surgeon introduces a catheter to exclude distal obstruction, the catheter passes through the new urethra and widens the narrow incised plate, giving the false impression that the new urethra is wide.

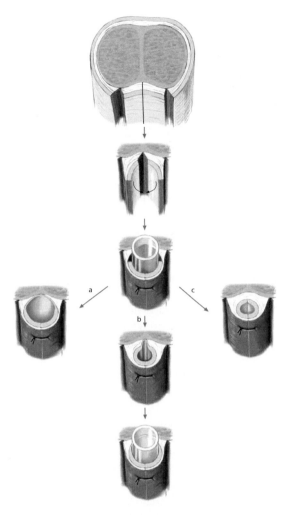

Figure 68.16 The incised urethral plate may heal in three possible pathways: (a) Wide groove resulting in the formation of a wide new urethra; (b) narrow deep groove that only yields to a sound or a catheter passing through the new urethra resulting in functional urethral obstruction (FUO); (c) linear scar resulting in urethral stricture (©Ahmed T. Hadidi 2021. All rights reserved.)

POSTOPERATIVE CARE

- Different surgeons prefer different dressing protocols, according to personal experience and local circumstances. The author prefers simple compression dressing to be removed together with the catheter 1–2 days after surgery in distal hypospadias and 7–10 days after surgery for proximal or perineal hypospadias.
- Most surgeons use oral antibiotic prophylaxis until the catheter is removed.

- Patients should be reviewed until 15 years of age. The standard protocol in the Hypospadias Center, Frankfurt, Germany, is to see the child 3 months after surgery, then after 1 year, then 3 years, then every 5 years until 15 years of age.
  - Control of micturition and urine stream.
  - Uroflowmetry is indicated usually if there is a problem or suggestions of back pressure on the bladder or kidney.

PROGNOSIS

- Good for penile forms of hypospadias without deep chordee in the hands of a fairly skilled surgeon.
- Good for the perineal hypospadias in the hands of an expert.

BURIED PENIS

GENERAL CONSIDERATIONS

- Buried penis (BP) is characterized by an abnormally long inner prepuce (LIP).
- Congenital **m**ega **p**repuce (CMP) was previously used to describe patients presenting with intermittent ballooning of the genital area; however, it should be included in grade I BP.
- Recent publications suggest that patients with BP have a shorter penis than normal, and it is possible that the buried penis does not grow normally as a normal penis may grow.
- Proper treatment is dependent on accurately diagnosing which entity is present.

CLASSIFICATION OF BURIED PENIS (FIGURE 68.17)

- BP may be classified into three grades:
  - *Grade I*: Where there is an abnormal LIP and loose attachment of skin and fascia to the corporal body. Excision of the loose areolar tissue and circumcision are usually enough.
  - *Grade II*: Where in addition of having LIP, there is abnormal distal attachment of the fundiform and suspensory ligament. The surgeon needs to fix the root of the penis in addition to excision of the loose areolar tissue and circumcision.

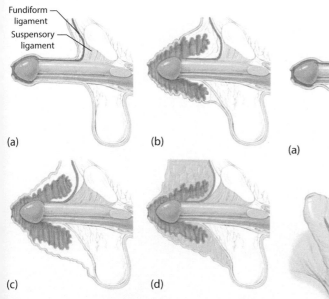

Figure 68.17 (a–d) classification of buried penis: (a) Normal penis with normal length of penile shaft, normal inner prepuce length (less than 1.5 cm), normal dartos fascia, and normal attachment of the fundiform and suspensory ligament. (b) Grade I. (c) Grade II. (d) Grade III. (©Ahmed T. Hadidi 2021. All rights reserved.)

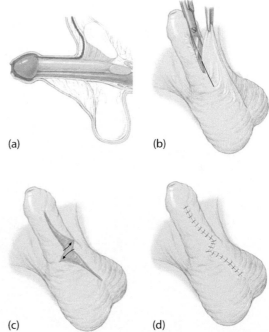

Figure 68.18 Webbed penis is due to abnormal penoscrotal junction. A V-shaped incision is made to bring the scrotum downward and is closed with a small Z-plasty. (©Ahmed T. Hadidi 2021. All rights reserved.)

- *Grade III*: LIP and distal attachment of the suspensory ligament and abnormal excess distribution of suprapubic fat in addition to the previous step.

The current accepted definitions are:

- BP is a congenital anomaly characterized by an apparent absence of a normal-sized penis buried beneath the integument of the abdomen, thigh, or scrotum.
- Concealed (hidden or inconspicuous) penis is an acquired condition presenting later in life due to abnormal excess fat accumulation in the suprapubic and genital area.
- Webbed penis is a different congenital anomaly that only involves the inferior penoscrotal junction, and surgical correction is achieved by a V-shaped midline incision that drops the scrotum down away from the penis. Circumcision is not required in webbed penis (**Figure 68.18**).
- Trapped penis is a term used to describe poorly designed circumcision in a child with

a buried penis and presents with a penis retracted behind the circular circumcision scar. Special care has to be taken, as in those children there is usually very limited skin and preputial inner mucosa. The surgeon may have to use the remaining inner mucosa to cover the defect in the penis due to the poorly designed circumcision.

SURGICAL PROCEDURE

- There are several techniques described to correct BP.
- A simple technique is shown in **Figure 68.19**.
  - Midline vertical incision with the advantage that this incision allows the surgeon to expand the approach according to the needs of each individual patient in consideration of the different grades, and the incision heals with minimal scarring and mimics the normal midline raphe.

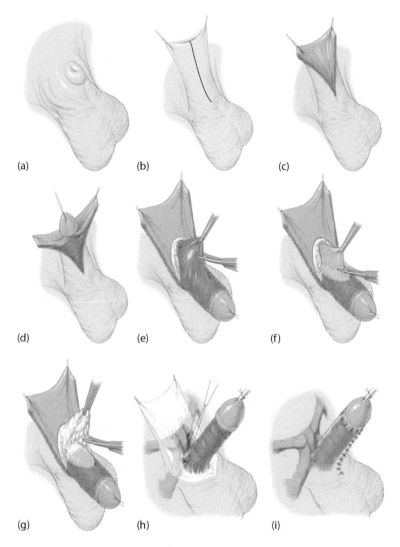

Figure 68.19 Operative steps. (From ©Ahmed T. Hadidi 2021. All rights reserved.)

- Two stay sutures and the ventral midline incision from the tip of prepuce down to the penoscrotal junction (**Figure 68.19b, c**).
- A stay suture at the tip of the glans (**Figure 68.19d**).
- Circumferential incision 0.5 cm from the coronal sulcus (**Figure 68.19e**).
- Distal attachment of the fundiform ligament and suspensory ligaments are divided in grade II and III (**Figure 68.19f**).
- Excess suprapubic fat is excised in grade III (**Figure 68.19g**).
- Two sutures fix the penile fascia to the periosteum (**Figure 68.19h**).
- The excess inner prepuce is excised and circumcision is completed (**Figure 68.19i**).

PENOSCROTAL TRANSPOSITION

GENERAL CONSIDERATIONS

- Penoscrotal transposition (PST) is a rare congenital genital anomaly in which the scrotum is positioned lateral to and above the penis.
- Early in human male genital development (8 weeks gestational age), the scrotal folds (labial folds in females) lie above and lateral to the genital tubercle. During normal development under testosterone influence, as the testes descend down, the two scrotal folds migrate downward and medially to fuse in the midline in normal males (**Figure 68.20**).

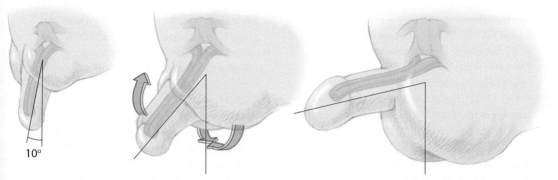

Figure 68.20 The scrotal fold develops lateral to the genital tubercle at about eighth week of gestation. It migrates downward and medially to fuse in the midline below the penis. (From ©Ahmed T. Hadidi 2021. All rights reserved.)

- PST is due to arrested downward migration of the scrotal folds, and it maintains the fetal position as in females.
- It is frequently associated with up to 90% urogenital (hypospadias, chordee, renal dysplasia) and/or up to 30% gastrointestinal malformations (predominantly imperforate anus).
- PST may present with a broad spectrum of anomalies ranging from simple shawl scrotum (doughnut scrotum) to very complex extreme transposition with craniofacial, central nervous system, cardiac, gastrointestinal, urological, and other genital (undescended testicles, hypospadias, and chordee) malformations. Growth deficiency and intellectual disability may also be noticed (60% of cases).

CLASSIFICATION

- Penoscrotal transposition is classified according to severity into three grades:
  - Partial penoscrotal transposition.
  - Complete penoscrotal transposition.
  - Penoscrotal transposition associated with bifid scrotum in perineal hypospadias.

SURGICAL PROCEDURE

- It is recommended to repair PST *ONLY* after correcting hypospadias if present so as not to interfere with the blood supply of the penis and the flaps used to reconstruct the neo-urethra.
- In infants, correction of hypospadias and correction of bifid scrotum usually drag the scrotal transposition down and correct the condition without the need of surgical correction.

- In older children, surgery is indicated to correct PST:
  - Two triangular incisions including the scrotal skin are made on either side of the penis.
  - The medial limbs of the two incisions are continued downward, under the penis to meet together in the midline, and the penis is lifted upward against the abdominal wall.
  - The two triangular flaps are elevated, freely mobilized, and brought together in the midline under the penis.
  - The resultant skin edges are sutured together.
- The operative steps are shown in **Figure 68.21**.

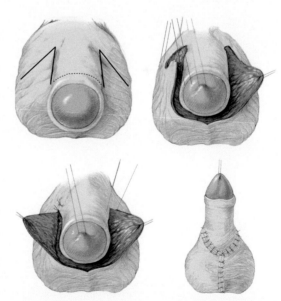

Figure 68.21 Operative steps for penoscrotal transposition repair. (©Ahmed T. Hadidi 2021. All rights reserved.)

BIBLIOGRAPHY

Hadidi AT (2012) Proximal hypospadias with small flat glans: The lateral-based onlay flap technique. J Pediatr Surg. https://doi.org/10.1016/j.jpedsurg.2012.06.027

Hadidi AT (2012) The slit-like adjusted Mathieu technique for distal hypospadias. J Pediatr Surg. https://doi.org/10.1016/j.jpedsurg.2011.12.030

Hadidi AT (2014) Perineal hypospadias; The Bilateral Based (BILAB) skin flap technique. J Pediatr Surg. https://doi.org/10.1016/j.jpedsurg.2013.09.067

Hadidi AT (2018) Perineal hypospadias: Back to the future chordee excision & distal urethroplasty. J Pediatr Urol. https://doi.org/10.1016/j.jpurol.2018.08.014

Hadidi AT (2010) Double Y glanuloplasty for glanular hypospadias. J Pediatr Surg. https://doi.org/10.1016/j.jpedsurg.2009.11.019

Hadidi AT (2017) History of hypospadias: Lost in translation. J Pediatr Surg. https://doi.org/10.1016/j.jpedsurg.2016.11.004

Hadidi AT (2022) Hypospadias Surgery: An Illustrated Textbook in Hadidi AT (ed), 2nd ed. Springer Nature.

Hadidi AT, Roessler J, Coerdt W (2014) Development of the human male urethra: A histochemical study on human embryos. J Pediatr Surg. https://doi.org/10.1016/j.jpedsurg.2014.01.009

Hadidi AT (2018) Hypospadias International Classification. 2nd Hypospadias International Society Congress, Frankfurt, Germany

Long C, Zaontz M, Canning D (2021) Hypospadias. In Partin AW, Dmochowski RR, Kavoussi CAP, LR (ed) Campbell-Walsh-Wein Urol., 12th ed. Elsevier, p 911

Mouriquand PDE, Mure PY (2004) Current concepts in hypospadiology. BJU Int Suppl. https://doi.org/10.1111/j.1464-410x.2004.04706.x

69

Bladder exstrophy and variants

PETER CUCKOW

Great Ormond Street Hospital for Children NHS Foundation Trust, London, UK

Question: A male new-born weighing 3.2 kg presents at delivery with a large midline abdominal wall lesion (see below figure). Describe this anomaly and your initial assessment and management plan for this baby.

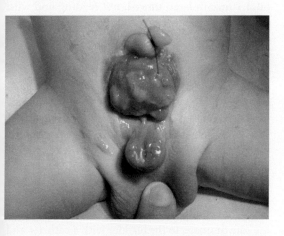

Answer: This is classic bladder exstrophy, which globally occurs in around 1 in 30,000–50,000 live births and seems to present more commonly in males than in females (2:1 ratio) [1–3]. Whilst over 50% cases are diagnosed in the antenatal period and suspected by a low-set umbilical cord, absence of a cycling bladder, a low midline abdominal wall thickening and a short wide penis, many bladder exstrophy malformations still first present in the delivery room. The exstrophied bladder sits below the low-set umbilical cord and between the two halves of the divided rectus muscle sheath which attaches to the pubic rami inferiorly. The pubic symphysis is open (diastasis), and the penis is located between them. The ureteric orifices are seen on the surface of the bladder and constantly dribble urine, although the volume may be low in the early postnatal period. In males, the verumontanum can be seen in the midline at the proximal end of the dorsal urethral plate which extends to the tip of the penis. In females, the vagina can be seen below the bladder and between the divided clitoral bodies – each attached to its ipsilateral pubic ramus and associated with the labia minora. Testes are usually descended in the scrotum, and the gender is self-evident. Inguinal hernias can occur later as patent processus vaginalis (PPV) and are more common in males but are latent at this stage. There are rarely any other associated abnormalities (unlike the rarer and more severe cloacal exstrophy variant).

Whilst attention is, of course, drawn to the dramatic bladder malformation, exstrophy is really a lower abdominal wall and anterior pelvic ring defect likely caused by embryonic failure of developing mesenchyme and rupture of the cloacal membrane to expose the bladder hidden beneath. Classical exstrophy is survivable without any treatment (as still seen in some underdeveloped countries), and this thought should contextualise initial emergent management. There is no need for resuscitation (so no IV lines), and whilst there is a theoretical risk of urinary tract infection, it is extremely rare in unoperated cases. The infant should be kept with parents and preferably breast feeding encouraged, as good nutrition is key to subsequent postoperative healing. The bladder plate is covered with a cling film dressing within the

DOI: 10.1201/9781003182290-77

nappy to protect its exposed mucosa, and the baby is administered routine vitamin K and started on low-dose prophylactic antibiotics.

Early investigations are usually limited to an ultrasound scan to establish the baseline (usually normal) upper renal tract anatomy and at the same time the spine can be scanned to easily rule out any co-existent anomaly; although these are very rare in classic exstrophy, they may include anorectal malformations, neural tube defects and skeletal anomalies [4–6]. From early on a conversation can be started with the specialist exstrophy centre, but it is not necessary to transfer the patient early, as primary bladder closure is rarely ever performed in the first week of life. The first few days of life should focus on feeding and establishing the parent-child bond, with transfer after a few days for the family to receive appropriate expert advice from the surgical team in a specialist centre familiar with treating the anomaly. Note: A well-nourished infant with bladder exstrophy has better surgical outcomes.

Question: What clinical issues are there to be considered for this baby? Discuss an initial surgical strategy to address these facts.

Answer: Apart from urinary incontinence and significant genital issues which are defined by the anomaly itself, other clinical issues for exstrophy patients may largely arise from its staged treatment. Treatment strategies are ideally tailored to re-establish the bladder as an internal container for urine with an ability to cycle a sufficient volume and empty completely, without compromising kidney function. Voiding continence is the goal, with various approaches described. Historically, most patients required an entero-cystoplasty, a bladder neck procedure, and emptied their bladder using intermittent catheterisation (usually via a Mitrofanoff channel conduit) in order to be dry. Whilst there are several procedures now available to perform all the surgery in a single stage, most paediatric urologists prefer to close the bladder shortly after birth and then later perform continence and genital surgery at a later date.

Most urology specialists treating bladder exstrophy now avoid an emergency closure in the neonatal period, and it seems sensible to wait up to a month to allow recovery from birth and delivery and for the baby at least to regain birth weight and be in positive nitrogen balance.

Technique: The bladder is carefully separated from the rectus muscle on either side, and this dissection is continued inferiorly to the level of the verumontanum, defining the proximal urethra/ bladder neck as a 1- to 2-cm midline strip. Deep dissection medial to the pubic rami releases the bladder neck to enable it to be adequately placed behind the abdominal wall. The bladder plate is then closed in two layers, with absorbable monofilament sutures such as Monocryl, and urinary drainage is provided with indwelling ureteric tubes and a urethral stent. The abdominal wall is closed with heavy interrupted sutures, and inferiorly these are placed in the pubic rami, closing the soft tissue medial to the pubic rami in front of the bladder neck. Bilateral inguinal herniotomy is performed routinely in males to avoid later presentation with clinical hernias, which are otherwise common. IV antibiotics are used routinely, and postoperative analgesia with an epidural catheter allows the infant to resume feeding soon after returning to the hospital ward. Primary closure in this way is usually achieved without bilateral pelvic innominate osteotomies, thus significantly reducing morbidity and achieving equal success.

Question: Following discharge after primary bladder closure, the infant presents to their local hospital 1 month later, unwell, not feeding and with a high fever. What scenario do you envisage here?

Answer: Following primary bladder closure, it is important to establish that the kidneys are draining adequately and that the outlet of the bladder is unobstructed. The vesico-ureteric junctions usually allow vesico-ureteric reflux, and this combined with outlet obstruction and infection is potentially very damaging to the kidneys. Routine ultrasound imaging surveillance is important in the early postoperative period. Urine cultures and ultrasound may confirm the diagnosis of infection in this acute scenario and its association with any hydronephrosis. Initial emergency treatment involves establishing safe drainage to the bladder with a catheter and treating urosepsis aggressively with IV antibiotics. A change of antibiotic prophylaxis and the option of intermittent catheterisation of the urethral stoma should be considered. The latter is well tolerated and can successfully stabilise the bladder outlet and help to re-establish adequate bladder cycling. Such intervention may be required in up to 10% of exstrophy patients, usually as a temporary measure.

Question: How would you address continence in this little boy who continues to dribble urine?

Answer: Patients with bladder exstrophy have a normally innervated bladder and normal detrusor muscle activity, so rearranging the anatomy has the potential to restore normal bladder function.

The goals and aims would be to enable 'normal' voiding continence through reconstruction of the bladder outlet as a second stage-operation scheduled during the second year of life or as part of a single-stage closure. Traditionally a Young-Dees-Leadbetter bladder neck reconstruction has been performed at this point in combination with an epispadias repair (see later), although the percentage of patients made continent is low, with persistent urine leakage and obstruction to the urinary outflow being common sequelae. Intermittent catheterisation and ultimately bladder reconstruction are common necessities with this approach.

The Kelly operation is a soft tissue reconstruction around the bladder outlet. The bladder is reopened and a bilateral ureteric reimplantation is first performed to prevent vesico-ureteric reflux and to help the bladder to gain capacity (rather than the upper tracts) following the surgery. The pelvic floor/levator ani muscles are released medial to their attachments to the obturator internus fascia, which then exposes Alcock's canal and the pudendal pedicle on its route to the base of the penile corpora on each side. Preserving this whilst separating the corpora by sub-periosteal dissection of their attachments to the inferior pubic rami allows the base of the penis and all the attached soft tissues to be brought together in the midline. The bladder neck is reconstructed and the urethra is then lifted off the corporal bodies and tubularised. The abdominal wall is then reclosed. The corporal bodies are brought together in the midline and usually rotated externally to reduce their dorsal curvature. The urethra is brought between them in the perineum to a ventral position on the undersurface of the penis. Here it can be wrapped proximally in the muscles of the perineum before being brought towards the glans, where it may terminate in a hypospadiac position. The glans penis itself is reconstructed and the base of the penis secured to the midline closure dorsally before replacing the penile skin cover.

In this way, both the penile reconstruction and continence are addressed by one operation. An analogous procedure is performed in females lifting the separated halves of the clitoris from the pubic rami, reconstructing the bladder neck and wrapping the perineal muscles around the urethra and the vagina.

Urinary continence takes some time to develop and depends on a combination of controllable bladder outlet resistance, compliance of the bladder wall and detrusor muscle activity. It may take some time for the exstrophy child to realise their full potential,

and when they are older biofeedback exercises can help attain this. The attainment of sufficient bladder capacity is fundamental and key to the development of firstly a dry interval, then followed with a further increase in daytime continence and in the next 5 years up to 70% of patients may later achieve this. Night-time continence will happen as the child matures and the bladder capacity approaches 70% of expected volume. The evolution of urinary continence is then followed with non-invasive bladder function assessments and surveillance urinary tract ultrasound, with prophylactic antibiotics together with aggressive treatment of any urinary infection.

For exstrophy patients who fail to develop enough bladder capacity or who are unable to adequately empty with a scarred outlet or detrusor failure, the final common pathway to continence (which used to be a primary treatment) is a tight bladder neck reconstruction combined with an ileo-cystoplasty and a Mitrofanoff catheteriseable channel conduit. This is still considered a very satisfactory outcome for exstrophy patients in whom it proves to be the only option. Persistent hypospadias in males can be addressed later by a staged urethroplasty, analogous to routine classical hypospadias repair.

Question: This 1-year-old male presents to your urology clinic for further treatment of this situation. What has happened here? How should this clinical state be treated? What can be done to prevent this?

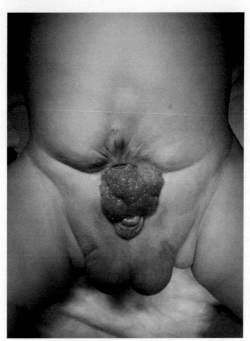

Answer: This is an all-too-familiar sight for bladder exstrophy surgeons term 'a failed exstrophy closure' with a dehiscence of the abdominal wall and pelvic ring leading to a recurrence of the exstrophy. Poor nutrition, infection, tension of the closure, ischaemia in the wound and a wide pelvic diastasis all contribute to this occurring, and undoubtedly the techniques and experience of the surgeon are also key important factors. Even in the world's best exstrophy centres the rate of dehiscence may be around 5–10% of cases. A delayed reclosure operation whilst establishing good nutrition support, scrupulous antibiotics, wound care and the addition of innominate osteotomies and postoperative immobilisation will be needed. This can return the patient to the exstrophy clinical care pathway once again, although the ultimate outcome may be worse.

Question: A baby boy has been diagnosed with an obvious penile abnormality. What are the features of this condition, how might they be assessed and what surgery may be needed?

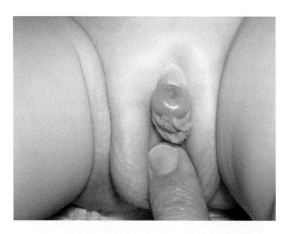

Answer: This is male primary epispadias, which occurs in around 1 in 100,000 births [7]. There is an open urethral plate on the dorsum of the penile corporal bodies, similar to the penis seen in classical bladder exstrophy. The foreskin is usually absent on the dorsal aspect of the penis, although when it is present the glans and the index diagnosis of epispadias may be concealed. In spite of the name suggesting an isolated penile condition, there is a variable association with dysplastic/hypoplastic development of the trigone and the bladder outlet which in severe cases will lead to intractable urinary incontinence.

The severity of the epispadias condition is generally considered related to the degree of bladder outlet abnormality and incontinence. The initial patient assessment together with clinical examination includes urinary tract ultrasound and scheduling cystourethroscopy. On examination, features may include a dorsally cleft glans and a urethral meatus proximal to this with a variable dorsal curvature of the penile corpora termed chordee. In severe cases the opening may be at the very base of the penis, and the verumontanum and a wide bladder outlet can be seen. There is little or no pelvic bone diastasis in epispadias, although a dip in the pubic symphysis indicates its dysplastic development. The foreskin is often found as a fringe hanging beneath the glans, but the scrotum and contained testes are usually normal and fully descended. Ultrasound imaging usually reveals normal upper renal tracts, and a clue to bladder function may be its ability to contain urine. Cystoscopy is performed within the first year of life to assess the bladder and bladder outlet. A well-formed posterior urethra with a distinct bladder neck above the verumontanum and a bladder capacity close to expected suggest the potential for future urinary continence. A wide-open bladder neck or one that completely relaxes in the early part of cystoscopic filling with the verumontanum within or everting into the base of the bladder suggests the very opposite. An abnormal bladder trigone with closely placed small ureteric orifices and a Y-shaped inter-ureteric bar, dipping towards the verumontanum, are pathognomonic of a dysplastic bladder outlet system and abnormal continence.

There is no need to commence treatment early, as boys are at little risk of complications and urinary tract infection is rare. Additional time for the family and medical staff to observe the baby is invaluable to help decide the appropriate surgical treatment. Does the patient dribble all the time or is he seen to void at intervals? Can the parents hold him upright without a nappy and not always get wet? Can the patient hold and void an appropriate volume of urine? A combination of these recorded observations, the physical findings and the endoscopic assessment are key to the decision making.

Boys with more distal epispadias tend to have favourable urinary continence parameters and are treated by Cantwell-Ransley epispadias repair, usually in the second year of life. In this operation the urethral plate is separated from the dorsum of the corpora, tubularised and transposed beneath the corporal bodies to reorientate normal penile anatomy. In the tip of the penis, the urethral meatus is moved further ventrally and the glans reconstructed behind it. The corporal bodies are rotated externally to correct the dorsal curvature, and the penile skin sleeve is reconstructed to leave a circumcised appearance. In some cases, in order to facilitate proximal reconstruction and to avoid any restriction to penile length, the urethral plate is completely separated and tubularised and the urethral meatus is left in a hypospadiac position.

More severe proximal epispadias cases with constant dribbling and evidence of poor bladder neck control are treated similarly to classical bladder exstrophy and require a bladder neck procedure, such as the Kelly operation, for continence. Because of the dysplasia of the bladder neck and associated abnormal physiology, their continence outcomes may not be as good, so many of the more severe cases may come to augmentation cystoplasty.

Question: A 4-year-old female presents with dribbling incontinence, and the appearance of the genitalia is seen here. What is this and how should this be treated?

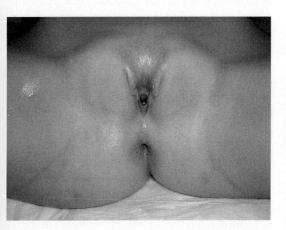

Answer: This image depicts primary female epispadias, which is much rarer than male epispadias and occurs in around 1 in 500,000 live births [8]. The anterior urethral wall and bladder neck above are deficient, and a midline cleft is seen anteriorly, with separated hemi-clitori and attached labia minora on either side with the vaginal orifice posteriorly. The rarity of the condition and a failure in routine clinical examination of the new-born female genitalia often contribute to the late presentation of many patients in childhood. All girls are destined to have intractable incontinence without surgical intervention. Many patients will have already been treated by incontinence clinics before they are referred to a paediatric urologist where the true diagnosis is then finally confirmed.

All patients will need a bladder neck continence procedure, and many of them ultimately find themselves on the final common pathway of a tight non-voiding bladder neck repair, augmentation cystoplasty and a Mitrofanoff for emptying the reconstructed bladder. The Kelly operation offers an alternative and is very similar to the operative procedure performed in classic bladder exstrophy females, without the difficulties posed by the scarring of the first surgery. Spontaneous voiding continence is a possibility in up to 75% of cases.

Question: You are called to the neonatal unit to review a premature baby with multiple abnormalities: A large exomphalos, imperforate anus, ambiguous genitalia and an odd-looking lobed mass in the lower abdomen. Describe your management strategy in childhood.

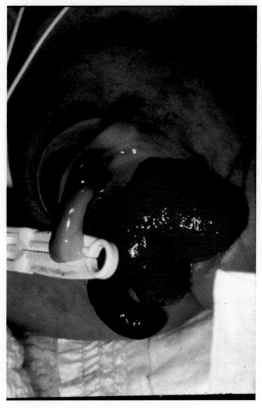

Answer: This is cloacal exstrophy, the most severe bladder abnormality found between 1 in 130,000 and 270,000 live births and notably slightly more common in males [9]. Survival and the urgent need to treat these vulnerable patients are relatively recent and brought about by advances in modern neonatal and surgical care. Many infants are born prematurely and, unlike in classic bladder exstrophy, there are significant associated co-anomalies, summarised in the table. Prematurity, myelomeningocele and severe cardiac defects take priority at birth and define early management, while the exstrophied segment is covered with cling film dressing to protect it and the associated exomphalos is allowed to dry and cicatrise, drawing the skin edges in and reducing the size of the abdominal wall defect. Early assessment includes cardiac, renal and spinal ultrasound imaging, and establishing early feeding helps to rule out small bowel atresia and secure adequate nutrition.

Renal anomalies of fusion or position	70%	
Sacral agenesis/spinal dysraphism	60%	
Myelomeningocele	50%	
Orthopaedic/limb anomalies	40%	
Small bowel atresias and malrotation	65%	
Cyanotic heart disease	<10%	
M – Severe epispadias		
F – Mullerian duplication 90%		
Vaginal agenesis	50%	
	[10]	

Examining the patient, there is often a significant midline abdominal wall defect filled by both the exomphalos above and the exstrophy lesion below. In the exstrophied segment there are usually two separated hemi-bladder plates on either side of the midline exstrophied hindgut with intussuscepted ileum and an imperforate anus. The genitalia in males may be a short, conjoined epispadiac penis or completely separate hemi-phalli and two conjoined or separated hemi scrotums, each containing a testis. In females there are hemi-clitori and labia minora and majora on either side and the vaginal orifice is often duplicated or absent. The pelvic diastasis is wide and usually over 5 cm.

Delayed closure is usual and may be significantly delayed for several months after birth if necessary, especially if cyanotic congenital heart disease or open myelomeningocele requires prior surgical attention. The hindgut segment is separated from the bladder plates and tubularised to establish continuity between the small bowel proximally and the variable length of distal hindgut. The latter is usually brought out as a permanent end colostomy in the left iliac fossa. The bladder plates are then joined together in the midline with a common incontinent urethral stoma, and the abdominal wall is closed over them. Occasionally a tense abdominal wall closure or a large defect requires the temporary use of a silo device as with classical gastroschisis to achieve closure.

As with bladder exstrophy patients, repair of the genitalia happens later in males, and a Kelly operation will achieve maximal penile length. Historically, it was common to assign female sex of rearing on the basis of a small penis, but development in our understanding of gender identity has thankfully changed this once-radical view. Continence is unlikely so this step is not used in females, who are left with divided clitori, whilst vaginal and Mullerian reconstruction is a variable and considerable challenge and often left until later life.

The final step towards continence (or rather dryness) is an ileo-cystoplasty, bladder neck repair and Mitrofanoff conduit; most patients have sufficient small bowel to achieve this. The surgery is usually performed after 5 years of age and varies considerably in this heterogenous patient group. They continue to remain a significant challenge, but patients may achieve near-normal milestones and quality of life with optimal treatment in specialist centres.

BIBLIOGRAPHY

1. Ebert, A.K., Zwink, N., Reutter, H.M. and Jenetzky, E., 2021. A prevalence estimation of exstrophy and epispadias in Germany from public health insurance data. *Frontiers in Pediatrics*, 9.
2. Nelson, C.P., Dunn, R.L. and Wei, J.T., 2005. Contemporary epidemiology of bladder exstrophy in the United States. *The Journal of Urology*, *173*(5), pp. 1728–1731.
3. Siffel, C., Correa, A., Amar, E., Bakker, M.K., Bermejo-Sánchez, E., Bianca, S., Castilla, E.E., Clementi, M., Cocchi, G., Csáky-Szunyogh, M. and Feldkamp, M.L. Bladder exstrophy: an epidemiologic study from the International Clearinghouse for Birth Defects Surveillance and Research, and an overview

of the literature. In *American Journal of Medical Genetics Part C: Seminars in Medical Genetics* 2011, November (Vol. 157, No. 4, pp. 321–332). Hoboken: Wiley Subscription Services, Inc., A Wiley Company.

4. Cadeddu, J.A., Benson, J.E., Silver, R.I., Lakshmanan, Y., Jeffs, R.D. and Gearhart, J.P., 1997. Spinal abnormalities in classic bladder exstrophy. *British Journal Of Urology*, 79(6), pp. 975–978.

5. Martinez-Frias, M.L., Bermejo, E., Rodriguez-Pinilla, E. and Frias, J.L., 2001. Exstrophy of the cloaca and exstrophy of the bladder: two different expressions of a primary developmental field defect. *American Journal Of Medical Genetics*, 99(4), pp. 261–269.

6. Ebert, A.K., Reutter, H., Ludwig, M. and Rösch, W.H., 2009. The exstrophy-epispadias complex. *Orphanet Journal of Rare Diseases*, 4(1), pp. 1–17.

7. Gearhart, J.P., Leonard, M.P., Burgers, J.K. and Jeffs, R.D., 1992. The Cantwell-Ransley technique for repair of epispadias. *The Journal of Urology*, 148(3), pp. 851–854.

8. Allen, L., Rodjani, A., Kelly, J., Inoue, M. and Hutson, J.M., 2004. Female epispadias: are we missing the diagnosis?. *BJU International*, 94(4), pp. 613–615.

9. Feldkamp, M.L., Botto, L.D., Amar, E., Bakker, M.K., Bermejo-Sánchez, E., Bianca, S., Canfield, M.A., Castilla, E.E., Clementi, M., Csaky-Szunyogh, M. and Leoncini, E., 2011, November. Cloacal exstrophy: an epidemiologic study from the International Clearinghouse for Birth Defects Surveillance and Research. In *American Journal of Medical Genetics Part C: Seminars in Medical Genetics* (Vol. 157, No. 4, pp. 333–343). Hoboken: Wiley Subscription Services, Inc., A Wiley Company.

10. Woo, L.L., Thomas, J.C. and Brock, J.W., 2010. Cloacal exstrophy: a comprehensive review of an uncommon problem. *Journal Of Pediatric Urology*, 6(2), pp. 102–111.

Preputial disorders: Phimosis, BXO and circumcision

SEMIU ENIOLA FOLARANMI
University Hospital of Wales, Cardiff, Wales

PAUL D. LOSTY
Institute of Systems and Molecular Biology, University of Liverpool, UK and
Ramathibodi Hospital, Mahidol University, Bangkok, Thailand

Scenario: A 4-year-old boy has ballooning of his foreskin on micturition and it is noted to be non-retractile. On examination at clinic he has a narrowed preputial orifice, with mild balanitis and no visible scarring (**Figure 70.1**).

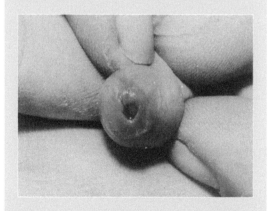

Figure 70.1 Phimosis. (From Rickwood AMK, Walker J. Ann RCS Eng 1989, 71: 275–277.)

Question: What is the diagnosis?
Answer: Phimosis.

Question: What treatment options are available in this case?
Answer: Often simple preputial hygiene measures may suffice with frequent showering/bathing. It's important to refrain from forcibly retracting the foreskin, as phimosis in young boys is often considered physiological or age dependent and notably will improve.

The application of topical corticosteroids (betamethasone or fluocinolone acetonide) has been shown to effectively treat phimosis successfully in up to 87% of cases where it is considered troublesome [1].

Scenario: An 8-year-old boy complains of spraying of urine, incomplete voiding and on occasions dribbling when making an effort to pass urine. On examination he has a scarred preputial orifice and his foreskin is firmly non-retractile (**Figure 70.2**).

DOI: 10.1201/9781003182290-78

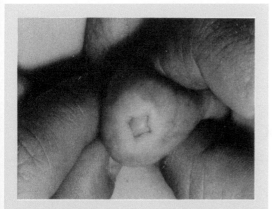

Figure 70.2 Balanitis xerotica obliterans (BXO). (From Rickwood AMK, Walker J. Ann RCS Eng 1989, 71: 275–277.)

Question: What is the diagnosis?
Answer: Balanitis xerotica obliterans (BXO). An alternative name for this condition is lichen sclerosus (LS).

Question: What are the management options for this boy?
Answer: Topical corticosteroids have been shown to have only a limited success in the definitive management of BXO with 0% success rates in some published series [2].

Foreskin preputioplasty and intralesional triamcinolone injection have been shown to be effective in the treatment of BXO. In a single-centre retrospective study, 81% of boys with BXO that underwent preputioplasty with intralesional triamcinolone injection had a fully retractile foreskin and no macroscopic evidence of BXO at a median follow-up of 14 months [3].

Circumcision remains the gold-standard therapeutic treatment of BXO.

Scenario: A 5-year-old boy attends outpatient clinic 6 weeks after undergoing circumcision for BXO, confirmed on histopathology. He is now complaining of difficulty passing urine.

On examination there is white plaque scarring evident on the glans penis around the external meatus, and a urine flowmetry study demonstrates poor urine flow.

Question: What is the diagnosis?
Answer: Lichen sclerosis (BXO) of the glandular external meatus resulting in urethral meatal stenosis.

Question: How would you manage this patient?
Answer: Topical corticosteroid with 0.1% betamethasone for a 2-week trial followed by a repeat course cycle if needed. If this fails, then a urethral meatotomy operation is needed. Up to 20% of boys have been shown to require a subsequent operation for meatal pathology after circumcision for lichen sclerosus (BXO) [4].

BIBLIOGRAPHY

1. Ashfield JE, Nickel KR, Siemens DR et al. Treatment of phimosis with topical steroids in 194 children. J Urol. 2003;169(3):1106–8.
2. Folaranmi SE, Corbett HJ, Losty PD. Does application of topical steroids for lichen sclerosus (balanitis xerotica obliterans) affect the rate of circumcision? A systematic review. J Pediatr Surg. 2018;53(11):2225–27.
3. Wilkinson DJ, Lansdale N, Everitt LH et al. Foreskin preputioplasty and intralesional triamcinolone: a valid alternative to circumcision for balanitis xerotica obliterans. J Pediatr Surg. 2012;47(4):756–9.
4. Homer L, Buchanan KJ, Nasr B et al. Meatal stenosis in boys following circumcision for lichen sclerosus (balanitis xerotica obliterans). J Urol. 2014;192(6):1784–8.
5. Rickwood AMK, Walker J. Is phimosis overdiagnosed in boys and are too many circumcisions perfomed in consequence? Ann RCSEng. 1989;(71)5:275–77.

Vesico-ureteric reflux

FABIO BARTOLI
Department of Medical and Surgical Sciences, Policlinico "Ospedali Riuniti", University of Foggia, Foggia, Italy

Scenario: An 8-month-old male infant is brought to the emergency room with a high fever (39°C), vomiting, abdominal distension and paleness. On clinical examination, the infant appears pale, lethargic and poorly reactive. The heart rate is 140/min, blood pressure 80/40 mmHg and respiratory rate 35/min. The abdomen is noted to be distended but without signs of an acute abdomen (soft on palpation). The stool history is normal, but the urine specimen is noted to be cloudy in colour. A urinary dipstick is positive for nitrites and registers pH 7.2.

Question: What is the most likely diagnosis in this child? What else will you now focus your examination on?

Answer: It is well known that urinary tract infection (UTI) may present as sepsis in infants. It is always useful to obtain a urine analysis and urine culture to confirm the diagnosis of UTI. In this specific situation, after the urine sample is sent to the laboratory, empiric antibiotic therapy with ampicillin in combination with IV fluid resuscitation may be started. In fact, the most common bacteria involved in UTI are *Escherichia coli* or *Proteus* species which are usually effectively treated with penicillin-related antibiotics. It is very important to realize that the diagnosis of UTI is not the end point of your examination, especially in the male infant. In fact, UTI is often the 'tip of the iceberg'

underlying a more complex problem affecting the urinary tract. It is important to achieve a correct interpretation of the urine culture results. In the first place, consider how the urine sample was collected by a urine bag or catheterization (in this very young age group, an intermediate micturition sample is not possible), as the only accepted result if urine is collected by a bag device is a negative culture report. In the case where the lab report is positive on the urine sample collected in the bag, you must confirm a 'true positive result' by undertaking a patient urine culture with sterile urethral catheterization. A urine culture positive for *Klebsiella* or *Pseudomonas* should always be considered a 'true positive' urine culture and the patient promptly treated with culture-specific antibiotics.

The following next steps should include an ultrasound imaging study of the urinary tract system to establish the presence of urinary tract dilatation and/or bladder anomalies (such as hydronephrosis/uretero-hydronephrosis, bladder volume before/after micturition and note any bladder wall filling defects).

In this male infant, urine culture is confirmed positive for *E. coli* with 100×10^5 colony-forming units/high power field, and the renal ultrasound report is as follows: 'Both kidneys are normal in location and dimension. On the right side, there appears to be a bifid pelvis which appears dilated with uretero-hydronephrosis. Also the left pelvis and ureter also appear somewhat dilated. The bladder is normal in its volume and at post

DOI: 10.1201/9781003182290-79

voiding evaluation, a persistent residual urine volume exists.'

Based on these imaging results, we can now diagnose left-sided vesicoureteral reflux (VUR) and a refluxing duplex reno-ureteral system on the right side.

A duplex renal system may also be complicated by an obstructing ureterocoele which affects the superior renal moiety unit (often the superior renal moiety has poor function with dysplasia), and VUR exists in the moiety draining the lower pole kidney unit.

After the UTI is properly treated and the infant is commenced on antibiotic prophylaxis, we will need to fully complete a diagnosis with additional investigations in the following weeks.

Our next objective is to confirm our working diagnostic hypothesis with a micturating cystourethrogram study (MCUG). The MCUG study report states: 'Filling phase; there is reflux evident on the left side with the ureter and renal pelvis appears dilated with calyces retaining their normal morphology. On the right side, there is a complete duplex renal system with both identified ureters and pelvis dilated. A bladder filling defect was not observed which would/may have been suggestive of a ureterocoele lesion. Micturating phase: After removal of the urethral catheter and with patient micturition there is free bilateral reflux grade 3 on the left and 4 on the right; the bladder is seen to empty properly with some residual urine volume noted. No urethral anomalies are observed' (**Figure 71.1**).

On the basis of the working classification system proposed by the International Commission

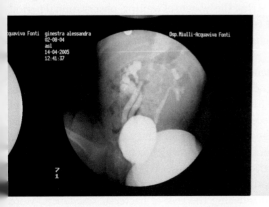

Figure 71.1 MCUG showing refluxing duplex renal system on the right side and moderate vesicoureteral reflux on the left side.

for Vesicoureteral Reflux Study Group, we can now make the following working diagnosis, notably left-sided moderate (grade 3°) VUR/right-sided duplex complete renal system with vesicoureteral reflux (grade 4°) and no ureterocoele lesion evident.

In fact, the classification of VUR is divided into five severity grades: Grade 1 – The reflux is limited to the ureter without dilatation; grade 2 – The reflux reaches the renal pelvis without dilatation; grade 3 – Reflux reaches the renal pelvis causing dilatation; grade 4 – Reflux reaches the pelvis with dilatation of both renal pelvis/calyces (retaining normal morphology) and the ureter which also appears slightly tortuous; and grade 5 – The ureteropelvic morphology is completely modified with gross marked dilation of the renal pelvis/calyces (abnormal morphology) and the ureter appears markedly dilated and tortuous [1] (**Figure 71.2**).

The next diagnostic challenges to consider are to address the impact on renal function and the characteristics of the reno-ureteral duplex system.

The gold-standard test to assess renal function in children with isolated VUR is a Tc-99 DMSA renal scan – static scintigraphy study. This examination provides useful information about residual renal function and the existence (or otherwise) of non-functioning areas of renal tissue notably due to scarring. However, when urinary tract obstruction is suspected associated with vesicoureteral reflux, the best examination is a Tc-99 MAG3 renal scan – dynamic scintigraphy study. This exam provides valuable information about renal tubular and urinary excretory function. Therefore, a full assessment of renal and excretory function is essential to fully establish the urinary tract malformation.

The results of the Tc-99 MAG-3 scintigraphy show the following: 'A split renal function of 60% on the left side and 40% on the right. Some scars are visible affecting both renal units. On the right side, the upper renal moiety is poorly functioning with a delayed excretory phase. The left and the right lower renal systems did not show excretory anomalies.'

The Tc-99 MAG3 scan thus confirms the right side has a complete duplex reno-ureteral system.

The next diagnostic challenge to consider is has a ureterocoele been missed. This lesion (if present) may cause obstruction to the bladder neck outlet or terminate at the prostatic urethra causing some degree of urinary incontinence/wetting. Of course, urinary incontinence in such a small male infant is

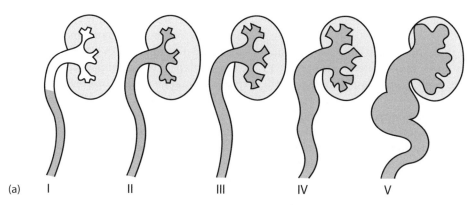

(a) I   II   III   IV   V

Grade	Description
I	Into a nondilated ureter
II	Into the pelvis and calyces without dilatation
III	Mild to moderate dilatation of the ureter, renal pelvis, and calyces with minimal blunting of the fornices
IV	Moderate ureteral tortuosity and dilatation of the pelvis and calyces
V	Gross dilatation of the ureter, pelvis, and calyces; loss of papillary impressions; and ureteral tortuosity

(b)

Figure 71.2 Classification of vesicoureteral reflux according to the international study group on vesicoureteral reflux.

difficult to confirm on a clinical basis, so further investigations are now needed.

These further investigations include a nuclear magnetic resonance (NMR) scan of the urinary tract system and operative cystoscopy. NMR in an infant will require general anaesthesia, so debate now exists for the paediatric urologist whether to request such a study. In fact, operative cystoscopy may provide most of morphological information required and at the same time may be therapeutic.

Urological malformations may be associated with genetic factors, so family relatives may harbour a 'sibling uropathy.' Furthermore, it is not infrequent that some children may present to the paediatric specialist with associated diseases of a urologic or non-urological origin. The most commonly found conditions are undescended testis, inguinal hernia and rarely complex gastrointestinal malformations such as oesophageal atresia and/or anorectal malformations.

Question: What would be the most appropriate treatment for children with vesicoureteral reflux?
Answer: This matter is a controversial debate between the paediatric urologist and medical nephrologist. These controversies are mainly based on two main factors: (a) The natural history of VUR is to improve spontaneously with age and over time and (b) slow progression of renal damage is thought to occur due to VUR.

Nowadays, most clinicians consider the following factors associated with the increased probability of spontaneous VUR resolution: (I) Early age at diagnosis, (II) low-grade VUR, (III) unilateral VUR, (IV) absence of bladder dysfunction and (V) absence of associated malformations. In these children, a more conservative approach is often advised for at least one or more years of early life. During the 'watchful waiting' observational period it is very important to monitor urine cultures and schedule surveillance as in renal ultrasound.

Another important factor to monitor is evidence of renal damage progression. Most clinicians underline the key importance of preventing UTIs, which play a major role in the development of ascending pyelonephritis and renal scarring. Here the nephrologist may have a different approach, the most common of which is to commence the paediatric patient on long-term antibiotic prophylaxis, while others may not prescribe antibiotic therapy considering the risk of bacterial resistance. More recent studies on urinary biomarkers of inflammation and renal damage progression have shown the significant value of monitoring inflammatory cytokines and markers of renal damage in children with VUR [2].

Question: When should we consider surgical treatment of VUR?
Answer: Indications for surgical intervention can be broadly divided into (1) relative and (2) absolute. Relative indications are:

a. Diagnosis of VUR at an older age.
b. Isolated grade 3 or IV VUR.
c. Persistence of VUR with long-term antibiotic prophylaxis.
d. Breakthrough UTIs.

Absolute indications are:

a. Recurrent UTI under antibiotic prophylaxis.
b. Grade 5 or severe bilateral VUR.
c. Progression of reflux nephropathy.
d. Intolerance to medical therapy from the patient and/or parents'/guardians' compliance to administer regular medication.
e. Associated complex urological malformations, e.g. posterior urethral valves.

Three options are available in terms of surgery:

a. STING endoscopic therapy: Performed as an ambulatory day care procedure. A sub-ureteric injection of a bulking agent is used to correct VUR. Several commercial agents are available on the market, most notably Macroplastique or Deflux – a dextranomer polymer. One, two or three hospital day care visits to have repeat injection sessions may be required to achieve complete success (**Figure 71.3a** and **b**).
b. *Open classical surgery*: The most common deployed are the (i) Cohen and (ii) Leadbetter-Politano ureteric reimplantation operations.
c. *Minimally invasive surgery (MIS)/robotic surgery*: A minimally invasive anti-reflux operation may be carried out laparoscopically or with robotic assistance, with the surgeon undertaking re-implantation of the ureters to correct VUR.

In conclusion, VUR is a common paediatric urological disorder which if untreated or poorly managed may progress to end-stage renal failure. Diagnostic care pathway algorithms play a key role in best practice management. The initial management

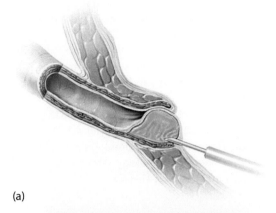

(a)

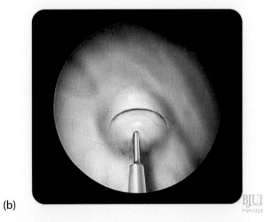

(b)

Figure 71.3 Endoscopic injection of the bulking agent, procedure and expected effect.

should always be medical therapy and watchful waiting surveillance monitoring in nearly all cases. Surgical interventions, including the STING, classical open, MIS and robotic operative correction, as stated, are best reserved only for those children who do not respond adequately to medical therapy [3–8].

BIBLIOGRAPHY

1. Lebowitz RL, Olbing H, Parkkulainen KV, et al. International Reflux Study in Children: international system of radiographic grading of vesicoureteric reflux. Pediatr Radiol 1985;15:105–109.
2. Pastore V, Bartoli F. Urinary excretion of EGF and MCP-1 in children with vesico-ureteral reflux. Int Braz J Urol 2017;43:549–555.
3. Mautouschek E. Treatment of vesicoureteral reflux by transurethral Teflon injection (author's transl). Der Urologe Ausg A 1981;20:263–264. (In German).

4. O'Donnell B, Puri, P. Treatment of vesico-ureteric reflux by endoscopic injection of Teflon. Br Med J 1984;289:7–9.

5. Malizia Jr AA, Reiman HM, Myers RP, Sande JR, Barham SS, Benson Jr RC, Dewanjee MK, Utz WJ. Migration and granulomatous reaction after periurethral injection of polytef (Teflon). JAMA 1984;251(24):3277–3281.

6. Solomon LZ, Birch BR, Cooper AJ, Davies CL, Holmes SA. Nonhomologous bioinjectable materials in urology: 'sizematters'? BJU Int 2000;85:641–645.

7. Bartoli F, Niglio F, Gentile O, Penza R, Aceto G, Leggio S. Endoscopic treatment of dilating vesicoureteral reflux in children with Macroplastique. BJU Int 2006;97:805–808.

8. Chertin, B, Kocherov S, Chertin L, Natsheh A, Farkas, A, Shenfeld OZ, Halachmi, S. Endoscopic bulking materials for the treatment of vesicoureteral reflux: a review of our 20 years of experience and review of the literature. Adv Urol 2011;2011:1–7.

72

Abnormalities of the vagina in childhood

PRINCE RAJ, ABEER FARHAN, AND MARTIN T. CORBALLY
King Hamad University Hospital, Kingdom of Bahrain, Bahrain

Scenario 1: A 14-year-old pre-menarche female attends the emergency department with a 1-week history of lower abdominal pain with no associated features of nausea, vomiting or fever. Abdominal examination shows no guarding or peritonism. A soft, non-mobile, suprapubic mass approximately 15 cm × 15 cm is evident A bulging hymen is further noted on perineal examination (**Figure 72.1**).

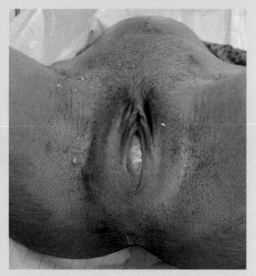

Figure 72.1 Perennial photograph showing a bulging hymen.

Question: What is the most likely diagnosis?
Answer: Imperforate hymen.

Question: What is meant by the term imperforate hymen?
Answer: Imperforate hymen is a minor anomaly of the female genital tract, which may – if complete – obstruct the genital opening. It arises from failure of normal canalization of the urogenital sinus. The hymen ring is located at the junction of the sinovaginal bulbs with the urogenital sinus and is usually perforated or fenestrated during fetal life. Failure of complete perforation results in an imperforate hymen of variant types.

Hymen variants:

a. Normal
b. Imperforate
c. Microperforate
d. Cribriform
e. Septated

Question: How can you diagnose this condition?
Answer: Diagnosis of an imperforate hymen may be readily established in the neonatal period if a bulging intraoitus is noted. This results in a mucocolpos from retained vaginal secretions secondary to hormonal stimulation by maternal estradiol. It may be wise therefore to re-examine female infants

DOI: 10.1201/9781003182290-80

at around 3–6 months of age to confirm such a diagnosis.

At menarche young girls may present with amenorrhea, cyclic abdominal or pelvic pain and hematocolpos, which may thus give the hymenal membrane a dark-bluish discoloration. Marked distension of the vaginal intraoitus may also lead to lower back pain, difficulties with stooling and/or urination.

Question: An ultrasound examination is performed. Can you interpret the imaging findings?

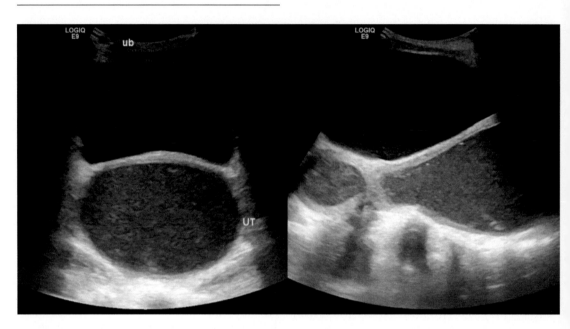

Figure 72.2 Ultrasound shows a large midline mass with hematometra.

Answer: Ultrasound scan shows a large, mid-line, sonolucent mass causing a forward displacement of the bladder with hematometra (**Figure 72.2**).

Question: What are the other potential causes for vaginal obstruction at this female age group?
Answer: Congenital vaginal obstruction may be caused by incomplete canalization of the vagina and can occur at different levels. The possible differential diagnosis therefore includes:

- Imperforate hymen (as listed earlier).
- Vaginal agenesis, also known as Müllerian agenesis or Mayer-Rokitansky-Küster-Hauser syndrome (MRKH), and refers to the congenital absence of the vagina with variable uterine maldevelopment. It results from agenesis or hypoplasia of the Müllerian duct system. Adolescent females often present therefore with primary amenorrhea.
- Transverse vaginal septum – Occurs due to failure of fusion and/or canalization of the urogenital sinus and Müllerian duct system.

- Anomalies of fusion may include vaginal duplication and obstructed hemivagina with ipsilateral renal anomaly (OHVIRA).
- Labial adhesions – Result from inflammation of the labia minora combined with low estrogen levels in the prepubertal female, which provides an explanation for the adhesions.
- Distal vaginal atresia (i.e. partial atresia or incomplete agenesis).

Question: What are the possible complications or morbidity consequences associated with this condition?
Answer:

a. Ascending infection
b. Impaired fertility
c. Endometriosis
d. Renal failure (in very rare cases)

Question: Outline the treatment options for this condition.
Answer: Surgical correction simply consists of an elliptical incision in the obstructed membrane close

to the hymenal ring followed by suction and relief of the obstructed contents. Extra-hymenal tissue is carefully excised to create a normal-size introital orifice, and the vaginal mucosa is then sutured to the hymenal ring to prevent re-adhesions and recurrence of the obstruction.

Hymen-preserving surgery methods such as a simple vertical incision and annular hymenotomy are tailored options to consider for some patients and respecting varied world racial cultures. Laser therapy ablation using a carbon dioxide laser is another option occasionally deployed by plastic surgeons.

> **Scenario:** A 15-year-old female presents to the ambulatory clinic with recurrent lower abdominal pain and primary amenorrhea. Secondary sexual characteristics are evident on clinical examination with normal breast development and pubic hair. On inspection the vestibule region appears normal, but there is no vaginal opening noted. A large, non-tender, mobile abdominal mass can be palpated. A radiological investigation is performed.

Question: Name the imaging study and now make an effort to interpret the findings (Figure 72.3).

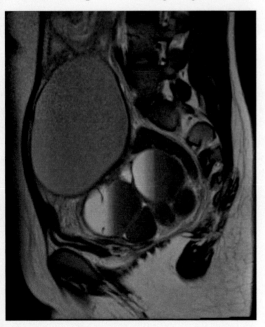

Figure 72.3 MRI scan showing multiple cystic pelvic lesions (chocolate cysts).

Answer: This is an MRI scan – sagittal view of the pelvis – showing multiple cystic pelvic lesions,

notably 'chocolate cysts' with hematometra, hydrosalpinx and vaginal atresia.

Question: What is the diagnosis when the vagina is completely absent?
Answer: MRKH syndrome is characterized by congenital agenesis of the uterus and the proximal portion (this female patient had no vagina) of the vagina which results from either complete agenesis or aplasia of the Müllerian duct system or failure of the para-mesonephric ducts to form the uterus and upper portions of the vagina.

These patients generally have acquired development of secondary sexual characteristics with a normal 46,XX karyotype. The first clue to the final clinical diagnosis is primary amenorrhea occurring in such patients with a normal female phenotype. Note these girls have normal functioning ovaries and no signs of androgen excess.

Question: What are the various types of MRKH syndrome?
Answer: Two different subtypes of MRKH syndrome have been described:

1. Isolated uterovaginal aplasia, referred to as type I (isolated) MRKH syndrome.
2. Incomplete aplasia and/or associated with other malformations, referred to as type II MRKH syndrome.

Associated malformations may include:

- Renal (unilateral agenesis, ectopia of kidneys or horseshoe kidney)
- Skeletal and, in particular, vertebral (Klippel-Feil anomaly; fused vertebrae, mainly cervical; scoliosis)
- Hearing defects
- More rarely, cardiac and digital anomalies (syndactyly, polydactyly)

Question: How may you diagnose this condition?
Answer:

1. History and a full clinical examination by an experienced pediatric gynecologist/surgeon. Findings include normal height, secondary sex characteristics and hair growth. Normal female external genitalia. Short blind-ending vagina (0–3 cm) with no cervix visible. No uterus detected by bimanual pelvic palpation.

2. Radiological examination:
   a. *Ultrasound of abdomen*: An ultrasound scan is the initial key imaging modality for Müllerian system anomalies. A partially developed small rudimentary uterine horn may be misinterpreted as a small tubular prepubertal uterus. Visualization of extra-pelvic ovaries may be challenging. Also the retro-vesicular quadrangular vestigial lamina may be misinterpreted as a hypo-plastic uterus.
   b. *MRI pelvis*: This is beneficial in discovering other MRKH-associated anomalies such as those in the skeletal or cardiovascular systems, which may be undetected with ultrasound imaging.
   c. Renal imaging to exclude nearly 30% association with MRKH.
3. Biochemical analysis.
   Serum follicle-stimulating hormone (FSH), luteinizing hormone (LH), estradiol and androgen status – all normal titer levels.
4. Chromosomal analysis: 46,XX karyotype.

Question: What are the definitive treatment options?

Answer: Before scheduling any treatment, it is of utmost importance to address the psychosexual challenges associated with an MRKH diagnosis. Counseling and allied support services with full assessment by gynecology teams should always be considered before embarking hastily into surgical corrections. The American College of Obstetricians and Gynecologists (ACOG) has recommended a dilatation therapy program as first-line treatment based on its high overall success rates (90–96%) with low complications and the economic cost. ACOG recommends that surgical operative correction be reserved for those females experiencing failure with dilatation therapy and herein emphasize that even with operation, there will still be required postsur-gical dilatation sessions to avoid future strictures.

Non-surgical: Vaginal dilatation is a valid effective alternative in females with a vaginal dimple anomaly. Daily vaginal dilatations over several periods of months with graded-size Hagar devices will yield a good-sized vagina to permit eventual intercourse.

Surgery: Innovative techniques for vaginal reconstruction in females with vaginal tract agenesis include construction of a skin neovagina and intestinal neovaginoplasty using the sigmoid colon or small intestine.

Surgical procedures:

a. *McIndoe vaginoplasty*: Split-skin graft covering a customized mold device is placed in a dissected pouch created between the rectum and bladder.
b. *Baldwin vaginoplasty*: Sigmoid colon neova-gina interposition graft.
c. Davydov vaginoplasty (peritoneal graft).
d. Williams vulvavaginoplasty (labia majora flaps).
e. Vaginoplasty using cultured autologous vulvar tissue and tissue-engineered biomaterials.
f. Minimally invasive surgery (MIS)–guided Vecchietti vaginoplasty in which a surgical traction device is anchored on the anterior abdominal wall with subperitoneal threads attached to a mold positioned in the vagina. Surgical corrective operations will still require continued use of vaginal dilators or regular sexual intercourse in the adult female to ensure good long-term outcome.

Question: What are the motherhood options for patients?

Answer: All patients with MRKH syndrome are 46,XX females but with absolute uterine factor infertility (AUFI). Motherhood options are:

i. Adoption
ii. Gestational surrogacy
iii. Uterus transplantation (UTX)

The world's very first live-birth after UTX took place in September 2014 in Gothenburg, Sweden, to a 35-year-old female MRKH patient. Approximately 75 UTX operations have now been successfully performed. Around 25 babies have been born world-wide, and MRKH females have delivered healthy babies twice.

Scenario: A 16-year-old female patient presents to the clinic with a history of cyclical lower abdominal pain for 10 months. The girl complains of difficulty in passing urine for 2 months, though there is no history of acute urinary retention. Menarche occurred at 13 years of age with a normal menstrual cycle for 2 years. Over the last year the patient has experienced increasing dysmenorrhea with lower abdominal discomfort. Clinical examination of the perineum and external genitalia was normal. Abdominal findings show a suprapubic mass inferior to the umbilicus.

Question: How will you proceed now with this patient?

Answer: As this adolescent female has attained menarche and is having normal regular periods for 2 years following that, we can easily rule out imperforate hymen, vaginal atresia and MRKH syndrome. EUA vaginal examination would yield helpful findings.

An ultrasound of the pelvis will aid determine the presence of a uterus, adnexal structures and a vagina (**Figure 72.4**).

Question: Interpret the ultrasound pelvis findings.

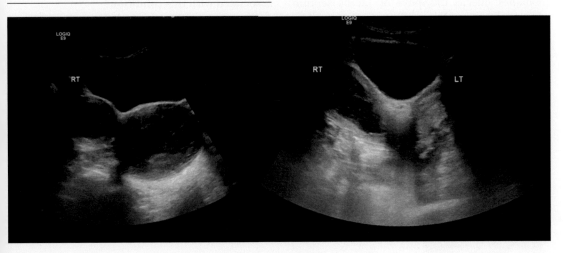

Figure 72.4 Ultrasound of pelvis showing uterus didelphys.

Answer: A ultrasound pelvis scan is consistent with uterus didelphys with a large amount of menstrual contents seen filling the right uterus and the right hemivagina. This is a hematometrocolpos likely due to an obstructed right hemivagina.

Question: In view of the ultrasound scan findings, what other systems would you like to evaluate and why?

Answer: In view of the uterus didelphys with obstructed right hemivagina it would be imperative to check the renal tract system, as this condition may occasionally be associated with an ipsilateral renal anomaly.

Question: Further imaging (Figure 72.4a and b) for a renal tract anomaly was performed and found the female patient to have ipsilateral renal agenesis. What is the name of the syndrome?

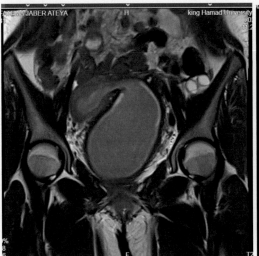
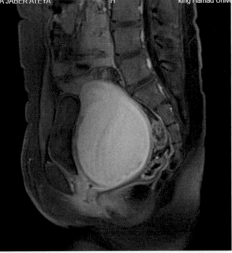

Answer: This female patient has Herlyn-Werner-Wunderlich syndrome (HWWS) which includes the syndrome triad of uterus didelphys, a blind hemivagina with ipsilateral renal agenesis. It is also referred to as OHVIRA syndrome when it includes at least two of the three main components of HWWS, which consists of different uterus anomalies (uterus didelphys or uterus septum) with a renal anomaly as well as renal agenesis or polycystic kidney.

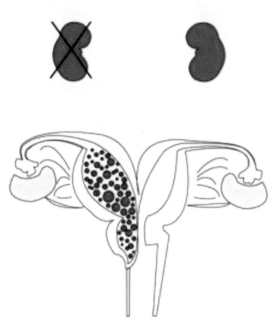

Figure 72.5 Schematic representation of HWWS.

Question: What is the embryological basis of this condition?
Answer: Uterine anomalies develop due to aberrations in vertical or horizontal fusion or arrest of the paramesonephric ducts during development. Earlier it was believed that the utero-cervical canal developed from the paramesonephric ducts, whereas the sinovaginal bulb from the urogenital sinus was thought to give rise to the lower vagina, whilst development of kidneys and ureters are from the Wolffian duct systems. However, some complex uterine anomalies like OHVIRA defied conventional doctrine until recently, when a new theory of urogenital development of the entire vagina from the mesonephric ducts was postulated.

Question: How will you manage this condition?
Answer: This disorder is best treated surgically by dividing the abnormal septum between the two hemivaginas and then draining the obstructed hemivagina into the patent vagina.

Question: What are the future concerns (if any) associated with this condition?
Answer: It has been reported that at least 25% of women affected by Müllerian duct system anomalies may present with obstetrical morbidity such as recurrent miscarriage of pregnancy, abnormal fetal presentation, postpartum hemorrhage, retained placenta, fetal mortality, fetal growth restriction and premature rupture of membranes. However, HWWS is considered to have a good obstetric prognosis, with nearly 87% of females achieving pregnancy and 62% achieving normal vaginal births. Rates of miscarriage in pregnancy are considered not significantly different from the general population. Cesarean-section rates may, however, be higher in view of fetal breech presentations and preterm delivery.

Scenario: A 16-year-old female patient presents to the clinic with recurrent lower abdominal pain with primary amenorrhea and is noted to have a hearing impairment. Secondary sexual characteristics show normal breast development and pubic hair. Her sister is known to have 17-OH progesterone deficiency. The patient was seen at another hospital and diagnosed as having an imperforate hymen, and a futile attempt was made at treatment by a perforation method. On clinical examination the vestibule region appears normal looking, but there is no vaginal opening readily seen and a surgical scar is noted inferior to the urethral opening. A large, non-tender, mobile pelvic mass is palpated. A radiological study is performed.

Question: Can you interpret the imaging study?
Answer: This is an MRI scan (sagittal and coronal pelvis view) (**Figure 72.6**) which shows a normal-size uterus markedly compressed and displaced to the left by a distended (10 cm × 9 cm × 8 cm) upper vagina suggestive of hematocolpos and hematometra. The lower vagina is not clearly visualized, with the imaging scans suggesting an absent vaginal segment or segmental vaginal atresia.

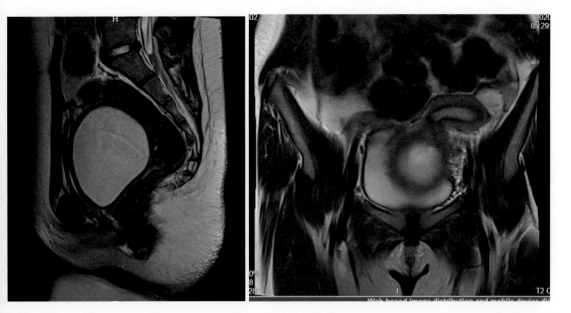

Figure 72.6 MRI scan showing distended upper vagina consistent with segmental vaginal atresia.

Question: What is the clinical impression?
Answer: This patient has a distal vaginal atresia. Selective agenesis of the lower vagina is a separate entity and usually associated with normal Müllerian system development. An experienced pediatric gynecologist or a pediatric surgeon should evaluate such index cases, as this disorder may be readily confused with a simple imperforate hymen and a patient may undergo unnecessary intervention, as was seen in this particular patient.

Question: What are the variant types of vaginal atresia?
Answer: Vaginal atresia is a rare disorder that may be classified as either complete or partial. Partial atresia is also sometimes termed segmental atresia and can be further classified into a distal atresia and proximal atresia. Usually, the distal atresia type lesion has a normal proximal vagina and good outcome following a pull-through vaginoplasty, and risks of vaginal stenosis are low. The complete and proximal atresia variant refers to an atretic lesion of the total and upper segment of the vagina which is usually accompanied by cervix malformations.

Question: How will you manage this patient?
Answer: Careful preoperative planning with imaging studies is essential to evaluate the anatomy and then a therapeutic tailored approach undertaken to restore functional anatomy and achieve reproductive potential.

Question: What is the surgical management therefore in this index case?
Answer: In cases of distal vaginal atresia presenting with amenorrhea and hematocolpos, a distal vaginal pull-through is a good option, as we have an adequate length of proximal dilated vagina. A transverse incision is created on the vaginal dimple and dissection is then proceeded carefully to reach the tense bulge of the hematocolpos. Thereafter the bulge is incised and 'chocolate colored' retained blood evacuated by suction. The upper vagina is visualized to rule out any other abnormalities. The mucosal margins of the upper vagina are then advanced to the intraoitus and repair completed.

BIBLIOGRAPHY

1. Shaw LM, Jones WA, Brereton RJ. Imperforate hymen and vaginal atresia and their associated anomalies. J R Soc Med. 1983;76:560–6.
2. Cetin C, Soysal C, Khatib G, Urunsak IF, Cetin T. Annular hymenotomy for imperforate hymen. J Obstet Gynaecol Res. 2016;42:1013–5.
3. Herlin M, Bjørn A-MB, Rasmussen M, Trolle B, Petersen MB. Prevalence and patient characteristics of Mayer-Rokitansky-Küster-Hauser syndrome: a nationwide registry-based study. Hum Reprod. 2016;31:2384–90.

4. ACOG Committee Opinion. Number 274. Nonsurgical diagnosis and management of vaginal agenesis. Obstet Gynecol. 2002;2002(100):213–6.

5. Brännström M. The Swedish uterus transplantation project: the story behind the Swedish uterus transplantation project. Acta Obstet Gynecol Scand. 2015;94:675–9.

6. Afrashtehfar CD, Pigña-García A, Afrashtehfar KI. Müllerian anomalies. Obstructed hemivagina and ipsilateral renal anomaly syndrome (OHVIRA) Cir. 2014;82(4):460–71.

7. Karag'ozov I. Herlyn –Werner-Wunderlich syndrome. Akush Ginekol (Sofia). 1983; 22(1):70–76.

8. Smith NA, Laufer MR. Obstructed hemivagina and ipsilateral renal anomaly (OHVIRA) syndrome: management and follow-up. Fert Steril. 2007;87(4):918–22.

9. Grigoris FG, Stephan G, Attilio DSS, et al. The ESHRE/ESGE consensus on the classification of female genital tract congenital anomalies. Hum Reprod. 2013;28(8):2032–44.

10. Leng J, Lang J, Lian L, et al. Congenital vaginal atresia: report of 16 cases. Zhonghua Fu Chan Ke Za Zhi. 2002;37(4):217–9.

73

Disorders of sex development

ABRAHAM CHERIAN AND NEETU KUMAR
Great Ormond Street Hospital for Children NHS Foundation Trust,
London, UK

Question: You have been asked to review a full-term baby delivered on the postnatal ward. Maternal antenatal scans were reportedly normal. The baby has passed urine and meconium since birth. On clinical examination the baby appears to have ambiguous genitalia. What is the initial management of this baby now?

Disorder of sex development (DSD) is the current term, adopted in 2006, to describe any congenital condition that suggests ambiguity of the external genitalia.[1] Ambiguous genitalia is a disorder in which the child's external genital appearance does not appear to be clear so as to confidently identify its sex of rearing as a girl or a boy. It is not a very common condition. The incidence is approximately 1 per 4,500 births[2]; however, some degree of male under-virilisation or female virilisation may be present in as many as 2% of live births.[2] Nevertheless, this disorder causes a great level of anxiety, concern and distress to parents, and extreme sensitivity is required right from the very outset of early management of these babies.

The primary aims of early assessment of the new-born are:

1. To rule out life-threatening conditions such as 'salt wasting' congenital adrenal hyperplasia (CAH).
2. To attain essential information for gender assignment.

This evaluation should include a detailed clinical history, physical examination and basic laboratory studies and imaging investigations.

Clinical history:

- **Antenatal history:**
  Maternal: Exposure/ingestion of androgens (e.g., Danazol – pharmacological agent used to treat endometriosis, fibrocystic breast disease), oral contraceptive pills (OCPs), soya products.
  Virilisation during pregnancy due to a deficiency of placental aromatase; luteoma of pregnancy; history of previous neonatal death/miscarriages (chromosomal abnormalities).
  Prenatal: Other known congenital abnormalities recorded on antenatal scans/investigations.
- **Family history:**
  Urological abnormalities, amenorrhea, precocious puberty, infertility, consanguinity of partners.

Physical examination:

- *General examination*: Observe for dysmorphic features (many syndromes e.g., Smith-Lemli-Opitz syndrome are associated with DSD[2]).
- *Genital examination*:
  - Hyperpigmentation (especially of genitalia/scrotum).

DOI: 10.1201/9781003182290-81

- *Phallus/genital tubercle*: Stretched length compared to normal ranges; a penis buried in fat may appear small; a clitoris may appear large in a pre-term infant or if there is minimal fat. Corporal consistency to palpate the phallus; absence/presence of chordee.
- *Labia or scrotal/labio-scrotal folds*: Observe development and rugosity.
- Presence (palpable/impalpable) and position (labial/inguinal) of gonads, gonad size (asymmetry) and consistency.
- *Number (N) of perineal openings*: Urethral anatomical position or degree of hypospadias; position/location of the anal margin.

The Prader classification is often used for 46,XX androgenisation. The I–V Prader Stages help describe the degree of virilisation.[2] The 'external masculinisation score' can be useful for 46,XY under-virilisation.[3] Documentation of all details should be clear and consistent so that any future/further changes can be correctly assessed (**Figure 73.1**).

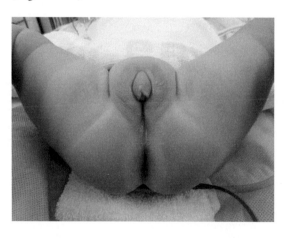

Figure 73.1 Ambiguous genitalia in an infant.

INVESTIGATIONS

Early investigations are usually performed within the first few hours or days of birth. The important key studies are:

Routine blood screening: Serum electrolytes and glucose level. Hypoglycaemia due to cortisol deficiency can be secondary to hypothalamic-pituitary or adrenocortical insufficiency.

Rapid fluorescent in situ hybridisation (FISH) genetic test to detect SRY/X chromosome followed by formal karyotype.

CAH: 17,OHP; cortisol; urinalysis; urinary electrolytes and steroid profile.

Hormone assay: Luteinising hormone (LH), follicle-stimulating hormone (FSH), serum testosterone.

Imaging studies: Pelvic ultrasound to look for presence of gonads and Mullerian system structures.

Question: A female infant has been diagnosed with CAH. What are the different types of CAH? What is the current management?

Answer: CAH is a group of inherited disorders that occur due to enzymatic defects at different points on the biosynthetic pathways to produce cortisol and aldosterone within the adrenal gland. There is then an overproduction of adrenal cortical hormone (ACTH) which further stimulates the increase in production of androgenic precursors by the adrenal glands (**Figure 73.2**).

CAH is the most common cause of 46,XX DSD. It accounts for nearly 85% of all infants with ambiguous genitalia in Western developed nations. The excess production of androgen is responsible for virilisation. The phenotype can range from mild clitoromegaly (Prader Stage I) to an appearance of normal male genitalia (Prader Stage V). There are three main variants of CAH.

1. **21-Hydroxylase deficiency (21-OHD deficiency)**
   Incidence: This is the most common type and forms nearly 90% of all types of CAH.[4] The estimated incidence is 1 in 15,000 births.

   Genetics: Autosomal recessive disorder and is associated with mutation of a gene located on the short arm of chromosome 6. The two subtypes are:

   Type 1: Virilisation with no 'salt wasting'.

   Type 2: (Classic) Virilisation with 'salt wasting'. The gene abnormality affects both the zona fasciculata and the glomerulosa zones of the adrenal gland. This results in deficiency of aldosterone and cortisol. It manifests as salt wasting with dehydration, or haemodynamic vascular collapse with or without hypokalaemia

Steroidogenic pathway

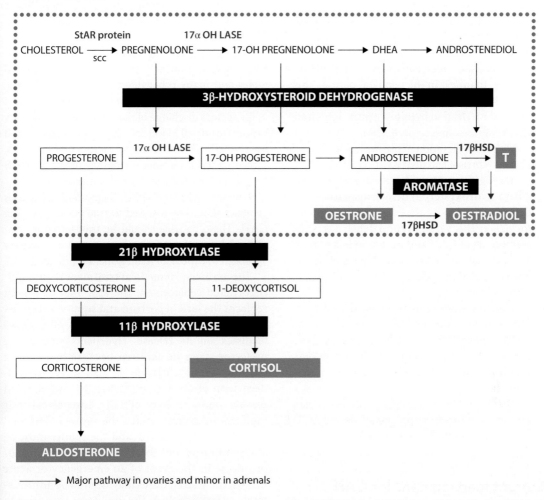

Figure 73.2 Steroidogenic Pathway. *Abbreviations*: StAR Protein: Steroid Acute Regulatory protein-steroidogenic regulatory protein (DESMOLASE). *Note*: CAH deficiency of-21β-OH-lase, 3β-OH-lase, 3β-HSD, 17α-OH-lase, StAR protein.

(low serum K+). This is considered one of the leading major neonatal medical emergencies and may be life-threatening.

Pathophysiology: The enzyme deficiency blocks the mineralocorticoid and glucocorticoid pathways leading to a deficiency of cortisol and aldosterone, which results in increased secretion of corticotrophin, which in turn leads to adrenocortical hyperplasia and overproduction of intermedullary biochemical hormone metabolites. Pigmentation of skin is due to increased ACTH and melanocyte-stimulating hormone (MSH).

Diagnosis: The classic diagnostic feature is elevation of plasma 17 hydroxy-progesterone (17-OHP).

Management: Glucocorticoid and mineral corticoid replacement therapy.

2. **11 Beta-hydroxylase deficiency**
Incidence: Also referred as the variant type 3 form. It is a less common cause of CAH.

Genetics: The gene has been mapped to the long arm of chromosome 8.

Pathophysiology: Decreased production of aldosterone results in extensive production of ACTH and leads to increased amounts of deoxycortisol, which causes hypokalaemia that may not manifest in the neonatal period. This condition leads to salt retention and potassium loss and can lead to hypoglycaemia, impaired stress response and hypertension.

Diagnosis: Elevation of plasma levels of 11-deoxycortisol and deoxycorticosterone (DOC).

Management: Steroid replacement therapy.

3. **3 Beta-hydroxysteroid dehydrogenase deficiency**

Incidence: This variant type 4 deficiency is the rarest form of CAH and occurs in less than 5% of all patients with adrenal hyperplasia. The estimated prevalence is less than 1 per 1,000,000 at birth.

Genetics: Autosomal recessive disorder causes mutation in the *HSD3B2* gene.

Pathophysiology: It results in decreased production of all three groups of adrenal steroids, i.e. mineralocorticoids, glucocorticoids and sex steroids.

Diagnosis: Elevation in plasma dehydroepiandrosterone, 17-hydroxy pregnenolone and ACTH.

Management: Like that of 21-hydroxylase deficiency.

Current management for CAH

The management of children with CAH has undergone significant change in recent years. With better understanding of pathogenesis and natural history, early and timely management of these children will lead to improved successful outcomes.

MEDICAL MANAGEMENT

Prenatal: Prenatal diagnosis is now possible in siblings and offspring of affected individuals. Chorionic villus sampling (CVS) and amniocentesis allows sex determination (karyotyping) and many other genetic studies with gene probes for CAH. External genitalia of the 46,XX fetus can be assessed to look for evidence of virilisation with the help of small-probed ultrasounds. Dexamethasone has now been reported for prenatal treatment of CAH. The long-term results are variable. A prospective, multicentre European study, PREDEX, is currently on-going.[5] It is therefore essential that antenatal counselling is informative about the potential risks and the benefits of treatment.

New-born screening: Screening new-borns for CAH is now routinely performed in the United States and many other developed countries in the world. A heel prick blood test is taken on day 1 or 2 of life (before discharge of the baby from the delivery unit).[6] This dried blood spot specimen is then tested for 17-OHP. There are several factors that limit this screening test for absolute accuracy including birth weight, gestational age, comorbidities, etc.

Postnatal: All babies with a diagnosis of ambiguous genitalia should be assessed to rule out salt wasting CAH. These patients should be transferred to specialised hospital services where a multidisciplinary approach to expedient management is provided.

The mainstay of medical treatment is with glucocorticoid replacement therapy. This treatment replaces the lack of cortisol and suppresses excessive androgen production by means of negative feedback on its release. Hydrocortisone is the preferred drug in children because of its short half-life. Fludrocortisone is also given to children with electrolyte disturbances and elevated plasma renin activity (PRA). Adrenal crisis is high risk in children under the age of 4.[7] Parental education is imperative, and the family must be advised to look out for any signs of illness and/or injury. In the event of an emergency or acute illness, the steroid doses may need to be administered intravenously or the oral doses may need to be 'doubled up'.

Adults: Hypertension may develop in adults with a diagnosis of classic 21-hydroxylase deficiency CAH, and hence such patients may need mineralocorticoid replacement to suppress plasma renin activity along with glucocorticoid therapy.[7] Adult women may suffer from polycystic ovarian syndrome (PCOS) and menstrual irregularity. This can be treated with OCPs. Acne and hirsutism in these patients can be treated with spironolactone.

SURGICAL MANAGEMENT

The role of surgical management in DSD is currently a contentious debate. New studies amongst adults with DSD have reported satisfactory genital appearance and function with early surgery, but there are reports of significant harm experienced by others.[8,9]

The main role of surgical intervention in CAH can be subdivided:

1. Emergency/urgent: To create an outlet/passage channel for stool and urine.
2. Elective: This mainly includes diagnostic procedures such as examination under anaesthesia (EUA), cystoscopy, vaginoscopy and laparoscopy. Definite genital surgery may involve feminising genitoplasty (cliteroplasty, labioplasty/monsplasty and/or vaginoplasty).

A compliant corticosteroid management in young girls will prevent clitoral pain and enlargement. This has consequently nearly obviated the need to perform any clitoral surgery. However, in some resistant and non-compliant cases, conservative tailored operation (with prevention of damage to the neurovascular bundle) known as cliteroplasty may be required.

Question: You are operating on an infant girl with bilateral inguinal hernias. You note at operation that the inguinal sac contains a gonad that appears to be a testis rather than an ovary with a fallopian tube. What is the next best management plan? What is the possible diagnosis?

Answer: In this scenario, the female child is having a surgical procedure for bilateral inguinal hernia. In a minimally invasive surgery (MIS) laparoscopic approach, the surgeon would repair the hernia as routine and can also take a detailed exam looking for the gonads and presence/absence of other Mullerian system structures (uterus). However, in the open classical inguinal approach, without prior parental consent, the most appropriate management steps would be to repair the hernia and then undertake an informative detailed discussion with parents after the hernia operation for further investigations. This will include blood lab studies for karyotype, abdominal-pelvic ultrasound, EUA of the external genitalia + cysto-vaginoscopy and diagnostic laparoscopy +/- biopsy of the gonads in consultation with the DSD multidisciplinary specialist team.

The most likely diagnosis is androgen insensitivity syndrome (ASI), also called testicular feminisation syndrome, first described in 1953.[10] The variant types are[11]:

1. Complete androgen insensitivity syndrome (CAIS).

2. Partial androgen insensitivity syndrome (PAIS).
3. Mild androgen insensitivity syndrome (MAIS) with typical male external genitalia.

CAIS: The incidence is approximately 1 in 20,400 to 1 in 99,100 genetic males.[12] It is an inherited X-linked recessive disorder which results from a point mutation in the androgen receptor gene, which is normally located on the long arm of the X sex chromosome.[13] The result then is that there is failure of the external genitalia and prostate in the 46,XY gonadal male fetus to respond to testosterone and/or DHT, which is produced in normal levels.[4] Some index cases are receptor negative and are found to have an inability of the cytosol receptor to bind DHT. Another variant is receptor positive, and the defect is post-receptor.

Clinical presentation: Index patients are raised as females, as the external genitalia (phenotype) is entirely that of a female. They often present with primary amenorrhoea or at the timing of surgery for an inguinal hernia, whereby a testis is found (like in the scenario). There is sparse/absent pubic or axillary hair. On examination they usually have normal female external genitalia with a blind-ending vagina. Non-palpable testes are usually present. No Mullerian structures are found, as the MIS levels are within normal range. Treatment includes either removal of the testes after puberty when feminisation is completed or prepubertal gonadectomy accompanied by oestrogen replacement therapy. Gonadectomy is scheduled to prevent testicular malignancy. The risk of malignancy is reportedly low in children; therefore, removal of gonads is again increasingly controversial at this age. However, studies have suggested an increased tumour risk of greater than 30% in late adulthood if gonadectomy is not performed early.[3] Patients with CAIS will require vaginal dilatation to assist with sexual intercourse and avoidance of dyspareunia.[11]

PAIS: This variant is less common where lesser degrees of insensitivity to androgens occur than the CAIS group. The disorder may be due to a receptor or post-receptor defects or due to qualitative defects, such as acceleration of dissociation of androgen receptor complex. Affected patients have a broad phenotype spectrum with varying degrees of virilisation, either the (1) female predominant type or the (2) male predominant type. Gender assignment and treatment are individualised.

Question: A 11-year-old female is being investigated for short stature. On examination, she has a web neck and no signs of secondary sexual characteristics. Karyotype reveals 45,XO genotype. What is the most likely diagnosis and when is the paediatric surgeon/urologist likely to get involved?
Answer: This young female has Turner syndrome (TS), also known as congenital ovarian hypoplasia syndrome.

It is one of the most common sex chromosomal disorders that affects females. It occurs in 1:2,500 female live births.[15] It is characterised by partial or complete loss (monosomy) of one of the secondary sex chromosomes. The features of TS were first described by Henry Turner in 1938, but the pathogenicity of the X chromosome monosomy was later identified in 1959.[16] Monosomy 45,X is present in about 45% of index cases; the remaining TS patients show a variety of chimeras/mosaicisms and structural abnormalities.[15] The incidence of TS is particularly noteworthy in China.[15] TS is highly variable and can present with a variety of clinical symptoms, which can differ from one affected person to another. Many different organ systems can be involved, including abnormalities of the eyes and ears, skeletal malformations, cardiac anomalies and kidney lesions. The most characteristic features are a short broad neck with webbing, low-set ears and down-slanted palpebral fissures with epicanthal folds affecting the eyes.[16] Common associations include short stature and premature ovarian failure, which can result in the failure to attain puberty. Most adult women with TS are infertile. Affected females may also experience certain learning disabilities.

TS may be diagnosed before birth or shortly after birth (20%)[17] or during early childhood. However, in some cases, the disorder may go unrecognised and not be diagnosed until well into adulthood, often as an incidental finding. Most affected cases do not occur genetically in families and appear to occur sporadically or randomly for no apparent reasons.

Apart from the congenital renal anomalies, notably horseshoe kidney, that may be associated with TS, some of the patients may also have the Y chromosome. This increases their risks of gonadoblastoma, which can be evident even at a very early age with the presence of streak gonads with Y mosaicism and may involve both gonads. Prophylactic MIS-guided laparoscopic gonadectomy of the streak gonads in index patients with TS who carry a Y mosaic genotype is thus recommended.[18]

Question: What is mixed gonadal dysgenesis (MGD)? What is the role of the paediatric surgeon/urologist?

MGD is most commonly the result of 45,XO/46,XY mosaicism. It is included under the term 'chimerism' as per the 2016 Updated Consensus Statement.[19] MGD is the second most common form of new-born ambiguous genitalia. A mixed gonadal phenotype usually consists of an inguinal testis (with limited endocrine function) on one side with a contralateral dysgenetic streak gonad with persistent Mullerian structure derivatives. The testis is most often palpable and commonly undescended (**Figures 73.3** and **73.4**).

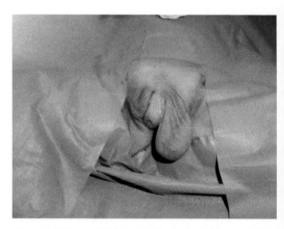

Figure 73.3 Impalpable right testis with asymmetry of the scrotum.

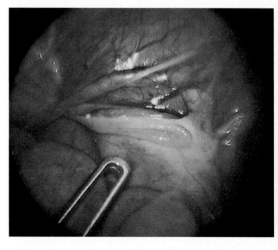

Figure 73.4 MIS laparoscopy showing the streak pelvic gonad (intrabdominal).

The external genital phenotype is variable with a predominant preference to female rearing of sex. Some cases may be sufficiently virilised to permit rearing as a male. The streaked ovary, if present, is characterised by increased connective tissue elements and diminution of primary follicles, which worsens with time. The Mullerian duct structures usually persist unilaterally or bilaterally. The testis is often accompanied with a fallopian tube rather than a vas and epididymis. The streaked gonad is usually drained by a Mullerian duct structure. A bicornuate or unicornuate uterus is usually present.

As mentioned in the scenarios, there is an increased risk of germ cell tumours (GCTs) in individuals with DSD where a Y chromosome is present. This risk may be notably high dependent on how much Y material is present. Some reports have documented the malignancy risk to be as low as 2%, while others have placed it as high as 35%.[20]

The age of the patient is also regarded as important for GCT development. There have been several reports of carcinoma in situ (CIS) discovered in infants as young as 3 months of age and GCTs encountered in children under 1 year of age.[21] The risks may be lower at the prepubertal age group, and gonadectomy may be deferred until much older with careful monitoring and risk surveillance assessments.[22] It has been suggested that tumour risk is increased in patients with poorly differentiated gonadal tissues.

There is also an increased risk of Wilms tumour in MGD patients. Five percent of patients will have Denys-Drash syndrome (ambiguous genitalia, Wilms tumour and glomerulopathy with associated hypertension).[23] A DSD MDT structured approach is thus highly recommended with a specialist team including paediatric endocrinologists, paediatric urologists, genetics, gynaecologists and clinical psychologists.[6,24]

BIBLIOGRAPHY

1. Lee, P.A., Houk, C.P., Ahmed, S.F., Hughes, I.A. and participants in the International Consensus Conference on Intersex organized by the Lawson Wilkins Pediatric Endocrine Society and the European Society for Paediatric Endocrinology (2006). Consensus statement on management of intersex disorders. Pediatrics, 118(2), pp. e 488–e500.

2. Ogilvy-Stuart, A.L. and Brain, C.E. (2004) Early assessment of ambiguous genitalia. Archives of Disease in Childhood, 89(5), pp. 401–407.

3. Ahmed, S.F., Khwaja, O. and Hughes, I.A. (2000) The role of a clinical score in the assessment of ambiguous genitalia. BJU International, 85(1), pp.120–124.

4. Dacou-Voutetakis, C., Maniati-Christidi, M. and Dracopoulou-Vabouli, M. (2001) Genetic aspects of congenital adrenal hyperplasia. Journal Of Pediatric Endocrinology & Metabolism: JPEM, 14, pp. 1303–1308.

5. Lajic, S., Nordenstrom, A., Ritzén, E.M. and Wedell, A. (2004) Prenatal treatment of congenital adrenal hyperplasia. European Journal of Endocrinology, 151(Suppl_3), pp. U 63–U69.

6. Eshragh, N., Van Doan, L., Connelly, K.J., Denniston, S., Willis, S. and LaFranchi, S.H. (2020). Outcome of newborn screening for congenital adrenal hyperplasia at two time points. Hormone Research in Paediatrics, 93(2), pp. 128–136.

7. Choi, J.H. and Yoo, H.W. (2017) Management issues of congenital adrenal hyperplasia during the transition from pediatric to adult care. Korean Journal of Pediatrics, 60(2), p. 31.

8. Gardner, M. and Sandberg, D.E. (2018) Navigating surgical decision making in disorders of sex development (DSD). Frontiers in Pediatrics, 6, p. 339.

9. Crouch, N.S., Liao, L.M., Woodhouse, C.R., Conway, G.S. and Creighton, S.M. (2008) Sexual function and genital sensitivity following feminizing genitoplasty for congenital adrenal hyperplasia. Journal of Urology, 179(2), pp. 634–638.

10. Morris, J.M. (1953). The syndrome of testicular feminization in male pseudohermaphrodites. American Journal of Obstetrics & Gynecology, 65(6), pp. 1192–1211.

11. Gottlieb, B. and Trifiro, M.A. (2017) Androgen insensitivity syndrome. Europe PMC plus. [Online]

12. Hughes, I.A., Werner, R., Bunch, T. and Hiort, O. (2012) Androgen insensitivity syndrome. In: Seminars in Reproductive Medicine (Vol. 30, No. 05, pp. 432–442). Thieme Medical Publishers.

13. Campbell MF, Walsh PC, Retik AB. Campbell's Urology. W B Saunders Company; 2002. p. 4082.

14. Hashmi, A., Hanif, F., Hanif, S.M., Abdullah, F.E. and Shamim, M.S. (2008) Complete androgen insensitivity syndrome. Journal of College of Physicians and Surgeons Pakistan, 18(7), pp. 442–444.

15. Cui, X., Cui, Y., Shi, L., Luan, J., Zhou, X. and Han, J. (2018) A basic understanding of Turner syndrome: incidence, complications, diagnosis, and treatment. Intractable & Rare Diseases Research, 7(4), pp. 223–228.

16. Ford, C.E., Jones, K.W., Polani, P.E., De Almeida, J.C. and Briggs, J.H. (1959) A sex-chromosome anomaly in a case of gonadal dysgenesis (Turner's syndrome).

17. Hemani, F., Niaz, S., Kumar, V., Khan, S., Choudry, E. and Ali, S.R. (2021) A case of early diagnosis of turner syndrome in a neonate. Cureus, 13(7):e16733.

18. Brant, W.O., Rajimwale, A., Lovell, M.A., Travers, S.H., Furness III, P.D., Sorensen, M., Oottamasathien, S. and Koyle, M.A. (2006) Gonadoblastoma and Turner syndrome. Journal of Urology, 175(5), pp. 1858–1860.

19. Lee, P.A., Nordenström, A., Houk, C.P., Ahmed, S.F., Auchus, R., Baratz, A., Dalke, K.B., Liao, L.M., Lin-Su, K., Looijenga 3rd, L.H. and Mazur, T. (2016) Global disorders of sex development update since 2006: perceptions, approach and care. Hormone Research in Paediatrics, 85(3), pp. 158–180.

20. Weidler, E.M., Pearson, M., van Leeuwen, K. and Garvey, E. (2019) Clinical management in mixed gonadal dysgenesis with chromosomal mosaicism: considerations in newborns and adolescents. Seminars in Pediatric Surgery, 28(5), p. 150841.

21. Manuel, M., Katayama, K.P. and Jones Jr, H.W. (1976) The age of occurrence of gonadal tumors in intersex patients with a Y chromosome. American Journal of Obstetrics and Gynecology, 124(3), pp. 293–300.

22. Cools, M., Pleskacova, J., Stoop, H., Hoebeke, P., Van Laecke, E., Drop, S.L.S., Lebl, J., Oosterhuis, J.W., Looijenga, L.H.J., Wolffenbuttel, K.P. and Mosaicism Collaborative Group (2011). Gonadal pathology and tumor risk in relation to clinical characteristics in patients with 45, X/46, XY mosaicism. The Journal of Clinical Endocrinology & Metabolism, 96(7), pp. e 1171–E1180.

23. Drash, A., Sherman, F., Hartmann, W.H. and Blizzard, R.M. (1970). A syndrome of pseudohermaphroditism, Wilms' tumor, hypertension, and degenerative renal disease. Journal of Pediatrics, 76(4), pp. 585–593.

24. Farrugia, M.K., Sebire, N.J., Achermann, J.C., Eisawi, A., Duffy, P.G. and Mushtaq, I. (2013). Clinical and gonadal features and early surgical management of 45, X/46, XY and 45, X/47, XYY chromosomal mosaicism presenting with genital anomalies. Journal of Pediatric Urology, 9(2), pp. 139–144.

PART 9

Neurosurgery

74

Neural tube defects

PRINCE RAJ AND MARTIN T. CORBALLY
King Hamad University Hospital, Kingdom of Bahrian, Bahrain

Neural tube defects (NTDs) are congenital malformations of the central nervous system due to faulty development and closure of the neural tube. This can result in a wide variety of abnormalities ranging from anencephaly to spina bifida occulta. Meningomyelocele (MMC) is the most common of all, characterized by the protrusion of the exposed spinal cord into a sac filled with cerebrospinal fluid, resulting in lifelong disability. Though the incidence is gradually falling due to increased antenatal diagnosis, folic acid fortification of food and elective termination, it remains a significant burden in developing countries with long-term impact on patients and the healthcare system.

Scenario: A 25-year-old prima-gravida is delivered of a full-term male baby who was antenatally diagnosed to have a 5 x 4 x 4 cm swelling in the back around lumbar region. The baby is vitally stable with a local soft cystic swelling at the L4–L5 level (**Figure 74.1**), which is disrupted by a small leak from the swelling and decreased power in both lower limbs. Both lower limbs are in fixed flexion position, and there is bilateral talipes. You are called immediately to assess the baby.

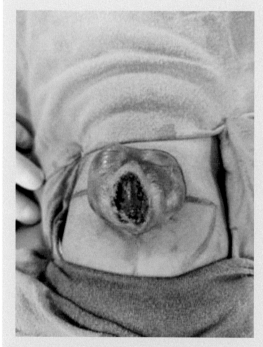

Figure 74.1 Neonate with open myelomengocele.

Question: How are you going to manage this case?
Answer: The baby has an open NTD MMC with an associated neurological deficit. He requires a thorough head-to-toe physical examination including

DOI: 10.1201/9781003182290-83

general vigor, baseline head circumference measurement, upper and lower extremity motor and sensory function, anal sphincter tone and reflexes. Note should also be made regarding the size, site, any cerebrospinal fluid (CSF) leak and the level of MMC. The clinical presentation is dependent on the site of spinal lesion, and in general the higher the level of the lesion, the greater the neurological deficit. He should also be evaluated for symptoms of an Arnold-Chiari malformation and any associated orthopedic conditions such as kyphoscoliosis and note taken of his talipes.

Skin-covered lesions do not require any urgent intervention, but open NTDs like MMC, as in this case, should be covered with sterile saline-soaked gauze and a plastic wrap placed over it to prevent heat loss and desiccation of the exposed neural plaque. The baby should be nursed in a prone or in the lateral position to prevent rupture of the sac and to avoid trauma to neural tissue. Prophylactic antibiotics (broad spectrum) should be started to prevent any impending central nervous system (CNS) infection.

Question: How are you going to evaluate this baby and proceed further?
Answer: It is pertinent for the primary treating team to set up a multidisciplinary team and discuss the management plan with the parents in a frank and empathetic manner. As the incidence of hydrocephalus associated with MMC is nearly 90%, head ultrasonography or computed tomography (CT) should be performed early to assess the ventricular enlargement and V:H ratio (ventricle to hemisphere ratio), which will give a baseline value to determine the need for possible future shunt placement. In some cases, the V:H ratio will be large enough at birth that a simultaneous placement of shunt along with MMC excision and closure are indicated. However, nearly 90% of patients will need a shunt after NTD closure. A spinal ultrasound or MRI of the spine is useful to determine any other proximal spinal anomalies. A renal ultrasound is also performed to determine the presence of any urinary tract abnormalities, as 5–10% of these babies would have hydronephrosis or reflux at birth.

Question: What are the other associated condition with MMC?
Answer: Open NTDs may be associated with following conditions:

a. Arnold-Chiari malformation (Chiari type 2) with hydrocephalus.
b. Clubfeet.
c. Kyphoscoliosis.
d. Congenital dislocation of the hip.
e. Neurogenic bladder.
f. Fecal incontinence.
g. Undescended testes.
h. Latex allergy.

Question: What are the steps of surgical management?
Answer: The MMC should be typically closed within 24–72 hours unless there is a severe lesion or other major cardiac condition precluding safe administration of anesthesia. The goal of the surgery is to close the exposed neural placode into the neural tube and achieve appropriate neuronal function.

Following are the important steps involved:

a. Adequate separation of neuronal plaque from the intermediate epithelial zone.
b. Reconstruction of neural plaque in tube form with preservation of all the available neural tissue.
c. Separation of the dura (whitish fibrous layer) from the epidural space at the lateral limit of the defect.
d. Watertight closure of dura over the newly created neural tube using a running 6-0 PDS or Maxon.
e. Reinforcement of dural cover with additional fascial cover obtained by mobilizing the fascia from the underlying muscle.
f. Midline approximation of the paraspinal muscle if possible.
g. Tension-free approximation of skin in midline (lateral releasing skin incision/complex flap repairs may be required only very rarely occasionally in case of a wide defect to achieve tension-free repair).

Question: What are the common complications following surgery?
Answer: Following surgery the baby should be nursed in prone or lateral position. Following are the common postoperative complications:

a. CSF leak,
b. Wound dehiscence,
c. Accelerated hydrocephalus,
d. Tethered spinal cord,

Question: Classify NTDs and comment on the etiology.

Answer: NTDs are broadly classified in two types: Open and closed. Open NTDs primarily occur due to faulty primary neurulation, whereas closed NTDs are due to faulty secondary neurulation.

Open NTD	Closed NTD
1. Anencephaly	1. Spina bifida occulta
	a. Lipomeningo-myelocele
	b. Lipoma
	c. Diastometamyelia
	d. Diplomyelia
	e. Neurenteric cyst
	f. Dermal sinus
	g. Tethered cord
	h. Sacral agenesis
2. Spinal raschicisis	
3. Encephalocele	
4. Spina bifida aperta	
a. Meningocele	
b. Meningomyelocele	
c. Myeloschisis	

Etiology: The exact etiology is yet to be ascertained but most likely it is multifactorial.

Possible factors playing a role:

a. Genetic.
b. Environmental.
c. Drugs and teratogens: Folic acid deficiency, valproic acid, carbamazepine, etc.

Question: How will you diagnose NTDs?

Answer: Open NTDs can be diagnosed by:

a. Measuring alpha-fetoprotein (AFP) in amniotic fluid and maternal bloodstream (15–20 weeks).
b. Amniotic fluid glial fibrillary acidic protein (AF-GFAP) – potential biomarker for open NTDs (considered better than serum AFP).
c. Fetal Ultrasound (operator dependent, requires skilled radiographer).
d. 3D ultrasound or fetal MRI may also be considered (reported sensitivity 94%).

Rapid strides have been made in last three decades, and almost all open NTDs are diagnosed in the antenatal period during the early second trimester around 15–20 weeks using anomaly scans and serum AFP levels. At the estimated gestational age of 20 weeks, maternal serum AFP level of more than 1000 ng/mL would be consistent with open NTDs. This has tremendously impacted the outcome, as the parents are counselled early regarding the condition and they can take an informed decision either to terminate the pregnancy in case of a severe defect and associated malformation or to continue with it. In case of continuation, they can be offered antenatal treatment (in centers that provide them) or postnatal treatment in tertiary care centers.

Question: Comment on antenatal management and the MOMS trial.

Answer: There has been growing advocacy for intrauterine repair of MMC, as it has been reported that the benefit of surgery outweighs the maternal risk. Neurological outcomes are improved as it reduces hindbrain herniation, and more than 50% will then not require a VP shunt. The hypothesis is that if the exposed neural tissues are closed early in the gestational period, it will prevent secondary damage to the neural placode and will also limit CSF loss and thus hindbrain herniation.

The Management of Meningomyelocele Study (MOMS) trial was a multicenter, prospective, randomized control trial started in 2003 in the United States to study the risk and benefit of intrauterine repair versus standard postnatal repair. Intrauterine repair was done between 19 and 25 weeks of gestation. This study provided the evidence that intrauterine repair of MMC can reduce the need for VP shunt and improved motor outcomes at 30 months when compared to standard postnatal repair.

Question: What are the outcome and prognosis of MMC?

Answer: Primary closure of MMC is just the beginning of medical care, and patients need a multidisciplinary team of medical, nursing and allied professions for their overall long-term management and to provide a good quality of life. With proper management these children can lead active and productive lives. The goal is to maintain stable neurological function, and the role of a pediatric neurosurgeon is important in recognizing these promptly. Neurological deterioration at any time can be either shunt malfunction or spinal cord tethering. As the child grows, the tethered spinal cord, which is fixed, is stretched and thus produces symptoms. It is pertinent to recognize those symptoms early. Symptoms of spinal cord tethering include new-onset leg weakness, back pain, gait abnormality, foot deformity, sensory loss, urinary incontinence or change in urodynamic data. These symptoms should alert the physician, as it may require surgical detethering. Upper urinary tract and bladder should be monitored on a regular basis with renal and bladder ultrasound and urodynamic studies (UDS). UDS should be done ideally in the neonatal period, as the presence of elevated detrusor filling pressure, high voiding pressure (more than 40 cm H_2O), poor compliance and capacity can result in upper urinary tract deterioration in as many as 63% of children. In these children early institution of clean intermittent catheterization (CIC) and anticholinergic drugs helps in maintaining a safe upper tract and renal function. In patients with neurogenic bowel quality of life can be improved by instituting a bowel washout program. In certain specific scenarios surgical intervention like Mitrofanoff's procedure or Malone antegrade colonic enema (MACE) procedure can be offered for the management of neurogenic bladder and bowel, respectively.

Question: How would you counsel this mother for future pregnancies?

Answer: Folate supplementation plays a vital role in the development of the neural tube during the first weeks of pregnancy, and hence any deficiency in folic acid increases the incidence of NTDs. The World Health Organization (WHO) has determined that folate concentrations >400 ng/mL are sufficient to prevent NTDs. The U.S Preventive Services Task Force currently recommends that women of childbearing age take 400 mcg daily of folic acid to prevent NTDs. It should be taken 1 month prior to and throughout pregnancy

As this mother already has a baby with NTD, the chances of having another baby with a similar defect is increased. She is in a high-risk group and should take high-dose folate supplements beginning 3 months before planning for the next pregnancy and should continue through the first 3 months of pregnancy. This high-dose folate (4 mg/day) reduces the risk of subsequent children with NTDs by 75% if started before pregnancy.

BIBLIOGRAPHY

1. Corbally MT. Neural tube defects. In: Losty PD et al. editors. Rickham's Neonatal Surgery. Springer; 2018. pp. 957–967.
2. Smith JL. Management of neural tube defects, hydrocephalus, refractory epilepsy and central nervous system infections. In: Coran AG et al. editors. Pediatric Surgery. 7th ed. Mosby: Elsevier; 2012. pp. 1673–1697.
3. Adzick NS, Thom EA, Spong CY, et al. A randomized trial of prenatal versus postnatal repair of myelomeningocele. N Engl J Med. 2011;364:993–1004.
4. U.S. Department of Health and Human Services Public Health Service Centers for Disease Control. Recommendations for the use of folic acid to reduce the number of cases of spina bifida and other neural tube defects. MMWR Recomm Rep. 1992;41:1–7.
5. Bauer SB. Neurogenic bladder: etiology and assessment. Pediatr Nephrol. 2008; 23:541–551.
6. Bibbins-Domingo K, Grossman DC, Curry SJ, et al. Folic acid supplementation for the prevention of neural tube defects: U.S. Preventive Services Task Force recommendation statement. JAMA. 2017;317:183–189.

75

Hydrocephalus and increased intracranial pressure

TALAL ALMAYMAN
King Hamad University Hospital, Kingdom of Bahrain, Bahrain

Scenario: A previously healthy 6-year-old girl presents to the hospital clinic with a headache and an unsteady gait. She has been noted to often hold on to things to walk for the past month. She is feeling tired all the time and is sleeping more often than usual. The girl has poor appetite with history of occasional vomiting that started a week before. On examination she looks sick, drowsy and lethargic. Both pupils are symmetrically reactive to light. The patient has horizontal nystagmus. Fundoscopy shows bilateral grade 2 papilledema. Her four-limb neurological exam shows normal tone, power, sensations and deep tendon reflexes. The Babinski plantar reflex is extensor. The girl has an intention and resting tremor, a positive Romberg's sign, dysdiadochokinesia and impaired tandem gait. The patient's neck is lax in tone, and cranial nerve examination unremarkable.

Last week she had a fall on her head and was seen to have abnormal movements with a change in level of consciousness that lasted a few seconds. The family medical history reveals a G6PD deficiency. She has had normal developmental milestones and an unremarkable postnatal history, is of normal intelligence and is socially interactive. Her vital signs are unremarkable, and she is afebrile.

Question: Explain the CT/MRI scan criteria for a diagnosis of hydrocephalus.

Answer: A dilated ventricular system on CT scan imaging requires further study to confirm the type, severity and cause of hydrocephalus. For example, a small tumor lesion obstructing the cerebrospinal fluid (CSF) pathway can be identified upon careful scrutiny. One should always look for the following features as shown in **Figures 75.4** and **75.5**.

1. *Ventricular ballooning*: Pattern of ballooning (tetra-, tri-, bi- or uni-ventricular) with or without ventricular distortion.
2. '*Micky mouse appearance*' of the frontal horns of lateral ventricles.
3. Obliteration of the **CSF basal cisterns**.
4. Obliteration of **cerebral sulci and gyri, Sylvian and interhemispheric fissures.**
5. **Dilatation of the third ventricle.** Normally this is a slit-like structure.
6. Dilatation of the **temporal horns** of the lateral ventricles (>2 mm is significant).
7. *Evans' index*: Is the ratio of the maximum width of the frontal horns of the lateral ventricles and the maximal internal diameter of the skull at the same level deployed in axial CT and MRI images. A normal Evans' index is less than 0.3.
8. *Trans-ependymal CSF permeation*: Is a highly sensitive feature for active/symptomatic disease, often seen in the frontal and occipital horns of the lateral ventricles.

DOI: 10.1201/9781003182290-84

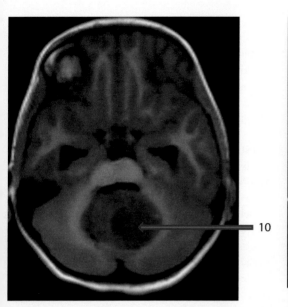

Figure 75.1

9. *Callosal angle*: Normally obtuse angle (100–120 degree); see **Figures 75.2** and **75.6**.
10. *Etiology*: For example, tumor, meningitis, trauma, hemorrhage, Dandy-Walker malformation. Contrast-enhanced imaging helps profoundly in this regard (**Figures 75.1–75.6**).

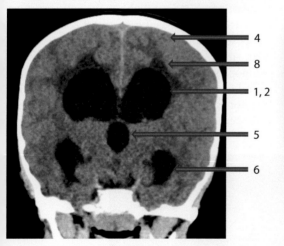

Figure 75.2

Question: How can the central nervous system (CNS) lesion be localized in this patient's case by the history and examination. How do you explain the girl's signs and symptoms?
Answer: The patient has clinical symptoms of raised intracranial pressure (ICP). Notably, the girl

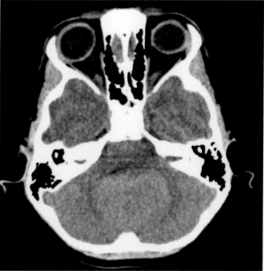

Figure 75.3

is also depicting cerebellar features and has had a history of seizures. Ataxia can be related to hydrocephalus because of the ballooned lateral ventricles and corona radiata compression. However, an intention tremor, nystagmus and dysdiadochokinesia are typical signs of a cerebellar lesion. Ataxia

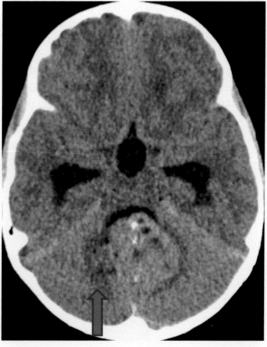

Figure 75.4

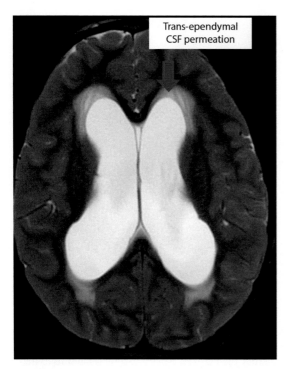

Trans-ependymal
CSF permeation

Figure 75.5

may also be the result of vermis compression or invasion by the lesion.

The offending lesion is likely to be located in the fourth ventricle and midline, as a vermis lesion involves a tandem gait. Additionally, cranial nerves closely related to the cerebello-pontine angle are intact.

Pertaining to the patient's progressive relatively short history of symptoms without fever, the girl most likely has a posterior fossa space-occupying lesion with associated hydrocephalus. The lesion is rapidly growing in size. Seizure activity could be related to the hydrocephalus.

This patient is in a typical age group for a pediatric posterior fossa tumor. The lesion may be a high-grade tumor; bleeding, edema or infarction in a benign/malignant/vascular lesion is also feasible.

Question: What are the most common pediatric brain tumors? What is medulloblastoma?

Answer: The most common pediatric brain tumors are related to the posterior cranial fossa, namely, medulloblastoma, cerebellar astrocytoma and ependymoma, respectively. Pilocytic astrocytoma is the most common form of cerebellar astrocytoma.

Medulloblastoma – the most common malignant brain tumor of childhood –was first described by Cushing and Bailey in the 1920s as a 'small blue cell tumor' of the cerebellum. These tumors are part of the PNET family (primitive neuroectodermal tumors) and comprise 12–25% of all pediatric CNS tumors. Often these tumors arise from embryonal remnant neuroepithelial cells sited along the roof of the fourth ventricle.

Medulloblastoma has four histopathology variant types: (1) Classic, (2) desmoplastic, (3) large-cell anaplastic and (4) medulloblastoma with extensive nodularity. The classic type is most common and composed of diffuse compact masses of highly cellular, small, undifferentiated oval or round cells. Desmoplastic medulloblastoma is an embryonal neural tumor characterized by nodular, reticulin-free zones and reticulin-rich internodular areas with densely packed, poorly differentiated cells.

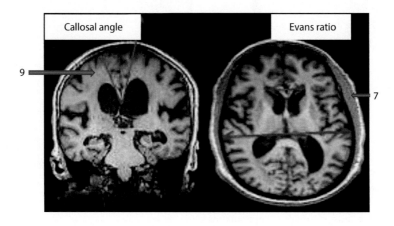

Callosal angle

Evans ratio

9

7

Figure 75.6

Table 75.1 Medulloblastoma: Molecular variant types

	WNT	SSH	Group C	Group D
Age group	Child	Infant/Adult	Infant	Child
Ratio (m: f)	1: 1	1: 1	2: 1	3 : 1
Outcome	Very good	Infants good, other intermediate	Poor	Intermediate
Anatomical location	Brainstem, fourth ventricle	Cerebellar hemispheres	Midline, fourth ventricle	Midline, fourth ventricle
Metastasis	5%–10%	15%–20%	40%–45%	35%–40%
Pattern of recurrence	Rare/local	Local	Metastatic	Metastatic
Genetic alterations	CTNNB1, DDX3X, SMARCA4, TP53 mutation, MYC,	PTCH1, SMO, SUFU, TP53, mutation, GL/2, MYCN amplification	GL/1, GFL1B activation, MYC, OTX-2 amplification, SMARCA4 mutation	KDM6A mutation, SNCAJP duplication, CDK6, MYCN amplification
Cytogenetic aberrations	Monosomy 6	3q gain, 9q, 1Oq, 17p loss	i17q, 1q, 7, 18q gain, 1O q, 11, 16q, 17p loss	I17q, 7q, 18q gain, 8p,11p, X loss

Desmoplastic/nodular medulloblastoma occurs in the cerebellar hemispheres and the midline (classic medulloblastomas are restricted to the midline).

Medulloblastoma may be classified as 'low risk' and 'high-risk' variants in terms of prognosis. Its four well-known molecular subtypes are WNT (wingless), SSH (sonic hedgehog), Group C and Group D.

High-risk lesions have a 5-year survival of <50% and include molecular group 3 and SSH with TP53 mutation, presentation typically at age <3 years. Metastasis to CSF/distant sites renders it high grade.

The standard risk group has a 5-year survival of 80%, diagnosed at >3 years old and M0 (no metastasis) (**Table 75.1**).

Question: Define hydrocephalus. How do we classify hydrocephalus?

Answer: Hydro = water/CSF; cephalus = head. Hydrocephalus is best defined as the excess or abnormal accumulation of CSF in the brain. Normally CSF cushions and plays a role in the physiological activities of the brain. When CSF is present in excess amounts, it exerts harmful pressure on the brain. Hydrocephalus can be classified as:

Congenital hydrocephalus: Aqueductal stenosis, Dandy-Walker malformation, atresia of the foramen of Monro/basal foramina, or co-associated with myelomeningocele (MMC) and the Arnold-Chiari type 2 malformation, encephalocele.

Acquired hydrocephalus: Prematurity and intraventricular hemorrhage, brain tumor, trauma, infections, arachnoid/dermoid/epidermoid cysts.

Communicating hydrocephalus: Also termed 'non-obstructive hydrocephalus', where the CSF flow pathway remains open, but there is an error of CSF absorption at the arachnoid granulations level, for example, secondary to scarring from hemorrhage or infection.

Non-communicating hydrocephalus: Also termed 'obstructive hydrocephalus' because there is obstruction in CSF flow at sites like the foramen of Monro (unilateral/bilateral lateral ventricle hydrocephalus), cerebral aqueductal obstruction (tri-ventricular hydrocephalus), fourth ventricular or basal foramina of Lushka or Magendie obstruction (tetra-ventricular hydrocephalus). This type of obstruction can be congenital (foramen of Monro/ cerebral aqueduct atresia or stenosis) or acquired (hemorrhage/infection/tumor/cyst).

Arrested hydrocephalus: Hydrocephalus can be progressive or spontaneously arrest in cases where it was previously progressive. In arrested hydrocephalus, the balance between production and absorption of the CSF is restored. Patients are mostly asymptomatic, and no surgical treatment is necessary for them.

Ex vacue hydrocephalus: A compensatory enlargement of the CSF spaces and a term used to describe the increase in the volume of CSF. It is characterized on imaging as an enlargement of the cerebral ventricles and subarachnoid spaces, caused by brain atrophy and volume loss.

Question: What is meant by the term 'raised ICP'? List common causes of raised ICP.
Answer: ICP is the pressure exerted within the craniospinal closed system that comprises a fixed volume of neural tissue, blood and CSF.

Normal adult ICP is defined as 7–15 mm Hg (10–20 cm H_2O). ICP exceeding more than the normal range value is considered high ICP. Normal ICP range in younger children is 3–7 mm Hg and in infants 1.5–6 mm Hg. ICP is noted to be relatively higher than the normal value range during recumbency and declines in the upright standing posture.

As ICP rises initially, it is compensated by CSF egress or outflow:

Stage I: Small increases in ICP are compensated by buffering, a process described by the Monro-Kellie doctrine, which states that, with an intact skull, the sum of the volumes of the brain, CSF and intracranial blood are constant. An increase in one component should therefore cause a reduction in one or both of the remaining two components.
Stage II: Moderate increase in ICP will cause midline shift, displacement/herniation.
Stage III: Markedly raised ICP will hinder the cerebral perfusion pressure (CPP) that will in turn activate compensatory autoregulation as cerebral vessel dilatation and systemic hypertension in an attempt to push the blood component strongly to the intracranial compartment and optimize CPP. Both, however, will initiate a vicious cycle leading to worsening of ICP (**Figure 75.7**).

Common causes of increased ICP include:

- Head Injury (moderate/severe traumatic brain injury, vasogenic brain edema)
- Cerebrovascular accident, aneurysm, arteriovenous malformation (AVM) (hemorrhage/infarct, brain edema)
- Hydrocephalus (communicating/non-communicating, brain edema)
- Craniocerebral disproportion (craniosynostosis)
- Brain tumor (supratentorial/infratentorial, brain edema)
- Benign intracranial hypertension (BIH)
- CNS infections (abscess/meningitis/cerebritis, brain edema)
- Metabolic encephalopathies such as hypoxic, ischemic, Reyes syndrome, hepatic coma, renal failure, diabetic ketoacidosis, hypernatremia, burns, near drowning.
- Status epilepticus

Question: Define the terms cerebral blood flow (CBF), cerebral perfusion pressure (CPP) and cerebral autoregulation. How are these parameters closely interrelated?
Answer:

CBF: Best defined as the blood supply delivered to the brain in a given period of time. In an adult, CBF averages 750 milliliters per minute or 15% of the cardiac output. This equates to an average perfusion of 50–54 milliliters of blood per 100 grams of brain tissue per minute.
CPP: The net pressure gradient causing cerebral blood flow to the brain (brain perfusion).

$$CBF = CPP/CVR$$

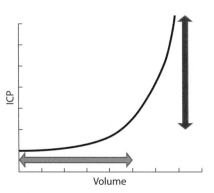

ICP Compliance curve

Compensated ICP (green)

Decompensated (rapidly raised ICP with small volume change (red)

Figure 75.7 ICP compliance curve.

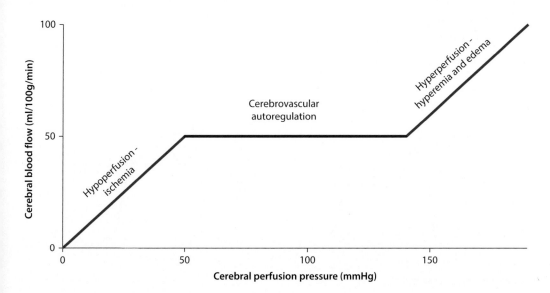

Figure 75.8 Cerebral autoregulation.

$$CPP = MAP - ICP$$

$$MAP = DBP + 1/3\,(Pulse\ pressure)$$

(MAP: Mean arterial pressure; DBP: Diastolic blood pressure; CVR: Cerebrovascular resistance.)

Cerebral autoregulation: That special ability of the cerebral vessels to maintain constant and adequate blood flow to the brain over a wide range of blood pressure variation (CPP of 50–150 mm Hg) (**Figure 75.8**).

Question: Elaborate what is meant by 'normal' and 'abnormal' ICP waveforms.

Answer: The ICP waveform consists of three components: (1) Respiratory waveforms associated with the respiratory cycle, (2) pulse pressure waveforms (frequency equal to the heart rate) and (3) slow vasogenic waveforms (e.g., fluctuation in blood pressure cause waves of 5–8/min (Traube-Hering waves) (**Figure 75.9**).

Each pulse waveform has three waves: P1, P2 and P3 (**Figure 75.10**).

Niles Lundberg described three patterns of abnormal ICP:

Lundberg A waves: Plateau waves, seen with very high ICP maintained for up to 5–20 minutes.
Lundberg B waves: Pressure pulses, are short, 30 seconds to 2 minutes. They show variation in breathing.
Lundberg C waves: Low- and high-amplitude waves, with a frequency of 4–8/min (**Figure 75.11**).

Question: What are variant types of cerebral edema?

Answer: Cerebral edema is a term which refers to increased water content in the cerebral parenchyma.

- *Cytotoxic*: Cell membrane pump failure (Na-K ATPase) results in a high intracellular sodium gradient with related fluid retention and cell swelling.
- *Hydrostatic*: Very high blood pressure and vigorous mannitol use will cause interstitial fluid seepage.
- *Vasogenic*: Vessel damage and blood-brain barrier damage related extravasation of fluid (**Figure 75.2**, blue arrow).
- *Hypo-osmolar*: Secondary to hyponatremia states.

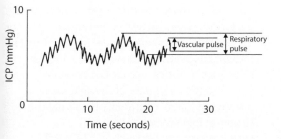

Figure 75.9 ICP waveforms.

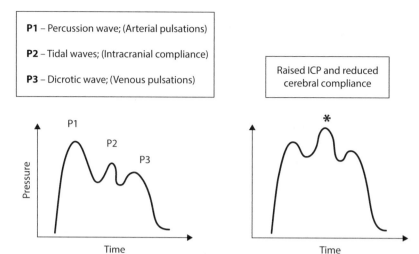

Figure 75.10 Pulse waveform.

Look for: *Increase in the mean pressure* – >20 mmHg – moderate elevation
>40 mmHg – severe increase in pressure
N.B. As ICP increases, the amplitude of the pulse pressure wave increases.

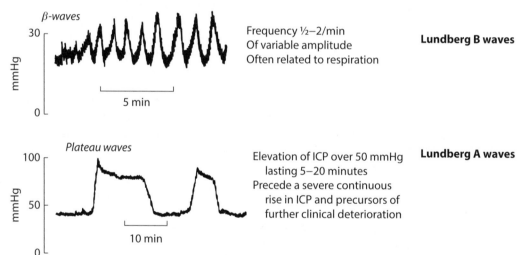

Figure 75.11 Abnormal Pressure Trace.

- *Interstitial*: High CSF pressure will initiate its permeation to the ependymal ventricular lining and onward into the cerebral parenchyma (**Figure 75.3**, red arrow).

Question: What is meant by the term high ICP–related cerebral herniation?
Answer:

Cingulate herniation: May displace or compress the anterior cerebral artery or internal cerebral veins.

Uncal herniation: Herniation of the uncus on midbrain, can lead to third cranial nerve or posterior cerebral artery compression. Patients may develop a 'comatose state' from brainstem reticular activating system (RAS) compression. Such a clinical scenario is typically observed with a unilateral sizeable space-occupying lesion, commonly involving the temporal fossa region.

Central transtentorial herniation: Shift of the diencephalon through the tentorial notch.

This is usually resultant from a massive hemorrhage with generalized cerebral edema.
Cerebellar tonsillar herniation: Compresses the brainstem and is usually a highly fatal event.

Question: What are the general measures adopted in clinical practice to manage ICP?
Answer:

1. Elevate the head end of the bed (HOB) to assist draining CSF into the spinal canal; this will help venous drainage outflow by a gravity effect. It has immediate effect.
2. Straighten the patient's neck region and remove any collar and clothing where it is safe and feasible to do so to assist with breathing.
3. Strict avoidance of hypothermia to prevent acidosis.
4. Hypotension must be prevented to optimize CPP.
5. Hypertension should be controlled to prevent further worsening of ICP.
6. Hypoxia, i.e. pO_2 <60 mm Hg should be corrected to avoid cerebral hypoxic injury.
7. Achieve normocarbia (pCO_2 = 35–40 mmHg). Hyperventilate patient if required.
8. Correct electrolyte imbalances and achieve glycemic (blood sugar) control.
9. Avoid seizures.

Question: How would you manage hydrocephalus? Explain the various surgical options. What different types of CSF shunts do you see in the CT scan?
Answer: See **Figures 75.12** and **75.13**.

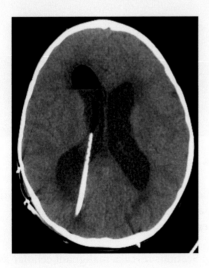

Figure 75.12 External ventricular drain (EVD).

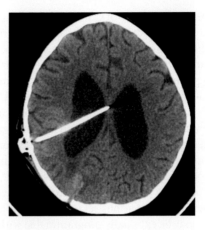

Figure 75.13 VP Shunt.

Hydrocephalus etiology should be looked for carefully and a management plan worked out accordingly with due consideration of the time period of onset and urgency of the clinical scenario. A rapidly deteriorating history within hours or days requires emergent action. This is usually assisted with the help of rapidly inserting a temporary external ventricular drain (EVD) with controlled CSF access for drainage, which can be manipulated according to the patient's clinical assessment. Further investigations (MRI brain imaging with contrast/or CSF dynamic flow analysis) are then scheduled for final diagnosis and complete workup, prior to definitive management of hydrocephalus.

Various options for therapeutic management of hydrocephalus include:

1. *Medical treatment*: Temporary adjuncts – furosemide diuretic therapy and mannitol or 3% saline can help to lower ICP while the definitive surgical plan is awaited.
2. *Lumbar or ventricular puncture and CSF aspiration*: An aid to diagnosis and temporary relief of raised ICP.
3. *CSF temporary diversion*: External ventricular drain (EVD): Usually in situations of acute or doubtful diagnosis prior to permanent CSF diversion. However, at times EVD is also used for temporary CSF drainage in obstructive hydrocephalus while tumor resection and CSF pathway reconstruction is being planned soon. EVD can also be used for a short period in the setting of intraventricular or subarachnoid hemorrhage.
4. *CSF permanent diversion: Ventriculoperitoneal shunt (VP shunt)*: A VP shunt is the most

common technique of CSF diversion surgery. The VP shunt kit consists of a soft ventricular catheter connected through a one-way pressure guarded valve system and reservoir to a draining peritoneal catheter. Operation is performed under general anesthesia. Small scalp and abdominal incisions allow the surgeon to access the ventricular system through a skull burr-hole and peritoneal cavity. The two incisions are connected by a subcutaneous created tunnel, through which the shunt tubing is passed. The opening pressure of the shunt valve system may be fixed at various set pressure settings, or it may be externally programmable with a device. A programmable VP shunt is more often used in pediatric practice and the older geriatric patient. Most common complications are notably shunt infection, obstruction and hemorrhage. Shunt catheter and tubing migration, mechanical kinks, allergy, skin excoriation, seizures, abdominal pseudocyst formation, intestinal obstruction, volvulus, ascites, sepsis, under-drainage and over-drainage are also not uncommon. Once VP shunted, patients are nearly always dependent on CSF diversion, as the arachnoid granulations scleroses.

5. *Ventriculoatrial shunt (VA shunt):* Apart from shunt system obstruction, infection, hemorrhage, sepsis, under-drainage and over-drainage, VA shunt nephritis and endocarditis are common complications.

6. *Endoscopic third ventriculostomy (ETV):* A minimally invasive procedure commonly used to treat obstructive hydrocephalus. The operation achieves CSF diversion by fenestration of the floor of the third ventricle with the help of an operating neuro-endoscope device. ETV has a relatively low complication rate and has many advantages in comparison to other CSF diversion techniques including the VP shunt.

The overall ETV complication rate was reportedly 8.5% by Bouras and Sgouros.

Immediate preoperative complications to consider include hemorrhage (subdural, intraventricular, intracerebral and epidural hematoma). Electrolyte and hormonal imbalances are reported in the literature. Syndrome of inappropriate antidiuretic hormone secretion (SIADH), diabetes insipidus (DI) and secondary amenorrhea are rare.

The most important late complication is the failure of the ETV. Seizures and neurological

morbidity are uncommon in less than 2% cases. Memory deficits may occur after ETV, and this may happen more often after a fornix injury during the operative procedure.

7. *Definitive treatment: Tumor resection:* This will restore the natural CSF pathway and hence absorption. This option is considered in obstructive hydrocephalus with a tumor mass lesion that can be safely excised.

8. **Other options include ventriculopleural shunt or other CSF diversion operations utilizing the gallbladder, urinary tract or appendix as conduits.**

Question: Can you describe the anatomy of the floor of the third ventricle?
Answer: The floor of the third ventricle is located within a thin portion of the hypothalamus region. The ventricle floor is bordered by the mammillary bodies posteriorly, the walls of the third ventricle laterally and the infundibular recess anteriorly. The third ventricle floor perforation is created with the help of a trocar device and Fogarty catheter in a 'safe zone' region just anterior of the midway junction between the infundibular recess and mammillary bodies (**Figure 75.14**).

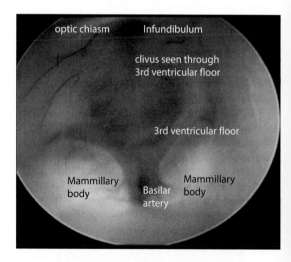

Figure 75.14 Third ventricular floor.

Question: Explain the findings in this patient's histopathology slides (see below figure).
Answer:

Slide a: Sections reveal a malignant cellular neoplasm showing features of a small, blue, round cell tumor composed of sheets and syncytial

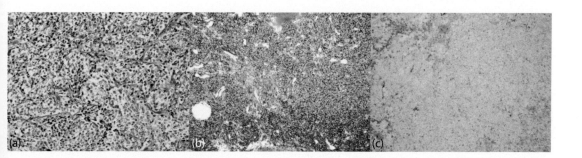

arrangement of densely packed undifferentiated cells (embryonal cells).

Slide b: Immunoreactive staining for synaptophysin.

Slide c: Immune-negative staining for Glial Fibrillary Acidic Protein (GFAP).

BIBLIOGRAPHY

1. Durinck S, Spellman PT, Birney E, Huber W. Mapping identifiers for the integration of genomic datasets with the R/Bioconductor Package Biomart. Nat Protoc. 2009;4: 1184–1191. doi: 10.1038/nprot.2009.97

2. Monro A. Observations on the Structure and Functions of the Nervous System. Creech and Johnson; Edinburgh, UK: 1783.

3. Frank E, Hall MA, Witten IH. The WEKA Workbench. 4th ed. Morgan Kaufmann: 2016. p. 553–71. doi: 10.1016/B978-0-12-804291-5.00024-6

4. Rekate HL. The definition and classification of hydrocephalus: a personal recommendation to stimulate debate. Cerebrospinal Fluid Res. 2008;5:2.

5. Kirkpatrick M, Engleman H, Minns RA. Symptoms and signs of progressive hydrocephalus. Arch Dis Child. 1989;64(01):124–128.

6. Del Bigio MR. Neuropathological changes caused by hydrocephalus. Acta Neuropathol. 1993;85(06):573–585.

7. Laurence KM, Coates S. The natural history of hydrocephalus. Detailed analysis of 182 unoperated cases. Arch Dis Child. 1962;37:345–362.

8. Leffert LR, Schwamm LH. Neuraxial anesthesia in parturients with intracranial pathology: A comprehensive review and reassessment of risk. Anesthesiology. 2013;119:703–718.

9. Zhang X, Medow JE, Iskandar BJ, Wang F, Shokoueinejad M, Koueik J, Webster JG. Invasive and noninvasive means of measuring intracranial pressure: A review. Physiol Meas. 2017;38:143–182.

10. Guiza F, Depreitere B, Piper I, Citerio G, Jorens PG, Maas A, Schuhmann MU, Lo TM, Donald R, Jones P et al. Early detection of increased intracranial pressure episodes in traumatic brain injury: External validation in an adult and in a pediatric cohort. Crit Care Med. 2017;45:316–320.

11. Rasulo FA, Bertuetti R, Robba C, Lusenti F, Cantoni A, Bernini M, Girardini A, Calza S, Piva S, Fagoni N et al. The accuracy of transcranial doppler in excluding intracranial hypertension following acute brain injury: A multicenter prospective pilot study. Crit Care. 2017;21.

12. Antes S, Stadie A, Müller S, Linsler S, Breuskin D, Oertel J. Intracranial pressure-guided shunt valve adjustments with the Miethke sensor reservoir. World Neurosurg. 2018;109:642–650.

13. Schick RW, Matson DD. What is arrested hydrocephalus?. J Pediatr. 1961;58: 791–799.

14. Bouras T, Sgouros S. Complications of endoscopic third ventriculostomy. J Neurosurg Pediatr. 2011;7:643–649.

15. Gilland O. Normal cerebrospinal-fluid pressure. N Engl J Med. 1969;280: 904–905.

76

Central nervous system lesions

TALAL ALMAYMAN
King Hamad University Hospital, Kingdom of Bahrain, Bahrain

Scenario: A 2-year-old female child has had repeated hospital admissions, outpatient clinic and emergency visits for drainage of a subcutaneous lesion in the natal cleft that has had recurrent episodic purulent discharge for the past year.

On examination, you note that the child has a tender swelling 2.5 cm × 3 cm in the lower midline close to the natal cleft. She is febrile, irritable with an ataxic gait and has lower limb hypotonia. The lesion is red, swollen and indurated with foul-smelling odor, oozing pus and an obvious dermal sinus apparent. There is a visible tuft of hair in the sacral area. Neurological examination is otherwise unremarkable.

Question: What is your leading working diagnosis? What are the other differential diagnoses?
Answer: The patient has spina bifida occulta/spinal dysraphism, which comprises a dermal sinus tract with an infected dermoid cyst and an early tethered cord syndrome.

The differential diagnosis will include:

- Pustule or boil/furunculosis
- Pilonidal cyst
- Sacrococcygeal teratoma (SCT)
- Sacral chordoma neoplasm
- Perianal fistula/abscess formation
- Lipomeningocele

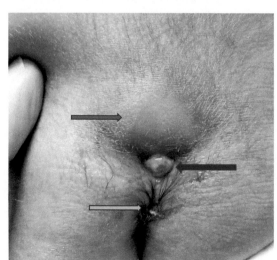

Blue Arrow: Lumbar subcutaneous lesion

Red Arrow: Dermal sinus oozing pus

Green Arrow: faun tail

DOI: 10.1201/9781003182290-85

Question: What is meant by spina bifida occulta? What are the other types of spinal dysraphism?

Answer: Spinal dysraphism is a variant type of neural tube defect where incomplete closure of the vertebral bony ring exists around the neural tube (spinal cord).

Variant types of spinal dysraphism also include:

Spina bifida cystica/aperta which may be a meningocele or myelomeningocele.

Spina bifida occulta, which is derived from Latin meaning 'hidden split spine'. This is the mildest form of spina bifida. The posterior structures of the spine fail to fuse properly, but unlike other severe forms, the spinal dura sac does not protrude into a large cyst, and the defect is typically covered by full-thickness skin.

Most patients will have notable certain external features that should raise suspicion to attending doctors and warrant further investigation:

- *Lipomeningocele*: Conus and caudal
- *Split cord malformation (SCM)/diastematomyelia*: SCM means two cords:
  - Type 1 (two dural tubes harboring a hemicord similar to pantaloons appearance)
  - Type 2 (single dural tube around a split cord)
- Dermal sinus tract
- Thickened filum terminale

Cutaneous stigmata are present that should raise a 'red flag' and a high index of suspicion:

- Hypertrichosis/faun tail
- Dimple (in the midline/large/2.5 cm from anal verge)
- Acrochordons/pseudo-tail
- Lipomas
- Hemangiomasmangiomas
- Aplasia cutis/scar
- Dermoid cyst
- Dermal sinus

A low index of suspicion may be encountered with telangiectasia, capillary malformation, hyperpigmentation, nevi and teratoma.

Question: How will you further investigate this patient?

Answer: Obtain a detailed history, family history, socioeconomic and drug history followed by clinical examination.

Tests to order will include:

Full blood count (FBC)
Inflammatory markers: Erythrocyte sedimentation rate (ESR), C-reactive protein (CRP)
Blood cultures
Wound culture and sensitivity
MRI lumbosacral spine with contrast and a screening MRI scan brain and whole spine
CT lumbosacral spine
Urodynamic studies
Nerve conduction studies (NCS) and electromyography (EMG)

These varied test investigations were performed, and the reports showed raised inflammatory markers and a culture swab positive for *Escherichia coli*.

MRI LUMBAR SPINE T2WI

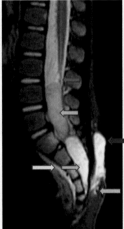

Blue: Low lying conus
Medullaris at L4 (Tethered cord)

Yellow: Intradural Dermoid
Cysts with variable infection

Red: Subcutaneous abscess

Green: Dermal sinus tract

White: Presacral inflammation
and sacral osteomyelitis

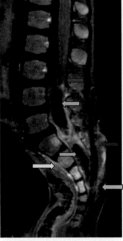

Blue: Low lying conus
Medullaris at L4 (Tethered cord)

Yellow: Intradural Dermoid
Cysts with variable infection

Red: Subcutaneous abscess

Green: Dermal sinus tract

White: Presacral inflammation
and sacral osteomyelitis

Question: What MRI scan findings are shown in the sagittal images? What are the typical MRI appearances of a dermal sinus tract with associated dermoid cyst?

Answer: MRI lumbar spine with contrast shows an infected lumbosacral dermal sinus associated with a cutaneous abscess, soft tissue inflammation and intraspinally two dermoid cysts extending up to the L4 vertebral body level.

MRI scan also reveals diffuse contrast enhancement in the paravertebral muscles, piriformis muscles and sacral alae suggestive of an extensive infective process due to spread of a spinal canal infection and the dermal sinus tract. A low-lying conus medullaris and filum terminale are connected to the dermoid cyst with thickened filum terminale.

Precontrast T1WI is hyperintense with high cholesterol content.
T2WI image is of variable intensity.
Post-contrast T1WI is a non-enhancing lesion or fade ring enhancing.

Diffusion weighted images show variable diffusion restriction as compared to an epidermoid cyst (hyperintense as compared to spinal cord). Differentiation from lipoma/lipomeningocele may be difficult in certain cases on the basis of MRI only.

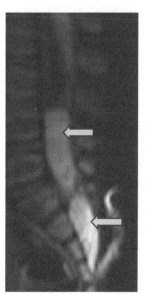

Diffusion weighted image

Shows restriction (hyperintense)

Question: Define the term dermal sinus tract.

Answer: Congenital dermal sinus was initially described by Walter and Bucy in 1932.[1] Spinal dysraphism may rarely present with a congenital dermal sinus tract as a result of failure of nondisjunction of the ectoderm from the actual neuroectoderm, during early neurulation (third to fifth week of gestation).[3,4] These tracts are often associated with other cutaneous and intraspinal pathologies.[5]

Congenital dermal sinus tracts are rare with an incidence of 1 in every 2,500 live births.[2] Dermal sinus tracts have been reported all the way along the midline neuroaxis from the ventral nasion, to dorsal inion/occiput caudally, to the lumbar and sacral spine. The majority are encountered in the caudal region of the neuroaxis.

Stratified squamous epithelium typically lines the sinus and connects the skin surface and may extend variably with deep tissues connections and co-existent anomalies. They may terminate superficially within the subcutaneous layers or may extend deeper through the fascia layers traversing normal vertebrae or via a congenital defect in the posterior spinal arches to communicate directly to the external surface of the dura mater or have an intradural component. They may occasionally terminate with the filum terminale and be abnormally thickened and/or associated with dermoid or lipoma lesion. The tract can therefore be associated with several pathological findings notably as inclusion tumors (e.g. epidermoid, dermoid, lipoma or teratomas).

MRI and CT imaging are the diagnostic studies of choice that greatly help to establish a diagnosis and plan surgical treatment.

Question: What is meant by the term tethered cord syndrome?

Answer: Tethered cord syndrome is a clinical diagnosis based on chronic neurologic progressive dysfunction involving the lower spinal cord. As the spinal column grows faster than the spinal cord during the initial years of life, tethering lesions result in progressive stretching of the spinal cord. Abnormal traction forces progressively lead to chronic ischemic changes and neuronal dysfunction. Patients may present with any combination of the following findings:

- Progressive leg weakness or sensory loss
- Bowel or bladder sphincter dysfunction
- Low back pain or sciatica
- Spinal deformities, usually scoliosis and kyphoscoliosis
- Foot deformities such as pes cavus
- Cutaneous stigmata of spinal dysraphism (hairy patch, dimple, subcutaneous lipoma, dermal sinus tract, dermoid)

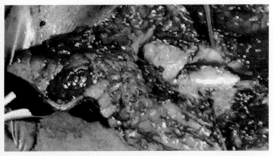

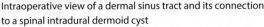

Intraoperative view of a dermal sinus tract and its connection to a spinal intradural dermoid cyst

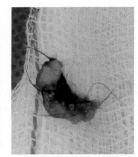

Content of L4-5, S1-3

Photograph - Intradural spinal dermoid cyst excised showing hair, pus, keratin and sebum contents

Question: What are the major differences in cauda equina syndrome, conus medullaris syndrome and tethered cord syndrome?

Answer: Please see the following table.

Table 76.1 Differences in cauda equina syndrome, conus medullaris syndrome and tethered cord syndrome

Characteristics	Cauda equina syndrome	Conus medullaris syndrome	Tethered cord syndrome
Onset	Acute-subacute	Acute-subacute	Chronic
Location of lesion	Below L1–2: Spinal level Below conus: Cord level	L2: Spinal (>5 years of age) Spinal and conus: Cord	Below L1–2 and conus
Pain	Common Back: Less often Legs: More often	Uncommon Back: Predominantly	Chronic legs stretching muscles pain and sciatic pain along with back pain are common
Sensory findings	Asymmetrical limbs and saddle anesthesia	Symmetrical limbs and saddle sensory loss Dissociative sensory loss	Asymmetrical, hypoesthesia and paresthesia
Motor findings	Asymmetrical	Symmetrical	Asymmetrical
Reflex changes	Usually both ankle and knee jerk loss	Ankle jerk loss commonly	Common, ankle and knee jerk usually exaggerated
Sphincters disturbance	Late presentation, starts as urinary retention	Common and early presentation with incontinent urine and faces	Common and late presentation
Onset	Relatively acute to subacute weeks to months	Subacute to chronic over moths	Chronic over years
Tone	Flaccid, may have twitches	Spastic	Spastic
Leg deformity/muscle contractions	Uncommon	Uncommon	Common
Lumbar dimple/lipoma/faun tail/skin color change	Nil	Nil	Common
Scoliosis	Nil	Nil	Common

Question: What is an intrathecal dermoid cyst? How will you differentiate such a lesion from a dermoid and epidermoid cyst?

Answer: Spinal dermoid and epidermoids are benign cysts in the spine. However, they may compress important neural structures, notably the spinal cord or spinal nerves, and they may eventually rupture. Spontaneous/intraoperative rupture may result in chemical or bacterial meningitis. Management involves surgical excision.

The lining of dermoid cysts may include skin appendages such as hair follicles and sebaceous or sweat glands in addition to stratified squamous epithelium. Diagnosis is confirmed with histopathology examination.

Both dermoid and epidermoid cysts contain skin material. Both lesions are lined with a layer of skin that naturally sheds dead cells. But instead of shedding to the exterior, shed skin cells accumulate inside the cyst. In this way such cysts gradually expand over months to years.

Dermoid and epidermoid cysts differ in their contents. Epidermoid cysts are lined with simple skin cells, and they thus contain only the products of skin cells (like the 'pearly 'white protein keratin) and an accumulation of shed skin cells. Dermoid cysts contain skin cells and their products plus many other skin components such as hair follicles, hair, sebaceous or sweat glands and may also have other material such as teeth, oily sebum or blood.

Question: What are the risk factors (if any) for dermoid cysts?

Answer: Dermoid and epidermoid cysts are rare in overall incidence but are much more commonly encountered in children than in adults. They may be either congenital (i.e., present at birth) or iatrogenic (arise later in life as a result of a medical procedure).

- Congenital cysts form early during embryonic development. They may be associated with dysraphism, a condition that will affect the developing spinal cord. This is the most common variant type of dermoid cysts.
- Iatrogenic: Iatrogenic cysts may be the result of the inadvertent introduction of skin cells into a space around the spinal cord. This may be a recognized sequela of dysraphism surgery or even a lumbar puncture. These will commonly result in an epidermoid cyst.

Question: How we can manage these patients?

Answer: Patients should be commenced on broad-spectrum intravenous antibiotics according to culture and sensitivity reports. Surgical excision should be scheduled to excise the cyst.

Microsurgical removal is the treatment of choice for most spinal cysts. MRI and the patient's neurological status help in surgical planning. If surgery will involve the spinal cord, its function is carefully assessed by intraoperative monitoring together with the use of somatosensory evoked potentials and motor evoked potential navigational guidance.

A laminectomy/laminoplasty is undertaken to gain access to the spinal canal. If necessary, the spinal dura is then opened to expose the spinal cord/nerves.

The goal of operation is complete cyst excision. However, if the cyst wall is densely adherent to the spinal cord or spinal nerves, its complete removal may not be safely possible. In such cases, a maximum safe resection is undertaken. Spillage of contents of a dermoid cyst and dermal sinus tract should be avoided at all costs and protected with sealing patties and immediate suctioning to prevent chemical and bacterial meningitis. Postoperatively antibiotics are administered to combat surgical site infection (SSI).

Question: Interpret the histopathology slide shown.

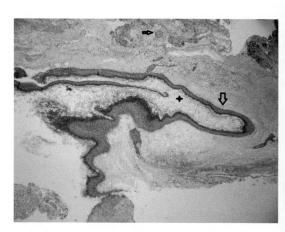

Answer: The histological slide examination reveals a cyst lined by stratified squamous epithelium (large arrow) with a cyst wall harboring hair follicles and pilosebaceous units (small arrow), and the lumen reveals keratin flakes (*).

BIBLIOGRAPHY

1. Amador LV, Hankinson J, Bigler JA. Congenital dermal sinuses. J Pediatr. 1955;47:300–10.
2. Ackerman LL, Menezes AH, Follett KA. Cervical and thoracic dermal sinus tracts. A case series and review of the literature. Pediatr Neurosurg. 2002;37(3):137–47.
3. Gupta RK, Yadav YK, Pandey S, Srivastava C, Jaiswal AK. Spinal dorsal dermal sinus tract: An experience of 21 cases. Surg Neurol Int. 2015;6(Suppl. 17):S429–S34.

4. Srivastava AK, Sibal AJ. Spinal dysraphism. J Pediatr Neurosci. 2011;6(Suppl. 1):S31–S40.

5. Hamill N, Grant JA, Myers SA. Congenital dermal sinus. 2008.

6. Davies SG, BChir SG, Chapman S et-al. Aids to Radiological Differential Diagnosis. Saunders Limited. 2009 ISBN:0702029793. Read it at Google Books - Find it at Amazon

7. Osborn AG. Diagnostic Neuroradiology. Mosby Inc. 1994. ISBN:0801674867. Read it at Google Books - Find it at Amazon.

8. Barsi P, Kenéz J, Várallyay G et-al. Unusual origin of free subarachnoid fat drops: a ruptured spinal dermoid tumour. Neuroradiology. 1992;34 (4): 343–4. Pubmed citation.

9. Van aalst J, Hoekstra F, Beuls EA et-al. Intraspinal dermoid and epidermoid tumors: report of 18 cases and reappraisal of the literature. Pediatr Neurosurg. 2009; 45(4):281–90. doi:10.1159/000235602

10. Kukreja K, Manzano G, Ragheb J et-al. Differentiation between pediatric spinal arachnoid and epidermoid-dermoid cysts: is diffusion-weighted MRI useful? Pediatr Radiol. 2007;37(6):556–60. doi:10.1007/s00247-007-0463-8

11. Goodrich A, Wolf CW, Allen MB. Intradural dermoid cyst. Spine. 1984;9:832–4.

12. Guidetti B, Gagliardi FM. Epidermoid and dermoid cysts. J Neurosurg. 1977; 47:12–18.

13. Mathew P, Todd NV. Intradural conus and cauda equina tumours: a retrospective review of presentation, diagnosis and early outcome. J Neurol Neurosurg Psychiatry. 1993;56:69–74.

14. Wilkins RH et al. Spinal intradural cysts. Handbook of Clinical Neurology. North-Holland: Amsterdam, 1976; 55–102.

15. Messori A, Polonara G, Serio A et-al. Expanding experience with spontaneous dermoid rupture in the MRI era: diagnosis and follow-up. Eur J Radiol. 2002;43 (1): 19–27. Eur J Radiol (link) - Pubmed citation.

16. McComb JG, Congenital dermal sinus. Pang D: Disorders of the Pediatric Spine New York: Raven Press, 1995; 349–60.

PART 10

Trauma

77

APLS and ATLS: Essentials of care

HUSSEIN AHMED HAMDY
Women's and Childrens Hospital, Kingdom of Bahrain, Bahrain

MARTIN T. CORBALLY
King Hamad University Hospital, Kingdom of Bahrain, Bahrain

The ability to recognize a seriously ill child can save a life. The main principle of APLS and ATLS is "what kills first should be managed first". Trauma is a major cause of morbidity and death in childhood.

Such trauma may be the result of motor vehicle accidents (MVAs), bike injuries, pedestrian injuries or other myriad activities resulting in injury in childhood. In general, the management of pediatric trauma follows the same general principles as in adult trauma (ATLS: Advanced Trauma Life Support) but recognizes the fundamental differences in physiology, anatomy and functional reserves. The ATLS protocol for emergent trauma management follows two distinct but inseparable pathways:

Primary survey:

A: Airway and cervical spine motion restriction
B: Breathing and ventilation support
C: Circulation and hemorrhage control
D: Disability and Glasgow Coma Scale (GCS)
E: Exposure and environment control

Secondary survey:

AMPLE history
Head-to-toe full clinical examination

Scenario: A healthy 8-year-old girl is involved in an MVA. She was an unrestrained (not wearing a seat belt) back seat passenger and has a GCS (refer to **Table 77.4**) of 14 on arrival to hospital. She is in pain, has extensive facial lacerations which are actively bleeding, her neck is obviously swollen and the child complains of abdominal pain.

Question: What are your initial thoughts before you see this emergency patient, and what do you feel needs key priority?
Answer: The scenario outlines a serious trauma accident to a previously healthy child. The mechanism of trauma is important, as it helps you to focus on critical aspects of emergent care that could be fatal if not corrected promptly.

The 8-year-old patient will have significantly different physiological responses to trauma, and this can influence the presentation and interpretation of injury. Given the accident history and mechanism of injury, the chances are that this child will have more serious injuries.

Question: Why?
Answer: The patient was unrestrained in the vehicle and could have more severe injuries from being

DOI: 10.1201/9781003182290-87

thrown about inside the vehicle cabin, or direct collision with other passengers, or she may have been ejected from the car. The trauma care provider must consider this and crucially determine the mechanism of injury in detail and also rule out head trauma, spinal injury, intra-abdominal injury, thoracic injuries and pelvic fractures. Any injury is therefore possible!

Normally a trauma code will be activated when the receiving hospital is made aware of the impending arrival of such a patient, and the trauma team will start resuscitation according to the ATLS protocol.

Question: How can we estimate the child's weight and surface area?

Answer: The child's weight is very important for management, as equipment, instruments, drugs and IV fluids will depend on the patient's weight.

A child's weight can be estimated based on age (**Table 77.1**).

Another way to assess the child's weight is by using the Broselow tape. This tape is based on the

Table 77.1 Estimated weight in different age groups

Age	Formula
0–12 months	Weight (in kg) = (0.5 × age in months) + 4
1–5 years	Weight (in kg) = (2 × age in years) + 8
6–12 years	Weight (in kg) = (3 × age in years) + 7

child's length and gives an approximate determination regarding the child's weight and drug doses (**Figure 77.1**).

PRIMARY SURVEY

A: Airway and cervical spine motion restriction

Question: How do we examine and manage the airway in this trauma patient?

Answer: Airway care management is the first key step in resuscitating a trauma patient because if

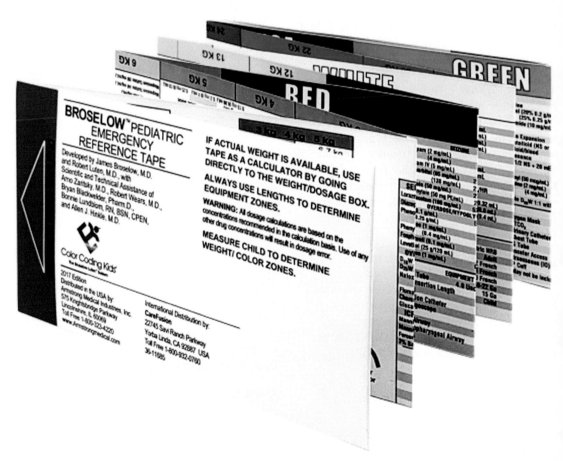

Figure 77.1 Broselow tape.

the patient doesn't have a stable patent airway (obstructed), then death is inevitable. The airway should be patent and protected at all times during emergent trauma management.

The easiest way to check airway patency is to talk to the patient. A patient who can talk has a patent airway. If the airway is obstructed by blood, vomitus or a foreign body, it should be cleared by a working suction device and an oropharyngeal airway (e.g. a Guedel airway) inserted. It is also critically important to assess if the airway is adequately protected or if it needs protection from aspiration. A fully conscious patient will generally have a protected airway, but an unconscious patient cannot safely maintain their airway for breathing. The GCS score will be later discussed during the D component of the primary survey.

Referring to our patient in this trauma scenario, the child has a GCS score of 14, which indicates that she is conscious, fully orientated and able to communicate. Her airway is currently secure and patent.

Given the clinical history of being an unrestrained vehicle passenger she could, however, have sustained injury to the spine, and every patient is therefore assumed to have a spine injury until proven otherwise. Cervical spine motion has to be restrained and protected, as uncontrolled movements in the presence of an unstable neck injury can significantly worsen spinal cord damage or cause sudden death. Cervical spine protection measures must be fully maintained during airway management assessment.

To establish cervical spine protection, a proper-sized cervical collar has to be securely placed and two sandbags to maintain immobilization laid beside the patient's head with two straps then placed across the forehead and chin. This limits any spinal motion for the moment while attention is now paid to other vital areas as part of the emergency primary survey exam.

Full examination of the cervical spine and back region and documenting the neurological status of the patient is part of the secondary survey. (Protection is primary and detection is secondary.)

Question: Is the patient's airway at risk of deterioration?

Answer: Since the patient is talking coherently to hospital emergency personnel, there is no immediate problem, but as the patient has extensive facial lacerations and soft tissue neck edema from the accident, the airway is at risk of impending compromise.

Be aware the patient's airway can deteriorate at any time during the resuscitation phase, so it is always better to intervene early and consider electively intubating a patient under controlled circumstances where this may occur and not be forced into a more urgent and less controlled airway intubation if the patient deteriorates suddenly.

Question: What should we expect next?

Answer: Intubating a pediatric trauma victim is not always straightforward. The unique anatomical differences between children and adults make intubation in children more difficult and require certain special precautions. Note that the head of a very young child or infant is proportionately large, and this leads to greater degrees of neck flexion when a child is in a supine position. Placing a bag or pillow under the shoulders will help to avoid this flexion and puts the pediatric patient in the "sniffing" position, which can make intubation easier. The larynx in children is located more anterior in anatomical terms, which also makes intubation difficult. A skilled anesthetist is required when dealing with the airway in a trauma child. Also the surgeon should always keep in mind the possible need for a surgical airway at any time and be ready to perform a cricothyroidotomy. Remember the key rule: The cervical spine must also be fully protected during intubation.

B: Breathing and ventilation support

Question: How will you assess the child's breathing?

Answer: Assessment of breathing is checked by:

1. Inspection: Ecchymosis, open wounds, lacerations, chest wall movement, etc.
2. Palpation: Tenderness, surgical emphysema, crepitation, and check that the trachea is central in location by neck palpation.
3. Auscultation: Decreased air entry on one side of the thorax may indicate hemothorax or pneumothorax. Absent air entry on one side of the chest indicates a tension pneumothorax, particularly if signs of shock are present, which will be discussed in "Circulation" management.
4. Percussion: Hyperresonance indicates a pneumothorax and dullness a hemothorax.

Table 77.2 Vital signs in different pediatric age groups

Age	Heart rate	Systolic blood pressure	Respiratory rate
Newborn	120–160	50–70	30–50
1–12 months	80–140	70–100	20–30
1–3 years	80–130	80–110	20–30
3–5 years	80–120	80–110	20–30
6–12 years	70–110	80–120	20–30
>12 years	55–105	110–120	12–20

Note: Any trauma victim may present in a state of shock.

Question: What are the most common thoracic injuries encountered in children?

Answer: Pulmonary contusions are the most common thoracic injury occurring in children. Rib fractures are not common, as the thoracic cage in children is very pliable, and this therefore leads to lung injury without evidence of rib fractures.

C: Circulation and hemorrhage control

The first steps for hemorrhage control are to apply direct pressure. Secure and apply a hemostat if there is visible arterial bleeding. Open weeping wounds should be covered by clean pressure dressings.

Vital signs: Monitoring and resuscitation should be done at this stage.

The trauma victim should have two large IV lines secured. If IV access is proving difficult to secure, then interosseous (IO) access can be deployed.

Blood should be sent for laboratory test evaluation including full blood count (FBC), urea and electrolytes (U&E), serum lipase and amylase estimation and cross-match (× 4 units). Note: Pediatric vital signs are different than adults. Moreover, vital signs in children vary according to age groups (**Table 77.2**).

Question: What is meant by the term shock?

Answer: Shock is best defined as a clinical state of tissue organ hypoperfusion. Hemorrhagic shock is the most common type sustained in trauma victims. A shocked patient will have abnormal vital signs according to the class of shock (category amount of blood loss – **Table 77.3**).

In a trauma patient, bleeding may be from open wounds, fractures of long bones, pelvic fractures or intrathoracic injury together with lung contusions or significant abdominal injury to the liver, spleen or kidneys.

Note that a traumatic head injury is not a major leading cause of hemorrhagic blood loss, although significant bleeding can occur from large scalp lacerations.

Resuscitation first commences with IV crystalloid solutions (normal saline 0.9% or Ringer's lactate/Hartmann's solution) at 20 mL/kg bolus rates over 15–20 minutes. Type-specific blood transfusion or O-negative blood 10 mL/kg should be deployed very early if the patient is considered a "non-responder" to crystalloid bolus volume resuscitation.

Table 77.3 Class of hemorrhagic shock

Parameter	Class 1	Class 2	Class 3	Class 4
Blood loss %	<15%	15–30%	30–40%	>40%
Heart rate	Normal	Normal or increase	Increase	Increase
Blood pressure	Normal	Normal	Hypotension	Hypotension
Pulse pressure	Normal	Decrease	Decrease	Decrease
Respiratory rate	Normal	Normal	Normal or increase	Increase
Urine output	Normal	Normal	Decrease	Decrease

D: Disability and GCS score

At this stage of trauma evaluation, the consciousness level of the patient should be evaluated. Head trauma is common in pediatric trauma victims. Many children with minor head injuries will vomit.

The GCS (**Table 77.4**) is used to assess the patient's level of consciousness and to broadly classify the severity of head trauma.

There are three main GCS components to evaluate. Eye opening (E), verbal response (V) and best motor response (M). The patient will be assigned a score in each component (EVM) based on the best response. The sum of all scores is then the total GCS (**Table 77.4**). The highest score is designated 15 and the lowest score 3.

Question: What is the GCS score if the patient's eyes open only in response to pain? They are not vocalizing appropriate words, and the trauma victim flexes only in response to pain.
Answer: The GCS is now 10.

Note: On the initial emergency hospital department evaluation, the GCS was equal to 14.

Head trauma may be classified into mild (GCS 14–13), moderate (GCS 12–9) and severe (GCS ≤8). Patients with GCS ≤8 should be intubated, as they cannot protect their airway.

In our scenario patient, the GCS when first evaluated was equal to 14, which indicates mild head trauma.

Mild head trauma needs observation, as the patient's consciousness level may later deteriorate. A CT head scan may be indicated after the primary survey.

Different types of intracranial injury may be seen on a head CT scan:

1. Epidural with bleeding due to an arterial injury outside the dura (termed extradural bleed).
2. Subdural
3. Subarachnoid
4. Intracranial
5. Intraventricular

The role of the trauma care provider is always to prevent secondary brain injury by avoiding hypoxia (early intubation and ventilation) and hypotension (fluid resuscitation) as discussed earlier.

Early referral to a neurosurgeon is key.

Table 77.4 Glasgow Coma Score

Behavior	Response	Score
Eye opening	Spontaneous	4
	To speech	3
	To pain	2
	No response	1
Best verbal response	Conscious	5
	Confused	4
	Inappropriate words	3
	Incomprehensible sounds	2
	No response	1
Best motor response	Obeys commands	6
	Localizes pain	5
	Flexion from pain	4
	Abnormal flexion from pain	3
	Abnormal extension from pain	2
	No response	1

E: Exposure and environment control

Every trauma patient should be exposed fully to allow for detailed examination and detection of all injuries. At the same time the patient should be protected against hypothermia. Warming the emergency room, use of warm IV fluids and covering the patient with heated blankets are all measures to protect against hypothermia.

Hypothermia in a trauma patient can be fatal, as it is considered part of the lethal triad (**Figure 77.2**).

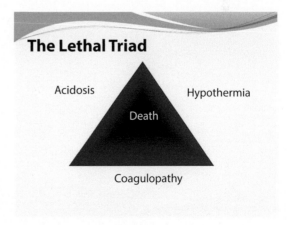

Figure 77.2 Lethal triad.

Question: What are the adjuncts to the primary survey?

Answer: These are tools to help during resuscitation of the trauma patient.

Pulse oximetry: Measures oxygen saturation in blood.

ECG: Monitors cardiac rate and rhythm and detects any arrhythmia.

X-rays: Chest and pelvic X-ray are part of the primary survey. Any other imaging can be scheduled only after first securing resuscitation and stabilization of the patient.

Focused assessment sonography for trauma (FAST) scan: An ultrasound scan examination which shows blood in four specific areas:

Hepatorenal pouch: Liver injury.

Lienorenal pouch: Spleen injury.

Pelvis: Pelvic fracture or pelvic organ injury.

Pericardial space: Hemopericardium
   (**Figures 77.3** and **77.4**).

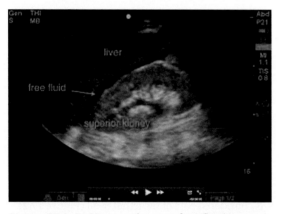

Figure 77.3 FAST scan showing free fluid around the liver.

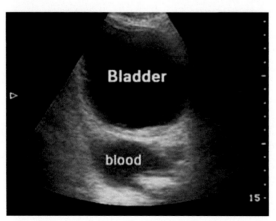

Figure 77.4 FAST showing free fluid (blood) in the pelvis.

A Foley catheter to decompress the urinary bladder and to accurately measure urine output should be considered. Before inserting the catheter, the surgeon must ensure there is no urethral injury. Signs to indicate a possible urethral injury are blood at the external urethral meatus, perineal hematoma ("butterfly sign") and perineal ecchymosis. The presence of a pelvic fracture is an indicator of possible urethral injury. If a urethral injury is suspected, a urethral catheter should thus be avoided and a suprapubic catheter deployed. A retrograde contrast urethrogram study can be used to diagnose urethral injury, which is notably more common in males.

A catheter will help to measure urine output, which indicates resuscitation status of the trauma patient. Urine output volume should be at least 1 mL/kg/hour (in an adult, this would be 0.5–1 mL/kg/hour).

Once the primary survey is completed, the patient should be re-evaluated and the primary survey should be repeated if the patient's condition deteriorates at any subsequent stage.

SECONDARY SURVEY

1. The history should be always obtained for a trauma patient. The AMPLE history is what we need to know about the trauma patient:
   Allergies.
   Medications.
   Past medical history.
   Last meal.
   Events before trauma.
2. Head-to-toe examination.
   A detailed examination of the trauma patient is very important to detect every possible injury.
      In our scenario, the female patient has sustained neck trauma, and examination to access for possible cervical spine fracture is thus very important.

If the patient is conscious, fully cooperative and has no other distracting injuries, we can ask the patient to help us to evaluate the status of the cervical spine.

1. Ask the patient about neck pain.
2. Ask the patient to voluntarily move their neck, as it will be limited by pain, and do not attempt to move the neck yourself.
3. Examine for tenderness over the cervical spine region.

If the patient has no pain on movement and no tenderness on palpation, the cervical spine can be cleared and the cervical collar removed.

If the patient has pain or tenderness, then a cervical spine X-ray (AP and lateral views) or CT scan should be scheduled to clear the cervical spine.

A detailed neurological examination should be performed to identify any neurological defects secondary to a spine injury. Early referral to orthopedic or neurosurgical services should be considered at this stage.

If the patient is unconscious, then the spine has to be protected until cleared by a spinal surgeon after undertaking X-rays and/or CT scan imaging.

Note: If the patient deteriorates, then the primary survey has to be repeated starting from the airway.

Question: What you should do now if the patient's heart rate slowed to 45 per min (heart rate was 85 on initial admission)?
Answer: Bradycardia should be addressed carefully in a pediatric trauma patient. Usually a trauma patient presents with tachycardia due to a shock state.

A patient with bradycardia may have sustained a cardiac injury or hemopericardium (blood in the pericardial space) or have raised intracranial pressure (ICP) secondary to a head injury.

ECG monitoring is important to detect arrhythmias, which may indicate cardiac injury.

The FAST scan can help detect hemopericardium. If hemopericardium is evident, then urgent pericardiocentesis should be undertaken by inserting a long hollow needle below the xiphisternum at 45° into the pericardial sac.

Note: Another important cause of bradycardia is neurogenic shock with spinal injury. Neurogenic shock is due to loss of sympathetic tone due to spinal cord injury sustained above the level of T6.

The injury will cause bradycardia and peripheral vasodilatation leading to hypotension. Fluid resuscitation and vasopressors will be needed to treat neurogenic shock.

Note: Always consider increasing raised ICP secondary to head injury as a cause of bradycardia.

- The patient's O_2 saturations have now dropped to 60% and she has difficulty breathing.

We should immediately re-evaluate the patient's airway and ensure it is patent and protected as discussed in airway management.

Breathing should be evaluated as discussed in breathing and ventilation.

Tension pneumothorax has to be considered always. This diagnosis has to be made urgently clinically without imaging. Signs of tension pneumothorax are:

1. Hypotension and tachycardia
2. Absent chest wall motion on the affected side
3. Absent air entry on the affected side
4. Hyperresonant percussion on the affected side
5. Trachea shifted to the opposite side
6. Congested neck veins

This is an emergency scenario and should be managed immediately by inserting a wide-bore needle into the second intercostal space at the mid-clavicular line to aspirate and decompress the pleura cavity. The needle thoracocentesis is immediately followed by scheduling insertion of a chest tube intercostal drain into the fifth intercostal space anterior to the mid-axillary line and connected to an underwater seal system. Check the chest tube for "fogging" and the water seal system for bubbling/water fluid movement indicating adequate functioning. Order a chest X-ray only after insertion of the drain.

BIBLIOGRAPHY

1. Advanced Trauma Life Support Manual 10th edition. American College Of Surgeons. 2018.
2. Advanced Pediatric Life Support - The Practical Approach - 5th edition. Australia and New Zealand. 2012
3. J Grant McFadyen et al. Initial assessment and management of pediatric trauma patients, Int J Crit Illn Inj Sci. 2012 Sep-Dec;2(3):121–127.
4. Committee On Pediatric Emergency Medicine Council On Injury And Violence And Poison Prevention, Section On Critical Care Section, Orthopaedics Section On Surgery, Section On Transport Medicine, Pediatric Trauma Society, And Society Of Trauma Nurses Pediatric Committee. Management of Pediatric Trauma. Pediatrics. 2016 August;138(2):e20161569.
5. Paneitz DC, Ahmad S. Pediatric trauma update. Mo Med. 2018 September/October;115(5):438–442.
6. Williams RF, Grewal H, Jamshidi R, et al. Updated APSA guidelines for the management of blunt liver and spleen injuries. J Pediatr Surg. 2023 Aug; 58(8):1411–1418.

78

Foreign body aspiration

HESHAM YUSUF SAAD

King Hamad University Hospital, Kingdom of Bahrain, Bahrain

Scenario: A 3-year-old male child is brought to the emergency department (ED) by his parents, who were very concerned as they noticed him choke and turn blue as he was running and chewing nuts whilst playing.

Upon evaluation by the ED physician the child is now pink, vitally stable, and maintaining his oxygen saturations at around 95% on room air. The boy is sitting comfortably and not in obvious distress or showing shortness of breath nor using any accessory muscles. The patient has no noisy breathing except for occasional episodes of dry coughing.

Question: What is your initial impression?

Answer: Foreign body aspiration (FBA) in view of the clinical history.

Question: What is the definition of FBA?

Answer: It is the accidental inhalation of solid and/or liquid debris material into the airway.

Question: What are the various types of foreign bodies that may be aspirated and the particular significance of each?

Answer: In general organic foreign bodies account for the majority (62%) of aspirated contents in the pediatric age group, as shown in one study. Among these nuts (mostly peanuts and pistachios) are the major offending objects in most studies. Unlike their inorganic counterparts (coins, toy parts, etc.)

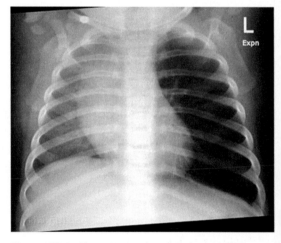

Figure 78.1 Chest X-ray showing hyperinflation of the left lung due to an obstructing inhaled foreign body.

that are often radiopaque, organic aspirated foreign bodies such as peanuts are mostly radiolucent on routine chest X-ray (CXR). They can therefore only be suspected indirectly by their resultant sequelae such as lung or lobar collapse or hyperinflation (**Figure 78.1**).

In addition, it should be noted that *all* types of foreign bodies, due to their mechanical effects, will cause atelectasis and/or hyperinflation, with a physiological reaction, most notably reactive bronchospasm. Organic foreign bodies are notably more likely to create secondary pathological changes in the form of inflammatory granulations and cicatricial bronchial stenosis in the long term.

DOI: 10.1201/9781003182290-88

Question: In the scenario the patient manifested a history of a choking episode followed by intermittent coughing. What other symptoms and signs might be anticipated in such condition?

Answer: Other predictors of FBA of significance would include noisy breathing/stridor/dyspnea, recurrent or persistent rhonchi of new onset, and abnormal suspicious radiological features on imaging or localized clinical findings.

Once a foreign body gets trapped in the upper airways, the associated clinical symptoms are usually well manifested, which highly suggests aspiration. However, in the vast majority of cases (75%–94%) the foreign body will then migrate to the lower airways with subsequent loss of the unique specific classic signs and symptoms, which can impose difficulty in the final diagnosis in the face of subtle or few symptoms.

Question: What is meant by the term penetration syndrome and how frequently is it encountered in FBA?

Answer: It is defined as a sudden onset of choking and intractable coughing with or without vomiting and is said to be identified on patient interview in as many as 81% of index cases. Other symptoms that may occur in isolation or in association are notably coughing, fever, breathlessness, and wheezing.

The diagnosis of FBA gets more challenging if penetration syndrome has ceased spontaneously or the attending physician has underestimated its key significance and consequent implications.

Question: What are the potential detrimental effects of FBA and those associated with the delay in its recognition and subsequent delayed management?

Answer: FBA is ranked as the fifth leading cause of accidental deaths in children aged 1–3 years and a major primary cause of mortality during infancy.

These facts and figures explain why FBA is recognized as a serious emergent medical condition with significant related mortality. It is also linked with significant morbidity if undetected, resulting in obstructive pneumonitis, atelectasis and lung abscess, pneumomediastinum, and pneumothorax. In the long term this may result in recurrent unresolved pneumonias, bronchiectasis, bronchial stricture, hemoptysis, and the development of inflammatory polyps and granulations at the site of impaction.

Delayed operative-related complications may include difficulty in foreign body extraction, especially beyond 24 hours of aspiration.

Question: What are the incidence and typical age distribution of FBA?

Answer: Seventy-five percent of FBA events are seen in children younger than 3 years of age. The peak reported incidence is typically 10- to 24-month-old infants.

Question: As in most cases, there are only subtle physical and radiological hints with regard FBA, and the dilemma often raised is "To bronchoscope or not to bronchoscope?" So what should the adopted diagnostic working algorithm be?

Answer: Refer to Mortinot (1997).

Rigid bronchoscopy shall be reserved for cases with asphyxia, radiopaque foreign bodies, and in the presence of localizing clinical signs, notably decreased air entry or obstructive emphysema. Otherwise, flexible bronchoscopy should be advocated as the initial diagnostic intervention modality (**Figure 78.2**).

Such a structured pathway approach will decrease the chances of a negative unnecessary rigid bronchoscopy to as low as 4% cases.

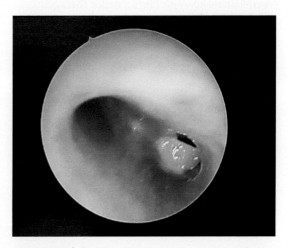

Figure 78.2 Organic foreign body at the orifice of the right main bronchus.

Question: Name the diagnostic investigations or workup that should be scheduled in suspected FBA.

Answer: They are as follows:

Chest X-ray: Radiolucent foreign bodies are the vast majority of aspirated agents (as high as 96%), and an expiratory anteroposterior (AP) plain film chest X-ray may highlight bronchial obstruction indirectly. Here it can show evidence of air trapping in the form of emphysema or hyperinflation due to a ball-valve effect exerted by the foreign body. Atelectasis is noted in up to 41% of foreign body cases due to distal collapse of lung parenchyma. Rarely, pneumothorax or pneumomediastinum can be seen if the foreign body penetrates and ruptures the airway.

Fluoroscopy: Can be useful to demonstrate decreased diaphragmatic excursion movement due to obstructive emphysema on the ipsilateral side of the inhaled foreign body. However, this investigation is operator-dependent, and its real value is surpassed by CT virtual bronchoscopy.

Chest CT: Multidetector CT scan has shortened the acquisition time to seconds and provides a refined quality image without sedation in a cooperative child with a sensitivity of almost 100%. However, specificity varies from 66.7% to 100%, that can be attributed to mucus plugging and possible artifacts. This modality will not only show the foreign body but also can confirm the presence of related pathological radiological findings. Additionally, 3-D CT scan reconstruction provides an invaluable tool of allowing virtual bronchoscopy (VB).

Flexible bronchoscopy: Plays a major therapeutic role in FBA with a sensitivity and specificity approaching 100%. Endoscopy may be carried as a diagnostic study under light sedation or general anesthesia. It allows the operator to retrieve small foreign body objects.

The most significant aspect of management is to consider the possibility of aspiration and have a low threshold for diagnostic bronchoscopy.

BIBLIOGRAPHY

White JJ, Cambron JD, Gottleib M, Long B. Evaluation and management of airway foreign bodies in the emergency department setting. J Emerg Med. 2023;64(2):145–155.

Wang ML, Hui Png L, Ma J, et al. The role of CT scan in pediatric airway foreign bodies. Int J Gen Med. 2023;16:547–555.

Wiemers A, Vossen C, Lucke T, et al. Complication rates in rigid vs. flexible endoscopic foreign body removal in children. Int J Pediatr Otorhinolaryngol. 2023;166:111474.

Freitag N, Mollenberg L, Wiemers A, et al. Preference matters: new aspects on how foreign bodies should and could be removed from a child's airway. Pediatr Pulmonol. 2023. Doi:10.1002/ppul.26411.

79

Chest trauma

ANDREW J. A. HOLLAND
The Children's Hospital at Westmead Sydney Medical School,
Faculty of Medicine and Health, The University of Sydney, Westmead,
New South Wales, Australia

Scenario: A 23-month-old male child falls from a first floor balcony onto a concrete wall. The child was alert and crying at the scene with bruising of the mid-anterior chest (**Figure 79.1**). Ambulance officers note that the pulse (P) was 147, respiratory rate (RR) 28 and blood pressure (BP) 85/40 mmHg. A cervical collar is applied and supplementary oxygen administered at 10–12 L/minute via a Hudson mask.

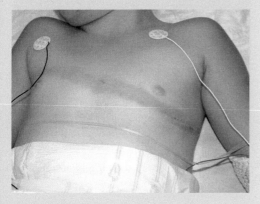

Figure 79.1 23-month-old child with marked bruising of anterior chest wall.

Question: What steps would you take to prepare for arrival of this child at a paediatric trauma centre (PTC)? What potential injuries would you consider?

Answer: The trauma team should be alerted and advised of the child's estimated time of arrival (ETA). Information on the mechanism of injury (MOI, M), injuries sustained (I), signs (S) and treatment (T) given should be supplied (MIST). Blunt trauma is much more common in children than penetrating trauma and typically occurs as a result of motor vehicle injuries, either as a pedestrian or passenger, or falls. In cases when the history is less clear, clinicians need to consider the possibility of non-accidental injury (NAI). In children, their compliant chest wall, together with reduced muscle mass and subcutaneous fat when compared to adults, results in greater transmission of forces through the rib cage to the underlying soft tissues. In the past rib fractures have been considered rare and indicative of massive trauma or NAI. More recently it seems that fractures, when carefully looked for, may occur in up to 60% of children and can be easily missed on a standard anteroposterior plain film chest radiograph.

Based on the MOI and signs, likely chest injuries would include pulmonary contusions (the most common thoracic injury in children), pneumo and/or haemothorax, rib fractures, flail chest and cardiac contusions. Rare injuries would include the airways (trachea and bronchi), sternal fractures, vascular (aortic arch), oesophagus and thoracic spine. Given the history of a fall from a height onto a solid surface, associated injuries of the head, cervical spine and limbs should be actively sought whilst maintaining appropriate spinal precautions.

DOI: 10.1201/9781003182290-89

The child arrives in the resuscitation room of the emergency department 90 minutes after their injury: P 155, RR 30 and BP 80/40. ECG monitoring is commenced, revealing a sinus tachycardia. The child is still crying with oxygen saturations of 96% on 12 L/minute via a non-rebreather mask and a Glasgow Coma Score (GCS) of 14 with equal and reactive pupils. His weight is 15.7 kg, and a 20-G cannula has been inserted.

Question: What would be your next steps in management? What investigations would you request, and when should these be performed?

Answer: Optimal care of the injured child involves practiced, co-ordinated team work to ensure that diagnosis and treatment occur in parallel using a standardised approach: Catastrophic haemorrhage control, airway (with cervical spine immobilisation), breathing (with oxygen), circulation (with haemorrhage control and IV access), disability (GCS, pupils and glucose) and exposure (keep warm). Although trauma remains the most common cause of death in children, major trauma requiring operative surgical intervention, especially involving the chest, remains infrequent (<5% of cases), particularly for first responders and clinical staff in non-trauma centres. The use of simulation, potentially in situ, to practice trauma care and teamwork, in conjunction with appropriate orientation, has been shown to enhance clinician confidence and decision making and improve adherence to trauma care protocols. The patient should have IV fluids commenced, preferably warmed normal saline with additional dextrose. Based on the patient's tachycardia and tachypnoea, a 10 mL/kg bolus should be given and the response assessed whilst continuing to give maintenance fluids.

In trauma, clinical examination should occur in parallel with investigations and treatment. Whilst chest trauma may be isolated and is less frequent than limb, head and abdominal trauma, accounting for approximately 10% of paediatric trauma admission, it is commonly associated with other injuries, especially head and torso. Chest trauma remains a marker for serious injury, with higher morbidity and mortality than more common forms of trauma in children.

Initial investigations should include a full blood count, urea and electrolytes, liver function tests, blood gasses, blood sugar and cross-match together with a standard trauma series of lateral cervical spine, chest and pelvic radiographs. Whilst CT of the chest or assessment of the chest as part of a multi-detector CT (MDCT) may be required in complex patients or those with a widened mediastinum, this involves much higher doses of radiation than chest radiography and requires transport of the patient to and from the CT scanner. Point-of-care (POC) ultrasound has been increasingly used in the care of children and may be useful particularly in the assessment of haemothorax and potential pericardial tamponade, but requires additional equipment and training.

Based on the MOI and initial clinical findings, it seems likely that this patient will have pulmonary contusions, possibly rib and/or sternal fractures and potentially cardiac contusions. In the case of pulmonary contusions, the initial chest radiograph may be normal or reveal only limited changes, with more obvious consolidation taking 6–8 hours to appear (**Figure 79.2**). Chest radiographs frequently underestimate the extent and severity of pulmonary contusions, whereas CT is more sensitive. Ultimately the patient will be managed based on their clinical status, so CT should be reserved for those patients when there is suspicion of an additional injury.

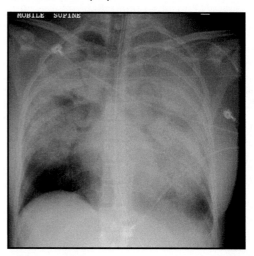

Figure 79.2 Chest X-ray showing bilateral pulmonary contusions.

The child's pulse rate falls to 140 with the fluid bolus and BP is now 85/44. At 3 hours post injury but still in the emergency department, the RR is 32 and saturation 92%. The lateral cervical spine and pelvic radiographs appear normal. A detailed secondary survey finds abrasions on the left hip and thigh but no other injuries. Haematological investigations are normal apart from a haemoglobin of 112 g/L. Urinalysis reveals microscopic haematuria only.

Question: How would you manage this patient's tachypnoea and low oxygen saturation? What further investigations would you consider?

Answer: The patient's respiratory status is likely to deteriorate further as the pulmonary contusions evolve. It is possible therefore that the patient will require intubation and ventilation for a period of time (perhaps several days) and a paediatric intensive care unit (PICU) admission will be required or at least admission to a high dependency or close observation unit following assessment by a PICU clinician. A careful clinical examination of the chest and chest radiograph should be performed to assess for the presence of rib fractures, sternal injury or flail chest, as appropriate analgesia in the form of a local anaesthetic rib blocks and/or an epidural anaesthetic may ameliorate some of the deterioration in respiratory function resulting from respiratory embarrassment or decreased chest wall excursion. Flail segment remains rare, and there appears limited evidence in the literature to either support or refute fixation in children.

The patient is transferred to the high dependency unit (HDU) and arrives there approximately 5 hours after their injury. On arrival the pulse rate is 145, BP 80/45, RR 34 and oxygen saturation 93%. A repeat chest radiograph reveals no significant further change. Following review by the PICU fellow, the patient is transferred to the PICU, intubated and ventilated. The patient's oxygen saturation improves to 98% with an FiO_2 of 0.7, a tidal volume of 6 mL/kg and positive end expiratory pressure (PEEP) of 10 cmH$_2$0. A CT scan of the chest is performed, revealing worsening bilateral pulmonary contusions and a small left haemothorax.

Question: How would you treat this patient's haemothorax? Are there any additional therapies you would consider if the patient deteriorates or fails to improve?

Answer: As the patient is on positive-pressure ventilation, drainage of the haemothorax would be appropriate, as this will allow for assessment of ongoing haemorrhage and may assist lung recruitment (although it could also increase the subsequent risk of a post-traumatic empyema). This should be performed at the bedside in PICU using an open technique with a standard 18–22 Fr intercostal catheter (ICC, generally size approximately corresponds to 4 times the size of the appropriate endotracheal tube for the patient's age) or by means of an interventional radiology approach with a 10–14 Fr pig-tail catheter depending on the status of the patient and local facilities. The ICC must be connected to an underwater seal and drainage carefully monitored. In patients with large haemothoraces, a chest drain collection device to allow auto-transfusion should be considered.

Surgeons need to carefully liaise with their ICU colleagues in relation to the patient's ventilator requirements to strike a balance between appropriate respiratory support and optimal oxygenation whilst minimising the risks of barotrauma, ventilator-induced lung injury and the development of acute respiratory distress syndrome (ARDS). Treatment with prophylactic antibiotics and/or steroids remains of unproven efficacy.

Scenario: A 12-year-old boy and his brother were fishing using a multi-pronged hand-spear. This was inadvertently fired, piercing the boy's right side just above the costal margin. The boy collapsed at the scene, and an ambulance was called. When the ambulance crew arrived approximately 35 minutes later, the boy was alert with a GCS of 14, P 124, BP 95/65 and RR 36.

Question: What injuries might have occurred with this mechanism? What treatment would you recommend to the ambulance officers if contacted for advice?

Answer: Penetrating chest trauma remains rare in children in a civilian setting in most countries outside the United States. Given the mechanism and location of the injury, trauma to both chest and upper abdominal viscera needs to be considered, in addition to musculoskeletal injuries, including rib fracture. Collapse at the scene raised the possibility of a tension pneumothorax (**Figure 79.3**), major vascular and/or hepatic injury.

Supportive measures should include high-flow supplementary oxygen via a non-rebreather mask and establishment of IV access with the administration of normal saline or Hartman's solution. Given the patient's tachypnoea, tachycardia and hypotension, an initial fluid bolus of 10 mL/kg should be given. A brief clinical examination at the scene should enable a tension pneumothorax to be detected and, if appropriate, temporarily relieved

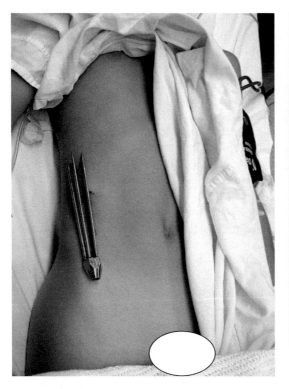

Figure 79.3 Child with penetrating chest trauma.

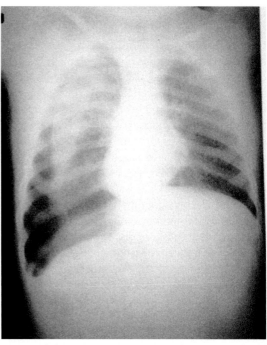

Figure 79.4 Chest X-ray showing pulmonary contusion and pneumothorax.

with a 14-gauge cannula placed in the second intercostal space in the midclavicular line.

Whilst classically patients develop a tracheal deviation to the contralateral side and an elevated jugular venous pressure (JVP, distended neck veins), these are late signs. Children are more likely than adults to develop a tension pneumothorax, and in the setting of penetrating trauma this should be considered a likely diagnosis. Whilst children are less likely to suffer a haemothorax than adults, blood loss into the chest may be more likely to account for haemodynamic compromise. In adult-sized or obese children, the pneumothorax may not be drained with a standard 4.5-cm cannula, so consideration should be given to using a longer cannula (8.25 cm) or inserting the cannula in the fifth intercostal space in the mid-axillary line until a formal ICC can be inserted.

The patient arrives in the PTC approximately 1 hour post-injury. He appears pale and sweaty, with vitals recorded as PR 120, BP 90/65, RR 32 and oxygen saturation of 94%. Clinical examination reveals a multi-pronged barb protruding from the right side (**Figure 79.4**). He has oxygen running at 12 L/min and has received 350 mL of normal saline. A 14-gauge cannula in the second intercostal space has been inserted by the ambulance officers in the field.

Question: What steps would you take next? What investigations should be performed?

Answer: Whilst trauma represents a life-threating situation, a concise history of the injury together with relevant past medical history should be obtained (allergies, medications, past medical history, last eaten, events leading – AMPLE). The patient's tetanus status should be determined, and if required, appropriate cover provided. Given that the foreign object would likely be contaminated, broad-spectrum IV antibiotics should be administered and include anaerobic cover. Investigations in the resuscitation bay should include basic haematological investigations, cross-match and a chest radiograph. Given the patient's clinical condition, an inadequately drained tension pneumothorax should be considered likely and an ICC catheter inserted in the fourth or fifth right intercostal space above the site of the foreign body.

A 22-Fr ICC is inserted into the fifth intercostal space with a rush of air. Following connection to an underwater seal drain, this is seen to swing and bubble with the patient's respiratory cycle. His PR falls to 100, BP improves to 100/75 and RR falls to 24, with oxygen saturation improving to 97%. A chest radiograph confirms satisfactory position of the ICC with a small, residual pneumothorax.

Question: When and where would you remove the foreign body?

Answer: Given the possibility of thoracic and abdominal injuries, the foreign body would be best removed in an operating theatre when, if necessary, a thoracotomy and/or laparotomy could be performed. Depending on local facilities, this would ideally be performed in a hybrid operating theatre, with access to interventional radiology, angiography and open surgical techniques. Preoperative imaging, in the form of a chest and abdominal CT scan with IV contrast, could be considered providing the patient is sufficiently stable. An MRI scan would be contraindicated given the metallic nature of the foreign body.

The patient is taken to the operating theatre to have the wound explored and the foreign body removed. The patient has a second 14-gauge cannula inserted and is intubated and ventilated. On removal of the foreign body, the patient deteriorates, developing a tachycardia and becoming hypotensive.

Question: What incision would you make to obtain control of the haemorrhage?

Answer: Given the location of the penetrating injury, trauma to chest wall vessels, pulmonary vasculature and intra-abdominal organs, especially the liver, should be considered. Depending on the degree of haemodynamic compromise, an initial exploration through an extension of the entry wound may be reasonable, with the option to proceed to a thoraco-abdominal incision. In a patient with uncontrolled haemorrhage, resuscitative endovascular balloon occlusion of the aorta (REBOA) may have a role in management in an adolescent as an alternative to resuscitative thoracotomy, with improved survival rates reported in adults. If available, cell salvage techniques that allow blood from an intercostal catheter or surgical suction to be collected in a sterile fashion, filtered and/or centrifuged and returned to the patient should be utilised.

At operation a laceration of an intercostal vessel and developing haemothorax is found. The vessel is ligated and a 14-Fr ICC placed for drainage. The patient's tachycardia settles, and their hypotension resolves in response to 1.2 L normal saline administered during surgery. The ICC drains approximately 500 mL of blood initially, with a further 20 mL over the next 24 hours. The ICC is removed after 72 hours, and the patient makes a full recovery.

BIBLIOGRAPHY

1. Samarasekera, S.P., et al., *Epidemiology of major paediatric chest trauma. J Paediatr Child Health*, 2009. **45**(11): p. 676–80.
2. Moore, M.A., E.C. Wallace, and S.J. Westra, *Chest trauma in children: current imaging guidelines and techniques. Radiol Clin North Am*, 2011. **49**(5): p. 949–68.
3. Holscher, C.M., et al., *Chest computed tomography imaging for blunt pediatric trauma: not worth the radiation risk. J Surg Res*, 2013. **184**(1): p. 352–7.
4. Tovar, J.A. and J.J. Vazquez, *Management of chest trauma in children. Paediatr Respir Rev*, 2013. **14**(2): p. 86–91.
5. Flynn-O'Brien, K.T., et al., *Mortality after emergency department thoracotomy for pediatric blunt trauma: analysis of the National Trauma Data Bank 2007–2012. J Pediatr Surg*, 2016. **51**(1): p. 163–7.
6. Wood, J.W., et al., *Traumatic tracheal injury in children: a case series supporting conservative management. Int J Pediatr Otorhinolaryngol*, 2015. **79**(5): p. 716–20.
7. Pearson, E.G., C.A. Fitzgerald, and M.T. Santore, *Pediatric thoracic trauma: Current trends. Semin Pediatr Surg*, 2017. **26**(1): p. 36–42.
8. Bayouth, L., et al., *An in-situ simulation-based educational outreach project for pediatric trauma care in a rural trauma system. Journal of Pediatric Surgery*, 2018. **53**(2): p. 367–71.
9. Vasquez, D.G., et al., *Lung ultrasound for detecting pneumothorax in injured children: preliminary experience at a community-based Level II pediatric trauma center. Pediatric Radiology*, 2020. **50**(3): p. 329–37.
10. Osuchukwu, O., et al., *Asymptomatic non-occult Pneumothorax in pediatric blunt chest trauma: chest tube versus observation. J Pediatr Surg*, 2021. **56**(12):2333–36.

11. Holl, E.M., et al., *Use of chest computed tomography for blunt pediatric chest trauma: does it change clinical course?* Pediatr Emerg Care, 2020. **36**(2): p. 81–86.
12. Killien, E.Y., et al., *Acute respiratory distress syndrome following pediatric trauma: application of pediatric acute lung injury consensus conference criteria.* Critical Care Medicine, 2020. **48**(1): p. e26–e33.
13. Fenton, S.J., et al., *Use of ECMO support in pediatric patients with severe thoracic trauma.* J Pediatr Surg, 2019. **54**(11): p. 2358–62.
14. Norii, T., et al., *Resuscitative endovascular balloon occlusion of the aorta in trauma patients in youth.* J Trauma Acute Care Surg, 2017. **82**(5): p. 915–20.
15. Campagna, G.A., et al., *The utility and promise of Resuscitative Endovascular Balloon Occlusion of the Aorta (REBOA) in the pediatric population: An evidence-based review.* J Pediatr Surg, 2020. **55**(10): p. 2128–33.

80

Abdomen and pelvic trauma

HUSSEIN AHMED HAMDY
Women's and Childrens Hospital, Kingdom of Bahrain, Bahrain

MARTIN T. CORBALLY
King Hamad University Hospital, Kingdom of Bahrain, Bahrain

Scenario: A 10-year-old boy is hit by a car while crossing the street and is brought to the emergency room (ER) conscious and oriented. His heart rate (HR) is 140/min, blood pressure (BP) 90/60 and O_2 saturation 97%. A focused assessment with sonography for trauma (FAST) scan showed free fluid in the abdomen and pelvis.

Question: What are your priorities in managing this child?
Answer: As discussed in Chapter 77, the first priority is resuscitation following ATLS protocols: Primary survey (ABCDE) and secondary survey.

Question: As the FAST scan shows free fluid in the abdomen and pelvis, what are the possible injuries that may be present in this child?
Answer: Abdominal trauma can cause injury to intra-abdominal and pelvic organs. The list may therefore include:

- Liver
- Spleen
- Kidney
- Pancreas
- Duodenum
- Small bowel

- Bladder
- Urethra

Question: Now that the child is resuscitated with IV fluids and blood and his vital signs are returning to normal, what is your next step in management?
Answer: As the child is stable, a contrast CT scan will be the best next investigation to identify the injured organs and the grade of injury. The child should be haemodynamically stable before taking him to CT scan.

Scenario: CT scan shows liver and spleen injury grade 2 (see table), with active bleeding seen as contrast leak. What are the grades of liver and spleen injury according to CT scan imaging?

Question: How you are going to manage this patient?
Answer: Management of children with liver and/or spleen injury starts initially with consideration of conservative (non-operative) care plans. The patient should be admitted to the surgical ward or paediatric intensive care unit (PICU) for close monitoring of vital signs. The decision as to the hospital care facility, i.e., ward or ICU to admit the child, and for how long is dependent on the grade of injury (**Figures 80.1–80.3**).

	Grade	Injury Description
I.	Hematoma	Subcapsular, nonexpanding, <10cm surface area
	Laceration	Capsular tear, nonbleeding, <1cm parenchymal bleeding
II.	Hematoma	Subcapsular, nonexpanding, 10 to 50% surface area
		Intraparenchymal nonexpanding <10cm in diameter
	Laceration	Capsular tear, active bleeding; 1–3cm parenchymal depth <10cm in length
III.	Hematoma	Subcapsular, >50% surface area or expanding;
		Ruptured subcapsular hematoma with active bleeding;
		Intraparenchymal hematoma >10cm or expanding
	Laceration	>3cm parenchymal depth
IV.	Hematoma	Ruptured intraparenchymal hematoma with active bleeding
	Laceration	Parenchymal disruption involving 25% to 75% of hepatic lobe
V.	Laceration	Parenchymal disruption involving >75% of hepatic lobe
	Vascular	Justahepatic venous injury (i.e., retrohepatic vena cava)
VI.	Vascular	Vascular avulsion

Figure 80.1 Liver organ injury grading.

Grade*	Type	Description of Injury
I	Hematoma	Subcapsular, <10% surface area
	Laceration	Capsular tear, <1 cm parenchymal depth
II	Hematoma	Subcapsular, 10%–50% surface area; intraparenchymal, <5 cm in diameter
	Laceration	1–3 cm parenchymal depth; does not involve a trabecular vessel
III	Hematoma	Subcapsular, >50% surface area or expanding; ruptured subcapsular or parenchymal hematoma
	Laceration	>3 cm parenchymal depth or involved trabecular vessels
IV	Laceration	Laceration involving segmental or hilar vessels and producing major devascularization (>25% of spleen)
V	Laceration	Completely shattered spleen
	Vascular	Hilar vascular injury that devascularizes spleen

Figure 80.2 Spleen organ injury grading.

	CT Grade*			
	I	II	III	IV
ICU stay (d)	None	None	None	1
Hospital stay (d)	2	3	4	5
Predischarge imaging‡	None	None	None	None
Postdischarge imaging‡	None	None	None	None
Activity restriction (wk)	3	4	5	6

Figure 80.3 Grade of injury.

Close monitoring of vital signs is essential in the non-operative management strategy care plan. Tachycardia and hypotension indicate ongoing bleeding, and serial haemoglobin measurement is important to indicate the need for blood transfusion. Complete bed rest and length of activity restriction are decided according to the grade of injury.

Question: What are your options if the non-operative management plan fails, and the child continues to bleed?

Answer: This is an uncommon scenario, as up to 95% of children with liver and/or spleen injuries generally respond to non-operative management. If the patient does not respond, then bleeding may be controlled by intervention radiology by embolisation or can be operatively managed by undertaking laparotomy.

Question: What are the surgical options to consider for management of splenic injury that fails to respond to non-operative management?

The spleen is an important immune organ for children. All efforts should therefore be deployed to preserve it. The specific vascular anatomy of the spleen makes partial splenectomy possible, as the splenic artery divides before entering the spleen. This operative technique will therefore help to preserve part of the spleen for immunity function. Embolisation techniques are also feasible if interventional radiology expertise is available.

Where total splenectomy is required, the child must receive pneumococcal, *Haemophilus influenzae* and meningococcal vaccine postoperatively.

Question: The patient has responded to conservative management and he is vitally stable, but on day 5 he starts to experience episodes of bile-stained and blood-tinged vomiting. What is the possible cause of his vomiting?

Answer: Duodenal hematoma is the most likely cause for his current symptoms. A haematoma developing in the duodenal wall can progress to cause partial or complete obstruction. Abdominal examination may reveal distension as a result of gastric outlet obstruction. It is important also to keep in mind the likelihood of duodenal perforation and a co-existent small bowel injury as a cause of his symptoms.

Question: How you will investigate this child now?

Answer: CT scan with oral contrast or upper gastrointestinal (GI) contrast fluoroscopy will help in making the diagnosis of duodenal haematoma and/or perforation and also small bowel perforation.

Question: What are the management options for duodenal haematoma?

Answer: Duodenal haematoma usually responds to conservative management in the form of nothing by mouth (NPO), nasogastric tube (NGT) and total parenteral nutrition (TPN). The patient can then be started on oral fluids and progressed to diet as tolerated. If the child does not improve with conservative management, then operative duodenotomy and evacuation of the haematoma and/or a duodenojejunostomy may be indicated.

If CT imaging shows a duodenal or small bowel perforation, then emergent laparotomy is indicated.

Question: What other injuries may be detected in this child?

Answer: Pancreatitis and pancreatic trauma are possible associated injuries. Serial amylase and lipase are important for timely diagnosis and follow-up.

Pancreatic pseudocyst may develop as a complication of pancreatic trauma. The cyst may usually resolve spontaneously, but endoscopic gastro-cyst drainage or percutaneous drainage or surgical management may be indicated.

> **Scenario:** A 7-year-old boy presents to the ER after an Road traffic accident (RTA). On presentation his HR was 120/min and BP 80/60. Pelvic examination (pelvic compression) showed marked tenderness and instability with blood evident from the urinary meatus.

Question: What are your key priorities in management?

Answer: Primary survey (ABCDE) and secondary survey as per Advanced Trauma Life Support (ATLS) protocols.

Question: What is an unstable pelvis?

Answer: An unstable pelvis indicates a pelvic fracture. A fractured pelvis can cause significant bleeding and shock. It is important to commence resuscitation with IV fluids and blood and seek to control the bleeding using a pelvic binder.

If the pelvic binder is unavailable, then a standard hospital bed sheet can be wrapped around the pelvis to control bleeding.

Question: Why is the patient bleeding from the external urinary meatus?

Answer: Urethral injury is commonly associated with pelvic fracture. The presence of blood from the meatus is a 'red flag' indicator of urethral injury.

Question: What other signs of urethral injury may be evident?

Answer: A perineal hematoma and butterfly ecchymosis are other signs that likely indicate urethral injury.

Question: If urethral injury is suspected, what is your management plan?

Answer: If you suspect urethral injury, then you should avoid inserting a Foley catheter, as this may

Grade	Type	Description
I	Contusion	Microscopic or gross haematuria. Urological studies normal.
I	Haematoma	Subcapsular, non-expanding without parenchymal laceration.
II	Haematoma	Non-expanding peri-renal haematoma confined to renal retroperitoneum.
II	Laceration	<1.0cm parenchymal depth of renal cortex with no urinary extravasation.
III	Laceration	>1.0cm parenchymal depth of renal cortex w/out collecting system rupture or urinary extravasation.
IV	Laceration	Parenchymal laceration extending through renal cortex, medulla & collecting system.
IV	Vascular	Main renal artery or vein injury with contained haemorrhage.
V	Laceration	Completely shattered kidney.
V	Vascular	Avulsion of renal hilum that devascularises kidney.

Figure 80.4 Renal organ injury grading

create a false passage or advance a partial urethral tear to a complete transection of the urethra. A suprapubic catheter should be inserted by the surgeon to avert further injury and monitor urine output.

To diagnose urethral injury and its grade severity, a contrast urethrogram will be needed. This can be performed with a (1) retrograde imaging study by gently inserting the tip of a catheter into the proximal external meatus and injecting contrast or (2) antegrade imaging study via the suprapubic catheter if already inserted.

The level and grade severity of the urethral injury can be carefully identified, and management planned accordingly with surgeon specialists.

Question: What are the management options for urethral injury?

Answer: This will depend on the level and grade of severity of the injury (partial or complete). Most urethral injuries are typically managed by suprapubic catheter drainage and delayed surgical repair of the urethra. Primary repair is an alternative option with risks of stricture which may require revisional surgery.

Question: What are the various types of bladder injury that may follow trauma?

Answer: Bladder rupture can be intraperitoneal or extraperitoneal.

Question: How would you manage bladder injury?

Answer: Bladder injury can be diagnosed with a cystogram study.

Extraperitoneal rupture can be managed conservatively with Foley catheter drainage. Intraperitoneal

bladder rupture requires exploratory laparotomy and bladder wall repair.

Question: What are the grades of kidney injury that may follow trauma?

Answer: Renal organ injury grading (**Figure 80.4**).

Question: What are the management options for kidney injury?

Answer: Renal injury may be managed non-operatively if the patient is haemodynamically stable. This will include bed rest, vital sign monitoring and serial evaluation of haemoglobin (Hb) level.

If the patient is haemodynamically unstable or conservative non-operative management strategies fail to control bleeding, then radiology embolisation techniques may be deployed or operative intervention for higher-grade injuries be used.

BIBLIOGRAPHY

Advanced Trauma Life Support Manual 10th edition. American College Of Surgeons. 2018.

Advanced Pediatric Life Support - The Practical Approach - 5th edition. Australia and New Zealand. 2012

McFadyen JG et al. Initial assessment and management of pediatric trauma patients. Int J Crit Illn Inj Sci. 2012 Sep-Dec;2(3):121–127.

Committee On Pediatric Emergency Medicine Council On Injury And Violence And Poison Prevention, Section On Critical Care Section, Orthopaedics Section On Surgery, Section On Transport Medicine, Pediatric Trauma Society, And Society Of Trauma Nurses

Pediatric Committee. Management of pediatric trauma. Pediatrics. 2016;138(2); e20161569.

Losty PD, Okoye BO, Walter DP, Turnock RR, Lloyd DA. Management of blunt liver trauma in children. Br J Surg. 1997;84(7):1006–8.

Godpole P, Stringer MD. Splenectomy after paediatric trauma: could more spleens be saved? Ann R Coll Surg Engl. 2002;84(2):108–8.

Stringer MD. Pancreatic trauma in children. Br J Surg. 2005;92(4):467–70.

Williams RF, Grewal H, Jamshidi R, et al. Updated APSA guidelines for the management of blunt liver and spleen injuries. J Pediatr Surg. 2023; March 23;58(8):1411–8.

Wong KY, Jeeneea R, Healey A, Abernethy L, Corbett HJ, McAndrew HF, Losty PD. Management of paediatric high-grade blunt renal trauma: a 10-year single-centre UK experience. BJU Int. 2018;121(6):923–7.

Coccolini et al. Kidney and uro-trauma: WSES-AAST guidelines. World J Emerg Surg. 2019;14:54.

81

Pediatric extremity injury

ABDULLA FAKHRO
King Hamad University Hospital, Kingdom of Bahrain, Bahrain

Scenario: A healthy vaccinated 7-year-old boy presents to the hospital emergency room following a traumatic injury to his finger. The family report the child's finger was caught in a door and bled profusely from the nail. Vital signs show a temperature of 37°C, pulse rate 100/min, respiratory rate 16 breaths/min, blood pressure 120/73 mmHg, and oxygen saturation (SO_2) 100% in room air with no other apparent injuries.

On examination the child is anxious and complaining of moderate pain. There appears to be a flexion deformity of the fingertip with soft tissue trauma to the nail fold and maceration of the fingertip. The avulsed distal phalanx is bleeding through the injured nailbed (**Figures 81.1** and **81.2**).

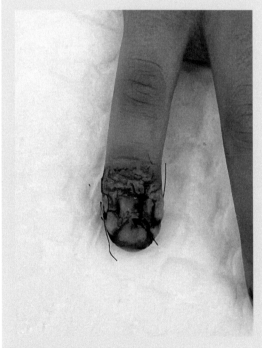

Figure 81.2 AP and lateral views of the injured finger.

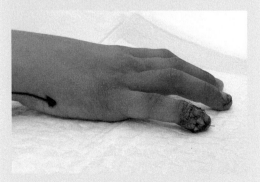

Figure 81.1 AP and lateral views of the injured finger.

Question: What is the working diagnosis in this child? What are some of the other findings you would expect to see with this injury?

Answer: The child presents with an open fracture of the fingertip, most likely typical of a Seymour fracture. The fracture is named after N. Seymour,

DOI: 10.1201/9781003182290-91

a Scottish orthopedic physician, who was the first to emphasize the significance of this juxta-epiphyseal fracture pattern in 1966. Seymour fractures are encountered in the pediatric population, usually in children aged 2–16 years; they are notably twice as common in males vs. females. Sensation of the fingertip is often preserved, and capillary refill is normal. There may be associated swelling and ecchymosis. The nail plate may appear longer than its counterparts, demonstrating obvious signs of avulsion or subluxation and occasionally lying superficial to the nail fold. The nail plate's proximal border rests on top of the eponychium fold rather than below it like the other fingernails. The distal interphalangeal joint appears to be in a position of flexion deformity, hence why many physicians confuse this injury with a mallet finger.

Question: How would you manage this child in the emergency room? What investigations would you seek to confirm your diagnosis?

Answer: As the severity of pediatric injuries vary, each child warrants a thorough trauma assessment exam and management in accordance with the Advanced Trauma Life Support (ATLS) ABCs protocol (airway, breathing, circulation). Once the trauma primary survey is complete and any life-threatening associated injuries identified and managed, the secondary survey exam should be commenced with attention to the injured extremity. It would be imperative to ensure tetanus vaccination is up to date. Analgesics and antibiotics should be administered as per protocol for open fractures. The most common oral antibiotics prescribed for an acute traumatic Seymour fracture are cephalexin, cefazolin, clindamycin, trimethoprim/sulfamethoxazole, and amoxicillin-clavulanate, among others.

The injured extremity should be exposed entirely, and the finger washed with warm saline irrigation. Patients who receive prompt antibiotic administration (within 24 hours after injury), irrigation, debridement, and fracture reduction will have a significantly reduced rate of infections.[1] A hand surgeon specialist should be consulted for early management of the injury; otherwise, the child should be transferred to the nearest specialist center. Given that open wounds are more likely to develop osteomyelitis and soft tissue infections, operation will be necessary.

Lateral and anteroposterior (AP) plain film radiographs should be obtained to assess the injury. The lateral radiograph will demonstrate a fracture through the physis of the distal phalanx or a fracture involving the proximal metaphysis 1–2 mm distal to the epiphyseal plate in conjunction with volar angulation of the diaphysis. There may be additional widening of the physis on AP projections, while lateral and oblique projections may better demonstrate the abnormal volar angulation (**Figure 81.3**). These findings confirm the diagnosis of the Seymour fracture, which is best defined as an open physeal injury of the distal phalanx. Since Seymour fractures are frequently the result of crush injuries, care should be taken to assess for retained radiopaque foreign bodies at the site of the fracture (**Figure 81.3**).

Question: What is the Salter–Harris fracture

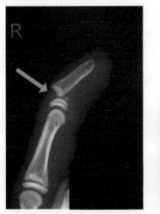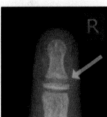

Figure 81.3 AP and lateral Seymour fracture.

classification of pediatric fractures, and what is the significance of each type? What kind of Salter–Harris fracture is a Seymour fracture, and what is the pathophysiology behind it?

Answer: The majority of fractures in the pediatric population result in predictable injury patterns specified in the Salter–Harris classification (**Figure 81.4**), named after Robert B. Salter and William H. Harris, who created and published this classification system in the *Journal of Bone and Joint Surgery* in 1963. These fractures typically occur in the brittle areas of the metaphysis, physis, and epiphysis. The mnemonic SALTR is best applicable to recall the different types of fractures:

Salter-Harris classification of physical fractures

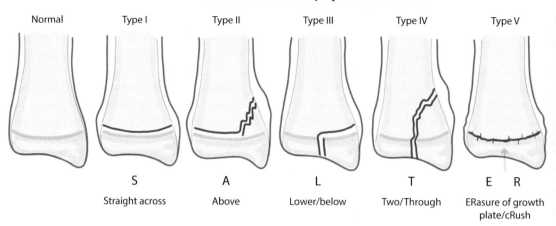

Figure 81.4 The Salter–Harris classification of fractures.

i. **Slipped** (i.e., through growth plate and not involving bone) = **Type I**.
ii. **Above** growth plate (i.e., through metaphysis) = **Type II** (most common).
iii. **Lower** growth plate (i.e., through epiphysis) = **Type III**.
iv. **Through** (i.e., through metaphysis growth plate and epiphysis) = **Type IV**.
v. **Rammed** (i.e., crush injury) = **Type V** (worst prognosis).

A proximal phalangeal fracture with a Salter–Harris type II structure is the most typical hand fracture encountered and is brought on by a deviating force. A finger's deviation in the plane of motion is typically acceptable, but deviation perpendicular to the plane of motion is not.

When a Salter–Harris type III or type IV fracture propagates into the articular surface, surgical reduction and stabilization are required to avoid intra-articular malunion and ensuing post-traumatic arthrosis. In Salter–Harris type V fractures, full growth stops and arrest of bone growth are then seen, which could lead to deleterious effects. Displaced apophyseal fractures necessitate early referral and treatment without delay and avoiding repetitive manipulation, which may worsen the prognosis and risk growth arrest of the bone.[2]

A Seymour fracture is a juxta-epiphyseal or Salter–Harris type I/II fracture of the distal phalanx with an associated nail bed laceration. The fracture usually occurs at the epiphyseal/metaphyseal junction as a result of a crushing injury to the fingertip. The distal bone fragment can be pulled into flexion by the flexor digitorum profundus (FDP) tendon, while the proximal portion remains extended by the terminal extensor tendon and the volar plate. Hence, the nail plate becomes displaced proximally and lies superficial to the eponychial fold. The germinal matrix, which is located closest to the fracture, might become lodged inside the fracture and obstruct the attempts to reduce it.

Question: Once the hospital emergency room management is complete, how would you then proceed with the management of this fracture? What happens if this type of fracture is misdiagnosed for a mallet finger?

Answer: Once a Seymour fracture is recognized, early referral to a specialist is best advised. First, the nail plate may be removed through relaxing incisions in the nail fold to allow for extensive irrigation and debridement of the injury. Before the fracture is reduced, any interposed soft tissue should be removed from the fracture line with maneuvers such as the hyperflexion of the digit or distal fragment retraction with a skin hook. Lastly, the nail bed is repaired using 6-0 or 7-0 absorbable sutures and the nail plate replaced again to act as a stent/splint to hold the nail fold open.

Pin fixation is required occasionally after the reduction of the fracture if the fracture is unstable or if the patient is likely to be poorly compliant. The fracture normally recovers rapidly. Antibiotics are continued between 4 and 10 days

The Distal Phalynx

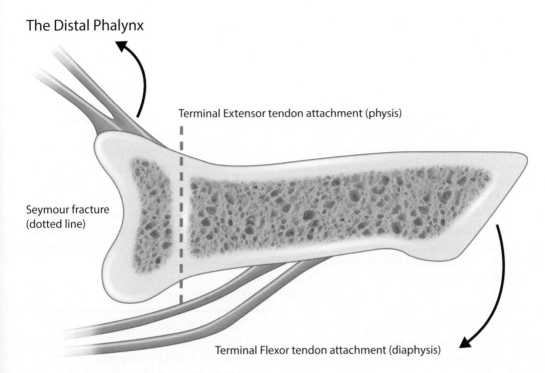

Terminal Extensor tendon attachment (physis)

Seymour fracture
(dotted line)

Terminal Flexor tendon attachment (diaphysis)

Figure 81.5 Cross-section of the Seymour fracture.

depending on the surgeon's practice. Patients who undergo prompt antibiotic administration (within 24 hours after injury), irrigation, debridement, and fracture reduction have significantly lower rates of infection. Additionally, antibiotic administration is also protective against nonunion or delayed union.

Mallet finger is the most frequent differential diagnosis for a Seymour fracture because both injuries result in a similar flexion deformity of the distal phalanx. As a result, there is a high risk of misdiagnosis and subsequent undertreatment with conservative management, which is how a mallet finger is typically managed. An osseous avulsion fracture of the extensor tendons in a mallet finger results in a Salter–Harris type III/IV physeal injury. The distal interphalangeal joint is where the fracture line enters. In a Seymour fracture, a Salter–Harris type I/II physeal injury results from the avulsion of the nail bed/germinal matrix; note the joint line is not involved by the fracture line (**Figure 81.5**).

Since this injury is frequently misdiagnosed as a simple nail bed injury or a mallet finger, treatment may be delayed, leading to substantial nail deformity In addition, chronic osteomyelitis or persistent non-union and physeal arrest may occur.

Imaging often will show osteomyelitis-related radiographic alterations, and serial imaging examinations should take into account delayed union, malunion, and non-union if suspected.

Question: How common are pediatric extremity injuries? How do you manage acute extremity trauma in children?

Answer: Trauma remains the leading cause of mortality in the pediatric population after neonatal deaths, with over half the mortalities in childhood being secondary to injury.[3] Multi-system injury is more common in children due to their anatomical and physiological traits and various mechanisms of injury. Children frequently experience trauma of the extremities, accounting for approximately 40% of all injuries. Significant difficulties may arise when treating lower extremity trauma where there are severe injuries or deformity. A scale termed the Mangled Extremity Severity Score (MESS) employs objective standards based on scoring four parameters: Skeletal/soft tissue injury, limb ischemia, shock, and age, to help with acute management of the injury. Scores for shock, age, skeletal/soft tissue injury, and limb ischemia are all assigned. For ischemia lasting longer than 6 hours, the score for limb ischemia is doubled. The results of the various parameters' ratings are then added. The MESS number ranges between 1 and 14. A MESS number of at least 7 has a 100% predictable value for amputation.[4]

Although the priorities and principles of acute management of injuries in the pediatric population are similar to their adult counterparts, pediatric patients are not young adults per se, and aggressive management therefore ought to be implemented promptly. Children's fracture incidence rates range from 1.2% to 5%. This variability may change depending on the condition, age, and social and environmental factors of the child.[2] As injured children present at different ages and stages of physical, cognitive, and social development, they experience traumas in myriad ways.[5] In addition to the financial burden incurred, injuries may lead to life-changing emotional trauma for children and their caregivers.

While many injuries can be treated first in an emergency department, severely affected children need to be transported immediately to specialist pediatric trauma centers. The severity of pediatric traumatic injuries often varies; therefore, each child warrants a thorough trauma evaluation by the ATLS ABCs protocol. Multiple fractures in an extremity may increase the risk of complications synergistically, and the presence of concurrent skeletal and visceral injuries raises overall morbidity and mortality even though individual extremity fractures may not endanger life or limb.[6] Severe intra-abdominal, thoracic, or head injuries should be attended to first and foremost. Early coordination between the trauma, thoracic, vascular, orthopedic, plastic, and neurosurgical services is pivotal to good outcomes.

It is important for healthcare professionals assessing and caring for pediatric extremity injuries to be aware of the unique characteristics and treatment considerations of pediatric trauma to provide the best possible care for these patients. Accurate diagnosis requires familiarity with musculoskeletal physical examination procedures as well as knowledge of typical injury processes.

Extremity trauma prevention measures are a key objective for both families and healthcare professionals. Several strategies can aid in lowering the risk of these injuries, including the use of safety gear like helmets and protective clothing during sports and leisure activities, careful kid supervision, and driving safety precautions such as the use of seat belts and car seats. It should be noted that pediatric patients recover sooner from most hand injuries and heal from them successfully with a good functional prognosis compared to adult patients.

Pediatric extremity trauma is a common occurrence requiring timely assessment and treatment to ensure a full recovery. The unique characteristics of the child's developing growing body and the potential for long-term effects make it important for healthcare providers to have a thorough understanding of pediatric extremity trauma. By involving the child and their family actively in the treatment process, providing education about injury, and taking steps to prevent these injuries, healthcare providers can assist children to recover from extremity trauma and return to normal daily activities as soon as possible.[7]

BIBLIOGRAPHY

1. Samade R, Lin JS, Popp JE, Samora JB. Delayed presentation of Seymour fractures: A single institution experience and management recommendations. Hand (N Y) 2021;16:686–93.

2. Levine RH, Thomas A, Nezwek TA, Waseem M. Salter Harris Fractures. 2022 Nov 23. In: StatPearls [Internet]. Treasure Island (FL): StatPearls Publishing; 2022.

3. Cunningham RM, Walton MA, Carter PM. The Major Causes of Death in Children and Adolescents in the United States. N Engl J Med. 2018 Dec 20;379(25):2468–75.

4. Helfet DL, Howey T, Sanders R: Limb salvage versus amputation. Preliminary results of the Mangled Extremity Severity Score. Clin Orthop Relat Res. 1990, 256: 80–6.

5. Jones IE, Williams SM, Dow N, Goulding A. How many children remain fracture-free during growth? a longitudinal study of children and adolescents participating in the Dunedin multidisciplinary health and development study. Osteoporos Int. 2002;13:990–5.

6. Guice KS, Cassidy LD, Oldham KT. Traumatic injury and children: a national assessment. J Trauma. 2007 Dec. 63(6 Suppl):S68–80; discussion S81–6.

7. Maheshwari, Sharma H, Duncan R. Metacarpophalangeal joint dislocation of the thumb in children. J Bone Joint Surg 2007; 89-B:227–9.

82

Munchausen by proxy, non-accidental injury and child abuse

AMPAIPAN BOONTHAI
Ramathibodi Hospital, Mahidol University, Bangkok, Thailand

PAUL D. LOSTY
Institute of Systems and Molecular Biology, University of Liverpool, Liverpool, UK
and Ramathibodi Hospital, Mahidol University, Bangkok, Thailand

Scenario: A 3-year old girl – a previously healthy child – had angioedema and repeated vomiting. She was brought to the hospital emergency department by her 30-year-old mother who provided medical staff with a history of seafood allergy affecting her child.

Physical exam findings noted a temperature 38°C, pulse rate 150/min, respiratory rate 40/min and blood pressure 90/60 mmHg. The patient was treated as having an anaphylaxis shock episode and later developed generalized oedema, which was thought to be resultant from a drug allergy. She was admitted to hospital subsequently for a few days before being discharged home.

A month later the young girl had another further illness with symptoms of vomiting, fatigue and dyspnoea. She underwent allergic skin testing, which revealed she had multiple allergies (wheat, egg white, peanuts, seafood, meat, dust mite, mosquito, insects, cotton and wool). Hospital records further showed the girl had undergone multiple admissions attributed to episodes of 'severe allergic reaction' during the next 4 months.

The young girl's illness later progressed further to extreme fatigue, a massive haematemesis, epistaxis and severe hypertension. Echocardiography showed cardiomegaly thought to be linked to hypertension. Endoscopy examination showed a severely inflamed oral cavity, oesophagus and stomach. The medical paediatric team scheduled a CT abdomen scan which showed a lesion in the right kidney. A diagnosis of 'reninoma' was made – a very rare disease with an incidence of 1 in 1,000,000.

During this time the mother posted many photos of her child on social media platforms and attempted to raise finances and funding for her daughter's hospital treatment. She also stated in social media that she was a 'single mom'.

Four months later, the young girl had a massive upper gastrointestinal (GI) haemorrhage which was notably associated with significant laryngeal and tracheal airway oedema. The girl was admitted to the intensive care unit but rapidly developed acute liver and renal failure. Sadly, she died on this last hospital emergency admission.

On the day the young girl died, her mother was by her hospital bedside all the time 'filming' herself reading books and singing for her daughter 'for the last time'.

DOI: 10.1201/9781003182290-92

Question: What (if anything) do you think seems unusual in this scenario?

Answer: The child's varied hospital admissions were dramatic and yet didn't always go with a definitive final diagnosis. The symptoms cannot be readily explained easily in 'illness pathway physiological ways' and only apparently occurred when the child was always with the mother who was a single parent. It is also undeniable that the mother's behaviour at times was not what we as treating clinicians would usually anticipate or witness during a child's illness, most notably frequently posting and seeking attention on social media platforms from the public.

The case fulfilled the working criteria for Munchausen syndrome by proxy (MSBP) child abuse, that is (1) physical or psychological symptoms or signs intentionally produced or invented by a parent; (2) the perpetrator often denies inventing or causing the symptoms or signs; and (3) the symptoms and signs of illness diminish or dramatically cease when the living child is separated from the offending perpetrator.

The term 'Munchausen syndrome' was first described in 1951 by Asher to characterise individuals who intentionally produce signs and symptoms of an illness or disease and who then tend to seek medical or hospital care. Later, in 1977, Meadow used the term 'Munchausen syndrome by proxy' (ICD-9-CM code 301.51) to describe children whose mothers produce histories of illness in their children and who then support such histories by fabricated physical signs and symptoms, even to extremes by altering laboratory test results in search of attention and personal gratification for themselves. MSBP therefore links to 'medical child abuse' – a cascading scenario in which the health service caregiver(s) 'overprovide medical services' and thus is seen as the very opposite of neglect.

The term has had many synonyms, i.e. factitious disorder imposed on another individual, Meadow's syndrome, paediatric falsification syndrome and Polle's syndrome.

Question: How common is MSBP?

Answer: MSBP cases are very rare compared with other types of child abuse. The incidence of MSBP in the UK was reportedly 2.8 per 100,000 children younger than 1 year of age and 0.5 per 100,000 per children under 16 years old. However, it is widely known that the incidence of MSBP is likely much higher than these grim statistics show, and there might yet be many undiagnosed 'at risk' cases.

MSBP typically affects children equally with respect to gender and birth order. Perpetrators are often mothers in 76% of cases, and sadly 55% of the paediatric victims may have other chronic illnesses. MSBP is therefore a gravely serious form of sinister child abuse with a high risk of repetition, and failure to diagnose it may result in the death of a child. The mortality rate of the victims is estimated as varying between 6% and 33%.

Question: How may a diagnosis of MSBP be established?

Answer: Making a diagnosis of MSBP needs a very careful structured approach – a meticulous history is therefore always key. Poor history taking or incomplete records have been implicated in contributing to misdiagnosis.

There is no single typical history, but there are certain 'warning signals' such as (1) persistent symptoms that are inappropriate or incongruous and occur only when the perpetrator (usually the mother) is with the victim, (2) inconsistency and ineffectiveness of the treatments which were poorly tolerated, (3) a calm perpetrator who is acceptant of all painful medical tests for the child and who is constantly with the ill child in hospital and happily at ease on the children's ward and who may also and often form unusually close relationships with staff, (4) family history may reveal sudden death of another child and (5) a history of similar illnesses in the family.

Common clinical presentations of the paediatric victims may include:

- Seizures
- Bleeding, e.g. GI tract haemorrhage, urinary tract haematuria
- Central nervous system depression
- Apnoea
- Vomiting or diarrhoea illness
- Fever
- Rash

These are always nearly present.
Investigations in MSBP follows several directions:

1. Study the history of illness to determine if it is 'real 'or 'fabricated'.
2. Look for a temporal association between illness events and the presence of the mother/other perpetrator.

3. Check fully details of the personal, social and family history that the mother (or perpetrator) has given.
4. Make contact with other family members if possible and take a history of the child's illnesses from them.
5. Study the previous episodes of illnesses. Think and consider possible Munchausen syndrome in the family (within the family).
6. Establish motives for the behaviour. Try to understand why the mother or other perpetrator behaves this way.
7. If the child is in the hospital, there are further manoeuvres such as:
   Keep the hospital charts and records clear from the mother/perpetrator.
   Retain any samples that may be useful for poison analysis/toxicological screening at any time in patients with unexpected coma, GI upset or other major events.
8. If there is haematuria, haematemesis or other bleeding, check if the blood is human or not (note that human red blood cells are enucleated vs animal blood, which is nucleated) or is it actually the child's blood rather than another person's.
9. Careful, often discrete, surveillance of the mother/perpetrator and child must be arranged. Be mindful that this action may cause a reluctant reflex human response from nursing ward staff to fully accept the possibility that the mother may be harming her child. Covert surveillance may at times be challenging to set up in a hospital paediatric ward in which mothers are resident and parents are welcome at any time. Surveillance by video technology is often deployed and will help provide conclusive proof of child abuse. Video surveillance can be arranged through police force agencies which have operational task force units and are ably prepared to use modern technology for crime solving and the right thereafter to prosecute offenders subsequently.

Criteria for MSBP include:

a. Psychological and physical signs and symptoms or induction of lesions, illness or disease on the other person are feigned in association with identified fraud.
b. Individual offenders present the other paediatric victim as ill, impaired or injured.

c. Fraudulent behaviour is evident even in the absence of obvious external rewards.

The perpetrator – not the child victim – receives the diagnosis of MSBP, and MSBP can amount to single or recurrent offending episodes.

The scenario we herein present represents MSBP in which a child receives unnecessary and harmful or potentially harmful medical care caused by the offending caregiver exaggerating or lying about the child's illness. Moreover, the caregiver in this scenario case is 'benefitting' from the patient's illness.

Unfortunately the diagnosis of MSBP in this tragic case illustrated was not made until the second child victim appeared some 3 years later to hospital with the same illness.

Scenario: A 4-year-old boy presented with haematemesis and multiple episodes of severe allergic reactions. This time the attending physicians raised early concerns and began to work up test investigations for the possibility of the child being a poison victim, and they discovered the alleged substance agent used by the mother.

The mother was finally caught on video camera surveillance while she was feeding her child the tasteless, odourless and highly alkaline noxious agent commonly used in the cleaning industry.

Question: What is the management in MSBP?
Answer: After making a diagnosis, it is crucially important to hastily protect the remaining other children of the family by separating them from the perpetrator. Management practices interlinking with social care services and multidisplinary health care teams – including law enforcement agencies – are vital to restore the victim's physical and psychological damage.

As for the offending perpetrator, custodial jail sentencing is commonplace. More often than not offenders do not readily accept their actions and behaviours, refusing to adhere to therapy programme rehabilitation or professional counselling.

Question: Does MSBP have any long-term consequences?
Answer: MSBP is associated with appreciable morbidity and mortality. In addition to the many

suicidal fatalities undertaken by offenders, the deception and the fabrication, if not uncovered, continue as the children victims become older, and there is then sadly a pathological tendency for them also to participate in the ongoing deception and to later become teenagers and adults with Munchausen syndrome by proxy. There is also evidence for paediatric victims to later become adults believing themselves as disabled.

MSBP therefore creates a significant burden to healthcare services as patients – as victims – often receive expensive and unnecessary investigations and tests.

Timely diagnosis involving senior experienced hospital staff early in all suspected MSBP cases will significantly reduce overloaded health care systems and save many lives.

MSBP: SUMMARY

It is crucially important for paediatric surgeons to be aware and promptly recognize MSBP, as many victims may first present to hospital services with fabricated surgical illness. Establishing a diagnosis of MSBP requires vigilant multidisciplinary teamworking and assistance from the social services community and law enforcement police agencies.

NON-ACCIDENTAL INJURY: CHILD ABUSE

Scenario: A 5-year-old girl is brought to the hospital emergency room by ambulance as the mother reported a fall at home. The young patient is assessed by the accident and emergency (A&E) medical staff and noted to have an 'acute abdomen', and the on-call surgeon is requested to assess accordingly. On examination the patient is alert, crying, conscious and in pain with peritonism. Vital signs record temperature 37.5°C, pulse rate 100/min and blood pressure 90/60 mmHg. Trauma care plans are followed with two IV cannulas secured; blood sampling for full blood count (FBC), group and cross-match; and urea and electrolytes plus serum amylase. After initial haemodynamic stabilization, CT imaging investigations are scheduled with the radiology department.

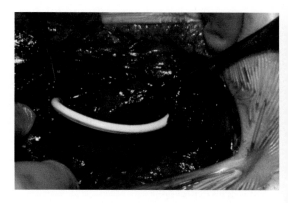

Figure 82.1 Transection of the duodenum. A tube stent is placed across the site of injury. Operative primary repair is undertaken.

En route to the radiology department the patient acutely deteriorates and is rushed to the operating theatre. At emergent laparotomy, the surgeon notes the following findings – bile-stained fluid in the abdominal cavity and transection of the duodenum (**Figure 82.1**).

Postoperatively the child makes a good recovery, although they are noted to be very withdrawn and non-communicative with hospital staff and nurses.

In an effort to better understand the emergency event that led to the child's hospital admission, the mother is later interviewed by surgeons and paediatricians on routine ward round visits. The surgeons are told the mother thinks the child fell down stairs. The paediatric team are informed the child fell outside in the garden from a swing whilst playing alone.

Question: What (if any) are your concerns?
Answer: The mother has provided two very different accounts to health care staff of how the child may have been injured. The injury is strangely not typical of a fall from a flight of stairs or a garden swing on to a grassy surface. There were no other injuries notably to the head/neck, chest, pelvis or bony extremities. Duodenal transection is a visceral injury typically sustained after a high-speed motor vehicle accident with a seat belt restraint or resultant from a bicycle handle bar accident whilst cycling. A blow, punch or fist to the abdomen likewise may cause such an injury.

Question: What will you do next?
Answer: A full history of events leading to hospital admission will need to be carefully documented – date, time, place of incident. Family and social

history needs to be examined. Family and social history reveals the mother is cohabitating with a new male partner following a divorce. Another older female child aged 16 years has moved away and is living now with grandparents. The mother is reluctant to co-operate with further questioning and becomes tearful, ending the interview with doctors. The nursing staff later that evening notice when bringing the mother a cup of tea on the ward that she is increasingly agitated and has bruises on her forearms and scarring that looks like cigarette burns.

Question: Is this significant?

Answer: The mother is clearly distressed. Bruising on the forearms and burn marks are unlikely to be self-inflicted. It's now approximately 3 days from emergent hospital admission, and the male partner has not visited.

When asked by nurses if the mother needs to get anything from home brought to the hospital, notably personal items or the child's underwear or clothing, she becomes tearful. Social services are notified. The mother claims she cannot contact the male partner who is not answering his mobile telephone or voicemail texts. The hospital child protection unit team are consulted for advice and raise 'red flag' alerts.

The grandparents, when interviewed on visiting the hospital, reveal the male partner is not at the home. Late that evening the mother informs the surgeons on a night ward round that her partner had been in the room at home with her daughter alone whilst she was having a shower and heard crying and screaming. She ran downstairs and found her daughter collapsed on the floor and called an ambulance. The partner, who had been drinking vodka and beer all day, quickly left the house. Police are consulted by the hospital child protection

services and search for the 'missing partner' on suspicion of assault.

The male partner was subsequently detained by police at a local train station, arrested, appeared in court and jailed for child abuse offences.

NON-ACCIDENTAL INJURY CHILD ABUSE: SUMMARY

Paediatric surgeons must be always vigilant and alert to promptly recognize non-accidental injury child abuse, as many victims of all ages may first present to hospital services with varied patterns of surgical illness or trauma: Head-neck injury, abdominal-pelvic injury, sexual abuse, extremity injury and burns.

BIBLIOGRAPHY

1. Lacey SR, Cooper C, Runyan DK, Azizkhan RG. Munchausen syndrome by proxy: patterns of presentation to pediatric surgeons. J Pediatr Surg. 1993;28(6): 827–32.
2. Meadow R. What is, and what is not, 'Munchausen syndrome by proxy'?. Arch Dis Child. 1995;72(6):534–8.
3. Meadow R. and Munchausenby Proxy. The hinterland of child abuse. Lancet. 1983; 13 Aug 1977, 310(8033):343–5.
4. Escobar Jr MA, Wallenstein KG, Christison-Lagay ER, Naiditch JA, Petty JK. Child abuse and the pediatric surgeon: A position statement from the Trauma Committee, the Board of Governors and the Membership of the American Pediatric Surgical Association. J Pediatr Surg. 2019;54(7):1277–85.

83

Burns and bites

AGATA PLONCZAK AND ADEL FATTAH
Alder Hey Children's Hospital, Liverpool, UK

BURNS

Question: What is the definition of a burn?

Answer: A burn is an injury to the skin or other organ tissue primarily caused by heat or due to radiation, radioactivity, electricity, friction or contact with chemicals. Thermal (heat) burns can be subdivided into:

- Scalds – caused by hot liquids.
- Contact burns – caused by contact with solids.
- Flame burns.

An estimated 180,000 deaths every year are caused by burns – the vast majority occur in low- and middle-income countries (1). In many high-income countries, burn death rates have been decreasing, and the rate of child deaths from burns is currently over 7 times higher in low- and middle-income countries compared to high-income countries (1). Survival is related to burn size, burn depth, age, comorbidities and co-existing inhalation injury. Children and the elderly remain the most vulnerable groups with the highest mortality.

Question: Talk me through how you would manage an acute burn.

Answer: Management of major burns follows the Advanced Trauma Life Support (ATLS) algorithm.

First aid consists of stopping the burning process (i.e. removing any clothing that may be burned, covered with chemicals or that is constricting) and cooling the wound (cooling any burn as soon as possible with cold tap water for at least 20 minutes and then carefully drying the patient). This is followed by covering the patient with a clean dry sheet or blanket to prevent hypothermia and then covering the burn injury with cling film (2) (**Figure 83.1**).

Primary survey

Airway and C-spine control:

- Give oxygen.
- Maintain the airway.
- Consider definitive airway (defined as an endotracheal [ET] tube device placed in the trachea with cuff inflated below the vocal cords) in cases of apnoea, inability to maintain the airway, to protect airway, impending airway compromise, Glasgow Coma Score (GSC) <8, unable to oxygenate by other means.

Breathing:

- A patent airway is of no use without adequate gas exchange.
- All patients should be given oxygen.
- Expose.
- Percuss.
- Palpate.
- Auscultate.

DOI: 10.1201/9781003182290-93

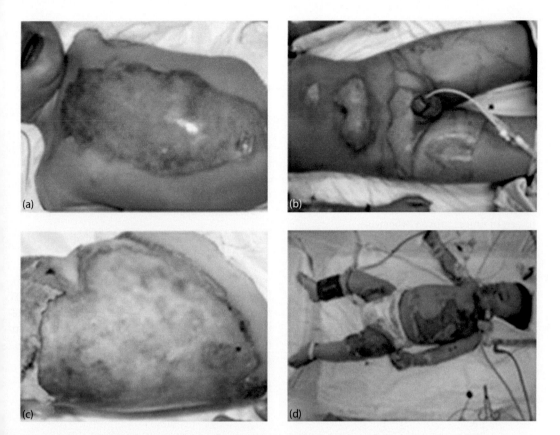

Figure 83.1 Burn appearances. (a) Superficial burn. Typical of hot drink pulled onto the child from a table: The distribution is on the chest. The wound is freshly cleaned (the blister has been wiped off with sponges) and the base demonstrated pink blanching dermis. This indicates capillary refill and a currently viable dermis, which will heal from epidermal elements around hair follicles. The burn can 'convert', i.e. get deeper if fluid resuscitation is inadequate or the wound becomes infected. Silver dressings here are a useful care plan (no bacteria species has resistance to colloidal silver). (b) Typical appearance of hot water knocked onto seated child. Notice the 'shorts' distribution and sparing around a tight waistband. Also note early catheter urinary diversion to protect the wounds from soakage and soiling. Note: Families sometimes use hot water with a dissolved nasal decongestant in a bowl to help children with blocked noses. This is also a superficial scald wound. (c) Mixed-depth burn at 5 days. The pinker areas are the more superficial burns that have started to re-epithelise. The yellow area is eschar: Full-thickness loss of dermis and epidermis and will require excision and skin grafting. The eschar and burn wound act as a nidus for infection and can be a source of sepsis. In children with mixed depth burns, requiring burn wound excision is often required in order to allow the injury to declare which areas are viable and which require debridement. (d) Child with mixed-depth scald burns in the typical distribution from pulling a hot drink or kettle onto themselves by accident: Mainly to one side, affecting the face, neck, chest and arm. Typically these are around 5–7% of injuries. The burn may be deeper in places due to delayed first aid or inadequate fluid resuscitation.

Aim to exclude 'ATOM FC': Airway obstruction, Tension pneumothorax, Open pneumothorax, Massive haemothorax, Flail Chest and Cardiac tamponade. Identify early need for escharotomy.

Circulation and haemorrhage control:

- Hypotension occurs in burns with hypovolaemia unless proven otherwise. Clinical assessment is based on the level of consciousness (reduced perfusion leads to confusion), skin colour and pulse rate. Note: Blood pressure in children is maintained until significant blood and fluid loss has occurred!

- Apply direct pressure to any bleeding points.
- Insert two wide-bore cannulae – obtain blood sampling for full blood count (FBC), electrolytes, glucose, group and save, COHb, arterial blood gas (ABG) and beta human chorionic

gonadotropin (bHCG) (pregnancy test) in females.

- Administer a fluid bolus and assess haemodynamic response.

Disability:

- Record AVPU (Alert, Verbal, Pain, Unresponsive) and GCS, check pupils.
- The most common causes of reduced consciousness level are hypoxia and hypovolaemia.
- Once cardiovascularly stable, a reduced level of consciousness should be considered traumatic in origin unless proven otherwise.

Exposure preventing hypothermia:

- Remove all clothing, ensure high ambient temperature.
- Remove all jewellery.
- Log roll to check the patient's back, check for scalp burns that are easily missed, consider shaving the head.

- Estimate total body surface area (TBSA) (using the 'Rule of Nines' - Wallace or Lund and Browder chart).
- Estimate depth of burns.
- Recognise the need for escharotomy (**Figure 83.2**).

Take clinical photography and seek a broad consent from family/carers/guardians for investigation and treatment.

Calculate and begin the formal fluid resuscitation protocol.

Parkland formula:

4 mL/kg/%TBSA = Total amount of crystalloid fluid during first 24 hours.

Delivery of half the volume is administered in the first 8 hours from the time of the burn (and NOT from the time of evaluation), and the remaining volume given over the next 16 hours. Hartmann's solution is the preferred choice of crystalloid resuscitation solution (3–4).

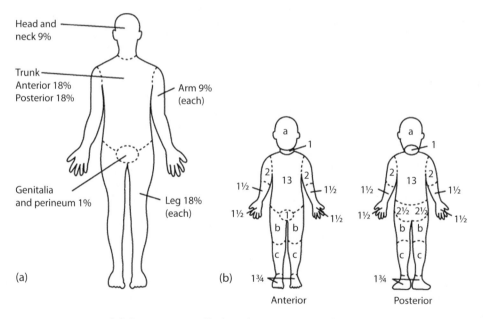

Relative percentage of body surface area (% BSA) affected by growth

Body Part	Age				
	0 yr	1 yr	5 yr	10 yr	15 yr
a = ½ of head	9½	8½	6½	5½	4½
b = ½ of 1 thigh	2¾	3¼	4	4¼	2½
c = ½ of 1 lower leg	2½	2½	2¾	3	3¼

Figure 83.2 Paediatric Lund and Browder chart. This chart is used to calculate the surface area of the burn in order to calculate IV fluid resuscitation. The chart highlights the different proportions of the child relative to the adult.

Adjuncts include:

- Observations
- ECG
- Urinary catheter
- Nasogastric tube (to decompress the stomach); nasojejunal tube to feed
- Plain X-ray radiographs as indicated

The patient is revaluated after the primary survey and 'AMPLE' history is taken.
Wound advice:

- Toilet with aqueous chlorohexidine solution.
- Cling film to be applied to wounds (allows regular inspection without disturbing sites of injury and therefore need for further analgesia).
- Make arrangements for transfer.
- Inform and support family and relatives.
- Tetanus at point of care; antibiotics at this stage are not indicated.

Secondary survey

Eyes:

- In case of concerns of eye involvement, fluorescein examination is warranted and referral to ophthalmology should be scheduled.
- Consider taping the eyes or tarsorrhaphy (especially in a sedated patient) in addition to lubrication.

Perineum:

- The key principles of care involve urinary diversion with catheter, prevention of infection, management of wounds with exposure and topical silver dressings. Conservative measures rather than radical surgical approach, consider vaginal stents, late release of contractures.

Escharotomies:

- Circumferential, full-thickness burns, whether on limbs or trunk, can produce a tourniquet effect which compromises circulation and reduces muscle movement. The eschar does not allow for the tissues to expand. If untreated, this can result in distal extremity ischemia, compartment syndrome, respiratory failure (if restricting respiratory excursion), tissue necrosis or death.
- An escharotomy is the surgical division of the tough, inelastic, nonviable eschar to release the constriction, restore distal circulation and allow adequate ventilation. The burnt skin is incised down to the subcutaneous fat and into the healthy tissues deep enough to release all restrictive effects from the eschar. Unlike fasciotomies, where incisions are made specifically to decompress tissue compartments, escharotomy incisions do not breach the deep fascial layer (5).

Question: When would you transfer a burn to a specialist unit?
Answer:

- Mid to deep dermal burns in adults >10% TBSA.
- Full-thickness burns in adults >5% TBSA.
- Mid-dermal, deep dermal or full-thickness burns in children >5% TBSA.
- Burns to the face, hands, feet, genitalia, perineum and major joints.
- Chemical burns.
- Electrical burns including lightning injuries.
- Burns with concomitant trauma.
- Burns with associated inhalation injury.
- Circumferential burns of the limbs or chest.
- Burns in patients with pre-existing medical conditions that could adversely affect patient care and outcome.
- Suspected non-accidental injury (NAI) including children, assault or self-inflicted.
- Pregnancy with cutaneous burns.
- Burns at the extremes of age – infants and frail elderly.

Question: What should you remember before transferring the patient?
Answer:

A, B – Secure airway, tube if needed.
C – Vascular access, IV resuscitation fluids running, urinary catheter.
G – Nasogastric tube (NGT) if >10% TBSA burn in a child (gastric dilatation more of a risk leading to unexplained hypotension, arrhythmia or aspiration).
C – Cover wound.
A – Analgesia.

T – Tetanus.

MAN – Appropriate and skilled personnel to transfer.

Question: What are the differences between paediatric and adult burns?

Answer: Over two thirds of paediatric burns are scalds (6, 7). A child with an uncomplicated 95% burn has a 50% chance of survival. Yet children under 1 year of age have a poorer survival from burns, and the causes are unclear, in contrast to burns in the elderly, where their age and comorbidities play a role (8).

Features in children that modify care:

- Different body proportions.
- Thinner skin.
- Higher metabolic rate.
- Greater evaporative loss (surface area:volume ratios).
- Greater heat loss.

Therefore:

- Increased risk of hypothermia.
- Increased depth of burn.
- Increased IV fluid requirements.

Differences are encountered during the acute phase and in the longer term.

During acute resuscitation

A: Airway differences.

The paediatric airway can develop a more rapid resistance to airflow given that a small amount of injury and swelling can have a significant impact in the smaller-diameter airway.

The airway is shorter, occluded by large tonsils, adenoids and floppy epiglottis, and is more prone to laryngomalacia and bronchospasm (9). An uncuffed ET tube is used in children under the age of 10.

B: Diaphragmatic respiration.

Abdominal burns, even if not circumferential, may impede ventilation and require escharotomy.

C: Larger circulating volume than adults (80 mL/kg vs 60 mL/kg in adult).

Heart rate is a poor indicator of volume, and blood pressure is generally maintained until very late before a precipitous cardiovascular collapse. Children need to maintain higher urine outputs, and intraosseous needles may be needed for circulatory access.

D: Less cooperative for neurological examination.

E: Surface area: Volume differences.

Thermoregulatory response is less effective in children (neonates have no shiver reflex). Thinner skin results in deeper burns. Children have much larger heads (approaching 18% TBSA) and smaller legs (approximately 14% TBSA), resulting in differences in the Rule of Nines. A child has less insulating fat and poor piloerector function.

F: Fluid is estimated as 4ml/Kg body weight/% burn area.

There is a significant risk of hypoglycaemia, so additional maintenance fluids are needed in children. Children should receive maintenance fluids in addition to their calculated fluid requirements (up to 40 kg):

- 100 mL/kg for the first 10 kg body weight.
- 50 mL/kg for the next 10 kg body weight.
- 20 mL/kg for the remainder of body weight (up to 40 kg).

AMPLE history

Children have different comorbidities, such as asthma rather than ageing cardiovascular diseases. NAI must always be considered.

Long term

Children have different calorie requirements. A major burn injury causes a hypermetabolic response in children, which markedly increases caloric requirements (10). In children with burn size greater than 40%, it is advisable to secure a nasoenteral tube and initiate enteral feeding within the first 12 hours of injury. The hypermetabolic response continues throughout hospitalisation and can last longer than 6 months post burn injury. Growth retardation is a significant comorbid issue.

Children's lungs continue to grow and develop with progressive alveolarisation up to the age of 8 years in addition to having a higher incidence of respiratory disease than adults. Hence, children are at increased risk for the development of acute respiratory distress syndrome (ARDS) and pneumonia, particularly after inhalation injury. They are also susceptible to long-term reductions in respiratory mechanics reserve following inhalational injury.

Children who survive massive burns will have major cosmetic and functional impairments that can never be completely corrected (11). Joint contractures can be problematic for them. Whilst breast development may be impaired in females by burns, circumferential burns to the trunk do not hinder later pregnancy. Although massively burned children cannot be fully returned to their pre-injury appearance and function, high-quality acute care combined with skilful multidisciplinary aftercare and positive family support can produce satisfying long-term outcomes for children with massive burns (11).

BITES

Question: What age groups are most likely to be bitten by a dog?

Answer: In the UK, about 25% of households own a pet, with an estimated dog population of 9 million dogs (12). This high number is therefore reflected in the common presentation of dog bites, being the most common mammalian bite injuries in children. The age groups of children most often bitten by dogs are those under the age of 2 years and those aged between 9 and 12 years old (13). Children are more likely to require urgent medical attention from those injuries than adults. Children under 5 years are significantly more likely to be bitten in the head or neck region (14) (**Figure 83.3**).

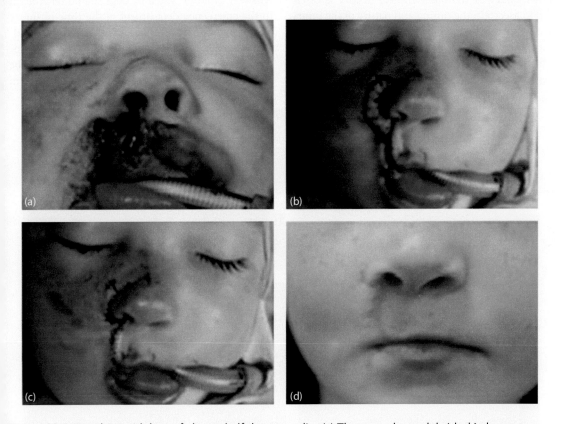

Figure 83.3 Dog bite with loss of almost half the upper lip. (a) The wound was debrided in layers to clean the edges. The philtrum, an important aesthetic landmark, was preserved. One may close a defect of up to one third of the upper lip directly. In this case, being greater than one third, the resulting puckering ('dog ear') would create a deformity at the base of the nostrils. (b and c) In this case, the scar was made longer but hidden between cosmetic subunits of the face in order to 'cheat the dog ear' and hide the eventual final scar. In this way, a flap reconstruction can be delayed until everything has healed. This strategy is a modification of the techniques used for cleft lip reconstruction. (d) Two-year follow-up. Note the nose and lip are pulled to the right. The scar has healed well but is most visible at the lip. Once growth is complete or if psychological morbidity has a significant impact, a lip-switch flap can be used to take lower lip tissue to improve asymmetry in the upper lip.

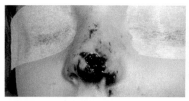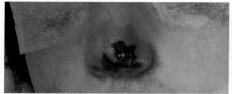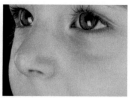

Figure 83.4 Not all dog bites need suturing or reconstruction. (a) Acute presentation after dog bite. (b) After cleaning and before application of dressing. (c) Result at 2 years following healing by secondary intention.

Question: What physical assessment would you perform?

Answer: Children presenting with dog bites should be assessed as for any trauma victim patient (15). A laceration may distract from associated fracture or other injury. A thorough clinical history is essential to ascertain the timing and nature of the injury, including any first aid given at the scene, screen for any potential need for tetanus or rabies prophylaxis and highlight any safeguarding concerns. Questions regarding adequate supervision and appropriateness of seeking medical attention should be asked. Our working practice is to advise all parents to report the incident of a paediatric dog bite to the police.

Question: How do you manage the wound?

Answer: Children bitten by dogs should be brought to the emergency department at the time of injury and receive appropriate initial management, including thorough irrigation, tetanus and antibiotic prophylaxis if appropriate. Any foreign bodies should be removed, and the wound well irrigated with warm

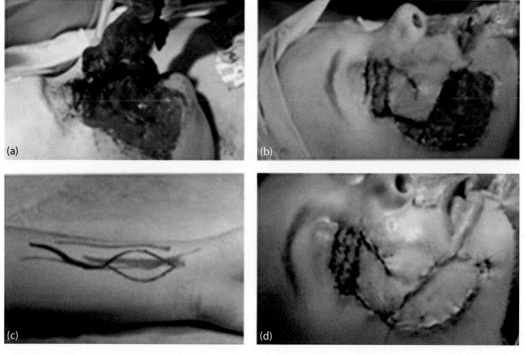

Figure 83.5 The most serious bites may require microsurgical free tissue transfer. (a) Facial bite has resulted in a medially based soft tissue flap and tissue loss. (b) After debridement a small skin graft was used to cover the area below the lower eyelid, and the remaining tissues were rotated to create a single defect. Missing from this defect was skin and fat. (c) Markings for a mini-radial forearm flap. The black ellipse is the skin that will be transferred, allowing direct closure of the defect. Red is the position of the radial artery, blue the superficial draining veins. (d) The flap was transferred to the face and microsurgically anastomosed to the facial vessels.

tap water. UK is a rabies-free country, and prophylaxis against rabies is not routinely indicated. Tetanus booster is not needed in children who are fully up to date with their immunisations. The National Institute for Health and Care Excellence (NICE) recommends antibiotic prophylaxis for any dog bites with deep penetrating injuries and associated structural damage, particularly for bites to high-risk areas such as the hands, feet, face, genitals and in immunocompromised children (16). Infected dog bite wounds were reported to yield a median of five bacterial isolates per culture, and most pathogens include a mix of aerobes (*Pasteurella* spp., *Streptococcus* spp., *Staphylococcus* spp., *Neisseria* spp.) and anaerobes (*Fusobacterium* spp., *Bacteroides* spp., *Porphyromonas* spp., *Prevotella* spp., *Capnocytophaga* spp.) (17). The UK National Health Service (NHS) working guidelines recommend co-amoxiclav as first-choice antibiotic prophylaxis where indicated, since this medication will cover all commonly expected organisms among the canine oral flora (16) (**Figure 83.4**).

Question: When do you operate, and what may you need to do?

Answer: Wounds with retained foreign material or heavily contaminated with the presence of devitalised tissue, tissue loss or in aesthetically and functionally important areas should be considered for surgical debridement and repair. Contrary to adults, most children will require general anaesthesia. In cases of fresh, non-infected wounds, adequate debridement and washout in the operating room allow for primary wound closure with interrupted absorbable sutures. Most children can be discharged the same day with a course of oral antibiotics. In already infected wounds, they may require to be left open and heal by secondary intention. Wounds with substantial tissue loss may require coverage with skin grafts/flaps and secondary revision once healed (**Figure 83.5**).

BIBLIOGRAPHY

1. World Health Organisation. Burns. [www.who.int; accessed 21.08.2021]
2. NHS Burns and scalds - Treatment - NHS (www.nhs.uk)
3. Haberal M, Sakallioglu Abali AE, Karakayali H. Fluid management in major burn injuries. Indian J Plast Surg 2010;43(Suppl):S29–36.
4. Zodda D. Calculated decisions: Parkland formula for burns. Pediatr Emerg Med Pract. 2018;15(Suppl 4):1–2.
5. Zhang L, Hughes PG. Escharotomy. 2021 Jul 18. In: StatPearls [Internet]. Treasure Island (FL): StatPearls Publishing; 2021 Jan 24.
6. Asena M, Aydin Ozturk P, Ozturk U. Sociodemographic and culture results of paediatric burns. Int Wound J 2020;17(1):132–136. doi:10.1111/iwj.13244
7. Hodgman EI, Burris A, et al. Epidemiology and outcomes of pediatric burns over 35 years at Parkland Hospital. Burns 2016;42:202–8.
8. Palmieri TL, Taylor S, Lawless M, et al. Burn center volume makes a difference for burned children. Pediatr Crit Care Med 2015;16(4):319–24.
9. Santillanes G, Gausche-Hill M. Pediatric airway management. Emerg Med Clin North Am 2008;26(4):961–75.
10. Jeschke MG, Chinkes DL, Finnerty CC, et al. Pathophysiologic response to severe burn injury. Ann Surg 2008;248(3):387–401.
11. Sheridan RL, Hinson MI, Liang MH, et al. Long-term Outcome of Children Surviving Massive Burns. JAMA 2000;283(1):69–73.
12. Pet Food Manufacturers' Association. Dog population 2019 [online], 2019. Available: https://www.pfma.org.uk/dog-population-2019
13. Fein J, Bogumil D, Upperman JS, et al. Pediatric dog bites: a population-based profile. Inj Prev 2019;25:290–4.
14. Loder RT. The demographics of dog bites in the United States. Heliyon 2019;5:e01360.
15. Jakeman M, Oxley JA, Owczarczak-Garstecka SC, Westgarth C. Pet dog bites in children: management and prevention. BMJ Paediatr Open 2020;4(1):e000726.
16. National Institute for Health and Care Excellence. Bites - human and animal: Scenario: managing a dog or cat bite, 2018.
17. Talan DA, Citron DM, Abrahamian FM, Moran GJ, Goldstein EJ. Bacteriologic analysis of infected dog and cat bites. Emergency Medicine Animal Bite Infection Study Group. N Engl J Med 1999;14:85–92.

Index

Note: Locators in *italics* represent figures and **bold** indicate tables in the text.